Unsatisfactory Results in Hand Surgery

Editorial Advisory Board

Douglas W. Lamb FRCS Chairman
Princess Margaret Rose Orthopaedic Hospital
Fairmilehead, Edinburgh, UK

Nicholas Barton FRCS
Department of Hand Surgery, University Hospital,
Queen's Medical Centre, Nottingham, UK

W. Bruce Connolly FRCS FRACS FACS
Hand Unit, Sydney Hospital, Macquarie Street,
Sydney, New South Wales, Australia

Lee W. Milford Jr BS MS MD
The Campbell Clinic, Madison Avenue,
Memphis, Tennessee, USA

Volumes already published

The Interphalangeal Joints
William H. Bowers

The Paralysed Hand
Douglas W. Lamb

Volumes in preparation

Fractures of the Hand and Wrist
Nicholas Barton

The Thumb
James W. Strickland

Microsurgical Procedures
Viktor E. Meyer and Michael J. M. Black

Joint Replacement in the Upper Limb
William A. Souter

Congenital Malformations of the Hand and Forearm
Dieter Buck-Gramcko

Skin Cover in the Injured Hand
David M. Evans

Dupuytren's Disease
R. M. McFarlane, D. A. McGrouther and M. L. Flint

THE HAND AND UPPER LIMB Volume 3

Unsatisfactory Results in Hand Surgery

EDITED BY

Robert M. McFarlane MD MSc FRCS(C) FACS

Professor of Surgery and Chief
Division of Plastic Surgery
Faculty of Medicine
University of Western Ontario and Victoria Hospital
London, Ontario
Canada

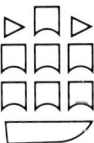

CHURCHILL LIVINGSTONE
EDINBURGH LONDON MELBOURNE AND NEW YORK 1987

CHURCHILL LIVINGSTONE
Medical Division of Longman Group UK Limited

Distributed in the United States of America by Churchill Livingstone Inc., 1560 Broadway, New York, N.Y. 10036, and by associated companies, branches and representatives throughout the world.

© Longman Group UK Limited 1987

All rights reserved. No part of this publication may be reproduced, stored in a retrieval system, or transmitted in any form or by any means, electronic, mechanical, photocopying, recording or otherwise, without the prior permission of the publishers (Churchill Livingstone, Robert Stevenson House, 1–3 Baxter's Place, Leith Walk, Edinburgh EH1 3AF).

First published 1987

ISBN 0-443-03387-0
ISSN 0269-4743; v. 3

British Library Cataloguing in Publication Data
Unsatisfactory results in hand surgery.—
    (The hand and upper limb. ISSN 0269-4743; v. 3).
    1. Hand—Surgery
    I. McFarlane, Robert M.   II. Series 617'.575059   RD559

Library of Congress Cataloging in Publication Data
Unsatisfactory results in hand surgery.
   (The Hand and upper limb; v. 3)
   Includes index.
   1. Hand—Surgery—Complications and sequelae.
I. McFarlane, Robert M.   II. Series: Hand and upper limb;
vol. 3. [DNLM: 1. Hand—Surgery. 2. Post-operative
Complications.   WE 830 U59]
RD559.U57   1987   617'.575059   87-6623

Typeset, printed and bound in Great Britain by William Clowes Limited, Beccles and London

Preface

There is a need for a book about unsatisfactory results simply because they are common. In each chapter of this book ways of avoiding, as well as methods of correcting, a bad result are discussed. Experienced surgeons are accustomed to dealing with problems, including those created by injury or disease as well as those created by inappropriate treatment. Authors have been chosen who can discuss these matters authoritatively.

Why do unsatisfactory results occur? A few are unavoidable but the majority can be prevented. We are all to blame. As teachers we often fail to impress our trainees about possible pitfalls, even of a minor nature, and assume that by observation alone they will learn. It is essential that young surgeons be forewarned so that they do not repeat all of the errors of their predecessors. In this regard I believe that a knowledge of the history of medicine, of surgery, and finally of hand surgery is valuable to place principles that should not be violated as well as those that should be changed, in perspective.

Medical students today do not receive much teaching in anatomy so our surgical trainees must make up for this deficiency. I am impressed that they do but it should be a continuum. Lack of anatomical knowledge is at the root of many surgical errors. Anatomy does not change but with advances in surgical technique our need for an understanding of various structures changes. The palmar aponeurosis was of little interest before Dupuytren nor the fascial spaces before Kanavel. The anatomy of the flexor tendons and their sheaths was straightforward before Doyle and Hunter. The veins were of no interest until Buncke spawned microsurgery. The detailed anatomy of the wrist joint and the carpal bones was beyond comprehension before Dobyns and Linscheid. With the computer and the arthroscope many young investigators are adding to our knowledge of this anatomical area.

Recently I was asked to sit on a committee of The International Federation of Societies for Surgery of the Hand to consider pitfalls in hand surgery. To gather data I wrote to a number of surgeons and have received valuable information, much of which is discussed in this volume. Dr Joe Boyes summarized his comments by stating that there are two kinds of errors: errors of judgement and errors of technique. He went on to say that errors of judgement are due to lack of knowledge whereas errors of technique are due to lack of proper training. Training in hand surgery today is universally available and it is uniformly good. There is no excuse for the untrained surgeon to perform hand surgery. However, as Dr Robert Carroll wrote in response to my letter 'It is more of a philosophical pattern how he applies this technology to judgement.' This 'application' applies to all of us, young and old, well trained, and not so well trained. We must continue to read, to discuss, and specially to listen and thus continue to improve.

I am grateful to the contributors for the thought they have put into the writing of their chapters. In every instance I sensed a dedication to help others in their discussion of unsatisfactory results.

London, Canada, 1987　　　　　　　　　R.M.McF.

Contributors

Loui G. Bayne MD
Clinical Associate Professor of Orthopaedics, Emory University School of Medicine, and Director, Hand Clinic, Scottish Rite Children's Hospital, Atlanta, Georgia, USA

Sidney L. Biddulph MB BCh(RAND) FCS(SA) FRCS(Eng) FRCS(Edin)
Hand Surgeon, Orthopedic Department, Johannesburg General Hospital and Natalspruit Hospital, Alberton; part-time Lecturer, The University of the Witwatersrand, South Africa

Douglas A. Bobb DO
Former Hand Surgery Fellow, New England Baptist Hospital, New England Medical Center, Tufts University, Boston, Massachusetts, USA

F. D. Burke MB BS FRCS
Surgeon-in-Charge, Hand Surgery Service, Derbyshire Royal Infirmary; Consultant Hand Surgeon, Derby and Harlow Wood Orthopaedic Hospitals, Derby, UK

W. Bruce Conolly FRCS FRACS FACS
Surgeon-in-Charge, Hand Unit, Sydney Hospital, Sydney, New South Wales, Australia

Richard G. Eaton MD
Professor of Clinical Surgery, Co-Chief Hand Surgery Service, St Luke's–Roosevelt Hospital Center and Columbia College of Physicians and Surgeons, New York, NY, USA

David M. Evans FRCS
Consultant Plastic Surgeon, Wexham Park Hospital, Slough, UK

Steven Z. Glickel MD
Instructor in Clinical Surgery, Columbia College of Physicians and Surgeons; Chief, Hand Surgery Clinic, St Luke's–Roosevelt Hospital Center, New York, NY, USA

Vincent R. Hentz MD
Associate Professor of Surgery, Chairman, Division of Hand Surgery, Stanford University, Stanford, California, USA

Geoffrey Hooper MMSc FRCS FRCS(Ed)
Senior Lecturer in Orthopaedic Surgery, University of Edinburgh and Clinical Research Unit, Princess Margaret Rose Orthopaedic Hospital, Fairmilehead, Edinburgh, UK

Francis M. Howard MD FACS
Clinical Professor of Orthopedic Surgery, Section of Hand Surgery, University of South Florida Medical School, Tampa, Florida, USA

Douglas W. Lamb MB ChB FRCSE
Department of Orthopaedic Surgery, University of Edinburgh, and Chief, Department of Hand Surgery, Royal Infirmary and Princess Margaret Rose Orthopaedic Hospital, Edinburgh, UK

Robert D. Leffert MD
Associate Professor of Orthopaedic Surgery, Harvard Medical School; Chief of the Surgical Upper Extremity Rehabilitation Unit and the Department of Rehabilitation Medicine, Massachusetts General Hospital, Boston, Massachusetts, USA

J. William Littler MD
Professor of Clinical Surgery, College of Physicians and Surgeons, Columbia University, Co-Director, Hand Surgery Service, St Luke's–Roosevelt Hospital Medical Center, New York, NY, USA

James A. McEwen PhD PEng CCE
Adjunct Professor, Department of Electrical Engineering and Clinical Engineering Program, University of British Columbia; Adjunct Professor, Faculty of Engineering Science, Simon Fraser University, and Director, Biomedical Engineering Department, Vancouver General Hospital and University of British Columbia, Health Sciences Centre Hospital, Vancouver, British Columbia, Canada

Robert M. McFarlane MD MSc FRCS(C) FACS
Professor of Surgery, and Chief, Division of Plastic Surgery, Faculty of Medicine, The University of Western Ontario and Victoria Hospital, London, Ontario, Canada

Robert W. McGraw MD FRCS(C)
Professor and Head, Department of Orthopaedics, University of British Columbia, and Head, Department of Orthopaedics, Vancouver General Hospital, Vancouver, British Columbia, Canada

Lewis H. Millender MD
Clinical Professor of Orthopaedic Surgery, Tufts University School of Medicine; Lecturer in Orthopaedic Surgery, Harvard Medical School; Assistant Chief, Hand Surgery Service, New England Baptist Hospital, Boston, Massachusetts, USA

Peter J. Millroy MB BS FRCS(Eng) FRCS(Ed)
Visiting Hand Surgeon, Princess Alexandra Hospital, Brisbane, Australia

James F. Murray MD FRCS(C)
Professor of Surgery, University of Toronto; Director of Hand Clinic, Sunnybrook Medical Centre; Consultant Hand Surgeon, The Worker's Compensation Board, Toronto, Ontario, Canada

Algimantas O. Narakas MD
Associate Professor, Faculty of Medicine, University of Lausanne; Surgeon-in-Chief and Chairman, Clinique Longeraie for Reconstructive Surgery of the Limbs, Hand and Peripheral Nerves, Lausanne; Consultant in Plastic and Reconstructive Surgery, University Hospital, Lausanne, Switzerland

George E. Omer Jr MD MSc FACS
Professor of Orthopaedic Surgery, and Chairman, Department of Orthopaedics and Rehabilitation; Professor of Surgery, and Chief, Division of Hand Surgery, Department of Surgery; Professor of Anatomy, University of New Mexico School of Medicine, Albuquerque, New Mexico, USA

Vincent D. Pellegrini MD
Assistant Professor of Surgery, Stanford University, Stanford, California, USA

R. G. Pulvertaft CBE MD MChir FRCS
Orthopaedic Surgeon Emeritus, Derbyshire Royal Infirmary and Harlow Wood Orthopaedic Hospital; Honorary Civil Consultant, Royal Air Force, Derby, UK

Douglas A. Campbell Reid FRCS
Honorary Consultant Plastic Surgeon to the Sheffield Health Authority. *Lately*, Honorary Lecturer in Surgery, University of Sheffield, Sheffield, UK

C. Christopher Reynolds RPT
Clinical Director, Hand Rehabilitation Unit, Glendale, Arizona, USA

Daniel C. Riordan MD
Professor of Clinical Orthopaedics, Tulane and Louisiana State University, New Orleans, Louisiana; Consultant in Hand Surgery, Shriners Hospital for Crippled Children, Shreveport, Louisiana, USA

Hugh G. Thomson MD MS FRCS(C) FACS
Professor of Surgery, Division of Plastic Surgery, University of Toronto, and The Hospital for Sick Children, Toronto, Ontario, Canada

Robert Lee Wilson MD FACS
Associate in Surgery, University of Arizona, Tucson, Arizona; Chief, Hand Surgery Service, Maricopa Medical Center, Phoenix, Arizona, USA

Eduardo A. Zancolli MD
Chief, Surgical Department of the Rehabilitation Centre of Buenos Aires and Professor of Orthopaedics and Traumatology of the Medical School of Buenos Aires, Buenos Aires, Argentina

Contents

1. General considerations 1
   R. M. McFarlane

2. The tourniquet 5
   R. W. McGraw and J. A. McEwen

3. Volkmann's ischaemic contracture 14
   G. Hooper

4. Joint stiffness 24
   R. L. Wilson and C. C. Reynolds

5. Minor surgical procedures and infections 40
   W. B. Conolly

6. Syndactyly 65
   H. G. Thomson

7. Club hand 89
   D. W. Lamb

8. Thumb duplication 101
   L. G. Bayne

9. Thumb reconstruction 109
   V. R. Hentz, J. W. Littler and V. D. Pellegrini

10. Amputations 140
    J. F. Murray

11. Skin grafts and pedicle flaps 158
    D. A. C. Reid

12. Burns 187
    D. M. Evans

13. Nerves 209
    G. E. Omer

14. Nerve compression 220
    R. D. Leffert

15. Flexor tendons 232
    F. D. Burke and R. G. Pulvertaft

16. Extensor tendons 250
    S. L. Biddulph

17. Tendon transfers 259
    D. C. Riordan

18. Tetraplegia 274
    E. A. Zancolli

19. Fractures and dislocations 281
    R. G. Eaton and S. Z. Glickel

20. Wrist injuries 301
    F. M. Howard

21. Rheumatoid arthritis 312
    L. H. Millender and D. A. Bobb

22. Osteoarthritis 336
    P. J. Millroy

23. Dupuytren's disease 348
    R. M. McFarlane

24. Brachial plexus 365
    A. O. Narakas

Index 373

R. M. McFarlane

1

General considerations

The purpose of this book is to help the surgeon avoid unsatisfactory results, but if they occur (and they are bound to occur in the practice of every surgeon from time to time), to help in solving the problem. In keeping with other disciplines of surgery there is great activity in hand surgery with the development of new fields of knowledge and new techniques. It is time to take stock, to re-emphasise basic principles, and to recommend standard procedures in the light of new knowledge. To accomplish this, surgeons with a wealth of experience have been asked to contribute to this book. I was pleased with their enthusiastic response which confirmed my initial impression that there was in fact a need for a book of this nature. Some of these surgeons chose to collaborate with a younger colleague and this has provided the best of the old and the new. As each chapter arrived I was impressed that the author(s) had given considerable time and thought to their subject. Dan Riordan said, 'it is the hardest damned chapter I ever wrote'. After reading his chapter you will realise that he has shared his vast experience with you, an experience that will never be matched. You may decide to use this book purely for reference and to read a certain chapter when the need arises. I recommend however that the book be read from beginning to end. There are many bits of information and tricks of surgery that have not appeared elsewhere.

Even though hand surgery is not yet officially recognised as a surgical speciality in some countries, hand surgeons realise that the speciality has become so extensive that not many surgeons are able to manage all of the problems. Even before being formally recognised as a speciality we are beginning to subspecialise! Conditions about the wrist caused by injury and disease demand an in-depth knowledge of anatomy and biomechanics beyond the scope of some surgeons. In the same way microsurgical techniques applied to nerve and vessel repair, replantation, and eventually transplantation is another area of special interest. All of us must be prepared to consult and refer to our colleagues—both young and old. The young surgeon will lack depth of experience in complex reconstruction whereas the older surgeon may not be familiar with the most recent techniques of treatment of acute trauma. It is indeed a luxury to practice within a group of hand surgeons who have a blend of young and old to solve the full spectrum of problems of hand surgery.

Early in my training it was drawn to my attention that, 'the bad results of surgery are the results of bad surgery'. There is merit in this statement but it is not entirely appropriate to hand surgery as it is practiced today. Other professionals are involved in the care of the patient. It is still true that the initial treatment of a hand injury will dictate the final result. With the development of emergency medicine as a speciality it is essential that we educate the emergency room physician to recognise serious hand injuries but also respect the so called minor injuries such as finger fractures and 'jammed' fingers and arrange appropriate and immediate attention. The surgeon is the central figure in the care of the patient but may not be the most important factor that determines the final result. The development of hand therapy has improved our results both objectively and in the quality of care provided to the patient. The contribution of an experienced hand therapist is needed to obtain a maximum result after most injuries and reconstructive procedures. The therapist therefore shares a good result with the surgeon and by the same token must accept a share of a bad result. Also, the patient influences the result of treatment. There is as much as 40 to 60% biologic variance in any clinical situation which is beyond the control of the surgeon and the therapist. This is expressed by the individual variation in the patient's response to injury and operation. For example, there is a great variation in the postoperative course in patients who have typical operations such as carpal tunnel release or palmar fasciectomy.

Reflex sympathetic dystrophy often occurs 'for no apparent reason'. We simply have not recognised the biologic mechanism. It is a complication that can occur after injury, either trivial or severe, and after an operation of any magnitude. This complication is mentioned and discussed in many chapters of this book. More often than not the problem is not recognised until the dystrophy is well established, that is, until the patient has severe burning pain, with swelling of the hand and digits and marked limitation of movement. In retrospect the pain and swelling were present for some time, perhaps from the time of operation. Reflex sympathetic dystrophy likely can be prevented as well as aborted in its early state. Elevation of the hand and forearm and control of pain and anxiety are the keys to prevention. We face a dilemma in this day of increasing hospital costs and pressures to perform more and more outpatient procedures. It is impossible to be sure that an outpatient keeps the hand elevated and it is difficult to estimate the amount of postoperative medication required. However it is now a reality that many of our elective hand operations will be performed on outpatients. There is a trend to perform more operations under local anaesthesia and distal nerve blocks. This in itself minimises immobilisation of the hand and arm and also permits useful movements of the digits during such procedures as tenolysis. Postoperative supervision can often be provided by hostel accommodation or a regional nursing service.

The initial examination of the patient is an important first step in avoiding an unsatisfactory result. One must evaluate both the injury and the patient. The history of injury is often ignored or recorded superficially but so many injuries are typical. Someone who falls (often a child) holding a drinking glass or a glass bottle usually divides a flexor tendon and/or a digital nerve. A human bite over the metacarpophalangeal joint can result in septic arthritis and must be treated accordingly even though the wound appears to be trivial. A knife laceration from trying to pry frozen meat apart is now a common cause of flexor tendon laceration. On the other hand some typical injuries are not easily diagnosed. In the act of catching a ball the patient may suffer a typical mallet or boutonniere deformity. However careful examination of injuries about the proximal interphalangeal joint is required to rule out pseudoboutonniere deformity and collateral ligament injury. As one's experience increases so does one's reliance on the details of the history of injury. The hand is easy to examine and damage to various structures will not be missed if the hand is examined in an orderly fashion from superficial to deep, from skin to bone and joint with evaluation of tendon nerve and blood vessel in between. The examiner requires a minimal knowledge of anatomy and a high index of suspicion. There is a tendency to assume that a structure such as a tendon or nerve is not cut. On the contrary, the examiner must assume that all structures passing through the site of a laceration are cut until proven otherwise. In the chapter on wrist injuries Frank Howard says, 'a shrewd sense of the possible will help prevent non-union of a fracture or a missed dislocation'.

At the time of an acute injury it is difficult to know how a patient will react both to the circumstances of the injury and to the proposed treatment but an attempt should be made to design the treatment to some extent according to the age, state of health and occupation of the patient. One should watch carefully for signs of unexplained pain, or lack of compliance to postoperative treatment such as failure to cooperate with the therapist or to keep appointments. These signs are often recognised only in retrospect when an unsatisfactory result is all too apparent. One should look for a reason for this lack of cooperation on the part of the patient and not simply blame the patient. There may be a social problem at home or at work that is the underlying basis for the patient's unfavourable response to injury and treatment. A social problem per se may have caused the accident. There is clearly a role for the social worker, the psychologist and the psychiatrist in the care of some patients. A system whereby a social worker can evaluate most patients after a hand injury is ideal and will uncover many correctable problems but unfortunately, in the hospital setting, social workers usually have a heavy case load and are not always available. The family physician is of inestimable value in the ongoing care of a patient who has suffered a severe hand injury whether or not the recovery and rehabilitation are uneventful or associated with excessive emotional response. There is always an emotional response from the patient to a hand injury regardless of the severity of the injury. Usually the patient copes with the situation but the surgeon must look for signs that the patient needs help. The family physician should be the first professional to be consulted. The present training of the family physician emphasises the emotional response to illness and disease and prepares them to provide support. This is exactly what is needed in many patients who suffer a hand injury.

Occasionally the patient's emotional response to injury or operation becomes pathological. The surgeon must constantly evaluate patients so that the occasional pathological state will be recognised. According to Sims (1985) psychiatric morbidity is extremely common in the general population and the commonest psychiatric diagnosis is neurosis. Neurosis is a psychological reaction to acute or continuous perceived stress expressed in emotional behaviour ultimately inappropriate in dealing with that stress (Sims 1983). It follows that many neurotic patients will suffer hand injuries or have other hand problems and these patients may require special support. The surgeon cannot make an accurate psychiatric diagnosis but is in the best position to recognise an abnormal state and seek psychiatric advice. The specific conditions that confront the hand surgeon are somatoform disorders, factitious disorders and malingering (DSM-III 1980). A brief description of these conditions may be helpful in drawing the hand surgeon's attention to the possibility that one or other is interfering with the recovery of a given patient:

1. Somatoform disorders include somatisation disorder (hysteria), conversion disorder, psychogenic pain and hypochondriasis. In this group the symptoms suggest a physical disorder but there are no organic findings and there is good evidence of psychological problems. Most important, the symptoms are not under voluntary control.

2. Factitious disorders include factitious oedema, infection and ulceration, Munchausen's syndrome, Secretans disease, and SHAFT syndrome (Smith 1975; Reading 1980; Cooper 1985; Wallace & Fitzmorris 1978). The essential features of these conditions are that they are under the voluntary control of the patient but there is no apparent goal other than to continue to be a patient. A factitious disorder always implies psychopathology, most often a severe personality disturbance.

3. Malingering is also under voluntary control but there is a recognisable goal such as to avoid work or to obtain financial or other compensation. Both malingering and factitious disorders are under voluntary control. They are differentiated by the physicians judgement as to whether or not the symptoms are produced in pursuit of a goal. Malingering is differentiated from somatoform disorders by showing that the symptoms are under voluntary control and there is a recognisable goal.

Factitious disorders are usually recognised by the hand surgeon but psychiatric treatment is often disappointing simply because the patients refuse treatment. It is characteristic of factitious disorders for the patient to refuse treatment. It is difficult for the psychiatrist to make an accurate diagnosis in most of the patients and often treatment, if accepted by the patient, is prolonged. Nevertheless a liaison with a psychiatrist who is interested in these problems is valuable, because it is occasionally helpful to the patient and always supportive of the surgeon's efforts to resolve the problem.

The problem of informed consent is ubiquitous to the practice of medicine. In hand surgery it is necessary not only to explain the proposed operation and outline the possible complications but also to predict the nature of the postoperative course. Almost always a course of postoperative therapy is advisable in order to obtain a good result. The patient should be informed of the time involved and also the added expense of travel, splints and other costs. The excision of a dorsal ganglion is a simple procedure, especially in the mind of the patient. Some patients experience pain and limitation of wrist movement postoperatively and are unable to return to work for many weeks. They should be forewarned. The repair of a flexor tendon laceration is a major undertaking for the surgeon and yet the patient usually considers the injury to be trivial. Particularly with secondary flexor tendon procedures the difficulty of the operation and the magnitude of postoperative therapy should be explained.

Long-term follow-up is not only instructive but is necessary for a good result following most hand operations. It is often necessary to follow a patient who has had a carpal tunnel release for several months before both patient and surgeon are satisfied. Tendon repair, tendon graft and tendon transfer require close attention in the immediate postoperative period to assure a correct balance of immobilisation and mobilisation. The hand therapist has assumed a central role and has added a valuable dimension but the surgeon should not lose contact with the patient. In fact the surgeon should communicate with the therapist as well as see the patient occasionally during the course of therapy. Physical and occupational therapy are essential to a good result but patients also need reinforcement of their efforts and this is best supplied by periodic visits to the surgeon.

Unsatisfactory results are bound to occur simply because we, those around us, and our patients are all human. We must strive to minimise them and throughout this book ways of doing so will be discussed: by taking a careful history and conducting a thorough examination, by careful planning of treatment and by monitoring the patient in the postoperative period.

REFERENCES

Cooper M A C S, Davies D M 1985 Charcot's Oedeme Bleu des Hysteriques. The Journal of Hand Surgery 10B:399

DSM-III. Diagnostic and Statistical Manual of Mental Disorders. 1980, 3rd edn. The American Psychiatric Association, Washington, DC

Reading G 1980 Secretan's Syndrome: Hard Edema of the Dorsum of the Hand. Plastic and Reconstructive Surgery 65:182

Sims A C P 1983 Neurosis in Society. Basingstoke, Macmillan

Sims A C P 1985 Editorial. The Journal of Hand Surgery 10B:281

Smith R J 1975 Factitious Lymphedema of the Hand. Journal of Bone and Joint Surgery 89A:94

Wallace P F, Fitzmorris C S 1978 The SHAFT Syndrome in the Upper Extremity. Journal of Hand Surgery 3:492

R. W. McGraw and J. A. McEwen

2 The tourniquet

The pneumatic tourniquet is a device essential to modern hand surgery. The primary goals of operative hand surgery, namely precision and atramautic technique, cannot be achieved optimally without a bloodless surgical field. The use of such a device to temporarily arrest all circulation in the operative field is not without hazard. It is the responsibility of the surgeon to minimise the possibility of a tourniquet related complication. The surgeon should select a modern tourniquet system and be familiar with its operative characteristics and maintenance requirements. The guidelines for safe inflation time and pressure settings must be known and observed. It is possible that with continued research even safer methods of regional circulatory arrest for surgical procedures will be developed.

HISTORICAL REVIEW

The history of the use of non-pneumatic tourniquets in surgery has been reviewed extensively elsewhere (Klenerman 1962). The first record of the use of a tourniquet is by the Roman surgeon, Heliodoris, who in the second century A.D. wrote, 'I have been accustomed to apply a bandage above the part to be amputated so as to compress the vessels as far as possible' (Kessler 1966). Thus, the original tourniquet use was synonymous with the surgical procedure of amputation. In 1817, the French surgeon, Jean Louis Petit, described his device for hemostasis and named the instrument the 'tourniquet' (Klenerman 1962). Three advances were to follow in the evolution of bloodless field limb surgery: the introduction of the elastic wrapped bandage for exsanguination in 1873 (Esmarch 1873) the introduction of a pneumatic tourniquet by Harvey Cushing in 1904 (Cushing 1904), and the introduction of microprocessor-based tourniquets (McEwen & McGraw 1979). The original 'Esmarch bandage' was a tube the thickness of a finger which was wound tightly around the limb after the blood had been expressed from it by bandaging. The flat rubber 'Esmarch bandage' used today was designed by von Langenbach. The Martin bandage, which is a similar device is made of cream coloured latex rubber. Cushing originally designed the pneumatic tourniquet to minimise bleeding during craniotomy. He also described the use of this tourniquet for 'cocaine operations' on the hand (Cushing 1904). Until recently, the pneumatic tourniquet underwent few if any significant modifications or improvements since its introduction by Cushing, except for the addition of a pressure gauge and the inclusion of mechanical pressure regulating mechanisms in the 1940s and 1950s. It was not until the late 1970s that the third significant advance occurred with the introduction by the authors of microprocessor-based tourniquets having improved safety and performance (McEwen & McGraw 1979, McEwen 1981).

HAZARDS OF TOURNIQUET USAGE

A 'tourniquet-related hazard' may be defined as a possible source of peril, danger, risk, or difficulty involving a tourniquet. In contrast, a 'tourniquet-related incident' may be defined as an unexpected outcome associated with the use of a tourniquet in which it is suspected that a possible malfunction, misuse or characteristic of the tourniquet may have contributed to the unexpected outcome. Table 2.1 contains a comprehensive summary of tourniquet-related hazards, clinical signs and possible causes of injury which have been reported in the literature (McEwen & McGraw 1982, McEwen & Auchinleck 1982).

To assess the actual types and frequencies of tourniquet-related hazards, the authors initiated a programme of periodic inspections of 12 pneumatic tourniquets with mechanical pressure regulators (Kidde Model 400 Pneumatic Tourniquets) in two teaching hospitals over a 30-month period beginning in 1981 (McEwen & Auchinleck 1982). During this period, the 12 pneumatic tourniquets were given 84 safety and performance inspections at scheduled intervals by a hospital-based biomedical engineering department. In addition to scheduled inspections, the 12 pneumatic tourniquets were also given 71 unscheduled inspections as a result of reported incidents, hazards or malfunctions. The test results revealed an unexpectedly high frequency of occurrence of a variety of significant hazards. For example, in 49% of these tests a very large hysteresis (Johnson 1980, McEwen 1981) or error in the pressure-regulating mechanism, of 200 mmHg or more was observed. Significant physical deterioration of one or more major elements was observed in 45% of the tests. In 10% of the tests, an error in the pressure gauge of more than 10% was noted. In 5% of the tests, a maximum cuff pressure of over 1100 mmHg could be generated; in 5% of the tests, cuff pressure drifted more than 10% from the set value over a 15-minute period; in 5% of the tests, leaks were observed which were sufficiently large to cause visible depletion of the compressed-gas reservoir;

Table 2.1 Summary of tourniquet-related hazards, clinical signs and possible causes of injury which have been reported in the literature.

Clinical signs	Possible tourniquet-related causes
Hazard 1: Overpressurisation	
Tourniquet paralysis	Malfunctioning pressure regulator
Postoperative muscle weakness	Excessive hysteresis in pressure regulator
Pain at cuff site	Inaccurate pressure gauge or sensor
Other compression injuries to blood vessel, nerve, muscle, or skin	Lack of audiovisual alarms
	Infrequent monitoring by staff
	Improper setting of tourniquet pressure
Hazard 2: Underpressurisation	
Blood in surgical field	Malfunctioning pressure regulator
Passive congestion of limb	Excessive hysteresis in pressure regulator
Shock	Inaccurate pressure gauge or sensor
Hemorrhagic infiltration of nerve	Lack of audiovisual alarms
	Infrequent monitoring by staff
	Improper setting of tourniquet pressure
	Kinking of hose to cuff
	Geometric mismatch of cuff and limb
	Cuff failure
	Loss of pressurised gas source
	Large leaks in cuff or hose
	Disconnection of cuff or hose
	Intraoperative increase in systolic pressure
Hazard 3: Excessive period of inflation	
Tourniquet paralysis	Infrequent monitoring of elapsed time
Postoperative muscle weakness	Lack of audiovisual alarms to warn of excessive inflation periods
Ischemic injury distal to cuff	
Excessive postoperative reactive hyperemia	
Hazard 4: Improper cuff application or perioperative procedures	
Venous congestion	Improper preoperative exsanguination
Soft tissue injuries (bruising, blistering, pinching, necrosis of skin)	Excessively slow inflation or deflation
	Incomplete or overly aggressive seal at cuff
Chemical burns at cuff	Pooling of preparation solutions
	Cuff geometry or physical characteristics

and in 4% of the tests it was noted that the pressure gauge did not return to zero between uses, resulting in erroneous readings.

Cuff-related hazards were examined in a second study initiated by the authors which involved the investigation of 55 tourniquet-related incidents over a 20-month period (McEwen 1983). Cuff-related hazards which were identified include: undetected kinking between cuff and controller, resulting in non-regulation of cuff pressure; sudden depressurisation due to telescoping, pop-off or rupture of the cuff during use; sudden depressurisation due to disconnections of hosing; pinching and necrosis of soft tissue under an inflated cuff; mismatch of cuff and limb shapes leading to possible nerve injuries; chemical burns to skin due to seepage of fluids under the cuff; and overly tight or loose application of the cuff resulting in inappropriate cuff/limb interface.

As the design of modern tourniquet systems has improved, the relative significance of the hazards listed in Table 2.1 with regard to tourniquet-related incidents has changed.

ELEMENTS AND CHARACTERISTICS OF MODERN TOURNIQUET SYSTEMS

The primary objective of a modern tourniquet system is to reliably maintain the minimum pressure necessary in a cuff which encircles a patient's limb to stop blood flow into the limb (Erlanger & Gasser 1937). Secondary objectives are to do so in a manner which minimises obstruction of the surgical field, and in a manner which minimises any tourniquet-related injury of the patient.

To accomplish these objectives, it is necessary that each component of a modern tourniquet system be effective and safe. The three basic elements of such systems are: 1. a cuff for encircling the patient's limb and pressurising to a pre-set value; 2. a pressure-regulating mechanism for initially pressurising the cuff, maintaining the pressure in the cuff at or near a pre-set value, and then depressurising the cuff; and 3. controls, indicators and alarms to provide the operator with means for controlling the function of the system, for displaying current values of parameters such as cuff pressure and elapsed time of cuff inflation, and for warning the operator of tourniquet-related hazards. Various suggestions regarding voluntary standards for desired characteristics of specific elements of modern tourniquet systems have been proposed (e.g. McEwen 1981, McEwen & Auchinleck 1982, AORN 1984, ECRI 1984) but no specific mandatory standards exist at present.

Desired characteristics of tourniquet cuffs which have been suggested include the following: the cuff should conform closely to limbs of different shape; the cuff should be capable of being pressurised to pressures up to 500 mmHg without becoming detached from the limb or moving distally down the limb; the cuff should not obstruct the surgical field; the cuff should distribute pressure uniformly to underlying tissue; and the cuff should be constructed to minimise the probability of failure of any fasteners employed during use, and to facilitate cleaning, and re-use when intended. Any tubing and connectors intended for connecting the cuff to a controller should be designed and constructed to be resistant to kinking and inadvertent detachment.

Desired characteristics of a pressure-regulating mechanism for a modern tourniquet system include the following key requirements: it should regulate pressure to within 5% of a set value; it should maintain a stable pressure, remaining within 10% of the set value over at least a 60-minute period; it should function reliably over long periods of operation; and it should not consume excessive amounts of supply gas in regulating pressure.

Desired characteristics of controls, indicators and alarms for tourniquet systems include the following: the controls should permit an operator to conveniently specify parameters for safe and desired functioning; indicators should provide the operator with accurate values of key parameters (such as cuff pressure and inflation time); and alarms should promptly advise the operator of any condition or malfunction which could be hazardous to the patient or operator. The indicators and alarms, combined with design characteristics of the tourniquet system, should assure that any malfunction or failure of a single component of the system will result in a situation 1. which is immediately obvious to the operator, and 2. which is not hazardous to the patient.

The types of pneumatic tourniquets currently employed in hand surgery may be grouped into four general categories: 1. manual systems with operator-controlled regulation of pressure and monitoring; 2. mechanical systems with entirely non-electronic regulation of pressure, controls and displays; 3. hybrid systems incorporating mechanical pressure-regulating mechanisms with some degree of electronic displays or controls, and 4. digital systems with microprocessor-based pressure regulators, indicators and controls. All four groups of systems currently employ cuffs having similar characteristics. Manual approaches to maintaining occlusive pressure have largely been supplanted by other systems having reduced labour-intensiveness. Entirely mechanical systems as summarised above are currently being supplanted by other systems because many of the desired characteristics of modern tourniquet systems cannot be achieved cost-effectively (McEwen 1981, McEwen & McGraw 1982, ECRI 1984). Hybrid systems are an improvement over the earlier generation of purely mechanical systems, but still have inherent limitations in the accuracy and reliability of pressure regulation, as well as in alarms and indicators, which are not present in digital systems. Digital systems are now widely gaining in popularity in hand surgery because many of the desired characteristics can be achieved with acceptable accuracy, reliability, safety and cost.

COMPLICATIONS OF TOURNIQUET USE

The pneumatic tourniquet is regarded to be an essential device in modern limb surgery. Its everyday widespread usage has generated the erroneous notion that it is intrinsically safe. However, there continue to be reports in the recent literature of well documented and often unexplained nerve injury (Rorabeck & Kennedy 1980, Rudge 1974, Weingqarden et al 1979).

While the spectrum of complications associated with tourniquet usage is wide and generally subdivided into categories of cutaneous, vascular, and muscular, the most serious is neurological. The nerve palsies have the greatest potential for permanent disability. Moldaver has reported that the typical tourniquet paralysis syndrome consists of loss of light touch, light pressure, vibration and position sense appreciation together with a loss of motor power (Moldaver 1954). The effected function would most likely correspond to the large nerve fibres described by Erlanger & Gasser, the large A fibres (Erlanger & Gasser 1937). Temperature and pain appreciation and sympathetic function are less likely to be influenced. Therefore, pin testing is inappropriate in the postoperative period. Though a controversy persists as to whether the pathogenesis of the nerve injury is compression or ischemia, most investigators favour excessive local pressure (Danta et al 1971, Parkes 1973, Rorabeck 1980, Rudge 1974). Denny-Brown and Brenner suggested that ischemia due to compression of blood vessels supplying the nerve bundles was the primary cause of nerve damage. It has been confirmed experimentally that there is a localised conduction block as a result of mechanical deformation of nerve fibres (Ochoa et al 1972). These lesions have been shown with electron microscopy to be a type of intussusception within an axon in which a node of Ranvier is displaced away from the site of compression (Ochoa et al 1972). Large myelinated fibres only are so damaged and the nodes on the smaller myelinated fibres remain uninjured. This explains the sensory sparing of some modalities as reported by Gilliatt (1975). In addition to the effect of direct pressure on the nerve, ischemia distal to the compression site may contribute to impaired nerve function, particularly as the duration of the ischemia increases (Yates et al 1981). However, the relative importance of ischemia in relationship to the direct mechanical injury to the nerve compressed by the tourniquet in the pathogenesis of tourniquet paralysis in man has not yet been established. Recovery from tourniquet paralysis will depend on the absence of irreversible damage to the nerve tissue and vessels. Although experimental evidence is still lacking, it has been generally assumed that a high pressure would more likely produce irreversible damage in a short time than a low pressure for a longer period (Griffiths & Heywood 1973). Therefore, though a recovering lesion may not be explicable on the sole basis of either the pressure level or its duration, a permanent paralysis will almost certainly be solely due to an excessive pressure (Flatt 1972).

Muscle injury

Patterson & Klenerman showed that the damage to muscle ultrastructure was more severe as a result of direct tourniquet pressure than that seen in the ischemic muscle distal to the tourniquet (Patterson & Klenerman 1979). The degree of muscle injury was related to the duration of tourniquet application. In Patterson & Klenerman's experiment it was found that a 5-hour period of ischemia invariably produced severe muscle damage, whereas a 3-hour period caused similar changes in only a quarter of the monkeys examined. There is no obvious reason not to believe that these findings would be similar to man.

Venous thrombosis

Whether the use of a pneumatic tourniquet increases or for that matter decreases the likelihood of the formation of venous thrombosis is controversial and in fact unknown. Kroese & Stiris (1974, 1975) carried out venography on patients undergoing surgery of the lower limb under tourniquet within 48 hours of operation. In the first series 10% showed radiographic evidence of thrombosis while a 17% incidence was noted in the second series. The authors reported that these figures were low compared to other reports of postoperative thrombosis and therefore concluded that the tourniquet did not seem to increase the incidence of thrombosis formation. Kroese & Stiris concluded by recommending that the use of a tourniquet should be avoided in patients who are in a high risk category for thrombus formation.

Cutaneous

Minor skin problems are seen usually due to the improper application of the tourniquet. Burns may occur due to the seepage of skin preparation materials beneath the tourniquet.

Fat

On occasion fat necrosis following the routine and apparently appropriate application of a pneumatic tourniquet has been observed.

CONTRAINDICATIONS TO TOURNIQUET USE

The use of a tourniquet in patients with known peripheral vascular disease carries an increased risk and therefore should be avoided if at all possible. Patients who have vasculitis also may be at risk, not only from the use of the tourniquet, but also the actual procedure being employed. The use of a tourniquet in an infected limb is not contraindicated but exsanguination by stripping should probably be avoided to prevent bacteriemia and possible septicemia. This same principle should apply to the surgical management of neuromusculoskeletal malignancies when a pneumatic tourniquet is employed. The application of a pneumatic tourniquet to the calf or forearm is considered contraindicated if the appropriate thigh or upper arm is available for application. The compression of clearly defined fascial compartments is to be avoided if possible.

EXSANGUINATION AND THE TOURNIQUET

Some form of exsanguination is generally practiced in association with pneumatic tourniquet use. The application of an Esmarch or Martin's bandage (latex) immediately prior to inflation of the tourniquet is an acceptable method of preventing engorgement of tissues. Simple elevation of the limb for 2 minutes prior to elevation of the tourniquet is regarded by many to be equally effective. Exsanguination of a limb results in an effective increase in circulating blood volume of up to 800 ml (Bradford 1969). It would therefore be unwise to exsanguinate more than one limb at one time in an individual with poor cardiac reserve (Klenerman & Hulands 1979). It is recommended that the tourniquet be deflated prior to the application of any rigid dressing as exsanguination and pneumatic tourniquet inflation may result in up to a 20% reduction in limb volume.

OCCLUSION TIME AND PRESSURE

There is a wide variety of opinion with regard to the optimum inflation pressure in the upper and lower extremities. It has been traditional for manufacturers of tourniquets in North America to recommend a pressure of 300 mmHg for the arm and 500 mmHg for the leg (Instruction Manual for Kidde Pneumatic Tourniquet (Model 400)). These figures and similar figures suggested in the literature and by tourniquet manufacturers appear to be entirely arbitrary and have no scientific basis. They presumably arose historically as 'safe' pressures necessary to assure a supersystolic pressure on the limb while at the same time compensating for typical errors in the tourniquet regulators, gauges and cuffs (McEwen 1981, McEwen & McGraw 1982, Sanders 1973). It has been shown that the slowing in conduction velocity and time required for it to return to normal after release of the tourniquet varies directly with the amount and duration of the pressure applied (Rorabeck 1980). Sanders has recommended that the tourniquet pressure for upper limbs ideally should be only 70 mmHg above systolic pressure (Sanders 1973). Klenerman & Hulands advise that the occlusive pressure for the lower limbs be estimated by doubling the systolic pressure taken in the arm, thereby providing the lowest effective occlusive pressure and allowing for fluctuation in blood pressure which might occur during the course of a normal operation provided the patient is normotensive and does not have a grossly hypertrophied or obese limb (Klenerman & Hulands 1979). These recommendations for the upper and lower extremity are considered safe and practical.

Most reports in the literature recommend that the period of time of tourniquet application should not exceed 90–120 minutes (Bruner 1970, Flatt 1972, Wilgis 1972) although some authors feel that up to 3 hours of tourniquet application is safe (Klenerman 1980, Parkes 1973). For practical purposes a duration of a 150 minutes in normal individuals should not be exceeded if possible.

CONCLUSION

A number of possible tourniquet-related complications have been reported in the literature. The two most frequent problems of concern are tourniquet paralysis (or paresis) and intraoperative bleeding. Regardless of whether a potential tourniquet-related complication is considered to be major or minor when it is identified, each such incident should be investigated promptly and thoroughly by appropriately qualified staff, in order to minimise both the probability of similar incidents in future and potential legal liability. To assist in the thorough and consistent investigation of such incidents, the questionnaire shown in Table 2.2 has been developed. In employing the questionnaire to investigate a potential incident involving a tourniquet, the surgeon and any assisting nurse or technologist who might have been involved in the operation of the tourniquet should attempt to answer the clinical questions which are posed in Table 2.2. An experienced biomedical engineer or similarly qualified individual should attempt to respond to the technical questions posed. The authors have found that a thorough review of the responses to the set of questions posed in Table 2.2, in conjunction with a review of the literature on reported tourniquet-related complications which was cited earlier in this chapter, is of significant value in the satisfactory and prompt resolution of such incidents. A brief elaboration of the content of Table 2.2 for the two most frequent problems of concern, tourniquet paralysis (or paresis), and intraoperative bleeding, is given below.

Tourniquet paralysis

In the event of postoperative tourniquet paralysis or paresis there is no definite treatment unless there is a co-existent compartment syndrome. Therefore the principal concern is one of prevention. Accordingly, a tourniquet incident such as postoperative weakness with sensory change must be promptly investigated. As suggested by Table 2.2, one should quickly ascertain that this is indeed an isolated event and not one incident of a yet unrecognised series related to faulty equipment or procedural errors. The time and pressure values

Table 2.2 Questionnaire for use in the event of possible tourniquet-related complications

A. *Event*

1. What was the nature of the complication?
   —What extremity?
   —Paralysis or paresthesia, intraoperative bleeding, soft-tissue injury, or other?
   —If bleeding was observed, was the blood dark in colour?

2. Was more than one patient involved?
   —If so, over what period of time did the cases occur?
   —If so, did the complication seem associated with a particular anesthetic technique?
   —If not, how many patients had been treated previously with the same complete tourniquet system?

3. Approximately how many minutes after cuff inflation was the complication first observed?
   —If the complication was not observed during the procedure what was the total duration of tourniquet application?

4. What was the status of the patient?
   —Did the patient have any pertinent abnormal conditions (e.g. atrophied or hypertrophied limbs, calcified blood vessels, steroid treatment, hypertension)?
   —What were the limb circumferences at the proximal and distal cuff edges?
   —What was the patient's systolic pressure throughout the procedure?
   —If bleeding was observed, was the patient's systolic pressure recorded at the time?
   —If a paralysis or paresthesia was observed, was a post-op EMG study done to identify and localise any possible lesion? Results?

B. *Equipment*

1. What tourniquet system was used?
   —Cuff: manufacturer, model number, length, width, dual or single bladder?
   —Connector and tubing: type and length?
   —Was a non-standard connector or adapter employed to match the cuff connector to the tubing or pressure controller?
   —Tourniquet pressure controller: manufacturer, model, serial number?
   —What was the configuration of equipment (sketch)?
   —Was a dual-cuff switch employed in a Bier's block mode?

2. What safety and performance-assurance testing of the equipment was performed?
   —At what time prior to the incident were specific, documented tests last performed on each element of the system involved (cuff, tubing and controller)?
   —What standards were employed?
   —What written test procedures were followed?
   —What were the qualifications and experience of whoever performed these tests?
   —At what time following the incident were each of the above-noted elements of the tourniquet system again tested?
   Standards? Procedures?
   Who did the testing? Documented results? Abnormal results?

C. *Procedure*

1. What application procedures were followed?
   —Who applied the cuff to the patient?
   —What was the experience of the applicator with that specific cuff?
   —How tightly was the cuff applied?
   —Was a soft bandage applied beneath the cuff?
   —Was a tape seal employed at the distal edge?
   —How was the limb exsanguinated?
   —If it was exsanguinated by elevation, how long was the limb elevated? At what angle?
   —If it was exsanguinated by rubber bandage, how tightly was the bandage wrapped? By whom? Experience?
   —What pressure settings were used?

2. What was the nature and extent of training of each of the staff who were involved in the testing and operation of the tourniquet system?
   —e.g., was training received by review of labelling and operating instructions, operating manual, audio-visual aids, vendor's presentation, institutional seminars, etc?

associated with the incident must be reviewed and compared to the acknowledged safe ranges. If the values of these parameters were recorded with acceptable accuracy and frequency, and if commonly accepted limits were not exceeded, the possibilities of faulty equipment, cuff-related problems or procedural errors must be considered. Table 2.2 offers guidance in this regard. For example, when any of the older mechanical types of tourniquet systems are used, the pressure gauge and the pressure regulator should be tested frequently to identify errors and possible malfunctions; a structured investigation will help determine whether the device met standards and whether pre-incident tests were adequately performed. Inaccurate pressure gauges and defective pressure regulators permitting excessive hysteresis were common causes of tourniquet injury in the past. In contrast, inaccurate pressure indicators and defective pressure regulators are much less likely to occur in digital tourniquet systems, and are much less likely to exist undetected by the operator when they do occur in such systems. Again, this can be confirmed by structured investigations of all pertinent incidents.

Intraoperative bleeding

Intraoperative bleeding in the presence of a pneumatic tourniquet is an annoying occurrence which unnecessarily delays the procedure. With rare exception, it is, of course, preventable. If bleeding occurs it is usually wise to stop the procedure, deflate the tourniquet and evaluate a number of factors prior to re-exsanguination and re-inflation: 1. the patient's systolic blood pressure should be re-assessed in relation to the patient's limb circumference and cuff size, and the tourniquet pressure selected accordingly; 2. if the patient's limb is hypertrophied, or if the possibility of major vessel calcification exists, a higher pressure might be considered; 3. the tubing and connections should be checked; and 4. in older mechanical systems containing an integral gas cartridge, the gas source must be determined to be adequate. If consideration of these factors does not permit identification and resolution of the problem, the possibility of device-related factors should be considered. As in the case of tourniquet paralysis, device malfunctions such as defective gauges and pressure regulators can be responsible for intraoperative failure of mechanical tourniquets. However, modern digital tourniquet systems generally have audio and visual alarms which alert the operator to unintended and significant alterations in tourniquet pressure, as well as excessive periods of inflation, making these factors much less significant. Inappropriate exsanguination procedures can cause minor oozing with a properly functioning tourniquet system. Alternatively, Furlow's 'tourniquet ooze' syndrome may be responsible (Furlow 1971). Any of a variety of cuff-related problems, as outlined earlier in the chapter, may also be factors. This emphasises the need for systematic and prompt investigation of all incidents of possible tourniquet-related complications along the lines suggested in Table 2.2.

In the latest generation of computer-based tourniquet systems now being developed and introduced, the tourniquet has the capability of constantly adapting the cuff pressure to the patient's ever-fluctuating occlusion pressure in the limb, so that the minimum effective pressure can routinely be employed.

In future, it is possible that tourniquet injury might be eliminated entirely by a combination of thorough investigation of pertinent incidents, improved design of digital tourniquets, improved design of occlusive cuffs, and adoption of safe and effective operating procedures.

REFERENCES

AORN April 1984 Recommended practices: preparation, utilization and maintenance of the pneumatic tourniquet. Journal Association of Operating Room Nurses 39:808–812

Bradford E M W 1969 Haemodynamic changes associated with the application of lower limb tourniquets. Anaesthesia 24:190–198

Bruner J M 1970 Time, pressure and temperature factors in the safe use of the tourniquet. Hand 2:39–42

Cushing H 1904 Pneumatic tourniquets with special reference to their use in craniotomies. Medical News 84:577–580

Danta G, Fowler T J, Gilliatt R W 1971 Conduction block after a pneumatic tourniquet. Journal of Physiology (London) 215:250

ECRI October 1984 Pneumatic tourniquets. Health Devices 14:299–320

Erlanger J, Gasser H S 1937 Electrical signs of nervous activity. University of Pennsylvania Press, Philadelphia

Esmarch J F A 1873 Ueber Lunstliche Blutleere bei Operationen. Sammlung Klinischer Vortrage in Verbindung mit Deutschen Klinkenn. Chirurgie 19(58):373

Flatt A E 1972 Tourniquet time in hand surgery. Archives of Surgery 104:190–192

Furlow L T 1971 Cause and prevention of tourniquet ooze. Surgery, Gynecology, Obstetrics 132:1069–1072

Gilliatt R W 1975 Peripheral nerve compression and entrapment. In: Lant A F (ed) Proceedings of a conference held at the Royal College of Physicians of London. Eleventh Symposium. Pitman Medical Books, London

Griffiths J C, Heywood O B 1973 Bio-mechanical aspects of the tourniquet. Hand 5:113–117

Instruction Manual for Kidde Pneumatic Tourniquet (Model 400 manufactured by Walter Kidde, Inc., Belleville, N.J., U.S.A.)

Johnson D L et al 1980 Hazards in single-stage regulation of pressure cuffs. Journal of Clinical Engineering 5:59–62

Kessler F B 1966 The brachial tourniquet and local analgesia in surgery of the upper limb. Journal of Trauma 6:43–47

Klenerman L 1962 The tourniquet in surgery. Journal of Bone and Joint Surgery 44B:937–943

Klenerman L 1980 Tourniquet time—How long? Hand 12:231–234

Klenerman L, Hulands G H 1979 Tourniquet pressures for the lower limb. (Abstract) Journal of Bone and Joint Surgery 61B:124

Kroese A J, Stiris G 1974 Does preoperative pneumatic tourniquet cause thrombosis? Journal of Oslo City Hospital 24:69–73

Kroese A J, Stiris G 1975 The risk of deep vein thrombosis after operations on a bloodless lower limb. A venographic study. Injury 7:271–273

McEwen J A July–August 1981 Complications of and improvements in pneumatic tourniquets used in surgery. Medical Instrumentation 15:253–257

McEwen J A 1983 Hazards and improvements in cuffs for surgical tourniquets. Proc. 18th Meeting of Assn for Advancement of Medical Instrumentation (Dallas, TX). p 79

McEwen J A, Auchinleck G F 1982 Recent advances in surgical tourniquets. Journal of the Association of Operating Room Nurses 36:889–896

McEwen J A, McGraw R W 1979 An automatic tourniquet for surgical applications. Proceedings 32nd Annual Conference Engineering in Medicine and Biology (Denver, Colorado). p 243

McEwen J A, McGraw R W February 1982 An adaptive tourniquet for improved safety in surgery. IEEE Transactions Bio-Medical Engineering 29:122–128

Moldaver J 1954 Tourniquet paralysis syndrome. Archives of Surgery 68:136–144

Ochoa J R, Fowler T J, Gilliatt R W 1972 Anatomical changes in peripheral nerves compressed by a pneumatic tourniquet. Journal of Anatomy 113:433–455

Parkes A 1973 Ischaemic effects of external and internal pressure on the upper limb. Hand 5:105–112

Patterson S, Klenerman L 1979 The effect of pneumatic tourniquets on the ultrastructure of skeletal muscle. Journal of Bone and Joint Surgery 61B:178–183

Rorabeck C H 1980 Tourniquet-induced nerve ischemia: An experimental investigation. Journal of Trauma 20:280–286

Rorabeck C H, Kennedy J C 1980 Tourniquet-induced nerve ischemia complicating knee ligament surgery. American Journal of Sports Medicine 8:98–102

Rudge P 1974 Tourniquet paralysis with prolonged conduction block. Journal of Bone and Joint Surgery 56B:716–720

Sanders R 1973 The tourniquet. Instrument or weapon? Hand 5:119–123

Weingarden S I, Louis D L, Waylonis G W 1979 Electromyographic changes in postmeniscectomy patients. JAMA 241:1248–1250

Wilgis E F S 1972 Tourniquet in reconstructive surgery of the hand. Hand Chirurgie 4:99–101

Yates S K, Hurst L N, Brown W F 1981 The pathogenesis of pneumatic tourniquet paralysis in man. Journal of Neurology, Neurosurgery, Psychiatry 44:759–767

G. Hooper

3 Volkmann's ischaemic contracture

INTRODUCTION

Richard von Volkmann drew attention to the deformity produced by ischaemic contractures of the forearm muscles and distinguished it from a deformity caused by damage to nerves (Volkmann 1881). The classic 'Volkmann's ischaemic contracture' (Fig. 3.1) compromises function of the hand because the extrinsic muscles are damaged. In 1920 Richardo Finochietto described a similar type of contracture affecting the intrinsic muscles of the hand, in a mechanic who had sustained a crushing injury (Boyes 1976).

It is now recognised that such ischaemic contractures are the end result of muscle damage due to raised tissue pressure within closed compartments. Raised intracompartmental pressure may be the result of many different kinds of insult (Table 3.1), but once it becomes established it cannot be relieved by removing the initiating factor; irreversible damage to muscles and nerves within the compartment can be prevented only if the condition is recognised at an early stage and proper steps are taken to reduce pressure within the compartment. Unfortunately patients are still seen with established ischaemic contractures, and these patients may need reconstructive surgery to improve function and cosmesis.

This chapter will review the pathophysiology, clinical features and management of raised intracompartmental pressure and established ischaemic contractures in the upper limb. These are fortunately uncommon complications of elective hand surgery but a surgeon treating upper limb problems will inevitably encounter a patient with an acute compartment syndrome sooner or later. The onus will then be on him to take action that will avoid that most unsatisfactory of results, an established ischaemic contracture.

PATHOPHYSIOLOGY

'A compartmental syndrome is a condition in which increased pressure within a limited space comprises the circulation and the function of the tissues within that space' (Matsen 1980).

The limited tissue space is usually a fascial compartment in a limb, containing muscles, blood vessels and nerves. Depending on circumstances however the boundary of the space may be the epimysium around a muscle belly, the skin, or a circumferential dressing or cast (Fig. 3.2).

There is still doubt about the exact nature of the changes in circulation to tissues within a compartment that initiate a compartment syndrome, and

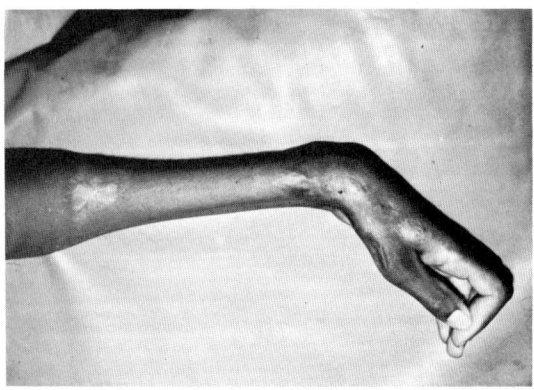

Fig. 3.1 Typical deformity in severe Volkmann's ischaemic contracture (Courtesy of Mr C Court-Brown)

Table 3.1 Causes of compartment syndromes

Decrease in volume of compartment	Tight closure of fascial defects

Increase in volume of tissue in compartment	Bleeding
	    Vascular injury
	    Bleeding disorder
	    Anticoagulation
	    Muscle avulsion
	Increase in tissue fluid
	    Reperfusion after ischaemia
	        Arterial repair
	        Embolectomy
	        Replantation
	        Lying on limb
	        Prolonged tourniquet
	    Trauma
	        Fracture
	        Contusion
	    Muscular activity
	    Burns
	    Cold injury
	    Intra-arterial drug injection
	    Surgery
	    Snakebite
	    Infiltrated infusion
	    High pressure injection injuries

External pressure	Tight casts or dressings Lying on limb

indeed they may vary with the original insult (Table 3.1). Exchange of oxygen and metabolites between capillaries and tissues depends upon blood flow, which in turn depends upon the pressure difference between the arterial and venous ends of the circulation. A direct arterial injury will result in ischaemia of tissues if the collateral circulation is inadequate. Ischaemia causes swelling and oedema which eventually obliterate the microcirculation. However most compartment syndromes are not associated with a major injury to a proximal artery but follow a direct insult to the compartment itself. This probably causes a rise in pressure at the venous end of the circulation within the compartment, so that there is a net outflow of fluid from capillaries to tissue; the result is increasing oedema of the tissues and again eventual obliteration of the microcirculation. Therefore, no matter what the original insult, be it an arterial injury (Type I injury) or direct trauma (Type II injury), once commenced the pathological process becomes a vicious circle of increased pressure within the compartment and diminished or absent capillary blood flow (Holden 1979) (Fig. 3.3). Where there has been no arterial damage the sequence of events can take place despite the presence of distal peripheral pulses and normal skin circulation. This is because blood flow in the major arteries, which are intracompartmental, ceases only when compartmental pressure is greater than arterial pressure (Parkes 1973) (Figs 3.4 & 3.5).

Muscles and nerves may be irreversibly damaged within a few hours of the onset of raised intracompartmental pressure unless fasciotomy is carried out. Although both tissues have some capacity for recovery and regeneration after ischaemic damage, it is rather limited (Sanderson et al 1975, Rorabeck & Clark 1978). Irreversible damage is followed by fibrosis of muscles and nerves and the establishment of a characteristic pattern of deformity which depends on the compartments affected and the extent of involvement.

Re-establishment of the circulation by fasciotomy may be followed by a further compartment syndrome. This is the result of swelling of muscles due to reactive hyperaemia, which may cause a muscle to be subject to increased pressure within its own epimysial sheath. The problem may also be encountered when a fasciotomy is performed through a small skin incision: the muscles swell and the skin eventually becomes the inextensible

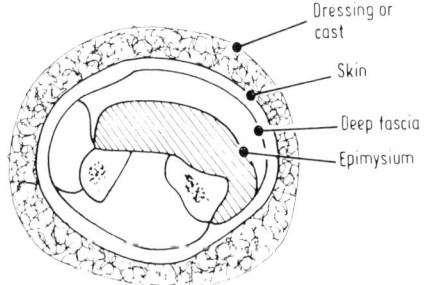

Fig. 3.2 The structures that may form the boundaries of compartments

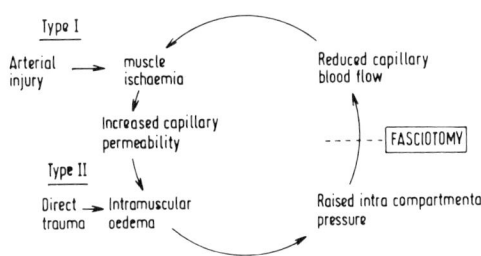

Fig. 3.3 The factors involved in the onset and perpetuation of a compartment syndrome

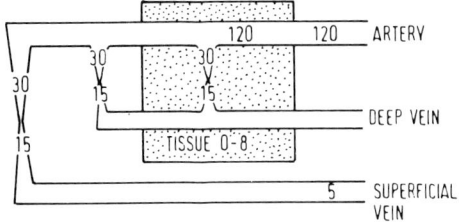

Fig. 3.4 The normal arrangement of blood vessels in a limb. Note that the venous blood from the compartment does not drain to superficial veins. Approximate pressures shown in mm of mercury

boundary of the compartment. This phenomenon is known as 'rebound ischaemia' or the 'double ischaemic insult'.

CAUSES OF COMPARTMENT SYNDROMES

A compartment syndrome can occur when there is a limited tissue compartment and a cause for raised pressure within that compartment. The frequency of the various causes of raised tissue pressure varies with different patient populations. Those most relevant to the hand surgeon are given in Table 3.1 which is derived from the exhaustive list given by Matsen (1980).

Prevention of compartment syndromes

It will be appreciated from the aetiological factors listed in Table 3.1 that an acute compartment syndrome can occur even when a patient has been managed with the greatest care. It is not usually

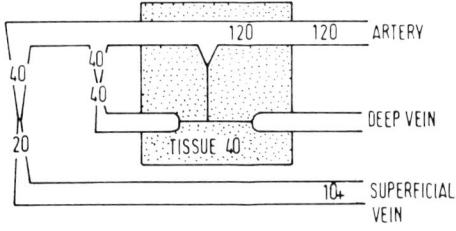

Fig. 3.5 When pressure is increased in the compartment the microcirculation is obliterated. Flow in the artery does not cease until the pressure within the compartment exceeds arterial pressure; until this happens there will still be flow in peripheral vessels. Approximate pressures shown in mm of mercury

the occurrence of a compartment syndrome but failure to recognise and treat it that reflects upon the patient's management. Having said this, there are certain factors contributing to compartment syndromes that are within the control of the surgeon and these are fairly obvious: tight bandages and casts must be avoided, as must prolonged tourniquet ischaemia; the likelihood of rebound ischaemia occurring after revascularisation and replantation procedures must be recognised and prophylactic fasciotomy performed.

DIAGNOSIS OF ACUTE COMPARTMENT SYNDROMES

Diagnosis rests almost wholly on history and clinical examination.

Clinical features

The surgeon should be alert to the possibility of the onset of a compartment syndrome, and especially when dealing with the problems listed in Table 3.1. He should also be aware that a compartment syndrome can follow an apparently trivial injury (Bennett 1965). Raised intracompartmental pressure usually develops within a few hours of the insult to the limb, but may occur up to three or more days later. Therefore the patient at risk must be examined regularly during this period.

The patient may experience a feeling of tightness in the forearm or hand, but *pain* is the major complaint. The pain is usually greater than expected from the clinical situation and increases despite being treated with analgesics.

The part affected is usually swollen. Swelling of the hand is often particularly marked even though the compartment involved is in the forearm and the hand tends to assume the 'intrinsic minus' posture, with the metacarpophalangeal joints extended and the interphalangeal joints slightly flexed (Spinner et al 1972, Wohlfort et al 1973). The involved compartment is tense and palpation may exacerbate pain.

Muscles in the affected compartments are weak and pain is increased when they are passively stretched. When testing the flexor muscles of the forearm the fingers should be extended fully before attempting to extend the wrist. The diminution in movement and the pain elicited are in proportion to the extent of muscle involvement; in severe cases it may not be possible to passively extend the fingers even with the wrist flexed. The intrinsic muscles of each finger are tested in turn by extending the metacarpophalangeal joints and then flexing the interphalangeal joints and deviating the finger in both radial and ulnar directions. If these passive movements elicit pain then pressure in the appropriate intrinsic compartment is raised, but frequently it is difficult to assess the significance of pain caused by muscle testing in the injured hand.

Neurological examination may reveal loss or diminution of sensation in the distribution of nerves passing through the compartment. When the forearm is involved the median nerve is usually affected, since it lies deep in the compartment. The ulnar nerve, which is more superficial, may be intact. Involvement of the intrinsic compartments does not itself cause sensory loss in the hand, since the digital nerves do not lie in the compartments. Nevertheless there is often numbness in the median nerve area, attributable to pressure on the nerve from the gross oedema that is often present in the palm.

In the absence of proximal arterial injury peripheral pulses and skin perfusion will be normal, since obliteration of arteries is a late feature of raised intracompartmental pressure. It must be stressed that the '4 Ps' of proximal arterial injury (*pain, pallor, pulselessness* and *paraesthesiae*) are *not* the diagnostic signs of an acute compartment syndrome, although of course some of them may be present.

In summary the most important clinical features of a compartment syndrome are pain aggravated by passive stretching of the muscles within the compartment. Disappearance of pain without recovery of muscle function is an ominous sign since it usually indicates severe ischaemic damage to nerves and necrosis of muscles.

Measurement of tissue pressure

Direct measurement of the tissue pressure within the compartment can be helpful diagnostically when the clinical picture is doubtful or the patient is unconcious. Pressure measurement is not indicated as a confirmatory investigation if the clinical signs are clear.

Three main methods are available: the needle manometer (Whitesides et al 1975), wick catheter (Mubarak et al 1978) and continuous infusion (Matsen et al 1980) techniques. Whichever technique is chosen, it must be used properly and the equipment calibrated accurately. An incorrect reading is worse then no reading at all as it will almost certainly lead to the wrong course of management.

A pressure of 40 mmHg or more (normal 0–8 mmHg) is an indication for fasciotomy in the forearm. This figure is only a guide since the measured pressure depends on the technique used and other factors such as the patient's blood pressure and peripheral circulatory volume.

There are conflicting reports about the reliability of direct measurements of tissue pressure in the intrinsic compartments of the hand (Garfin & Mubarak 1980, Halpern & Mochizuki 1980). This is a pity because clinical signs of raised intracompartmental pressure are often difficult to interpret in the injured hand and an objective test would be most useful.

Angiography

Angiography is not helpful in making a diagnosis of compartment syndrome. Surgical exploration rather than angiography is indicated if a suspected compartment syndrome is accompanied by absence of the peripheral pulses. This will allow direct inspection of the artery as well as decompression of the compartment.

Nerve stimulation

Occasionally it may be difficult to distinguish between paralysis due to compartment syndrome and paralysis due to proximal injury to a nerve. If the nerve is electrically stimulated close to the muscle and contraction occurs then paralysis is due to proximal nerve injury; if there is no contraction a diagnosis of compartment syndrome is more likely.

TREATMENT OF ACUTE COMPARTMENT SYNDROMES

Non-operative treatment

There is little place for conservative management of most compartment syndromes and time should certainly not be wasted on futile treatments with vasodilator drugs and sympathetic blocks. However it is of course mandatory to open encircling dressings or casts *widely* down to skin (Bingold 1979). It is sensible to treat systemic hypotension (e.g. due to hypovolaemia) if this is present, since local arterial hypotension contributes to the fall in arteriovenous pressure difference and also potentiates the effect of such a fall. Of direct importance to the hand surgeon is the fact that elevation of the upper limb above heart level diminishes pressure in the arterial side of the circulation; therefore at the first suspicion of a compartmental syndrome the arm and hand must be lowered to the patient's side.

The patient's general condition may require expert medical management. For example, an increasingly common cause of acute compartment syndromes is prolonged lying on a limb whilst unconscious, often as a result of drug overdosage. When pressure is taken off the limb toxic products of muscle breakdown are released into the circulation and may cause acute renal failure (Schreiber et al 1972).

Surgical treatment

Unless conservative measures such as splitting dressings and lowering the arm result in complete reversal of symptoms and signs within a few minutes, and they seldom do, urgent surgical decompression of the involved compartments is indicated.

Surgical aphorisms are usually based on hard experience and two are apposite here—'If you're wondering if you should do a fasciotomy you should do a fasciotomy' and 'No surgeon ever regretted doing a fasciotomy, but plenty regretted not doing a fasciotomy'.

Forearm

When making the skin incision care should be taken not to divide cutaneous nerves and superficial veins. The incision should be so designed that late skin contractures at wrist and elbow are avoided and it should be compatible with further incisions for future tendon transfers (Fig. 3.6). The deep fascia is divided, as is the bicipital aponeurosis at the elbow, allowing inspection of the brachial artery if indicated. The carpal tunnel is opened. The three main fascial compartments of the forearm (volar, dorsal and 'mobile wad' compartment containing the radial extensors) are interconnected, so that decompression of the volar compartment will usually relieve pressure in the others (Gelberman et al 1978). If it does not do so, or there is any doubt, then decompression of the dorsal compartment is performed through a straight dorsal incision.

After fasciotomy individual muscle bellies are inspected, particularly those of the deep flexor group, and local epimysial release is carried out if the bellies are tense. Debridement of muscles is avoided at this stage.

The skin incision is left open (Fig. 3.7). Exposed nerves are covered with soft tissue if possible. An absorbent dressing is applied and the forearm and hand are splinted. It is permissible to elevate the arm after adequate decompression. The wound is inspected at 5 days and can often be closed partially as the swelling will have gone down quite dramatically. Complete closure should be left until 10 days after injury. If the wound cannot be closed completely without tension the skin defect is covered with a split skin graft.

The scar of a forearm decompression is always unsightly (Fig. 3.8) but it is a small price to pay for regaining function (Fig. 3.9).

Hand

The intrinsic muscle compartments in the hand are separate and releasing one will have no effect on tension in the others (Fig. 3.10). A single

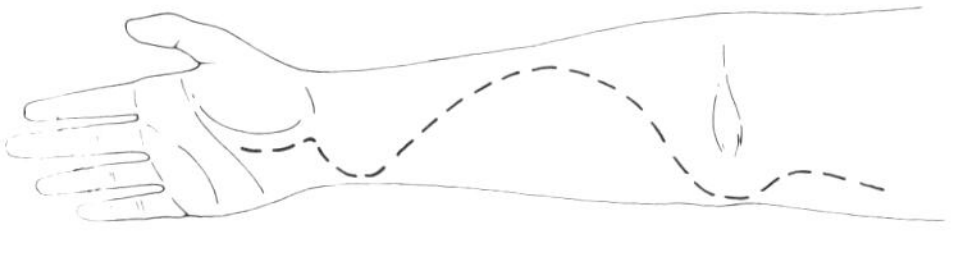

Fig. 3.6 A suitable skin incision for fasciotomy in the forearm

VOLKMANN'S ISCHAEMIC CONTRACTURE

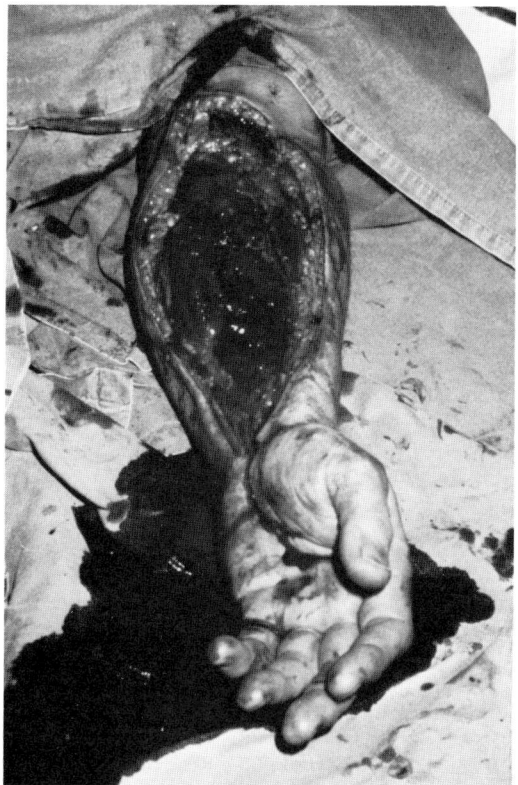

Fig. 3.7 Immediately after fasciotomy the muscles bulge out through the incision

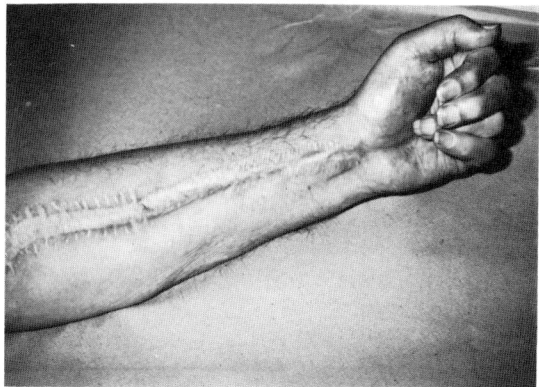

Fig. 3.9 Range of finger flexion. Grip strength and sensation were both excellent (same patient as Fig. 3.7).

compartment may be affected, or several (Spinner et al 1972, Reid & Travis 1973, Monteleone et al 1985). The compartments to be released can be identified by clinical testing of passive movements and palpation for locally increased tension, but these signs are often difficult to interpret in the injured hand. Therefore it is safest to decompress *all* the interosseous compartments and the adductor compartment of the thumb. Increased pressure in the thenar and hypothenar groups is easier to detect clinically and these compartments are decompressed if necessary.

The interosseous compartments can be released via a transverse dorsal incision or two longitudinal incisions over the index and ring finger metacarpal bones. The compartments are opened by incisions in the fascia on either side of the metacarpal bones (Fig. 3.10). Blunt dissection through the interossei on the ulnar border of the index finger metacarpal bone will allow release of the adductor pollicis compartment. If decompression of the thenar and hypothenar compartments is indicated they must be opened through further skin incisions on the radial and ulnar borders of the hand.

Skin incisions are left open and the hand is

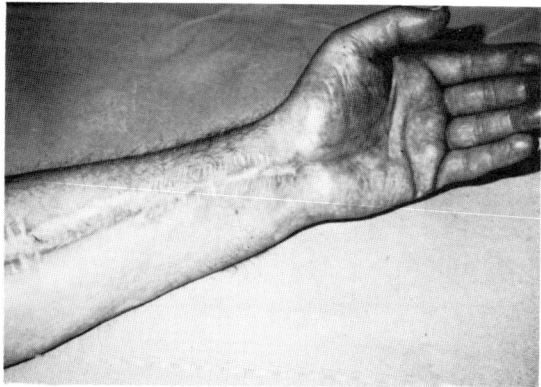

Fig. 3.8 Forearm scar several months after fasciotomy. Incision closed 10 days after decompression (same patient as Fig. 3.7).

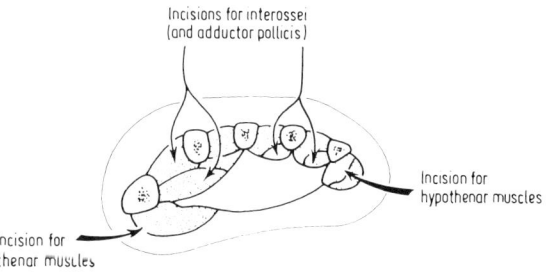

Fig. 3.10 The surgical approach to the intrinsic compartments of the hand

splinted in the standard position of immobilisation. The hand should be elevated to diminish swelling. Skin is closed 5–10 days after fasciotomy, using split skin grafts if necessary. Mobilisation of the hand is encouraged as soon as the primary condition permits.

Delayed fasciotomy

The earlier fasciotomy is done the better the end result is likely to be (Sheridan & Matsen 1976). Nevertheless, fasciotomy can be worthwhile, even at a late stage, particularly in children. Excellent recovery has been recorded after fasciotomy carried out between 3 days and 16 weeks after injury (Spinner et al 1972, Eaton & Green 1975, Geary 1984).

MANAGMENT OF ESTABLISHED ISCHAEMIC CONTRACTURES

Deformities affecting the hand may be caused by ischaemic contractures of forearm or intrinsic muscles, paralysis due to ischaemia of motor nerves, or a combination of these factors. It is usually possible to identify the main cause of the deformity by clinical examination.

Generally speaking, reconstructive procedures should be left for 3–6 months after the original episode to allow time for any recovery and regeneration to take place. During this time, if the patient is under observation, attention is directed towards minimising contractures by appropriate splinting.

Contractures of extrinsic muscles

Muscle degeneration and fibrosis are most marked in the middle of the mass of the forearm muscles and decrease towards the periphery, producing an 'ellipsoid infarct' which is variable in size (Seddon 1956). The median nerve is surrounded and compressed by this tissue whereas the ulnar nerve at the periphery is relatively spared.

Tsuge (1975) has classified Volkmann's ischaemic contracture into three groups, based on the clinical features and the extent of the infarct.

1. *Mild (localised) type.* There is degeneration of part of the belly of flexor digitorum profundus causing contractures of two or three fingers. Neurological signs are absent or minimal.

2. *Moderate type.* The damage affects virtually the whole of the muscle bellies of flexor digitorum profundus and flexor pollicis longus, and there is some involvement of the superficial muscles. Median nerve signs are present, but the ulnar nerve is not usually damaged.

3. *Severe type.* There is degeneration of all flexor muscles and some of the extensors, together with loss of function in the median and ulnar nerves. In addition there are often secondary joint contractures, skin cicatrisation and bony deformities if the condition was precipitated by a fracture.

Treatment

Mild type. If the patient is seen early after injury good results can be expected from a program of splinting, physical therapy and functional training.

Surgical treatment is indicated if the deformity does not respond to these measures. This takes the form of simple release of the involved muscle. In more severe cases a flexor muscle slide may be necessary. This is done through a volar zig-zag incision, with an additional ulnar incision to gain access to the interosseous membrane. The flexor muscles of the fingers are released at their origins and attachments to the interosseous membrane, taking care to avoid damage to the interosseous nerves and vessels. Adequate release is indicated when the fingers can be extended passively. The median nerve should be inspected and released from any scar tissue.

After surgery the forearm is splinted in supination with the wrist dorsiflexed, the metacarpophalangeal joints in slight flexion and the fingers extended. Splintage should not be maintained for more than 2–3 weeks. Early mobilisation is started in a dynamic splint.

Moderate type. The hand assumes the 'intrinsic minus' posture, with hyperextension of the metacarpophalangeal joints and flexion of the interphalangeal joints. As noted, the median nerve is involved, causing sensory and motor impairment.

Treatment is by the muscle-sliding procedure which needs to be more extensive than that described for the mild type of deformity. The digital flexors are released as before and flexor pollicis longus and pronator teres are stripped from the radius using additional radial incisions if necessary. The median and ulnar nerves are explored and transposed to unscarred beds. Postoperative management is as described for the mild type.

The muscle sliding operation tends to weaken grip and it may be necessary to combine it with appropriate tendon transfers, either at the same time or later. If there are joint contractures tendon transfer should be deferred until the range of movement in the joints is improved by physiotherapy.

Severe type. If the patient is seen within a few months of injury the infarcted muscles should be excised to prevent the onset of severe contractures. This should be combined with neurolysis of the median and ulnar nerves to try and restore sensation and intrinsic muscle function. As a second stage tendon transfers are done to restore finger and thumb flexion, using brachioradialis and available wrist extensors.

In old cases with established severe deformity, virtually no muscle function and no prospect of nerve regeneration it is doubtful if surgery has much to offer. Every case must be considered on its individual merits. It may be possible to regain some function by procedures such as tendon transfer, flexor tendon tenodesis and thumb stabilisation, although the gains are likely to be small. Free muscle transplantation using microsurgical techniques has been used, but its role is not yet established (Ikuta et al 1976).

Contractures of intrinsic muscles

In mild cases the extent of involvement may be gauged by the Bunnell test for intrinsic tightness: when the metacarpophalangeal joint is held extended with the proximal phalanx in line with the metacarpal bone, intrinsic tightness is present if the interphalangeal joints cannot be flexed passively. This tightness of the intrinsic results in weakness of the hand in gripping large objects.

Severe involvement of the interossei causes the hand to take up the characteristic 'intrinsic plus' posture with the metacarpophalangeal joints held flexed and the proximal interphalangeal joints extended (Bunnell 1953, Harris & Riordan 1954) (Fig. 3.11). The hand cannot be opened for grasping. It should be noted that this posture does not occur if there is a co-existent contracture of the forearm muscles, because the interphalangeal joints are pulled into flexion by the contracted extrinsics.

The thenar and hypothenar muscles may be affected with the interossei or alone. Involvement of the adductor pollicis is common, causing an adduction contracture of the first web space (Newmeyer & Kilgore 1976, Quigley et al 1981).

Treatment

Mild type. In mild forms of intrinsic contracture passive movement of the metacarpophalangeal joint is full but there is an extension contracture of the proximal interphalangeal joint and the test for intrinsic tightness is positive. To mobilise the proximal interphalangeal joint it is necessary to perform a distal intrinsic release by resecting the oblique fibres of the lateral bands (Harris & Riordan 1954, Smith 1971) (Fig. 3.12). The operation is done through a longitudinal incision in the midline of the proximal phalanx. The transverse fibres of the intrinsic aponeurosis are preserved, as are the central slip and lateral

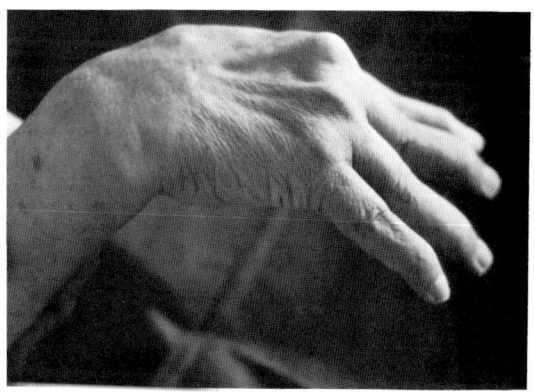

Fig. 3.11 Typical posture of the hand with ischaemic contracture of the intrinsic muscles

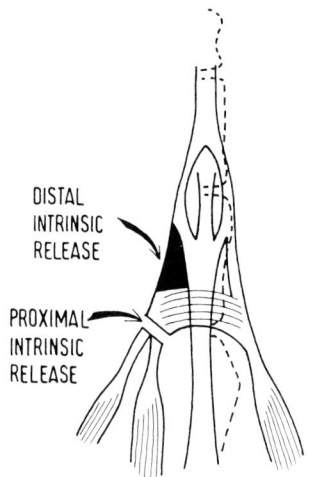

Fig. 3.12 Intrinsic release. The two levels of intrinsic release are shown. Both sides of the extensor apparatus are released but for clarity the releases are shown on one side only.

slips arising from the long extensor tendon. Active and passive movements of the interphalangeal joints are begun immediately after surgery, using a splint to keep the metacarpophalangeal joints extended.

Severe type. The metacarpophalangeal joints are held flexed and the proximal interphalangeal joints are extended (Fig. 3.11). Function of the hand can be improved by a proximal intrinsic release, dividing the tendons of the interossei at the level of the metacarpophalangeal joint (Smith 1971) (Fig. 3.12). This usually allows the metacarpophalangeal joints to extend. If it does not the volar plate and collateral ligaments may be contracted and, if so, should be released. Clawing of the hand due to hyperextension of the metacarpophalangeal joints is rarely a problem even after extensive release. Postoperative management is as described for the mild type of deformity.

REFERENCES

Bennett J 1965 Expanding forearm haematoma after apparently minor injury. Plastic and Reconstructive Surgery 36:622–625

Bingold A C 1979 On splitting plasters. Journal of Bone and Joint Surgery 61B:294–295

Boyes J H 1976 On the shoulders of giants. J B Lippincott Company, Philadelphia

Bunnell S 1953 Ischaemic contracture, local, in the hand. Journal of Bone and Joint Surgery 35A:88–101

Eaton R G, Green W T 1975 Volkmann's ischaemia. A volar compartment syndrome of the forearm. Clinical Orthopaedics 113:58–64

Garfin S R, Mubarak S J 1980 Treatment of rattlesnake bites—letter to editor. Journal of Hand Surgery 5:619

Geary N 1984 Late surgical decompression for compartment syndrome of the forearm. Journal of Bone and Joint Surgery 66B:745–748

Gelberman R H, Zakaib G S, Mubarak S J, Hargens A R, Akeson W H 1978 Decompression of forearm compartment syndromes. Clinical Orthopaedics 134:225–229

Halpern A A, Mochizuki R M 1980 Compartment syndrome of the interosseous muscles of the hand. Orthopaedic Review 9:121–127

Harris C, Riordan D C 1954 Intrinsic contracture of the hand and its surgical treatment. Journal of Bone and Joint Surgery 36A:10–18

Holden C E A 1979 The pathology and prevention of Volkmann's ischaemic contracture. Journal of Bone and Joint Surgery 61B:296–300

Ikuta Y, Kubo T, Tsuge K 1976 Free muscle transplantation by microsurgical technique to treat severe Volkmann's contracture. Plastic and Reconstructive Surgery 58:407–411

Matsen F A 1980 Compartmental syndromes. Grune & Stratton, New York

Matsen F A, Winquist R A, Krugmire R B 1980 Diagnosis and management of compartmental syndromes. Journal of Bone and Joint Surgery 62A:286–291

Monteleone M, Montorsi A, Luchetti R, Rovesta C 1985 Ischaemic isolated retraction of the abductor digiti minimi. Journal of Hand Surgery 10B:57–59

Mubarak S J, Owen C A, Hargens A R, Garetto L P, Enneking W F 1978 Acute compartment syndromes. Diagnosis and treatment with the aid of the wick catheter. Journal of Bone and Joint Surgery 60A:1091–1099

Newmeyer W, Kilgore E 1976 Volkmann's ischaemic contracture due to soft tissue injury alone. Journal of Hand Surgery 1:221–227

Parkes A 1973 Ischaemic effects of external and internal pressure on the upper limb. The Hand 5:105–112

Quigley J T, Popich G A, Lanz U B 1981 Compartment syndrome of the forearm and hand: a case report. Clinical Orthopaedics 161:247–251

Reid R L, Travis R T 1973 Acute necrosis of the second interosseous compartment of the hand. Journal of Bone and Joint Surgery 55A:1095–1097

Rorabeck C H, Clarke K M 1978 The pathophysiology of the anterior tibial compartment syndrome: an experimental investigation. Journal of Trauma 18:229–304

Sanderson R A, Foley R K, McIvor G W D, Kirkaldy-Willis H 1975 Histologic response of skeletal muscle to ischaemia. Clinical Orthopaedics 113:27–35

Schreiber S, Liebowitz M R, Bernstein L H 1972 Limb compression and renal impairment (crush syndrome) following narcotic and sedative overdosage. Journal of Bone and Joint Surgery 54A:1683–1692

Seddon H 1956 Volkmann's contracture. Treatment by excision of the infarct. Journal of Bone and Joint Surgery 38B:152–174

Sheridan G W, Matsen F A 1976 Fasciotomy in the treatment of the acute compartment syndrome. Journal of Bone and Joint Surgery 58A: 112–115

Smith R J 1971 Non-ischaemic contractures of the intrinsic muscles of the hand. Journal of Bone and Joint Surgery 53A: 1313–1331

Spinner M, Aiache A, Silver L, Barsky A J 1972 Impending ischaemic contracture of the hand. Early diagnosis and management. Plastic and Reconstructive Surgery 50: 341–349

Tsuge K 1975 Treatment of established Volkmann's contracture. Journal of Bone and Joint Surgery 57A: 925–927

Volkmann R 1881 Die ischaemischen Muskellähmungen und-Kontrakturen. Zentralblatt für Chirurgie 8: 801–803 (Translated by Bick E 1967 Clinical Orthopaedics 50: 5–6)

Whitesides T E, Haney T C, Morimoto K, Harada H 1975 Tissue pressure measurements as a determinant for the need of fasciotomy. Clinical Orthopaedics 113: 43–51

Wohlfort F G, Cochran T C, Filtzer H 1973 Immediate interossei decompression following crush injury of the hand. Archives of Surgery 106: 826–828

R. L. Wilson and C. C. Reynolds

4 Joint stiffness

The development of stiffness and contracture in the hand is the most serious complication that can arise following trauma or elective surgery to the upper extremity. While destruction of an articular surface from injury or disease will inevitably produce loss of motion, stiffness in the hand develops primarily through deposition of scar within the connective tissues. Realising that any injury or surgery will incite cicatrisation, the surgeon and therapist must try to control the factors associated with the healing process that are the most detrimental. Although stiffness is defined as loss of normal motion, one should not think of this as limited to joint involvement alone. All the tissues in the hand can be implicated and should be individually considered when evaluating the stiff hand.

The major cause of stiffness in the hand is immobility (Arem 1981). Following an injury, individual tissues require different periods of immobilisation to achieve healing. For instance, the patient with a crushed hand, including two fingers with unstable fractures, must be managed with a dual program. Internal splinting of the fractures with Kirschner wires allows early protected motion which can prevent joint stiffness (Wilson & Carter 1984a). However, more vigorous mobilisation can be carried out for those digits which are crushed but not fractured. Later, external splinting may be required to maintain proper joint position, to protect the fractures or to correct the deformity. Nevertheless, prolonged splinting from incorrect instruction to the patient will defeat the original purpose and promote stiffness. This problem may be prevented by better communication between the physician or therapist and the injured individual.

Stiffness in the hand is also related to several factors which can be influenced by the patient. The first is edema which restricts small joint motion and is related to increased scar deposition. If pain is associated with motion, the individual may be less inclined to move the joint and stiffness will occur. Finally, misunderstanding of basic instructions or exercises will compound the problem.

In addition to these factors, other problems lead directly to joint stiffness and are part of a vicious cycle (Fig. 4.1) (Lankford 1983). Edema results from vascular engorgement of the wound, a transduate leaking from the capillary bed into the interstitial tissue. This coagulum of protein encases normally mobile structures. Dorsal swelling tents the lax skin on the back of the hand, drawing the fingers into hyperextension at the metacarpal phalangeal joints (MP) and reversing the longitudinal arch of the hand. The wrist drops into flexion; extension may be prevented by a pain reflex. The proximal interphalangeal (PIP) joints assume a flexed position due to the increased long flexor muscle tone. Paralysis of the intrinsic muscles may aggravate this deformity.

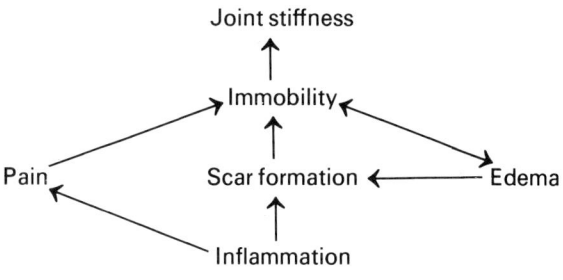

Fig. 4.1

Stiffness of the small joints in the hand can be directly related to anatomical changes in a number of important structures. The most important alterations occur in the capsuloligamentous structures surrounding the joints. The collateral ligaments, stabilising the interphalangeal joints, originate proximal-dorsal and insert distal-palmar. Ligament tension for these joints is constant throughout the arc of motion. However, the ligaments of the MP joints are under maximum tension in flexion and become lax in extension because of the volar flare of the metacarpal head. The dorsal capsule of the small joints in the hand is normally thin and supple, being lined with synovium, enclosing a large potential space. The volar plate envelops the palmar aspect of the joint and serves as a gliding surface for the proximal condyles on one side and flexor tendons on the other. This thick, fibrocartilagenous structure is anchored to the base of the phalanx distally and becomes attenuated proximally. A synovial recess between the palmar aspect of the joint and the volar plate assures mobility of this structure during joint flexion. At the PIP joint the volar plate has a thick proximal attachment to the phalanx which prevents, or check reins, hyperextension (Kuczynski 1968, 1975). This connection is absent at the MP joint, the junction to the metacarpal neck being a thin, weak membrane. The accessory collateral ligaments are situated between the volar plate and the lateral ligaments and relax with joint flexion. With injury, edema or immobility, the ligaments remodel and shorten and the dorsal capsule becomes thickened.

Joint immobilisation can produce changes on the articular surface by interfering with cartilage nutrition (Field & Hueston 1970). Compression of the joint surface with movement assists diffusion of nutrients through the cartilage (Salter & Field 1960). The unopposed surface of a joint fixed in a contracted position will demonstrate pitting, erosion and eventually cartilage loss. In addition to articular changes, prolonged immobilisation results in formation of adhesions within tendon systems. Digital motion is controlled by three groups of tendons: the long flexors, the extrinsic extensors and the intrinsics. Each pass in close proximity to the joints. At the PIP joint level, for example, the oblique retinacular ligament helps coordinate digital balance. Any abnormality of the tendon or retinacular arrangement may disturb this balance and promote finger stiffness. The sheaths surrounding the flexor tendons change shape with finger movements. If the digit is held flexed, the pliable cruciate portions may shorten. Remodeling of the skin can occur from prolonged immobility. This is most frequently seen in the web spaces and dorsally, particularly at the PIP joint. In a stiff hand, all tissues may be implicated, including fascia, subcutaneous tissues and muscles, as well as those previously mentioned. With severe contractures, even the neurovascular bundles become involved.

PREVENTION

To avoid joint stiffness, techniques are employed that can influence the factors under our control, namely edema, immobility and pain. Early wound closure following adequate debridement and hemostasis should insure primary healing and reduce the likelihood of infection (Adamson 1970). When evaluating any wound, a time table must be established for healing. Normally, hand wounds heal within 10 to 14 days. However, crush injuries resulting in small areas of skin and soft tissue loss or flap lacerations with partial devascularisation may heal more slowly. If a wound is not closed by the time that has been preselected, one must find a cause for this—necrotic tissue, dead tendon or devascularised bone. Infection should be prevented, but once present must be controlled and eliminated. A smoldering infection will lead to persistent edema and the recognised secondary effects.

Elevation of the extremity will promote wound healing and decrease edema. While relatively simple, the concept of sustained elevation is often misunderstood and forgotten by the patient a few days after injury or surgery. It is essential that an individual keep the extremity raised with the elbow above the heart at all times, whether they are standing, sitting or in a supine position. When standing, the hand can be placed on top of the head to prevent the arm from falling into a dependent state. When reclining, the patient is encouraged to rest the arm on a stack of pillows. Raising the hand over the head with the elbow and shoulder extended for 30 seconds, at least 50 times per day will hasten a reduction in swelling.

Early active protected motion will pump edema from the hand and restore gliding functions to the tendons and periarticular tissues (Wilson & Carter 1984b). How much stress can be applied and at what time will be determined by the structures that have been repaired. An individualised remobilisation program must be developed for each individual and provided in a supportive environment. It is essential that the patient become involved and eventually be responsible for his own rehabilitation program.

The hand must be splinted properly to decrease pain and protect any surgical repair. Therefore, it is placed in the intrinsic-plus or 'clam digger' position. This protected position places the wrist in slight extension, the MP joints flexed at least 70°, the PIP and DIP joints in full extension and the thumb abducted. In this manner the effects of stiffness are minimised and the establishment of the three most common contractures (PIP flexion, thumb adduction and MP extension) prevented. In the past, immobilisation of the hand has been recommended in the 'position of function'. Unfortunately, this position is more likely to facilitate small joint stiffness than prevent it (Fig. 4.2).

The development of pain may limit a patient's ability to participate actively in any exercise program. If analgesic medication does not adequately reduce the individual's pain, then various therapy modalities should be attempted. Transcutaneous electrical nerve stimulation (TENS) is one technique which may provide lasting relief. Other therapeutic modalities include the use of hot compresses or ice packs. When pain becomes disproportionate to the severity of injury, the possibility of a reflex sympathetic dystrophy must be considered. Abnormal edema, possibly produced by constrictive dressings may be the factor which initiates this reaction. Circulation is often decreased. The hand may feel cool and appear pale or splotchy. The reaction to touch may be exaggerated. The patient may complain of burning pain as well as increased sweating and the inability to tolerate extremes of temperature. Early recognition is essential for successful management of a reflex

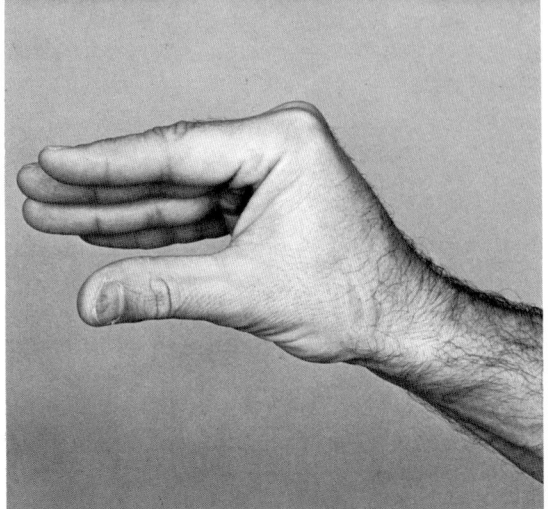

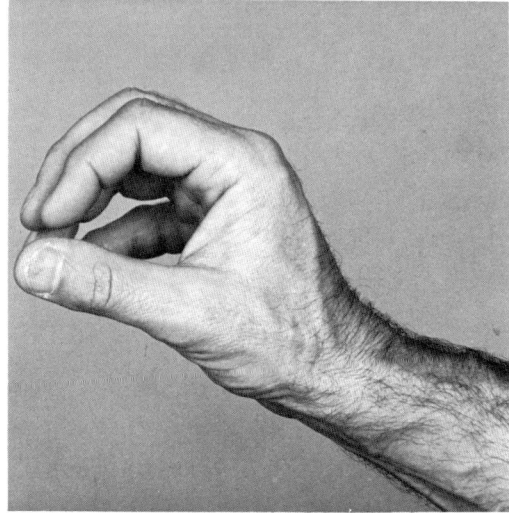

Fig. 4.2 (a) Intrinsic-plus or 'clam digger' position. (b) Prolonged immobilisation in the 'position of function' will produce small joint contractures

sympathetic dystrophy. Management with active use of the hand, TENS and contrast baths should be initiated promptly. Medical treatment often consists of sympatholytic drugs, trigger point anesthetic injections and stellate ganglion blocks.

EVALUATION

If preventative measures have failed to suppress the development of the stiff hand, certain guidelines must be established for further management.

Before treatment, the patient must be carefully assessed, evaluating which structures have been injured and which are normal. The examination should be tissue oriented and can be broken down into five categories (McCormack 1964, Weeks & Wray 1978).

1. Skin and subcutaneous tissue

Adherence can occur between the skin and underlying tissue particularly with severe involvement of the skin at the time of the original injury or in areas that have a minimal amount of subcutaneous tissue. Loss of skin may evoke further stiffening even with satisfactory tissue replacement. Contracture of normal skin or even a skin graft can occur, especially with a longstanding deformity. Hypertrophy of the palmar fascia from trauma may limit digital extension.

2. Periarticular tissues

The collateral and accessory collateral ligaments are usually involved in joint contractures. Joint stability must be tested and the pliability of the ligaments carefully assessed by the application of passive stress. The volar plate and the proximal check rein attachments are evaluated in the presence of a PIP flexion contracture. Equally important with extension contractures, is the ability of the volar plate to migrate proximally beneath the condyles of the metacarpal or proximal phalanx. The dorsal capsule is usually a flimsy tissue but may be thickened and limit joint flexion.

3. Joints and bones

Articular fractures, even when accurately reduced, can produce adhesions within joints. Osteochondral fractures involving the joint surface are more difficult to diagnose. The patient often presents with chronic synovitis unresponsive to medical treatment and demonstrates pain and limited motion. A previous subluxation or dislocation may not be appreciated at the time of examination, as the joint has a normal appearance on X-ray. To dislocate a joint, a significant periarticular soft tissue injury must occur and the articular surface may be injured (Wilson & Liechty 1986). At least three X-ray views (A/P, lateral and oblique) are required to evaluate a joint adequately. Special projections, such as the Brewerton view, will help localise an occult bony injury (Lane 1977). Healed fracture fragments may form a bony prominence and limit motion by trapping collateral ligaments or mechanically blocking joint motion. Displaced fractures may heal only to produce angulation, rotation or a collapse deformity. An individual with a malunited proximal phalanx fracture and a stiff PIP joint is especially difficult to assess. One cannot determine the exact amount of deformity caused by the fracture until the joint is fully mobile. Treatment should emphasise obtaining full joint motion, either nonoperatively or operatively, at a later stage correcting any rotational deformity through an osteotomy, if possible at a more proximal level. The presence of joint disease in association with pain also must be recognised as a frequent cause of stiffness.

4. Tendons and muscles

Adhesions between either the flexor or extensor tendons and adjacent tissue can produce secondary joint stiffness. Flexor tendon excursion may also be limited by triggering either from trauma or coincidental flexor tenosynovitis. Adherence of retinacular structures, i.e. the oblique retinacular ligament, can also disturb tendon balance and limit joint motion (Watson et al 1974). Extensor tendon entrapment in scar can produce a tenodesis effect distally. With dorsal adhesions between the extensor tendon and the metacarpal, passive flexion of the MP joint will produce prompt interphalangeal joint extension. Scarring of digital extensors in the forearm will result in limited wrist joint flexion. Contracture of the flexor fibrosseous sheath from injury or position should not be overlooked as a contributing factor in flexion deformity.

While the intrinsic-plus position is recommended for prevention of serious joint contractures, it will promote shortening of the intrinsic muscle-tendon units (Bunnell et al 1948). Treating the patient with the potential for developing a stiff hand requires removing the protective splint and performing intrinsic stretching exercises. Intrinsic tendon tightness must be evaluated in the patient presenting with an established stiff hand (Harris & Riordan, 1954). Unfortunately, joint stiffness will limit the ability to fully assess the contribution of the intrinsics. Ischemic contracture can occur not only in the intrinsic musculature of the hand but also in the forearm and be a major contributing factor to hand stiffness (Newmeyer & Kilgore 1976).

5. Nerve

Motor paralysis from a nerve injury can limit joint motion and produce secondary stiffness. Loss of sensibility will decrease perception and may diminish use of the hand. Nerve injuries may result in the establishment of pain patterns that can promote stiffness due to protection and a lack of activity. Unfortunately, trauma to even a small nerve can lead to stiffness in areas of the hand never involved in major trauma.

PRINCIPLES OF TREATMENT

Once established, treatment of joint stiffness should begin with a nonoperative therapy program. Appropriate modalities and procedures should be used to improve motion before surgery is considered. To achieve an optimal result, a goal-directed program must be designed for each patient. Patient education, edema control and a structured mobilisation program including specific exercises, activities and splinting techniques are the basis of nonoperative treatment.

An important aspect of this program is the team relationship and ongoing personal communication between the physician and the therapist. The physician provides the guidance necessary for the therapist to formulate treatment objectives. In turn, the therapist provides vital information which may assist the physician in determining when an operative course is indicated or if the patient is capable of performing his regular work. Finally, the therapist should be capable of motivating the patient to maximise his rehabilitation potential (Laseter 1983).

Controlling edema is the first component of the nonoperative program. Elevation, retrograde massage and active range of motion exercises will reduce swelling. The concept of sustained elevation has already been described. Deep manual massage performed in a distal to proximal direction will promote venous and lymphatic drainage in the swollen hand. The therapist instructs the patient to practice this technique using the uninvolved hand several times daily. Active range of motion exercises will diminish edema by compression of the fascial compartments to promote fluid movement. A specific exercise program is outlined to the patient with exercises for each of the three joints in an involved digit performed three to five times each hour.

If the conventional methods have not been effective in reducing edema completely, then mechanical means may be helpful. These include the Jobst pump, compression wraps and garments. In concept, tissue pressures can be altered to prevent fluids from accumulating outside circulatory routes. External compression enhances resorption of fluids. A compression unit is especially helpful for patients with pitting edema who do not respond rapidly to other measures. The Jobst pump is used for one hour daily, the sleeve inflated on the arm to 40–60 mmHg. Volumetric of circumferential readings are taken before and after each treatment. This program is terminated when the volume remains unchanged twice in a row. The patient then receives a compression garment which should not be constrictive nor interfere with circulation. Special care must be taken in the individual with a history of a vascular injury.

For edema localised distally, a variety of gloves are available and can be worn most of the day. They should be removed for range of motion exercises and skin care. For single digit edema, Coban wrapping may be beneficial. This elastic bandage must be applied with extreme care as the potential for excessive compression is present. Spiral or figure-8 wrapping reduces the likelihood of a constrictive application.

Heat or cold modalities such as paraffin, hot packs, or the whirlpool used in conjunction with elevation may be helpful in limiting edema. Since the circulatory response may be variable, close observation is necessary to insure effectiveness. Contrast baths, alternating heat and cold, are very effective in reducing edema and often decrease the subjective level of pain. Application of ice to a local area may reduce edema and pain but must be carefully monitored.

Increasing motion in the stiff hand is achieved by regaining the elastic quality in the tissues and promoting active movement by the patient. Heat, passive range of motion, dynamic and static splinting, functional activities as well as resistive exercises are the basic means to overcome stiffness and contracture.

Thereapeutic heat modalities are used as a warm-up prior to exercising and will improve tissue compliance. Specific heat modalities recommended include hot packs, paraffin baths and fluidotherapy. Choosing the right modality is dependent on several factors including patient preference. At home, the patient is instructed to apply moist heat two-to-three times per day for 20–30 minute periods, using warm, damp towels with the hand in an elevated position. Soaking the hand is discouraged as this tends to increase edema.

Gentle passive stretching or joint mobilisation can help restore range of motion. These techniques also help to prepare the patient's hand for active exercises and functional activities. The therapist passively stretches the patient's joints, mobilising them through their normal range of motion, as well as through accessory motions which the patient cannot perform by himself. Accessory motions include lateral-medial tilting, volar-dorsal gliding and in some cases, rotation. The techniques applied are dependent on the anatomical configuration of the joint and the structures involved (Fig. 4.3). Passive stretching must be gentle and forceful manipulations avoided. Painful stretching can lead to microscopic tears of the tissues, more bleeding into the joint, increased swelling and further stiffness.

An essential part in managing a program for hand stiffness is the correct application of static and dynamic splints. Nonmoving static splints are used to protect newly repaired structures from reinjury, to position the hand for rest, to maintain gains made by exercise and to apply serial stretch of a part over a period of time. Dynamic splints help to mobilise joints by assisting weak or absent muscles, as well as by stretching contracted tissues by mechanical means. Splint application will be described in more detail with discussion of specific contractures.

As motion returns the patient is encouraged to become involved in functional activities. This program begins early in the rehabilitative process, starting with very light activities and advancing to heavier, more difficult ones as progress is made. Many of the standardised tests that help document and evaluate functional recovery such as the

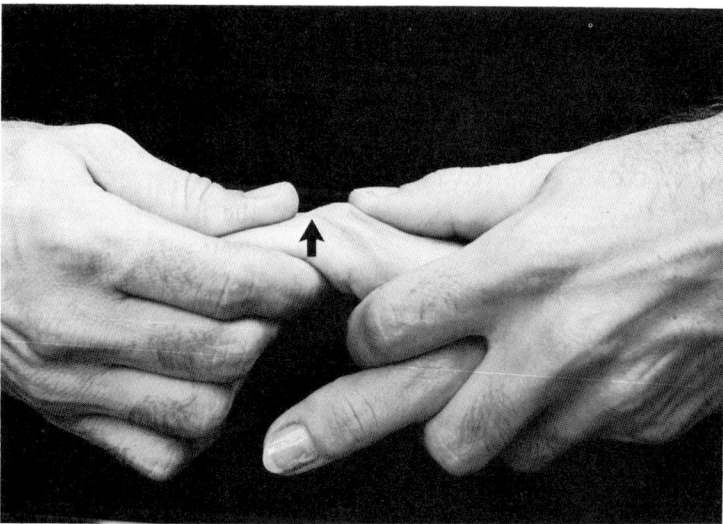

Fig. 4.3 Joint mobilisation techniques are performed by the therapist to stretch restricted portions of the joint capsule, and enhance flexibility. Dorsal gliding of the proximal phalanx with the metacarpal firmly stabilised stretches tight dorsal structures and improves MP joint flexion

Minnesota Rate of Manipulation Test, are used to initiate this part of the treatment program. This test involves a very light activity promoting shoulder motion and basic prehensile manoeuvres. If a specific pattern of movement needs improvement, a custom piece of equipment may be used. Gaining finger flexion to the palm, for example, can be promoted by using plastic tubing of various diameters. As the patient improves, he is able to grasp smaller diameter pipes. The patient is also encouraged to use the hand at home for activities of daily living whenever possible and report the progress to the therapist.

As mobility and function return and edema is no longer a problem, heavy resistive exercises and activities are incorporated in the treatment program. This is the transitional phase between the acute stage and the patient's ability to return to work. Strength and endurance exercises are promoted. Progressive resistive exercises for the major muscle groups of the upper extremity are outlined to the patient. A work simulator may also be beneficial (Fig. 4.4). This is a resistive exercise machine used for strengthening and improving endurance and work hardening. Tools attached to the shaft of the machine can exercise various muscle groups or can be used to simulate specific work-related tasks (Reynolds 1984).

When the patient's progress with the therapy program has leveled off, consideration must be given to whether further treatment is indicated. If the individual's motion is insufficient to permit important functional activities, then surgery may be entertained. The prime consideration is how much motion can be gained by the surgical release of a stiff joint and how this will translate into improved function for the patient. The end result will be proportional to the degree and severity of tissue involvement with the contracture. The patient with an MP extension contracture following a severe crush injury involving skin loss, metacarpal fractures, and extensor tendon injuries may not be a candidate for surgery because the improvement following an operation might be minimal. Lastly, the patient's ability to actively participate with a postoperative therapy program must be fully understood.

When planning surgery, the first consideration should be the structures involved in the contracture

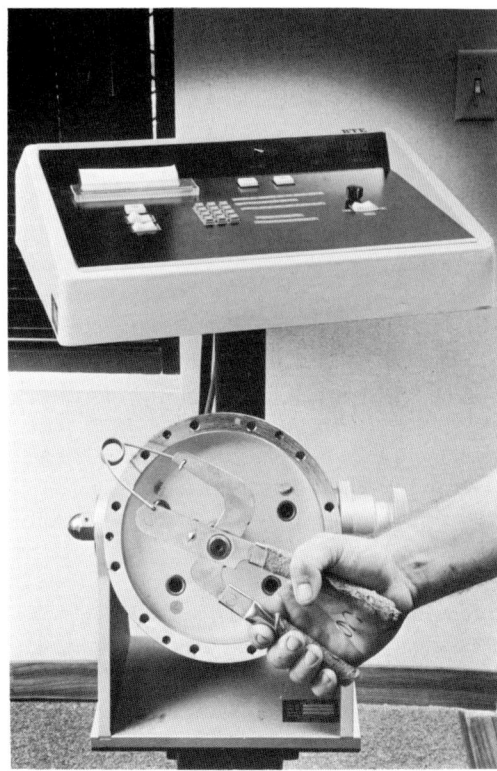

Fig. 4.4 The Baltimore Therapeutic Equipment (BTE) work simulator is a restrictive exercise device for strengthening upper extremity musculature and simulating various work related tasks

and how they are to be approached surgically. Incisions that can be extended are outlined. If both the flexor and extensor surfaces are to be approached, usually only one incision can be used on the finger. However, this may compromise exposure of the important structures. The surgeon should beware performing surgical procedures that will require contradictory postsurgical management. Should a z-plasty be required to revise a scar as well as a tenolysis, performance of both simultaneously may not yield a satisfactory result. Z-plasty flaps should be rested for 5–7 days to allow soft tissue healing, while a tenolysis requires rapid, vigorous mobilisation.

While joint involvement is usually central to stiffness in the hand, the contribution of the skin is often relegated to a minor role except in obvious cases, like burns. However, skin closure after a surgical release often serves to diminish the gains obtained from the operation. Relaxing incisions and rotating skin to cover important structures while leaving other areas open may be helpful in maintaining motion.

When operating on a contracted joint, exposure and release of the involved tissues is the prime consideration. An insufficient release will produce a suboptimal gain in motion. An over-zealous release may allow subluxation and introduce a deformity not present preoperatively (Harrison 1977). The gain anticipated from the surgical release of stiff joint is not that demonstrated by the surgeon forcefully manipulating the joint into the desired position. Rather, it is the motion obtained by gentle, passive flexion and extension of the joint.

Release of tendon adhesions requires a thorough understanding of the local anatomy, especially that pertaining to the retinacular structures. Lysing 90% of the adhesions about a tendon may improve motion to a degree, but complete release is usually necessary to gain full motion. The surgeon should prove himself willing to 'go to the last mile' by careful planning of incisions, time and energy.

While joint release procedures may be performed under general anesthesia, a block provided by infiltration or an intravenous perfusion of local anesthetic is more advantageous. At the completion of the operation, the tourniquet is released and the adequacy of the procedure determined by having the patient actively move the hand. If motion is not satisfactory, a further surgical release can be performed. Importantly, the patient can observe the gain and realise it is his responsibility to maintain this improved motion.

TREATMENT OF ESTABLISHED CONTRACTURES

Usually a stiff joint can be categorised as a contracture in either the flexed or extended position. While all the structures previously mentioned can contribute, each contracture will characteristically involve particular components.

Metacarpal phalangeal joint extension contracture

When the MP joint becomes contracted in the extended position, a number of structures are usually involved. The collateral ligaments which normally lengthen 20% during a 60° arc of flexion, shorten and adhere. Forceful flexion of the joint will cause the volar lip of the proximal phalanx to abut the metacarpal head preventing further flexion. Rather than glide the joint hinges open dorsally producing a depression which is evident clinically. The dorsal capsule is the primary tissue involved. In an extension contracture it may be the only one. The palmar pouch beneath the metacarpal head can collapse and prevent the volar plate from advancing proximally. The presence of a skin contracture or adhesions between the extensor tendon and the skin can be diagnosed if finger flexion produces blanching. Extensor tendon scarring can be localised by placing the more proximal joint in both flexion and extension and observing the effect on the more distal joints. Intrinsic paralysis will eliminate active MP joint flexion allowing unopposed extension and possibly creating joint stiffness.

Established MP joint extension contractures can be treated effectively with a program of exercises and splinting (Weeks et al 1978). The examiner must learn to recognise the 'end feel' of the stiff joint as this is a prognostic indicator for treatment. A soft, springy feel at the end of passive flexion indicates the contracture may respond well to an exercise program. However, if the joint has little give with full passive flexion conservative management will probably be less successful.

If the dorsal capsule and collateral ligaments are tight with an MP extension contracture, exercises to mobilise these structures are imperative. The therapist uses joint mobilisation techniques distracting the proximal phalanx in a distal direction and applying an upward gliding pressure to stretch the dorsal capsule. In a similar fashion, the collateral ligaments are distracted and tilted laterally. When extensor tightness or adherence limits MP joint flexion, the therapist passively flexes the MP joint, then flexes the IP joints further both passively and actively. All passive exercises must be performed slowly and without pain.

Active isolated MP joint flexion and extension with the IP joints alternately held flexed or extended are performed to mobilise the extrinsic extensors and intrinsic tendons. To promote MP flexion, motion at the more distal joints can be blocked with metal splints. In this fashion, the forces provided by the long flexor tendons are transferred proximally. Grasping and manipulating plastic pipes with an increasingly smaller diameter will encourage improved MP flexion. The patient is encouraged by visualising this progress.

Dynamic flexion splinting should begin as soon as swelling in the hand subsides. A custom dorsal forearm splint is fabricated from a thermoplastic material with a volar outrigger adjusted to provide a 90° flexion pull on the proximal phalanges (Fig. 4.5). A palmar bar maintains the arch of the hand and helps to stabilise the wrist (Laseter 1984). Traction is adjusted so the patient experiences mild to moderate tension. It is recommended that the splint be worn for 20 minutes each waking hour of the day. Static rest splints help maintain the gains made in MP flexion.

Surgical release of a metacarpal phalangeal joint extension contracture may be indicated if less than 65° flexion is present (Curtis 1984). Often all four digital joints are involved to varying degrees. The joints are approached through two or four longitudinal dorsal incisions. The extensor tendon is incised in the midline for three-to-four centimeters to the proximal phalanx base. The tendon and hood are separated from the underlying capsule which is thickened and confluent with the collateral ligaments. A rectangular portion of the dorsal capsule is excised from the level of the metacarpal neck to the base of the proximal phalanx and laterally to both collateral ligaments. Adhesions between the ligaments and metacarpal head are released and motion is tested. Further release may be gained by excising selectively and sequentially the dorsal 30–50% of the collateral ligaments. The palmar pouch is restored by lysing adhesions found between the condyles and the volar plate (Tubiana 1984). If the joint suddenly snaps on passive flexion a ligament contracture still remains and must be released. When the desired amount of flexion is achieved, hemostasis is obtained and the extensor tendon is reapproximated with interrupted, inverted nonabsorbable mattress sutures. The MP joints are immobilised in at least 75° of flexion. In the case of a severe injury or a difficult release, transarticular K-wires may be used to maintain this position.

Complications can include releasing an excessive amount of radial collateral ligament producing ulnar drift and detaching the interosseous insertion on the proximal phalanx, thereby weakening active MP flexion. Extending the tendon incision distal to the MP joint may produce button-holing and prevent closure. Disruption of the extensor repair may be aggravated by extreme flexion position in the immediate postoperative period. Recurrence of

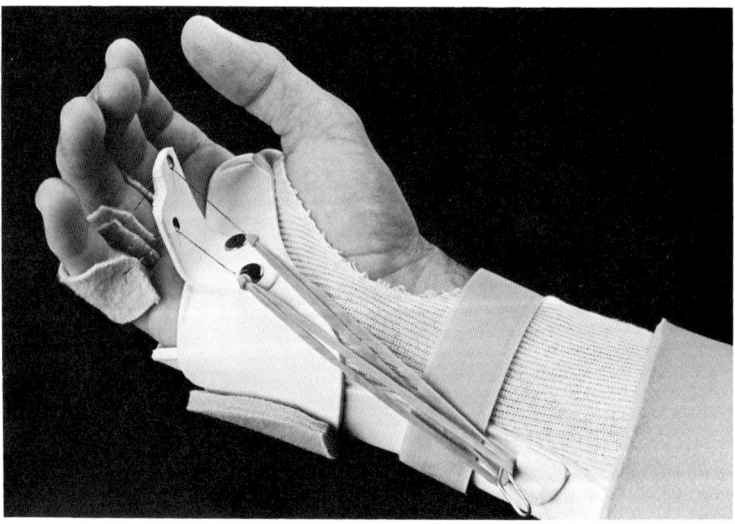

Fig. 4.5 A low profile rubberband traction device promotes MP joint flexion. Tension is adjusted to provide a gentle 90° flexion pull on the proximal phalanx.

the contracture can occur from incomplete release or noncompliance with the treatment program.

The mobilisation program following release of MP joint extension contractures begins 3 days after surgery. While the primary emphasis is on achieving maximum flexion, full extension of the MP joint must be maintained and pain and swelling controlled. In the first week, ice packs and elevation followed by retrograde massage are performed to reduce edema and provide analgesia. TENS assists in relieving the pain throughout the postoperative period. A light gauze dressing which does not restrict motion is applied to the wound until healed. The passive and active exercises, as previously described, are performed to prevent reformation of binding adhesions.

A gentle dynamic MP joint flexion assist is worn whenever the patient is not engaged in other aspects of the postoperative program. A static plaster splint is worn at night to maintain daytime flexion gains.

At 7 to 10 days after surgery, as pain and swelling subside, the exercise and splinting program is intensified. Ice packs are replaced with moist heat to facilitate soft tissue flexibility prior to stretching. After suture removal, friction massages are initiated to mobilise the dorsal scar. Three to four weeks after surgery, the flexion potential is usually achieved. However, changes in motion may occur for 3–6 months following surgery. Therefore, the patient's progress must be carefully monitored.

Continuous passive motion (CPM) devices have been employed recently in several rehabilitation centres following surgical joint releases. A pressure bar mobilises the finger through a tolerable arc of motion and is used by the patient three to four times daily for 2-hour periods. The initial response has been encouraging, but controlled follow-up studies will determine the actual efficacy.

Proximal interphalangeal joint flexion contractures

The most serious and difficult contractures to treat are those involving the PIP joint in the flexed position. The volar plate becomes adherent proximally with obliteration of the palmar pouch. The accessory collateral ligaments and the adjacent oblique retinacular ligaments contract. The flexor tendons may adhere within the sheath and the pliable tissue between the annular portions of the fibrosseous sheath can shorten. Joint erosions, especially with a longstanding deformity and secondary skin contractures are frequent.

Conservative management of PIP joint flexion contractures requires the same structured exercise and splinting program employed with other stiff joints. However, a higher level of patient motivation is required because of their slow rate of recovery.

The joint mobilisation program aims to stretch the contracted volar structures. Stabilising the proximal phalanx with one hand, the therapist uses the other hand to distract and apply a force on the middle phalanx. The accessory collateral ligaments are stretched in a similar manner by distraction, lateral and medial tilting. If the oblique retinacular ligament is contracted, stretching exercises will be necessary (Fig. 4.6). Active motion exercises are performed by encouraging IP joint extension with the MP joint stabilised in flexion. This transfers the power of the long extensors to the PIP joint and promotes activity in the intrinsic muscles (Laseter 1984). Dynamic splints to promote PIP joint extension are varied. A multitude of prefabricated splints are available and may be effective depending on the type of contracture present. The contracture that is not fixed responds well to splints which apply minimal pressure. These include the reverse finger knuckle bender, LMB wire foam splint or the Capener splint. Contractures that are fixed or firm require a splint with more dynamic tension such as the Joint Jack. Fixed contractures of 45° or more are not usually manageable with prefabricated splints. Custom splints utilising thermoplastic materials with rubberband traction or progressive serial casting of a digit with plaster are helpful in these cases (Colditz 1984). Recommended wearing time for dynamic splints is 20 minutes for each waking hour of the day. Serial plaster splints can be removed and reapplied every few days extending the PIP joint several degrees more. A static rest splint is necessary to maintain daytime gains except when serial casting is utilized. A three-point static splint constructed of alumifoam with a Velcro strap around the PIP joint

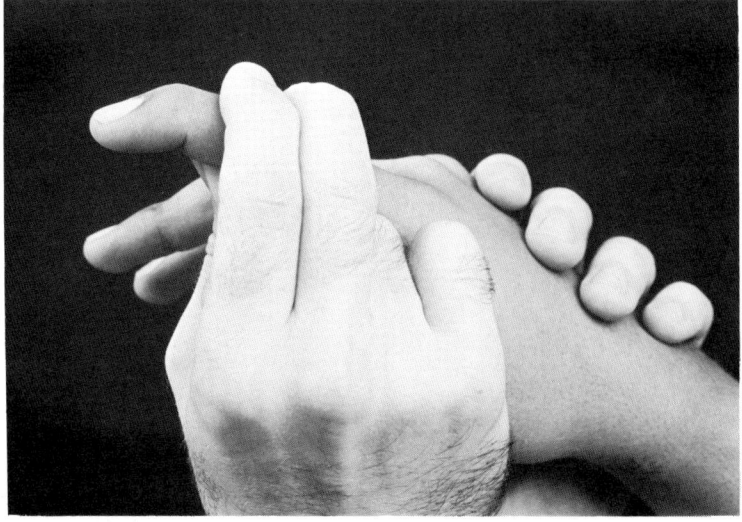

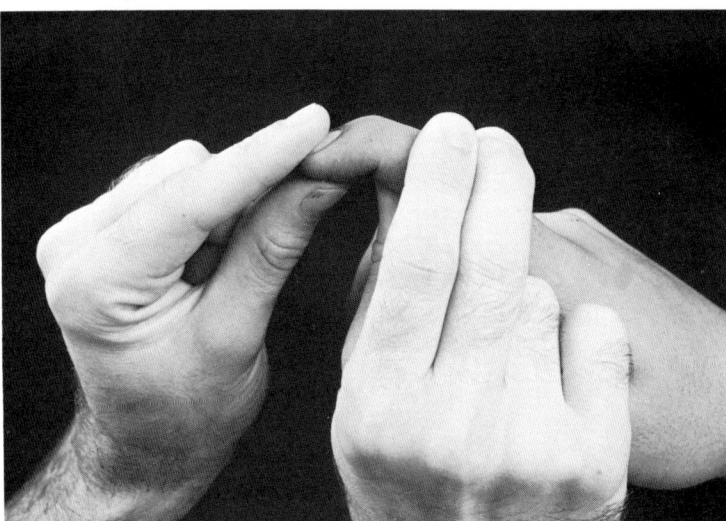

Fig. 4.6 The oblique retinacular ligament is put on stretch by maintaining the PIP joint in full extension and actively or passively flexing the DIP joint

holds this joint in maximal extension while the patient is at rest (Fig. 4.7).

Release of a PIP joint flexion contracture is technically more difficult and will invariably result in a persistent flexion deformity to some degree. The joint is approached through a mid-lateral incision with exposure of the volar plate-collateral ligament complex on one side of the digit (Curtis 1954). A second smaller incision on the opposite side will be necessary if release cannot be completed through the first one. The volar skin is separated from the flexor sheath and any restricting digital fascia is resected. The check rein of the volar plate and any fibrotic tissue laterally is resected bilaterally and the joint manipulated into extension (Watson et al 1979). If the joint release is not complete, the accessory collateral ligaments and a portion of the volar plate on each side are resected (Fig. 4.8). Should a further release be required, the volar one-third of the collateral ligament is excised. Other structures possibly involved in the treatment are as follows: 1. Release of the retinacular ligaments from the lateral aspect of the joint capsule may provide improved DIP joint flexion.

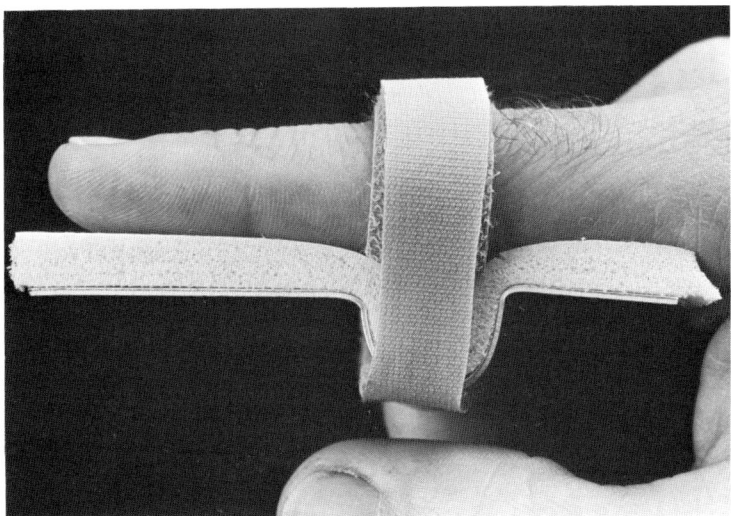

Fig. 4.7 A custom splint which provides static extension of the PIP joint can be constructed from alumifoam. An I-beam configuration allows three points of pressure while the PIP joint is drawn into the splint's recess with a Velcro or tape strap

2. Flexor tendon adherence or muscle contracture may be released through tenolysis, superficialis resection, or tendon lengthening. 3. Flexor sheath contracture will require partial sheath excision and elongation. However, if the sheath is resected widely over the volar portion of the PIP joint, tendon bowstringing will increase the lever arm of the flexor tendons biomechanically and add to the flexion force. 4. Skin releases; a minimal contracture can be treated with an L-shaped incision proximally or distally, rotating the skin towards the joint and closing the defect with a skin graft. Marked contracture with skin loss must be treated with a cross finger flap. If skin and soft tissue are inadequate, planning incisions for tissue replacement are required before the joint release. When extending the PIP joint with force, passively at surgery, the MP joint should be held in flexion to eliminate tension on the neurovascular bundles and flexor tendons.

After a maximal release has been obtained, the ability to actively extend the digit on the part of the patient should be tested. Prolonged PIP flexion will stretch out the extensor mechanism making active extension difficult or incomplete. Postoperatively, the joint is immobilised in extension for 3–10 days with a K-wire. Following pin removal, a therapy program is started. The primary goals in therapy are to maximise extension of the joint and prevent recurrence of the contracture. Often pain and swelling are more pronounced after PIP joint releases. This is dependent upon the extent of surgical dissection. Techniques similar to those employed after an MP joint capsulectomy are utilised here. Wrapping the effected area with Coban tape is especially helpful. Passive extension

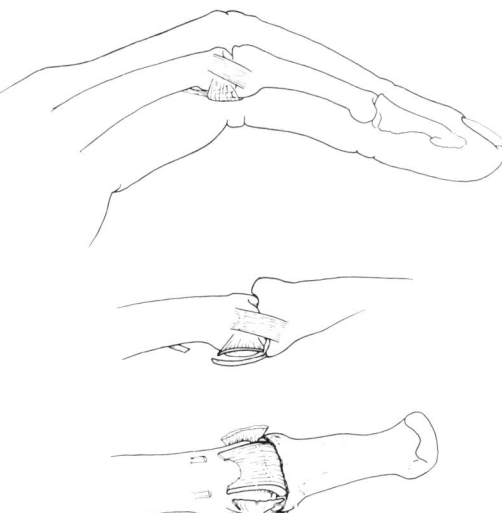

Fig. 4.8 Bilateral resection of the accessory collateral ligaments with a portion of the volar plate will release an established PIP flexion contracture

is generally not difficult to achieve. Following surgery, if an extension lag is present, active exercises must be emphasised with splinting in full extension. The splint should be worn at all times except during exercise sessions. The active exercise program includes extension of the PIP joint with the MP joint held in flexion as well as abduction and adduction exercises to encourage intrinsic function.

Over-zealous flexion will increase the likelihood of an extension lag. Only gentle active flexion to promote flexor tendon excursion is incorporated in the initial postoperative program. When pain and swelling subside and extension is maintained (at 3 weeks) a flexion program is intensified with passive exercises and dynamic splinting.

Use of the CPM unit is contraindicated until full PIP joint extension is achieved. The CPM may be appropriate only when more PIP joint flexion is needed and an extension lag will not recur.

Proximal interphalangeal extension contractures

The dorsal capsule and the dorsal one-third of the collateral ligaments are the most important structures associated with PIP joint stiffness in extension. Scarring about the extensor tendons and lateral bands, particularly after a compound injury, may limit PIP joint flexion. Contracture of the intrinsic muscles will further limit interphalangeal joint flexion. Stabilising the MP joint in varying positions while attempting passive PIP flexion will determine the intrinsic contribution (Smith 1975). While decreased PIP flexion secondary to burns or skin loss over the dorsum of the digit is usually obvious, nontraumatised skin can undergo a contracture from prolonged lack of flexion. When planning a surgical incision and its later closure, skin shortening must be taken into consideration.

Specific exercises and splinting techniques are the basis for nonoperative management of PIP joint extension contractures. A joint mobilisation program attempts to stretch the restrictive dorsal structures. Because the PIP joint is smaller than the MP joint, joint mobilisation techniques may be more difficult. Gentle passive joint flexion is often more appropriate for this problem. If intrinsic muscles are involved, they are stretched passively extending the MP joints and flexing the IP joint simultaneously. An active exercise program should include blocking for isolated motions of flexor digitorum profundus and sublimis as well as abduction and adduction for individual intrinsic motion. Active intrinsic stretching is also helpful. Functional activities that encourage flexion of the IP joints are incorporated into the program.

Dynamic splints to facilitate PIP joint flexion must be customised to be effective. A piece of padded banding metal is utilised for dorsal support with Velcro 'rings' around the wrist and proximal phalanx (Carter 1985). The traction apparatus consists of a rubber-band attached to the wrist cuff proximally and a mole skin loop over the middle phalanx distally. This splint is helpful in gaining the first 90° of flexion of the PIP joint (Fig. 4.9). To obtain the last 30°, elastic or Velcro web straps will be needed. Static rest splints can be fashioned to maintain flexion obtained during the day utilising tape or Velcro to hold the PIP joint in maximum flexion.

PIP joint extension contractures are easier to release surgically than flexion deformities. However, all the elements need to be evaluated in sequence. The joint is approached through a midlateral incision which may curve proximally to the centre of the digit on the dorsum. Any adhesions between the skin and tendon are released. If the

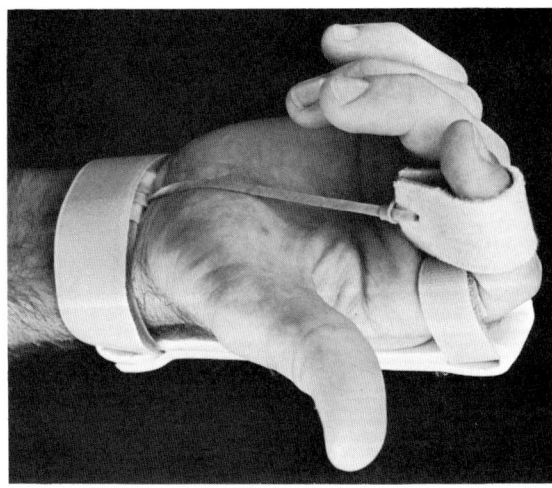

Fig. 4.9 A custom splint is the most effective means of providing dynamic flexion to the PIP joint. Velcro cuffs around the proximal phalanx and wrist stabilize the splint on the hand as elastic traction is applied to flex the PIP joint

collateral ligaments are felt to be major contributors to the extension contracture, it is necessary to retract the transverse retinacular ligament and excise the dorsal thirds bilaterally (Fig. 4.9). Care should be taken to preserve the extensor attachment onto the middle phalanx base dorsally. The dorsal capsule is incised and the extensor tendon is freed over the proximal phalanx bluntly, care being taken not to disturb the periosteum (Young et al 1978). With improved flexibility of the PIP joint, the contributions of the intrinsic tendons are evaluated and a selective release is performed as needed. Often, only one intrinsic is contracted and the contralateral side should not be indiscriminately incised. As improving flexion of the finger is achieved, any shortening of the skin will be appreciated. Lastly, when maximum passive flexion of the PIP joint is obtained, the amount of active joint flexion needs to be determined either by having the patient flex the finger on his own volition or with a traction flexion check. Hemostasis is achieved and the wound is closed. If skin closure limits finger flexion, a distal skin release with proximal rotation of the tissue may prove helpful (Fig. 4.10). The joint is immobilised in 45° of flexion and motion is started 18 to 48 hours postoperatively.

The postoperative program following release of PIP joint extension contractures is initiated 1–3 days following surgery. Management techniques to reduce pain and edema are similar to those previously mentioned. The primary emphasis is to maximise joint flexion while maintaining extension. To achieve full motion, the patient is instructed in active tendon gliding exercises for the long flexors, extrinsic extensors and intrinsic muscles. Mass finger flexion and extension exercises are performed. Intrinsic stretching as well as passive flexion and extension of the PIP joint are incorporated into the program.

The CPM program plays an important role here because the PIP joint is not sensitive to passive exercises following release of an extension contracture. The CPM protocol is the same as described for the MP joint extension release.

Initially, a dynamic flexion assist is worn by the patient during the daytime between exercise sessions. At night, the PIP joint rests in extension to prevent an extension lag. Careful observation and monitoring of the patient's change in motion indicate what splinting approach is appropriate. Alternate splinting in flexion, extension or the intrinsic stretch position may be necessary.

As with other capsulectomy procedures, most gains are made in the first 3 weeks following surgery and the patient must be involved in a daily therapy program to achieve full potential. The individual is gradually weaned from the exercise program over the next several months as his condition becomes stationary.

First web contracture

The fascia spanning the thumb-index web space distally, volarly, and surrounding the major muscles (adductor pollicis and first dorsal interosseous) is the tissue primarily involved in a first web space contracture. Crush injuries and burns produce marked edema in the loose dorsal tissues drawing the thumb into extension, adduction and supination. The skin will become secondarily contracted, and the ligaments at the trapezial metacarpal joint will shorten. The muscles may undergo myostatic contracture. Injury to the median and/or ulnar nerves can paralyze the thumb intrinsic muscles while the intact long extensor will create a supination-adduction deformity.

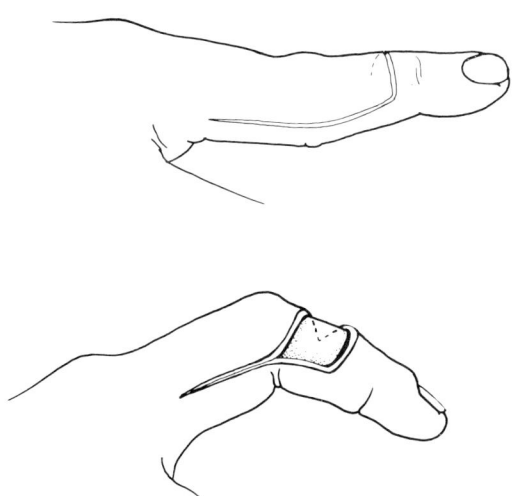

Fig. 4.10 Top: Closing contracted skin will limit the motion gained from surgery. Bottom: The skin is released through a transverse incision with proximal rotation and closure. The open area is allowed to heal by secondary intention.

Without an early therapeutic program, first web space contractures may be difficult to overcome nonoperatively. Problems with conservative management are related to difficulty in mobilising the intervening soft tissues between the base of the thumb and index finger. Often, passive exercises or dynamic splints in this area are misdirected and forces are applied to the MP joint ulnar collateral ligament. Consequently, active exercises and progressive serial splinting are the most appropriate treatment methods for first web space contractures.

A program of active exercises should include circumduction, as well as palmar and radial abduction. The first web space can be effectively stretched with molded thermoplastic splints which hold the thumb in palmar abduction and are widened every 4–7 days. Wrapping the splint with stockinette roll instead of Velcro straps distributes pressure evenly and holds the splint firmly in place.

A fixed adduction contracture of the first web space will require surgical release. Minimal contracture from skin contracture will require a dorsal rotation flap and skin graft. Extensive contracture will necessitate resurfacing the first web with a distant flap. Fascia present dorsally between the extensor tendons as well as over the first dorsal interosseous and adductor pollicis must be released and excised. Any fibrous tissue between these muscles should be resected as well as any abnormal palmar fascia (Tubiana 1985). Further release can be obtained by incising the first dorsal interosseous attachment onto the first metacarpal and recession of the adductor pollicis insertion proximally on the metarcarpal shaft. Persistent contracture or a malposition can be treated with a rotational osteotomy of the first metacarpal or even excision of the trapezium. Postoperatively, the web space is maintained with internal or external Kirschner wires. After healing for several weeks, exercise and splinting programs are instituted.

Following release of the first web space contracture and the removal of wire supports, a therapy program to maintain the first web space, soften the scar and mobilise stiff joints in the thumb is initiated.

A web space splint with elastomer insert is constructed to hold the thumb in maximal palmar abduction (Malick 1984). Pressure is applied over the scarred areas to prevent hypertrophy. The splint is worn between exercise sessions and while the patient rests. Moist heat followed by friction massage will mobilise and soften the first web space scar. Passive and active exercises are necessary to improve motion in the thumb and fingers. The index finger may develop an intrinsic contracture as a result of the incision in the first dorsal interosseous. Adherence of the thumb and index finger extensor will require an individualised exercise program as well.

Functional activities are initiated as soon as possible to encourage palmar abduction and pronation of the thumb. These include rolling theraputty balls with the pad of the thumb to index finger and middle finger, as well as twisting lids on jars or containers.

Pain and swelling are less problematic following this procedure than after release of the small joints. Scar hypersensitivity is a bigger problem and can be managed with various modalities including TENS, fluidotherapy and the use of progressively coarser materials to desensitise the skin.

The program following release of a first web space contracture is continued until full motion and functional use is returned to the radial aspect of the hand, motion is complete in the adjacent digits and the scar is pliable as well as pain free.

CONCLUSIONS

The results following the release of stiff joints have not been widely reported but Gould & Nicholson (1979) reported: (a) for MP extension contractures, the patient should demonstrate 25° improvement in motion and a 40° recovery in flexion towards the palm; (b) for PIP extension contractures, 40° of improved motion has been reported postoperatively, the individuals being able to flex 28° closer to the palm; (c) PIP flexion contractures have the least improvement in motion with an 18° correction in the flexion position. These authors demonstrated a satisfactory understanding of the pathological factors and an appropriate surgical approach. Furthermore, they incorporated therapy and splinting in their postoperative program.

Before one commits a patient to a surgical program specific needs and goals must be established. The patient must be motivated and cooperative. The surgical and rehabilitation programs must be carefully coordinated. Any complications will negate the efforts of all parties.

REFERENCES

Adamson J E 1970 Treatment of the stiff hand. Orthopedic Clinics of North America 1:467–480
Arem A J 1981 The stiff hand; an approach to prevention and treatment, Contemporary Orthopedics 3:501–514
Bowers W H 1983 Small joint injuries. Orthopedic Clinics of North America 14:793–810
Bunnell S, Doherty E W, Curtis R M 1948 Ischemic contracture local in the hand. Plastic and Reconstructive Surgery 3:424–433
Carter M S 1985 Therapeutic management of the proximal interphalangeal joint, In: Bowers W H (ed) The hand and upper limb; the interphalangeal joints. Churchill Livingstone, Edinburgh
Colditz J 1984 Dynamic splinting of the stiff hand In: Hunter J et al (eds) Rehabilitation of the hand 2nd edn. C V Mosby, St Louis. ch 19, p 231–240
Curtis R M 1954 Capsulectomy of the interphalangeal joints of the fingers. Journal of Bone and Joint Surgery 36A:1219–1232
Curtis R M 1984 Management of the stiff hand In: Hunter J et al (eds) Rehabilitation of the hand, 2nd edn. C V Mosby, St Louis. ch 17, p 209–215
Field P L, Hueston J T 1970 Articular cartilage loss in long-standing immobilisation of interphalangeal joints. British Journal of Plastic Surgery 23:186–191
Gould J S, Nicholson B G 1979 Capsulectomy of the metacarpophalangeal and proximal interphalangeal joints. Journal of Hand Surgery 4:482–486
Harris C Jr, Riordan D C 1954 Intrinsic contracture in the hand and its surgical treatment. Journal of Bone and Joint Surgery 36A:10–20
Harrison D M 1977 The stiff proximal interphalangeal joint. Hand 9:102–108
Kuczynski K 1968 The proximal interphalangeal joint. Anatomy and causes of stiffness of the fingers. Journal of Bone and Joint Surgery 50B:656–663
Kuczynski K 1975 Lesser-known aspects of the proximal interphalangeal joints of the human hand. Hand 7:31–33
Lane C S 1977 Detecting occult fractures of the metacarpal head: the Brewerton view. Journal of Hand Surgery 2:131–133
Lankford L L 1980 Reflex sympathetic dystrophy In: Omer G E Jr, Spinner M (eds) Management of Peripheral Nerve Problems. W B Saunders, Philadelphia. ch 12 p 216–244
Laseter G F 1983 Management of the stiff hand: a practical approach. Orthopedic Clinics of North America 14:749–765
Laseter G F 1984 Postoperative management of capsulectomies In: Hunter J et al (eds) Rehabilitation of the hand, 2nd edn. C V Mosby, St Louis. ch 21, p 246–252
Malich M H 1974 Manual on dynamic splinting with thermoplastic materials. Harmaville Rehabilitation Center Pittsburgh, p 2.
McCormack R M 1964 Stiffness of the injured hand: analysis, prevention and treatment. Journal of Trauma 4:581–591
McIntee P M 1984 Therapists management of the stiff hand. In: Hunter J M et al (eds) Rehabilitation of the hand, 2nd edn. C V Mosby, St Louis. ch 18, p 216–230
Newmeyer W L, Kilgore E S Jr 1976 Volkmann's ischemic contracture due to soft tissue injury alone. Journal of Hand Surgery 3:221–227
Reynolds C C 1984 The stiff hand. In: Malich M H, Kasch M C (eds) Manual of management of specific hand problems. Amer. Rehab. Educ. Network, Pittsburgh. ch 4, p 88–110
Salter R B, Field P 1960 The effects of continuous compression on living articular cartilage: an experimental investigation. Journal of Bone and Joint Surgery 42:31–48
Smith R J 1975 Intrinsic muscles of the fingers: function, dysfunction and surgical reconstruction In: AAOS Instructional Course Lectures. C V Mosby, St Louis. vol. 25, p 200–220
Tubiana R, Roux J P 1974 Phalangisation of the first and fifth metacarpals. Journal of Bone and Joint Surgery 56A:447–457
Tubiana R 1985 The treatment of stiffness of the fingers In: Tubiana R (ed) The Hand, vol II, W B Saunders, Philadelphia. ch 108, p 1040–1053
Watson H K, Ritland G D, Chung E K 1974 Post-traumatic interosseous-lumbrical adhesions. Journal of Bone and Joint Surgery 56-A:79–84
Watson H K, Light T R, Johnson T R 1979 Checkrein resection for flexion contracture of the middle joint. Journal of Hand Surgery 4:67–71
Weeks P M, Wray R C Jr, Kuxhaus M 1978 The results of nonoperative management of stiff joints in the hand. Plastic and Reconstructive Surgery 61:58–63
Weeks P M, Wray R C Jr 1978 Management of the stiff hand. In: Management of Acute Hand Injuries, 2nd edn. C V Mosby, St Louis. ch 12, p 329–379
Wilson R L, Carter M S 1984a Management of hand fractures. In: Hunter J M et al (eds) Rehabilitation of the hand, 2nd edn. C V Mosby, St Louis. ch 15, p 180–194
Wilson R L, Carter J S 1984b Joint injuries in the hand; preservation of proximal interphalangeal joint function. In: Hunter J M et al (eds) Rehabilitation of the hand, 2nd edn. C V Mosby, St Louis. ch 16, p 195–205
Wilson R L. Liechty B W 1986 Complications following small joint injuries. Hand Clinics 2: 329–345.
Young V R, Wray C R Jr, Weeks P M 1978 The surgical management of stiff joints in the hand. Plastic and Reconstructive Surgery 62:835–841

W. B. Conolly

5 Minor surgical procedures and infections

An operation for a relatively minor condition for example a trigger finger which becomes complicated by a wound problem, can result in stiffness not only of that finger but also of the normal fingers and the entire hand. The final result may be severe loss of function and the patient and his hand may be far worse off than before the operation (Figs 5.1 and 5.2). The outcome of any hand operation, and therefore the complications of such a procedure, depends on factors relevant to the patient, the operating surgeon and the pathology of the condition. A poorly motivated patient who ignores routine post-operative instructions such as elevation and joint exercises, can develop persistent swelling and stiffness. Many complications are generated by factors relevant to the surgeon—ignorance, neglect, indifference, inexperience, poor operative technique and poor judgement.

There is considerable variation in the tissue response of a particular individual to the injury of operation. Troublesome *scarring* is unpredictable and can follow *any* operation in *any* patient.

HOW TO AVOID THE UNWANTED RESULT

Preoperative

Assess the patient's motivation and need for the operation and the prognosis. A surgical procedure itself is an injury and can cause a disability. In a particular patient with a moderately severe carpal tunnel syndrome, conservative treatment might be safer than operative treatment. Check the diagnosis. Obtain X-rays in three planes for a radiopaque foreign body. Is postoperative infection likely? Has there been previous infection in this operation area? Are antibiotics indicated?

Operative

A full hand surgical technique is as necessary for these minor hand operations as other more major ones. A bloodless field and magnification are essential for any safe hand surgical procedure. Incision and exposure must be adequate to avoid operative damage to the vital deeper structures. If there is a risk of bleeding it may be safer to release

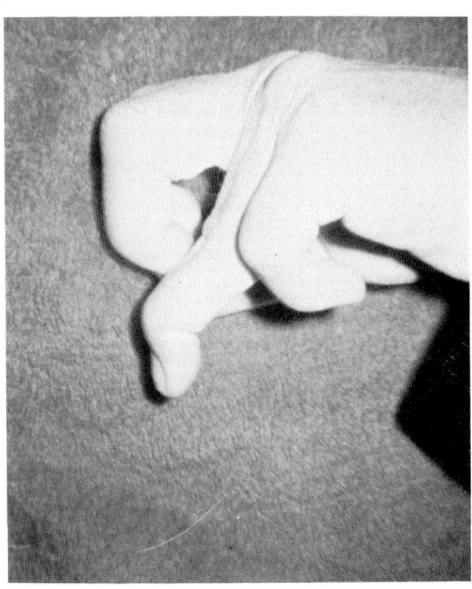

Fig. 5.1 The sequelae of a postoperative haematoma. Intrinsic contracture of the left ring finger from ischaemia and fibrosis of the intrinsic muscles. This followed a postoperative haematoma. This man's finger was eventually treated by amputation

MINOR SURGICAL PROCEDURES AND INFECTIONS 41

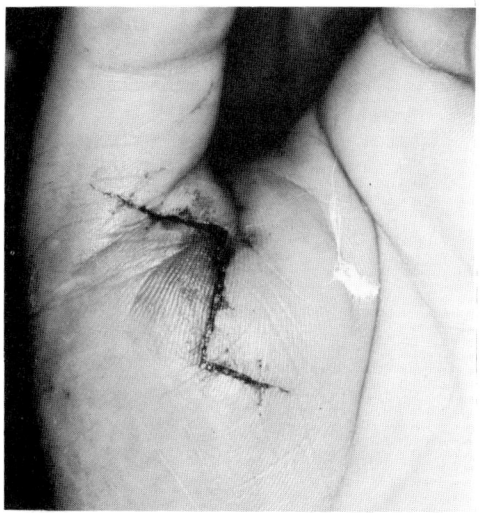

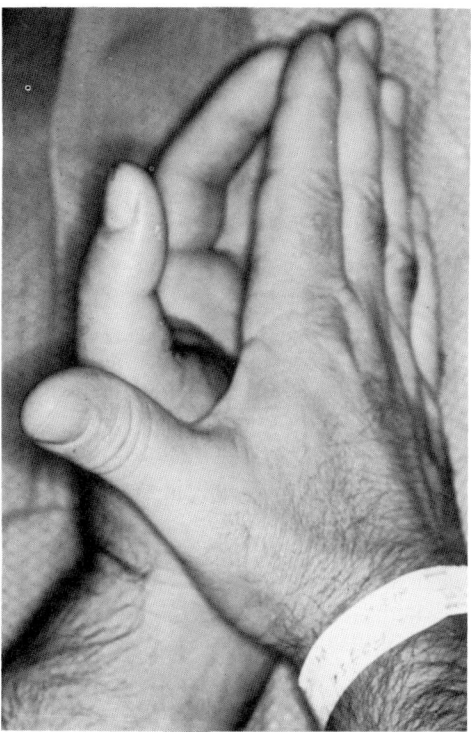

Fig. 5.2 Haematoma complicating removal of a ganglion from the palmo-digital area of the thumb (top). There followed stiffness of the thumb and a first web contracture (bottom)

the tourniquet and obtain haemostasis prior to wound closure. Suture only the skin. Avoid any tension which might impair the circulation. The key to optimal healing is an adequate blood supply.

Dressing and splintage

It is a wise practise to splint the wrist, the key joint of the hand, even for a few days.

Postoperative

The patient and staff must be aware of the significance of postoperative pain, which should be relieved in the first instance by mechanical and physical measures and not by drugs. Postoperative pain may be due to a tight plaster, dressing, or suture line or of course tension in the wound from a haematoma or infection. To minimise postoperative stiffness, exercise unsplinted and unoperated joints from the beginning, and exercise the injured or operated part according to the stage of healing.

Operations in children

In children who are naturally apprehensive and often unable to cooperate, diagnosis is difficult. A poor diagnosis may lead to complications, failures, and unsatisfactory results. Resolution of oedema, fibroplasia, remodelling and softening of the scars all occur more rapidly in children than in adults. However, contraction of wound scars during growth tends to be more troublesome. It is therefore even more important to place incisions correctly when operating on infants and children. Magnification is essential. Close postoperative supervision by both surgeon and parents will be required, and extra care is necessary to prevent dressings and splints from being dislodged. A long arm plaster with the elbow at right angles may be necessary. There is little fear of joint stiffness even if exaggerated positions of joints are required to relieve the tension on repaired nerves and tendons. Return of function is usually rapid and formal physiotherapy is less often required.

HAND INFECTIONS

Because the infective process itself distorts tissues and predisposes to hand oedema and stiffness, there is a higher risk than normal of the complications listed in Table 5.1. The following considerations will minimise the development of these complications.

42 UNSATISFACTORY RESULTS IN HAND SURGERY

Table 5.1 Complications following incision and drainage of hand infections

Intraoperative
Iatrogenic damage to nerves etc.
Spread of infection beyond the local site.

Postoperative
  Early
  Delayed healing, wound infection and necrosis
  Persistent oedema

  Late
  Hypertrophic scar, tender scar
  Stiffness of fingers and entire hand
  Persistent or recurrent infection
  Psychosocial and economic problems occur in cases of severe or prolonged infection

Preoperative

Assess and correct if possible factors predisposing to infection such as diabetes mellitus and steroid therapy.

Operative

Avoid local anaesthetics near the infection or its draining area to avoid spreading that infection. Use a general anaesthetic or a distant regional nerve block. Inadequate incision under inadequate anaesthesia produces inadequate drainage. A bloodless field is essential, but avoid risking the spread of infection by forced exsanguination with a circumferential Esmark bandage. Rather, drain the hand of blood by elevation and then apply a pneumatic cuff around the upper arm.

Incision (Fig. 5.3)

Do not incise for cellulitis. This should be treated medically by splintage, elevation, and antibiotics. Lymphangitis and haemorrhagic blisters indicate streptococcal infection and the need for medical rather than surgical treatment.

Incision is indicated once increased tissue tension or pus is diagnosed and localised. If there is a 2- or 5-day history of progressive throbbing pain or one sleepless night, pus can be anticipated. The critical sign is inflammatory brawny oedema with localised tenderness. Do not wait for pointing and fluctuation which are often late signs. Incise over the site of maximal tenderness or fluctuation (Fig. 5.3). Reduce the chance of damage to nerves and blood

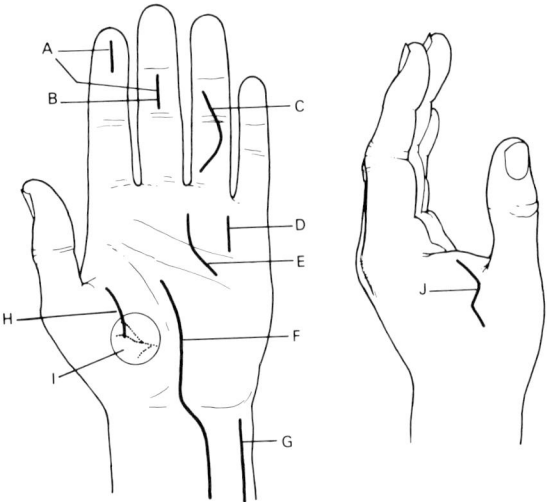

Fig. 5.3 Incisions for hand infections. (A) For pulp abscess (felon) if pointing there. (B) For distal tendon sheath. (C) For more extensive infection (avoid incision at right angles across a flexion crease). (D) For web abscess; a dorsal incision may also be required. (E) Proximal tendon sheath. (F) To expose radial and ulnar bursa. (G) For space of Parona (behind the flexor tendon sheaths). (H) For thenar space infection (beware of thenar branch of median nerve). (I) Thenar branch and proper palmar digital nerves to thumb across F.P.L. (J) Dorsal incisions for thenar web infection. For dorsal hand infections, incise longitudinally over the infected area

vessels and tendon sheaths by incising parallel to these structures. Use longitudinal incisions except across a flexion skin crease where a zigzag approach is used. Keep in mind that the wound may need extending. Use a scalpel to cut only the skin. Then use a blunt instrument, preferably sinus forceps in the deeper tissues to avoid cutting nerves and blood vessels. Remember that pus can occur at various levels (Fig. 5.4)—intraepidermal, intradermal, subcutaneous, and remember that there may be a combination of levels as in a collar stud abscess. After removing the pus, curette all slough and granulation tissue lining the abscess cavity. Complete excision of non-viable tissue is an absolute essential. Failure of wounds to heal is due to granulation of a sinus or a small part of the incision. Be careful not to injure or spread the infection to the tendons, periosteum, epiphysis or joint such as in draining a distal pulp space infection.

Take a swab of the pus for culture and sensitivity. An antibiotic should be injected parenterally before and during the procedure so that when the

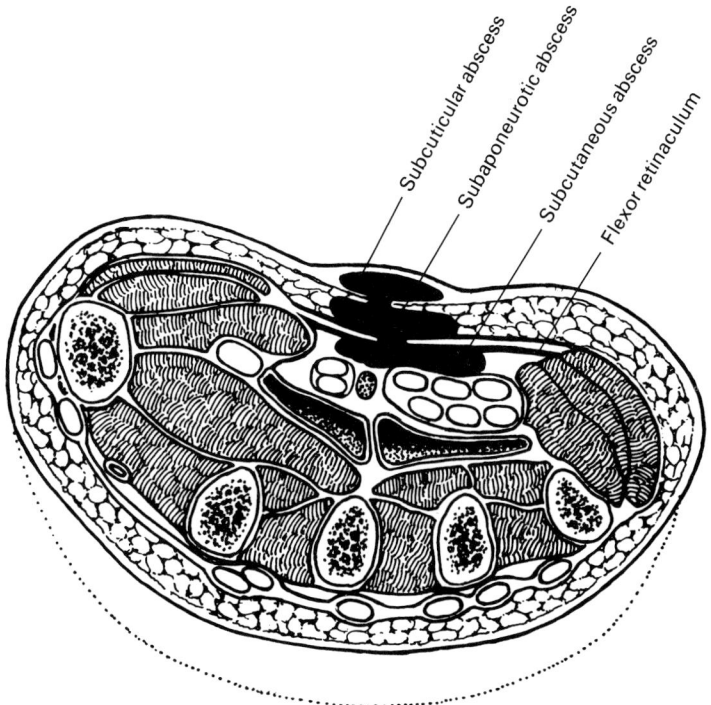

Fig. 5.4 Levels of abscess formation in the hand

tourniquet is released, blood containing the antibiotic oozes into the cavity. If there is necrotic skin cut it away and leave the wound open. Drains may be necessary to prevent haematoma and the formation of another abscess. Wet dressings or zinc oxide ointment facilitate wound drainage. Most of these wounds should heal in 7–10 days. If the infection has been well localised and all dead tissue has been excised and the skin cover is healthy, the wound may be closed without tension around a drain. This closed method (Scott & Jones 1952) results in less postoperative pain and quicker healing. Such a method is not to be used when infection is poorly localised and where the dividing line between dead and living tissue is poorly demarcated.

SPECIFIC INFECTIONS

Paronychia, eponychia and subonychia
(Fig. 5.5)

An eponychial abscess, confined by the adherence of the eponychium to the base of the nail is inclined

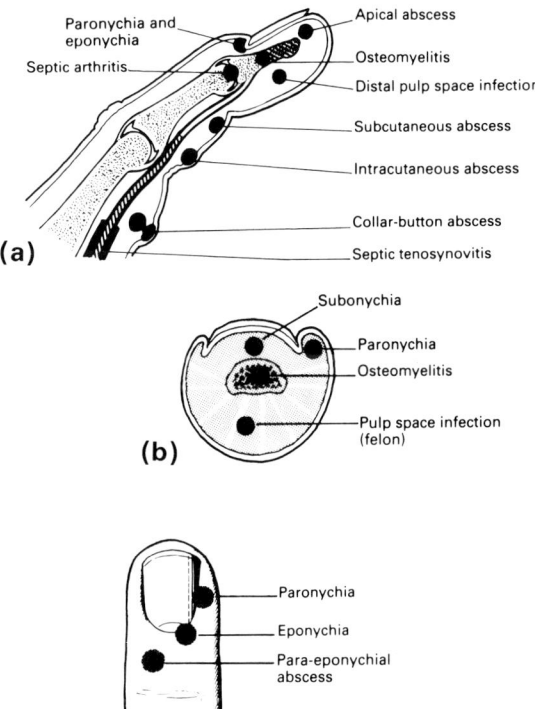

Fig. 5.5 Sites of infection in the finger and hand

to run around the nail fold and form a paronychia, and sometimes pass under the nail to form a subonychia. An acute paronychia should be differentiated from a lateral pulp space infection. A faulty surgical approach can cause scar and ridging of the nail fold and nail plate, and gross deformity of the nail plate (Fig. 5.6).

Operation

If the abscess lies just beneath the eponychial fold, lift the nail fold with fine pointed scissors (Fig. 5.7a) a scalpel blade or an elevator and maintain drainage by wet dressings or zinc oxide ointment. If the abscess is in the nail fold itself and will not drain under the free edge of the nail fold, incise longitudinally (Fig. 5.7b), but direct the scalpel blade away from the nail bed matrix. If there is an abscess under the proximal part of the nail plate, make two parallel incisions to elevate the eponychium to expose and remove the proximal part of the nail plate (Fig. 5.7c).

Skin infections

These include furuncle, pyogenic granuloma, pyoderma and collar stud abscess. The same principles apply as in other infections. The main complication is persistence or recurrence of the infection from inadequate drainage and removal of dead tissue. This occurs especially where there is a deeper component or components of the abscess (Fig. 5.4), and where there has been failure to find a foreign body.

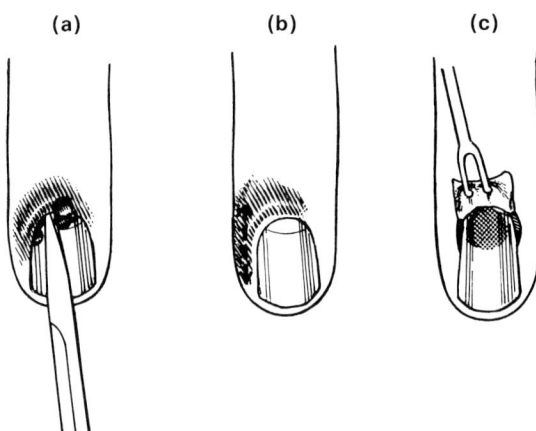

Fig. 5.7 Drainage of infections around the nail. (a) Drainage of an epo and paronychial abscess which is pointing beneath the nail fold. Keep a fine flat probe or fine flat scissors flat on the nail, lift up the nail fold and drain pus without drawing blood or causing pain. (b) Incision to drain a paronychial abscess which is not pointing beneath the nail fold. (c) Elevation of the eponychial fold preparatory to excising the proximal one third of the nail to drain a subonychial abscess

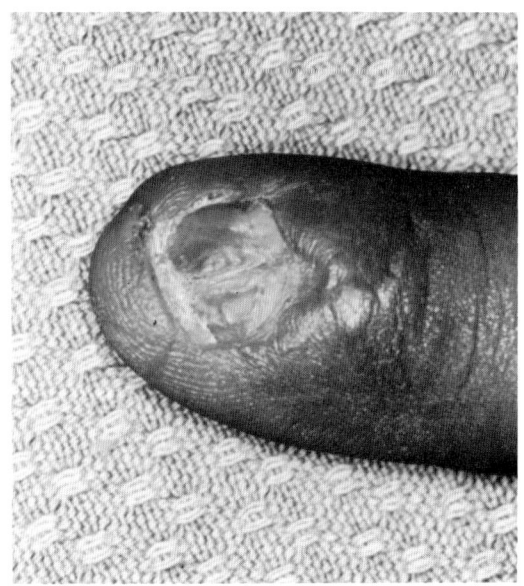

Fig. 5.6 Deformity of the nail fold and nail plate from operative damage to the nail fold and matrix when draining a paronychia

Space infections

The skin and fascia form compartments in certain areas of the fingers, hand, and forearm (Fig. 5.5). Infection of one of these compartments frequently follows a staphylococcal infection of a minor wound. Cellulitis can give a rapid increase of tissue tension, and this often results in suppuration and abscess formation. The swelling is most marked in the loose dorsal subcutaneous tissue of the hand. Incision and drainage is indicated if conservative measures fail to stop the progression of a space infection within 12 to 24 hours. If when first seen the space is already tense, incision and drainage should be performed. In the early stages there may be no more than a drop or two of pus, but the decompression relieves tissue tension and pain and the infection should rapidly resolve.

Felon

A felon is a subcutaneous abscess of the distal pulp of a finger or thumb (Fig. 5.8a). This space is bounded by the thick pulp skin, the distal flexion crease, the nail folds dorsally and the bony phalanx with the insertion of the profundus tendon. The digital neurovascular bundles traverse the space longitudinally arborising towards the centre and tip. The skin is stabilised by many fine fascial strands that tether it to the bone, but there are no strong septa as such. The fascial strands are most dense at the junction of volar and dorsal skin, at the flexion crease and the tip of the digit. They are least concentrated in the centre of the fat pad. There are multiple globules of fat among the strands.

Complications of operations to drain a felon

These include:
Operation area. Damage to the neurovascular bundle with anaesthesia of the pulp and painful neuroma. Spread of the infection to the tendon sheath, bony phalanx (Fig. 8.9) and joint. Instability of the fat pad from surgical incision of the fascial strands.
Wound. Sloughing of the skin.
Scar. Tender scarring of the fingertip.

To avoid these complications (Kilgore et al 1975): Because the incision should be over the site of maximal tenderness and pus formation, differentiate between a lateral pulp space infection and paronychia from a true felon. Most of the complications arise from faulty placement of the incision. Make a short longitudinal incision over the area of maximal tenderness in the midline where most of these abscesses form and point (Fig. 5.8b). Avoid lateral incisions which may damage the neurovascular bundles, causing ischaemia and anaesthesia, and avoid transverse incisions which may also cut the neurovascular bundle (Fig. 5.8c). Avoid the fish-mouth incision which again may leave a dorsal area of ischaemic skin, and which may sever the fascial strands or septa, creating an unstable fat pad. Advance the scalpel blade in search of an abscess. If pus is found, enlarge the incision to the proximal and distal limits of the abscess. Do not divide vertical fascial strands because those that are part of an abscess will be sequestrated spontaneously with the core as healing progresses. Curette the abscess space and remove devitalised fat. Be careful not to penetrate through to the phalanx or tendon sheath or joint. Irrigate the abscess cavity and decide on the most appropriate form of drainage which may be:

(a) Spontaneous drainage aided by a hygroscopic application of zinc oxide.
(b) A soft, small penrose or latex drain which might need suturing to the wound edge.
(c) A fine 16 or 18 gauge polyethylene catheter placed in the wound and sutured to the wound edge.
(d) Avoid solid packing of the wound which maintains rather than reduces dead space.
(e) Apply a loose, moist dressing, splint the wrist, and include the infected digit and an adjacent one, and elevate the hand above heart level.

Postoperatively, maintain splintage and elevation and antibiotics (to cover staphylococci and streptococci). Remove the drain after drainage has ceased, usually at about 2 days, and arrange for daily dressings. Check that there has been no persistence or recurrence of the abscess. The midline wound will heal spontaneously. Wound and scar complications are rare with this technique.

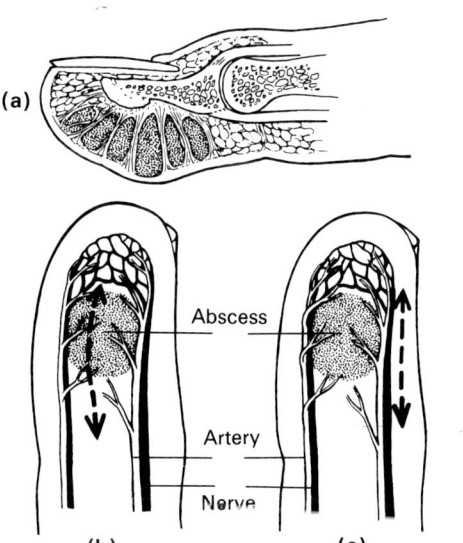

Fig. 5.8 (a) Diagrammatic representation of a felon. (b) correct and (c) incorrect types of incision for draining a felon

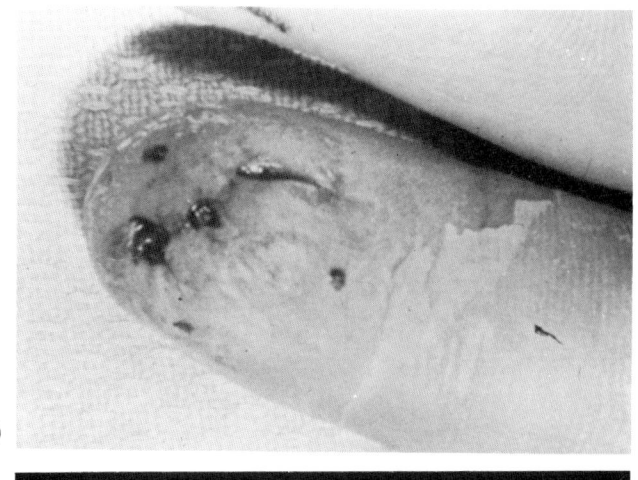
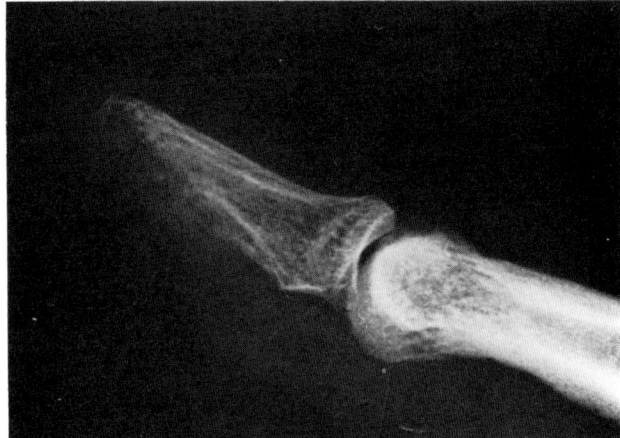

Fig. 5.9 Distal pulp space infection. (a) Three inadequate incisions over a 3-week period produced only temporary relief of pain on each occasion. (b) X-ray showed osteomyelitis

Deep space infections

The deep spaces include the web space, the midpalmar space, the thenar and hypothenar spaces, and the distal forearm space (Fig. 5.10a). The complications associated with the surgical drainage of these spaces and ways of avoiding them are as follows.

Scar contracture

Avoid transverse incisions in the web. Not only will these scars contract but they give poor access to the longitudinal running neurovascular bundles.

Operative damage to nerves

These include the palmar branches of the median and ulnar nerves, and the dorsal superficial sensory branches of the radial and ulnar nerves. Deep to the deep fascia there is risk to the major nerve trunks, median and ulnar, and their muscular and digital sensory branches. After incising the skin longitudinally, use a dissector or probe in the inflammatory area when looking for pus, rather than using sharp instruments which run the risk of cutting these structures.

Spreading of the infection

Deep space infections can be easily spread into surrounding tendon sheaths or joint structures by inappropriate incision. Again, blunt dissection is advised when seeking the abscess cavity.

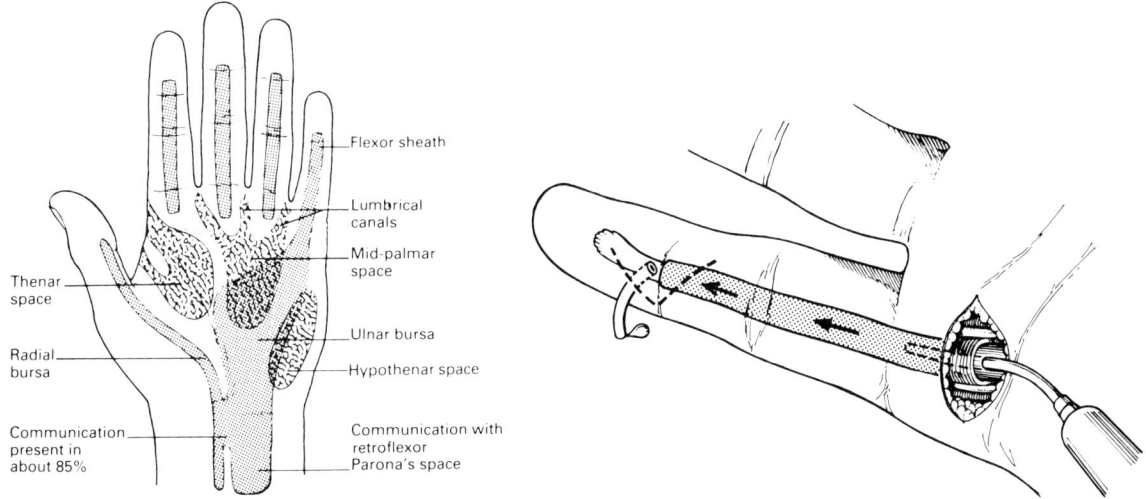

Fig. 5.10 (a) Fascial spaces of the palm and fingers. (b) Drainage of a flexor tendon sheath infection (see text)

Persistence and recurrence of the infection

Beware of a double abscess or a collar stud extension of an abscess into a deeper or more superficial plane. It is often necessary to make a separate incision on the dorsal or the palmar surface. Remove all devitalised tissue, especially fat, and if there has been an abscess cavity thoroughly curette all granulation tissue. Drainage must be adequate. One effective method is to place a catheter (16 gauge polyethylene) in the palmar wound and suture this to the skin to prevent accidental removal. If the remaining palmar wound has healthy skin margins this can be sutured and a small penrose or latex or silastic drain can be placed in the exit wound on the dorsum. Irrigate this system with saline to check its patency. Afterwards, irrigation with sterile saline can be maintained or intermittent irrigation with antibiotic solution for 48 hours. When the inflammatory signs have subsided the catheters can be removed. If there has been skin necrosis the wound can be left open to heal secondarily.

Slow wound healing

The closed catheter system enables most infected wounds of the hand to heal primarily. Second intention healing is of course slower.

Finger and hand stiffness

During the stage of cellulitis and severe infection the whole hand must be rested, but when that has subsided unsplinted and unoperated areas can be exercised, and when the catheters have been removed all joints can be exercised gently.

Septic tenosynovitis

This infection more than any other in the hand can lead to stiffness and loss of finger and hand function. An infection which can begin in the tendon sheath in the finger can spread along that tendon sheath to the palm, across to the other tendon sheaths and through the carpal tunnel to the distal forearm. Infection within the sheath destroys the gliding mechanism of the tendon, causing flexor tendon adhesions and occasionally even tendon necrosis. It is an uncommon but a potentially devastating condition of the hand.

Faulty operative technique can damage the neurovascular bundles, favour spread of infection to other tissues such as bone and joint, proximal spread in a deep palmar space, damage tendon blood supply causing necrosis, and inadequate drainage may allow persistence of the infection. Any of these complications may result in stiffness of the finger and the hand, and lead to amputation.

Treatment

The patient should be admitted to hospital and parenteral antibiotics given immediately. Splint the entire hand, wrist and forearm in the position of function and elevate the entire upper extremity. If the pain and tenderness are not improved within 6 to 24 hours, incision and drainage of the wound and of the proximal and distal parts of the tendon sheaths may be necessary.

Surgical treatment consists of closed tendon sheath irrigation according to Neviaser (1978). Make a zigzag incision over the proximal end of the tendon and open the proximal margin of the A-1 pulley (Fig. 5.10b). Make a second 'V' incision over the distal interphalangeal crease to expose the distal fibro-osseous tunnel, avoiding damage to the neurovascular bundle. Resect the distal end of the tendon sheath. Insert a drain and suture it to the skin. Make a single opening in the end of a 16-gauge polyethylene catheter and pass the tip of this catheter under the A-1 pulley for a distance of 1.5 to 2.0 cm. Suture the catheter to the skin and close the wound around it. Irrigate the tendon sheath with saline which should exit at the drain at the distal interphalangeal joint area. Dress and splint the hand and bring the catheter out of the dressing and connect it to a 50 ml syringe. Arrange the dressing so that the drain can be seen distally. Check the irrigation system prior to the patient leaving the operating room. Postoperatively, flush the sheath with 50 ml of sterile saline every 2 hours for 48 hours. Then inspect the digit. If the signs of infection have abated, remove both the catheter and the drain. Dress the wounds lightly and begin gentle exercises. If any doubt exists continue the irrigation for an additional 24 hours. A near normal range of movement should be regained at about a week.

Septic arthritis

The main complications of operations for this infection are:

1. Persistence of infection from inadequate drainage.
2. Spread of infection to cause osteomyelitis and septic tenosynovitis.
3. Operative damage to the articular cartilage or to the central extensor tendon slip. This may result in a buttonhole deformity.
4. Unless there has been prompt drainage, joint stiffness will occur.

The best approach to a metacarpophalangeal or proximal interphalangeal joint is a dorso-lateral one between the dorsal extensor apparatus and the posterior part of the collateral ligament (Fig. 5.11). After incising the capsule irrigate the joint with a fine catheter. Gently curette or use mosquito forceps to remove inflamed synovium, and depending on the severity of the infection, either leave the wound open or preferably close the wound around a very fine catheter. Irrigate the cavity of the joint for about 48 hours. Leave a small exit drain on the other end of the incision to allow the fluid irrigated through the catheter to escape from the wound.

If there has been erosion of the central slip by the disease process or if the central slip is cut during the operation, maintain splintage with the proximal interphalangeal joint in extension for 6 weeks.

Bite wounds of the hand

The main complication of the treatment of these injuries is persistence of infection and spread of the

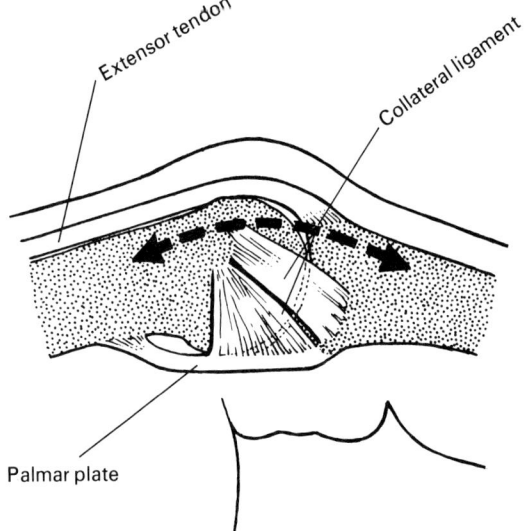

Fig. 5.11 Line of incision to drain septic arthritis between the extensor tendon and the dorsal part of the collateral ligament

infection to involve the joint and produce a septic arthritis. Bite wounds should not be sutured primarily. Mostly the wound requires extension and excision. Thoroughly cleanse the skin around the wound with soap. Thoroughly irrigate the bite wound. Remove all damaged tissue and send this for culture. Suture a catheter in place for irrigation but leave the wound open. Check that there has been no extension of the wound into the joint (Fig. 5.12). Bite wounds should only be closed secondarily, when all evidence of infection has subsided.

Osteomyelitis

The main complications are persistence or recurrence of infection and operative damage to the nerves. The best approach for metacarpal infections is a dorsal one and for phalangeal infections a lateral one, posterior to the neurovascular bundle. The aim of the operation is to remove all infected bone and sequestrae and either to pack the wound and to allow secondary healing, or to use a catheter and drainage system.

Amputation of the digit may be the best treatment for severe osteomyelitis. Protracted treatment for severe osteomyelitis of a digit can result in stiffness of adjacent digits and the hand itself.

Chronic infections

These include infections due to mycobacteria and fungi. Mycobacterial infections include *Mycobacterium marinum, avium, cansasii* and *intracellularis*. Mycobacterial infections, both tuberculous and atypical, show a predilection for synovial tissue of joints or tendon sheaths. Mycobacterial tenosynovitis usually requires tenosynovectomy of the thick infected hypertrophic synovium with preservation of the pulleys. Antituberculous medicines are important but because cultures can take up to 6 weeks to be positive, therapy should be started at the time of synovectomy on a presumptive basis. Mycobacterial involvement of joints requires joint synovectomy. Leprosy usually manifests as ulnar neuropathy at the elbow and median neuropathy at the wrist.

Fungal infections

Sporotrichosis can manifest as chronic skin ulcers, lymphangitis or arthritis. Coccidiomycosis can present as tenosynovitis or as bone infection. Candidiasis can cause chronic paronychia. Actinomycosis can present as a granuloma, skin ulcers or sinuses. Brucellosis can present as low grade septic arthritis or osteomyelitis. Boeck's sarcoidosis can present as granulomas involving the distal phalanx.

HAND TUMOURS

Tumours of the hand can be classified according to their site—skin, subcutaneous soft tissues, and skeleton. They can also be classified as pseudo, benign or malignant tumours (Table 5.2) (Conolly 1980). Most tumours of the hand are not true neoplasms, but the result of classic disease states such as trauma, infection, inflammatory disease, metabolic disorder, degenerative disorder or congenital anomaly. Almost all hand tumours require surgical removal. Biopsy is rarely needed because mostly the tumour can be completely removed for microscopic study. Standard hand surgical techniques are practised, but if there is any chance of malignancy do not use an Esmark bandage for exsanguination because of the risk of tumour spread. Recommended incisions are shown in Fig. 5.20 below. There is little potential free space in the hand and as tumours enlarge they distort and compress the nerves and other structures, and

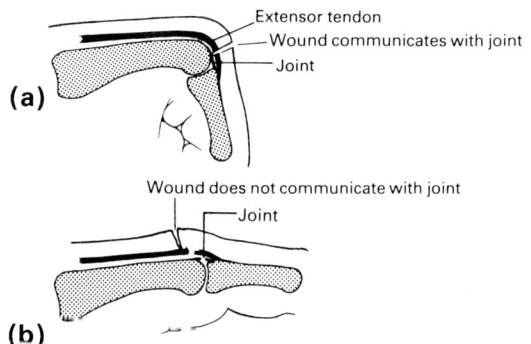

Fig. 5.12 The trapdoor effect of bite wounds of the metacarpophalangeal joint. Note in (a) when the joint is flexed the wound leads directly to the joint and in (b) when the joint is extended it becomes sealed off by the extensor tendon

Table 5.2 Tumours of the hand

Tissue	Pseudo-tumours	Benign tumours	Malignant tumours
Skin	Wart Sebaceous cyst Hypertrophic scar Epidermoid inclusion cyst Pyogenic granuloma Rheumatoid nodule	Keratosis (seborrhoeic, solar, senile) Dermatofibroma Kerato-acanthoma	Bowen's disease Basal cell carcinoma Squamous cell carcinoma Melanoma
Subcutaneous tissue, fat	Gouty tophus Haematoma, seroma Foreign body granuloma	Lipoma	Liposarcoma
Fascia	Dupuytren's nodule Knuckle pads	Fibroma	Fibrosarcoma Epithelioid sarcoma
Tendon	Tendon stump Rheumatoid nodule Tendon ganglion Synovitis	Giant cell tumour (Fibrous histiocytoma)	Malignant giant cell tumour of tendon sheath
Muscle	Anomalous muscle bellies Haematoma	Leiomyoma Rhabdomyoma	Leiomyosarcoma Rhabdomyosarcoma
Blood vessel	Aneurysm and arteriovenous fistula Lymph cyst Aberrant radial artery Varix	Haemangioma Haemangiolymphoma Glomus tumour	Haemangiosarcoma
Nerve	Neuroma	Neurilemmoma Neurofibroma Neurofibromatosis Neurofibrolipoma	Malignant neurilemmoma
Joint	Ganglion Mucous cyst Knuckle bursa	Giant cell tumour of joint synovium	Synovial sarcoma
Bone	Heberden's node Exostosis and callus Carpo-metacarpal boss Multiple hereditary exostosis Dislocated joint	Enchondroma Osteochondroma Giant cell tumour Aneurysmal bone cyst Osteoid osteoma Periosteal chondroma Bone cyst	Osteogenic sarcoma Chondrosarcoma Ewing's tumour Metastatic carcinoma
Miscellaneous	Paraffinoma Myxoma		

make them more liable to operative injury. The main complications are iatrogenic injury to nerves (Fig. 5.13) and vessels in the operation area, and persistence or recurrence of the tumour. In this section ganglion, giant cell tumour, lipoma, and nerve tumours will be discussed, together with skin cysts and tumours of fibroblasts.

Ganglions of the hand and wrist

Ganglia are mucin filled cysts usually attached to underlying joint capsule or tendon sheath. They represent about two-thirds of all soft tissue swellings in the hand and can arise from any joint or tendon sheath in any age group. Most have a communication via a one way valve mechanism to the underlying synovial sheath of the joint or tendon mechanism. Recurrences are common unless this communication is excised.

Complications (Table 5.3)

Ganglia may persist or recur from inadequate excision. There may be iatrogenic damage to superficial sensory nerves such as the palmar branch of the median nerve, the superficial branch of the radial nerve or the lateral cutaneous nerve of the forearm. Failure to ligate the bleeding vessel

MINOR SURGICAL PROCEDURES AND INFECTIONS 51

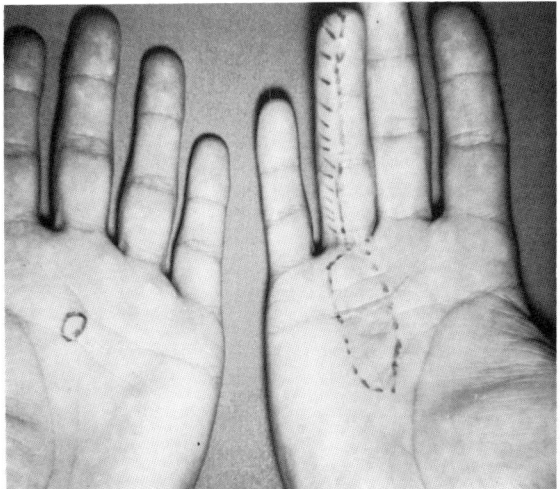

Fig. 5.13 Operation to remove an asymptomatic nodule in the palmar fascia was complicated by intraoperative division of the ulnar digital nerve to the ring finger. A similar small nodule is present in the left palm

Table 5.3 Resection of wrist ganglion—complications

Intraoperative complications
Iatrogenic damage to adjacent sensory nerves
Injury to radial artery

Postoperative complications
  Early
  Wound haematoma and infection
  Wrist stiffness

  Late
  Hypertrophic scarring or scar contracture from badly placed incisions
  Persistence or recurrence

on a joint capsule may result in a haematoma (Fig. 5.14). Do not attempt to close the joint capsule. Large or small capsular defects do not lead to joint infections or recurrences (Angelides 1982). Closure of the capsule can result in prolonged immobilisation and subsequent joint stiffness.

The radial artery is liable to injury during resection of a volar wrist ganglion. These ganglion often impinge upon and adhere to radial artery, even to the extent that the cyst wall becomes virtually one with that of the vessel. Lister & Smith (1978) describe a technique for protecting the radial artery during resection of an adherent ganglion. They recommend dissection of the vessel proximal and distal to the ganglion, incising the ganglion parallel to the arterial wall, leaving an adherent portion of the cyst wall with the artery and removing the remainder of the ganglion. They release the tourniquet to check there is good flow through the intact artery. Although ligation and division of the radial artery will not compromise survival of the hand, the incidence of cold intolerance is increased (McEvedy 1962).

Operative treatment for a ganglion

The aim is to resect the ganglion and its communicating pedicle and valve mechanism, and an area of joint capsule. Such an exposure and dissection is liable to complications unless full hand surgical facilities are available. A tourniquet, magnification, and an assistant are all essential. Because the tourniquet may need deflation to allow haemostasis prior to wound closure, an intravenous regional anaesthesia is not sufficient. A regional block or

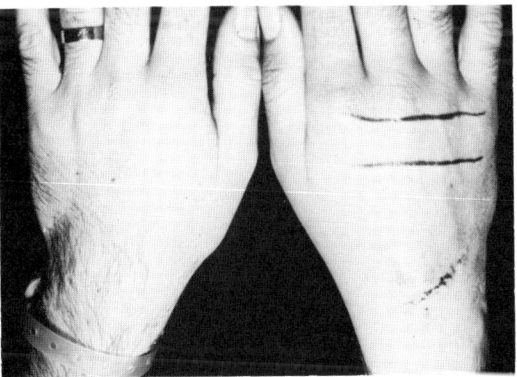
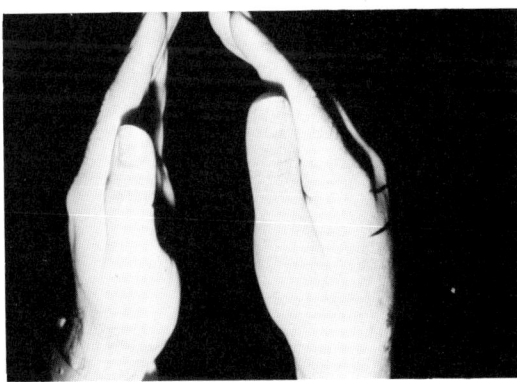

Fig. 5.14 (a) Haematoma complicating removal of a dorsal wrist ganglion. This patient was re-admitted for incision and drainage of the haematoma. (b) He did not regain a normal range of wrist movements for ten weeks

general anaesthetic is preferable. Do not close the joint capsule.

Dorsal wrist ganglion

Preoperative

Check the diagnosis. Exclude rheumatoid synovitis, a carpometacarpal boss and the dorsal prominence of the proximal pole of the scaphoid secondary to intercarpal instability.

Operative

Avoid hypertrophic or keloid scars by using a transverse or oblique incision over the proximal carpal row. After incision of the skin, dissect longitudinally in the subcutaneous tissues and look for the sensory branches of the radial and ulnar nerves which lie deep to the superficial veins, and so avoid damage to them and possible neuroma formation. Dissect between the extensor pollicis longus and the extensor digitorum communis around the ganglion capsule down to the pedicle and underlying wrist capsule. Incise the wrist capsule and expose the capsular attachments of the scapho-lunate ligament (Fig. 5.15). Most dorsal ganglion arise from the scapho-lunate ligament. Excise all attachments of the ganglion and pedicle to the scapho-lunate ligament and leave a defect in the joint capsule of about 1–1.5 cm in diameter. Leave the joint capsule open. It is safer to release the tourniquet and secure haemostasis prior to wound closure.

Postoperative care

Splint the wrist in neutral or gentle flexion for about five days. Then begin wrist movements, especially palmar flexion.

Management of recurrent dorsal ganglion

If there was previously a longitudinal incision and the scar is hypertrophied, a Z-plasty might give a better scar. Otherwise dissect and approach as for the primary operation, but taking extra care because of the surrounding scar which distorts the anatomy, especially of the sensory nerves.

Volar wrist ganglion

Most of these present under the volar wrist crease between the flexor carpi radialis and abductor pollicis longus tendons. They may be single or multiloculated cysts and may extend into the carpal tunnel, along the dorsal radial artery as far dorsally as the first web space or under the thenar muscles (Fig. 5.16).

Preoperative

Try and determine preoperatively by palpation, the extent of this ganglion. Assess the patency of

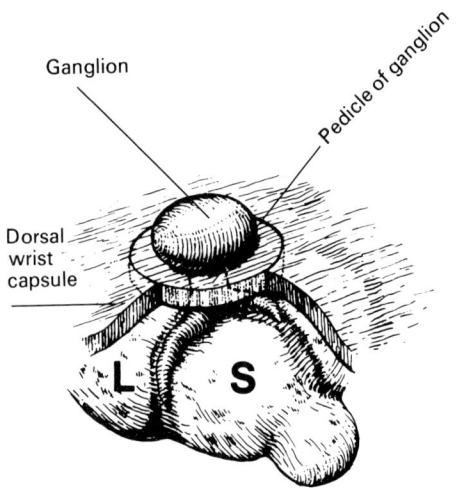

Fig. 5.15 A schematic representation of the attachments of a dorsal wrist ganglion (after Angelides 1982). L—lunate; S—scaphoid

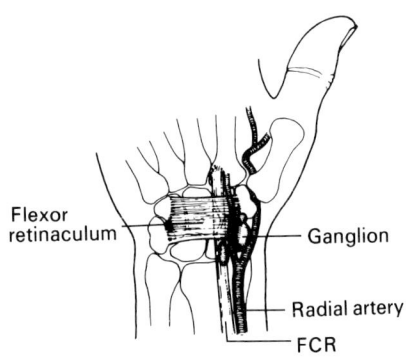

Fig. 5.16 The relationships of a volar wrist ganglion to the radial artery, flexor carpi radialis tendon and wrist joint capsule

the radial and ulnar artery by Allen's test, to check that there is sufficient circulation from the ulnar artery, in the event that there is operative damage to the radial artery.

Operative

Use a volar zigzag approach over the ganglion and be prepared to extend the incision to the thenar muscles or carpal tunnel (see Fig. 5.20 below). Incise the forearm fascia longitudinally and be on the look-out for the palmar branch of the median nerve. Dissect and protect the radial artery, which may be intimately attached to the wall of the ganglion and may even be completely encircled by the ganglion (Fig. 5.16). Trace the ganglion pedicle down to the volar wrist joint capsule—usually the radio-carpal or scaphotrapezial ligament. Open the wrist joint, explore the capsular attachments and excise about 5 × 10 mm of capsule. Look for and resect extensions of the ganglion or separate pedicles. Secure haemostasis and close only the skin.

Postoperative care

Splint the wrist in neutral or slight extension for 3–5 days and then begin wrist exercises, especially wrist extension.

Complications

As well as those complications common to operations for dorsal wrist ganglia there is always the likelihood of injury to the radial artery. Some surgeons prefer leaving a portion of the ganglion cyst wall attached to the artery to avoid arterial injury (Lister & Smith 1978). If when the tourniquet is released there is significant bleeding from the defect in the radial artery, the surgeon should decide whether he has the experience to repair that defect. If not he should ligate the artery. A vein graft should only be carried out by a surgeon experienced in microvascular techniques. Wound infection and breakdown are more liable if corticosteroids have been injected into the ganglion or surrounding tissue prior to operation. Hypertrophic scarring can occur in any wound. They are more common in longitudinal wounds.

Volar retinacular ganglion

This is usually a small, firm, tender, pea-like mass palpable under the palmo-digital crease. It arises from the fibro-osseous sheath, being attached to and having a communication with the synovial tendon sheath (Fig. 5.17).

Complications

Inadequate exposure may lead to damage of the neurovascular bundle. These ganglia may be single or multiple and a second cyst may be overlooked or the first cyst may recur, if there has been inadequate removal of tendon sheath.

Preoperative

Check that there is no associated triggering of the flexor tendon mechanism.

Operative

Incise transversely in the palmo-digital crease or through a curved or angular incision over the cyst. The exposure must allow dissection and retraction of the radial and ulnar neurovascular bundles. Dissect around the ganglion down to the tendon sheath and excise a 0.5–1 cm area of tendon sheath containing the communication with the ganglion.

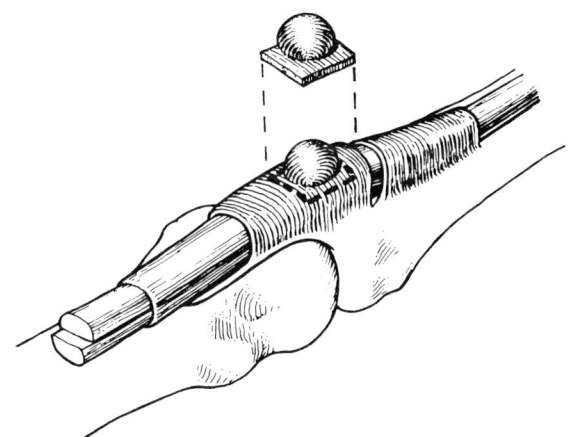

Fig. 5.17 A volar retinacular ganglion arising from the proximal annular ligament (A-1 pulley) of the flexor tendon sheath (after Angelides 1982). The specimen is excised with a surrounding margin of tendon sheath

54 UNSATISFACTORY RESULTS IN HAND SURGERY

Postoperative

Use a compression dressing for 24 hours and then begin finger movements.

Mucous cyst

These are ganglia arising from the dorsum of the distal interphalangeal joint, often associated with an osteophyte of the joint and often pressing on the nail bed and presenting under the dorsal nail fold (Fig. 5.18). There may be grooving of the nail, very thin skin over the cyst and inflammatory changes or infection of the area from previous steroid injection or needling. Resection of the cyst and the underlying bone spur requires careful dissection through thin and delicate tissues in a semi-rigid space containing the distal interphalangeal joint, the nail bed and the extensor tendon insertion. Previous inflammation around the joint and cyst and previous steroid injections make even more likely the possibility of wound congestion, ischaemia and infection, which might then spread to involve the joint and the nail bed (Fig. 5.19).

Preoperative

An antibiotic cover might be indicated if there has been previous inflammation.

Operative

Make a curved or oblique incision over the cyst and extend this proximally to the distal interphalangeal joint. Very thin skin over the cyst might be better excised. Avoid incision across the epony-

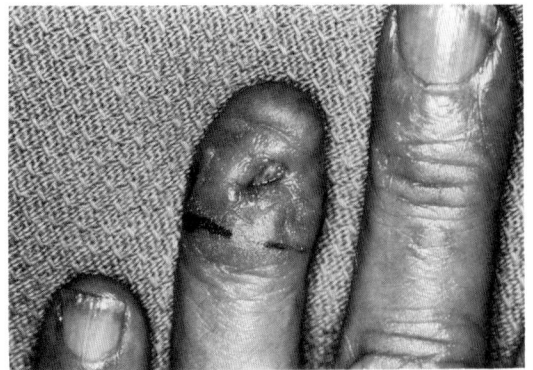
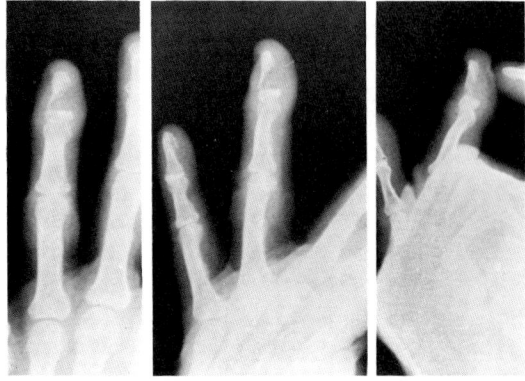

Fig. 5.19 Soft tissue and bone and joint infection complicating operative removal of a mucous cyst

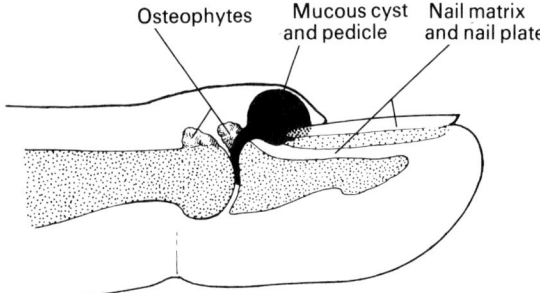

Fig. 5.18 A mucous cyst arising from the distal interphalangeal joint presenting under the nail fold. Such a cyst causes longitudinal grooving of the nail from pressure on the nail matrix

chium to avoid scarring and ridging of the nail fold and nail plate (Fig. 5.6). Very gently dissect the thin skin from over the cyst, dissect around the cyst down to the joint capsule and look for a small pedicle into the joint. Excise the capsule at the base of the cyst, taking care not to damage the extensor tendon insertion or nail matrix. Remove osteophytes with a sharp dissector or rongeur and remove hypertrophic synovial tissue from the distal interphalangeal joint. Closure of the skin wound may be by loose gentle suture, a skin graft or a local flap.

Postoperative

Protect the wound by a compression dressing and a finger and hand splint for 2 or 3 days to minimise wound problems and infection. When inflammatory responses have subsided begin distal interphalangeal joint exercises.

Complications

Recurrence occurs from inadequate excision of the capsular attachments of the cyst and bone spur, and failure to recognise extension of the ganglia under the extensor tendon to the other side.

Giant cell tumour

This tumour is also known as pigmented villonodular synovitis, pigmented nodular tenosynovitis, giant cell tumour of tendon sheath, fibrous xanthoma, benign synovioma or fibrous histiocytoma. This is a benign encapsulated tumour of unknown aetiology. It arises from the white tissue of the hand, most commonly from the tendon sheath or collateral ligament, but also from the joint synovium. It may also arise from fascia or bone. It is subcutaneous, the skin moving freely over it, but it is firm and fixed to deep fibrous structures. It is distinguished from a ganglion in that it does not transilluminate and does not yield fluid on aspiration. It is most common on the volar and lateral aspects of the digit. It grows insidiously extending between tissue planes and through narrow windows between anatomical structures. It can present as a dumb-bell tumour with one part on one side of the finger and the other extending beneath the extensor tendon apparatus and arising from the distal joint through a small space in the collateral ligament and extensor tendon. It has a fibrous consistency and is brownish yellow in colour, it is not invasive and can usually be dissected from the surrounding tissues. It can grow and displace nerve, artery and even tendon; it can cause erosion of bone ends. It may occupy any part of the flexor tendon sheath and involve any of the digital joints.

Complications

Unless completely removed these tumours tend to recur.

Preoperative

Try and determine by palpation the likely extent of the tumour. X-ray to show any bone or joint change.

Operative

Plan a longitudinal approach which can be extended. These tumours may require dissection on both volar and dorsal aspects of the finger, and even on both sides of the finger. Trace the neurovascular structures from normal tissue through the tumour, and retract these gently to avoid them being damaged. Be prepared to open the tendon sheath or interphalangeal joint. Curette the subcutaneous and osseoligamentous surfaces to minimise the chance of recurrence.

Lipoma

Lipoma is a relatively uncommon benign tumour of the hand—less than 5%. It occurs most frequently in the palm; it may be subcutaneous or subfascial. If subcutaneous it presents as a smooth, soft, fluctuant swelling. Sub-fascial lipoma may be difficult to diagnose before operation, but X-rays show the relative radiolucency of fat. They arise from the retro-flexor panniculus and grow from there along the paths of least resistance, bounded by the fascia and tendons. They may completely surround or displace nerves, vessels, and tendons. They can extend and present superficially in the distal palm or follow the interosseous tendons to appear on the dorsum between the fingers.

Complications

Most lipoma are encapsulated and may be shelled out. The complications occur from intraoperative damage to adjacent vessels and nerves. These can be avoided by longitudinal exposure and appropriate hand surgery facilities. Post-operative problems relate to bleeding and dead space. Recurrence of lipoma is rare.

Tumours of fibroblasts

These include dermatofibroma, juvenile aponeurotic fibroma, desmoid and fibrosarcoma.

Dermatofibroma

This benign tumour arises from the corium and represents a proliferation in response to minor trauma, for example insect bite. It is usually a pigmented reddish or yellowish raised small round (less than 1 cm) firm nodule. It may be mistaken for a ganglion.

Recurring digital fibrous tumour of childhood

This rare tumour develops in the fingers and toes in early childhood and may involve several digits, producing diffuse cutaneous swellings.

Juvenile aponeurotic fibroma

This is usually confined to children and occurs most commonly in the palms and soles as an ill-defined cellular fibrous proliferation involving the subcutaneous tissue and deep fascia. It may recur locally but never becomes malignant. Treatment should be conservative, consisting of local excision with preservation of important structures.

Desmoid tumours and fibrosarcomas

These are very rare. Close consultation with a pathologist is essential to help make such a diagnosis and plan appropriate treatment.

Epidermoid cysts

These are also known as inclusion cysts, epidermal cysts, dermal cysts, implantation dermoid or post-traumatic epidermoid. They can occur after injury or after operation. These cysts are round or ovoid, have thick walls of fibrous tissue with an inner lining of squamous epithelium. They contain white thick material, high in cholesterol and low in fat, thus differing from sebaceous cysts. They occur most commonly on the palmar aspect of the hand and finger. Rarely they can occur at the distal phalanx.

Complications

These cysts are not usually adherent to other structures. They rarely become infected. Recurrence is unlikely if there has been complete surgical resection of the cyst and its lining.

Sebaceous cyst

Sebaceous glands and cysts do not occur on the palmar surface, but do occur on the dorsum of the hand and fingers.

TENDON AND NERVE ENTRAPMENTS
(Fig. 5.20)

—de Quervain's syndrome
—Trigger finger and thumb
—Median and ulnar nerve compression at the wrist

de Quervain's syndrome

This is a stenosing tenosynovitis or entrapment of the tendons of abductor pollicis longus and extensor

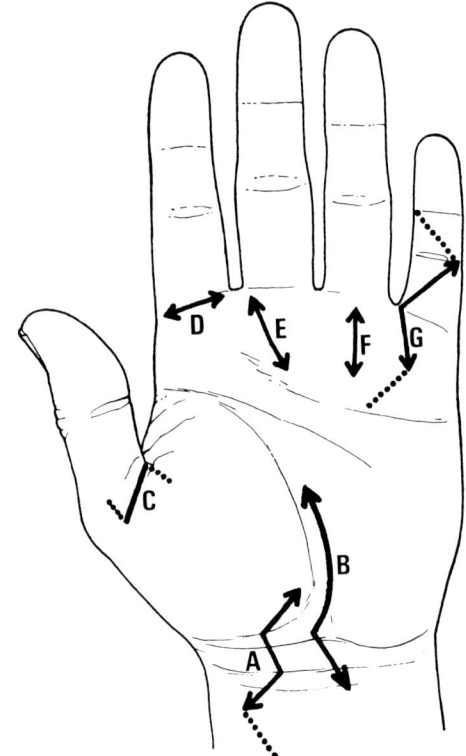

Fig. 5.20 Incisions for decompression of nerve and tendon entrapments in the hand. (A) For a volar wrist ganglion. (B) For carpal tunnel decompression (including ulnar neurolysis in Guyon's space). (C) For trigger thumb with dotted lines for synovectomy. (D), (E), and (F) transverse, oblique, and vertical incisions over the A-1 pulley for decompression of a trigger finger. (G) for a volar retinacular ganglion or for synovectomy in association for release of a trigger finger

pollicis brevis in the first dorsal compartment at the wrist. These tendons may occupy one or two or even three compartments. It may be primary, occurring in middle age, or secondary to rheumatoid synovitis. Occasionally a ganglion arises from the roof of the first compartment. Branches of the radial nerve run superficial to this compartment (Fig. 5.21).

Complications of surgical treatment

The most serious complication is a neuroma of one of the superficial branches of the radial nerve, which may follow complete or partial accidental section of the nerve or damage by vigorous retraction. Other complications include hypertrophic scar from a longitudinal incision and persistence of the entrapment from unrelieved compression of one of the tendons (Fig. 5.22). Most commonly, the extensor pollicis brevis tendon has its own compartment and this compartment is not released. Dislocation of the decompressed tendons can follow excision of too much sheath.

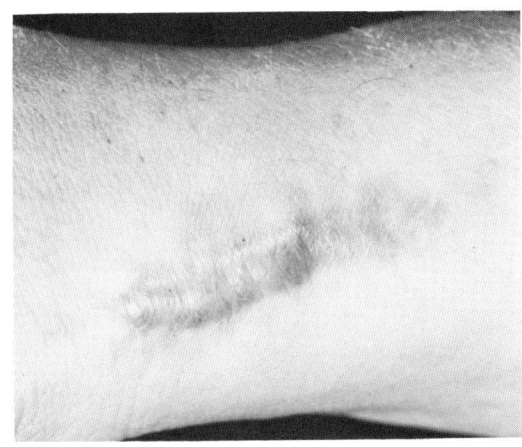

Fig. 5.22 Hypertrophic scar from a longitudinal incision to decompress the 1st extensor compartment

Prevention of the complications

Preoperative. Enquire whether there have been preoperative corticosteroids, in which case the wound should be supported by suture or tape for about 3 weeks.

Operation. Make a 2-cm transverse, oblique or Z-incision over the first dorsal compartment about 1 cm proximal to the tip of the radial styloid. Although a longitudinal approach gives safer access, it may be followed by hypertrophic scar. Identify and gently retract the radial sensory nerve branches which lie in the subcutaneous space deep to the superficial veins. Dissect down to the fibro-osseous sheath which is usually about 1 cm long. The synovial sheath extends proximal and distal to the tunnel. Incise longitudinally the sheath on its ulnar side and check the contents of the tunnel. With the thumb abducted and the wrist flexed lift abductor pollicis brevis, abductor pollicis longus, and extensor pollicis brevis, from their groove, check for a second and even third tunnel and make sure that the retracted tendons do in fact abduct the thumb metacarpal and extend the metacarpophalangeal joint independently. Lift the tendons by a hook or a blunt retractor out of the tunnel so that the entire unit from the muscle tendon junction to a point 1 cm distal to the tunnel can be seen (Fig. 5.23). If there is proliferative synovitis as in rheumatoid disease a tenosynovectomy may be carried out.

Postoperative. A compression dressing and splint

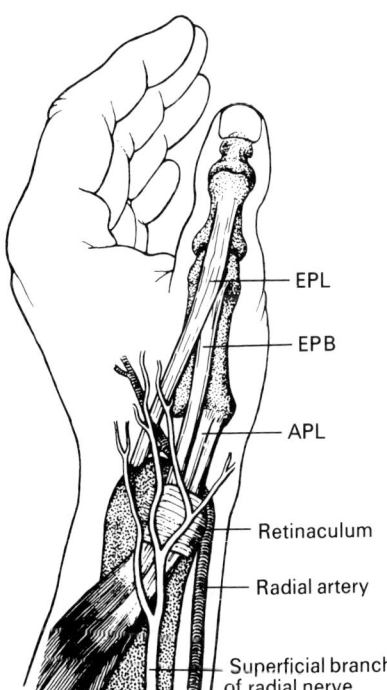

Fig. 5.21 The surgical anatomy of de Quervain's syndrome

58 UNSATISFACTORY RESULTS IN HAND SURGERY

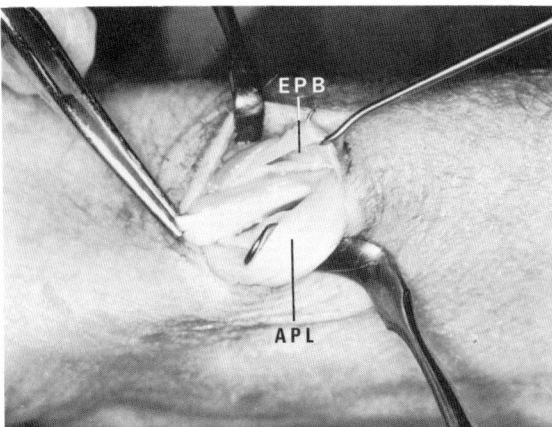

Fig. 5.23 Persistence of de Quervain's syndrome from unrelieved decompression of the extensor pollicis brevis tendon in its own compartment

should immobilise the thumb and wrist for 2 or 3 days. Then begin gentle exercises.

Treatment of the complications

If it is recognised that one or more of the branches of the superficial radial nerve are accidentally cut during operation, immediate microneural repair is recommended provided the surgeon has the necessary experience and facilities that will minimise further trauma to the nerve. Otherwise, the divided nerve is best left alone as not all divided nerves will develop a symptomatic neuroma.

If the nerve injury is not noticed at the time and/or the patient presents later with a radial neuroma, this is probably best dealt with initially by simple resection allowing the cut end of the nerve to retract into healthy soft tissues where local trauma will be minimal. Treatment of recurrent radial neuroma is beyond the scope of this chapter.

Hypertrophic scar. This can be improved by resection and Z-plasty.

Persistence of the syndrome. Re-explore according to the operative principles outlined above. Mostly a second or third tunnel will be found.

Trigger digit (fingers or thumb): stenosing tenovaginitis

Triggering occurs from disproportion between the flexor tendons and the tendon sheath. It may be primary, occurring in middle age, or secondary to connective tissue disorders (rheumatoid arthritis, gout), synovitis, nodule in the tendon or post-traumatic nodule. It may occur in association with other entrapments such as carpal tunnel syndrome and de Quervain's disease. It may occur in one or several digits on one or both hands. It may also be congenital.

Complications

The most severe disability follows iatrogenic digital nerve damage (Fig. 5.24). The commonest complication is stiffness; i.e. failure especially of full extension at the proximal interphalangeal joint or failed full flexion from incomplete section or postoperative flexor tendon adhesion. Persistence of the condition follows incomplete section and recurrence follows flexor tendon adhesions. Bow stringing or an ulnar deviation deformity follow section of the second annular (A-2) pulley. Wound problems such as haematoma and infection do occur occasionally with severe impairment of hand function.

Prevention of complications

Preoperative. Assess the patient and the healing potential. Has the patient had cortico-steroid injections? Is there a proximal interphalangeal joint flexion deformity?

Operative. Incise obliquely or longitudinally over the A-1 pulley. Be prepared to make a volar zigzag approach when a tenosynovectomy is indicated (Fig. 5.21). Retract the incised skin and incise through the palmar fascia and subcutaneous tissues

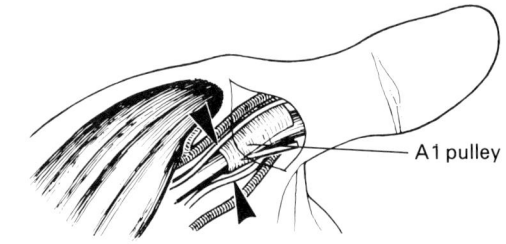

Fig. 5.24 The surgical anatomy of a trigger thumb. The arrows point to the proximal part of the A-1 pulley. Note the close association of the digital nerves

to expose the flexor sheath. Protect the neurovascular bundles with small right angle retractors. Identify the thick proximal edge of the A-1 pulley and divide this pulley longitudinally on the radial side to maintain the ulnar support for the flexor tendon. Incise as far as the palmo-digital crease. Inspect and retract from the wound, first the flexor digitorum superficialis and then flexor digitorum profundus to ensure their complete glide and to check that there is no associated tendon nodule or synovitis (Figs 5.25 and 5.26). After retraction of the tendons move the three joints of the fingers into full extension and full flexion to confirm that the triggering or locking has been abolished.

Postoperative. Apply a compression dressing for 1 or 2 days and then begin exercises to ensure full glide of both the flexor digitorum profundus and flexor digitorum superficialis tendons. If there is delay in full extension of the proximal interphalangeal joint a small splint at night may be required. If there has been preoperative corticosteroid injection leave the sutures for wound support for three weeks.

Carpal tunnel syndrome

The syndrome results from compression of the median nerve within the carpal tunnel. Any condition which reduces the capacity of the carpal tunnel may compress the median nerve, and so cause the syndrome; the commonest cause is swelling or thickening of the flexor tenosynovium. The terms 'spontaneous median neuropathy' or 'idiopathic median neuropathy' are used when there is no discernible cause. The syndrome occurs in adults of any age, but mostly in those 30 to 60 years of age. It is five times more common in females than males, and occurs more frequently in the dominant hand, although both hands are often involved.

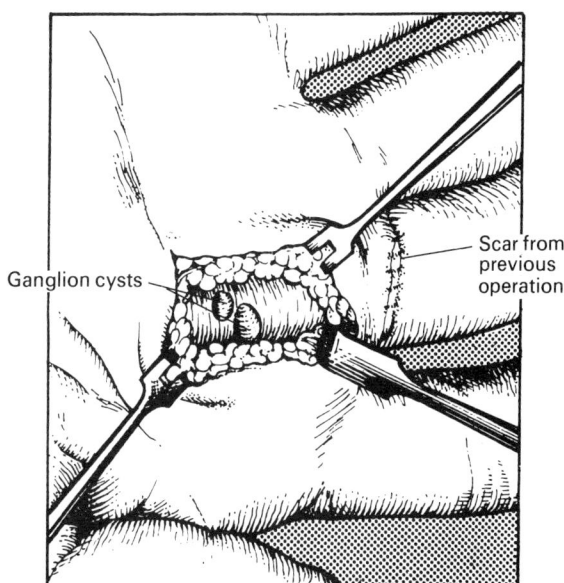

Fig. 5.26 Re-operation for persistent triggering. The first operation had been through the palmo-digital crease. Note the intact A-1 pulley in which two ganglion cysts are arising

Applied anatomy

The carpal tunnel is a rigid osteo-ligamentous canal bounded by the flexor retinaculum anteriorly and the carpal bones posteriorly (Fig. 5.27). At its upper border the flexor retinaculum is continuous with the deep fascia at the wrist, and superficially it has fused to it the distal edge of the volar carpal ligament. These two fascial layers can be responsible for compression of the median nerve proximal to the flexor retinaculum; e.g. after Colles' fracture. Ten structures pass through the carpal tunnel: the median nerve, the flexor pollicis longus tendon and the eight flexor tendons to the four fingers. The tendons are enveloped by the synovium of the radial and ulnar bursa. The median nerve is the softest and most volar structure in the carpal tunnel

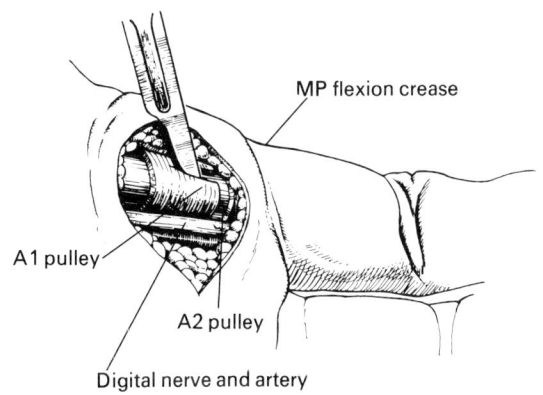

Fig. 5.25 Decompression of the A-1 pulley in trigger finger. Note the close relationship to the neurovascular bundle

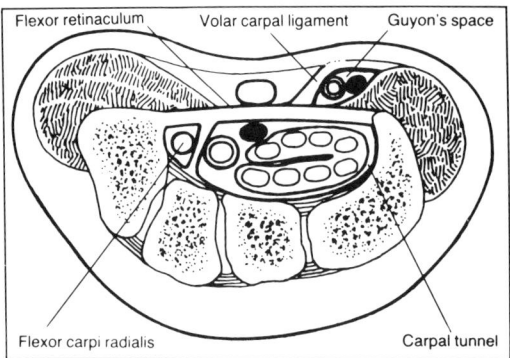

Fig. 5.27 Cross section at the level of the wrist showing the three tunnels. 1. The tunnel for flexor carpi radialis tendon. 2. The carpal tunnel. 3. Guyon's space or loge

lying directly beneath the flexor retinaculum and superficial to the nine digital flexor tendons.

There are considerable variations in the median nerve, its motor and sensory branches and its palmar branch. Figure 5.28 shows the variations in anatomy of the palmar branch. This branch usually

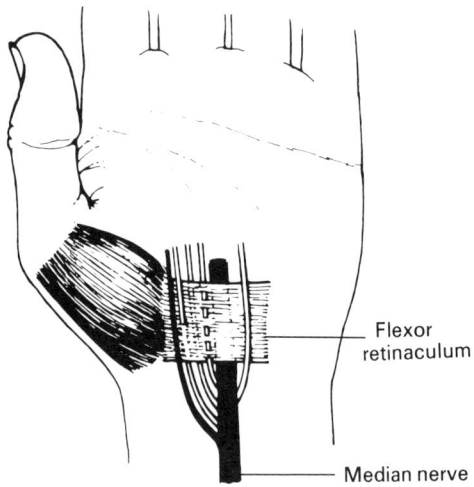

Fig. 5.28 Variations in the anatomy of the palmar branch of the median nerve. Palmar branch of the median nerve (arrow) penetrating the flexor retinaculum. The palmar branch arises usually from the radial aspect of the median nerve as it emerges from the radial margin of the flexor digitorum superficialis, usually 5 cm proximal to the radial styloid. It separates from the nerve trunk but runs parallel to it along its radial border to a point 1 cm proximal to the flexor retinaculum where it passes through its own tunnel within the flexor retinaculum just ulnar to the flexor carpi radialis tendon. There it divides into its terminal branches. These pass through the palmar fascia to supply a variable degree of skin overlying the thenar eminence at the base of the palm

arises from the radial aspect of the median nerve about 5 cm proximal to the radial styloid, running parallel along its radial border to a point 1 cm proximal to the flexor retinaculum where it passes through its own tunnel within the flexor retinaculum just ulnar to the flexor carpi radialis tendon. There it divides into its terminal branches. These pass through the palmar fascia to supply a variable degree of skin overlying the thenar eminence at the base of the palm.

The recurrent thenar motor branch usually arises as a single branch from the radial side of the median nerve just distal to the retinaculum (Fig. 5.29). It recurs back over the retinaculum into the thenar muscle. It may also arise at more proximal levels from the volar, ulnar or dorsal aspect of the median nerve. It may run superficial or deep to the flexor retinaculum. It can be absent, and the thenar muscles all supplied by the ulnar nerve. Aberrant thenar muscles such as enlargement of the superficial head of the flexor pollicis brevis may be a clue to an aberrant thenar muscle branch. The recurrent branch is extra ligamentous in 46%, sub-ligamentous in 31%, and trans-ligamentous in 26% (Lanz 1977). The median nerve may have a high division into medial and lateral divisions in the low forearm, in which case there is often a persistent median artery lying between the two divisions.

Complications

Carpal tunnel decompression is associated with one or more complications in about 10% of patients (Macdonald et al 1978). The complications are outlined in Table 5.4. There may be incomplete recovery, recurrence of symptoms following surg-

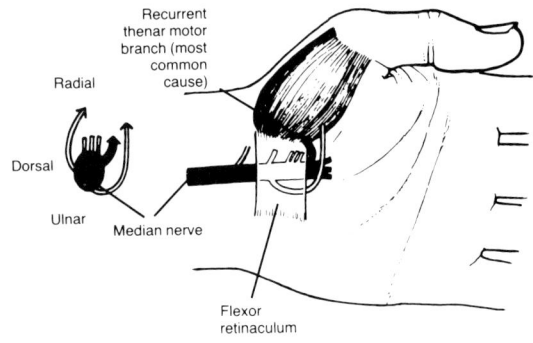

Fig. 5.29 Recurrent thenar motor branch (see text)

Table 5.4 Complications of carpal tunnel decompression—one or more of the following appear in about 10% of patients (Das & Brown 1976, Hybbinette et al 1975)

Intraoperative
1. Iatrogenic injury to
   —median nerve trunk
   —palmar branch*
   —recurrent thenar branch
   —digital branches
2. Inadequate carpal tunnel decompression from inadequate division of the flexor retinaculum

Postoperative
1. Early
   —haematoma (from damage to the superficial palmar arch)
   —oedema
   —wound complications (infection and dehiscence have occurred in those patients treated preoperatively by corticosteroid injection)
2. Later
   —weakness of grip (may last months)
   —stiffness of the fingers, wrist, and shoulder†
   —pain (in the wound from cutaneous nerve entrapped in scar in the retracted edges of the flexor retinaculum, and in the wrist from loss of carpal support) (Cseuz & Das)
   —scar hypertrophy and contracture from incision perpendicular to the wrist crease
   —palmar fasciitis
   —sympathetic dystrophy (causalgia all too frequently results from minor trauma to the median nerve) (Macdonald)
3. Recurrent carpal tunnel syndrome from fibrosis around the median nerve or hyperplasia of the tenosynovium (Fig. 5.31)
4. Other complications
   —bowstringing of the flexor tendons
   —adhesions of the flexor tendon after flexor tenosynovectomy

* Neuroma of the palmar branch can lead to disability far greater than the original disorder of carpal tunnel syndrome.
† Stiffness of the non-operated parts of the hand from pain, swelling or scar can be more disabling than the original sensory signs (McCormack 1960).

ical decompression or complications of the actual operation (Figs 5.30 and 5.31). The commonest problems are inadequate surgical decompression, postoperative fibrous proliferation or incorrect diagnosis (Conolly 1978). Re-operation may be successful where the original operation was inadequate (Langloh 1972).

Prevention of complications

Preoperative. Check for an underlying cause such as rheumatoid arthritis, space occupying lesion, flexor tenosynovitis.

Operative. Incise on the ulnar side of the thenar crease between the palmar branches of the median and ulnar nerves (Fig. 5.32). Blind carpal tunnel decompression through a transverse incision is dangerous and may result in cutting the median nerve or its branches, or incomplete division of the flexor retinaculum. Blind dissection makes inspection of the carpal tunnel impossible. Extension of the incision proximal to the wrist crease may be necessary to relieve median nerve compression by the volar carpal ligament or deep fascia of the forearm or for flexor tenosynovectomy. To avoid scar contracture of this extension, incise at an angle of about 45° in an ulnar direction. Incise vertically through the skin and subcutaneous fat to the level of the palmar aponeurosis, and minimise the dissection of the skin and subcutaneous tissues to prevent denervation of the skin flap or neuroma formation. If the palmar branch is cut dissect it proximally and section it at its origin from the median nerve. Do not attempt to repair the palmar branch because a disabling neuroma will almost certainly occur.

Incise the palmar aponeurosis and expose the fatty tissue distal to the flexor retinaculum around the superficial palmar arch. This should be the distal limit of dissection, because any nerve compression will be proximal to this point. Expose the distal part of the flexor retinaculum which is about 1 cm proximal to the arch. Protect the median nerve which lies to the radial side of the midline and in close contact with the deep surface of the retinaculum. Beware of the variations of anatomy of the median nerve or especially an anomalous recurrent thenar motor branch. Incise the retinaculum on the ulnar side of the midline. Retract the edges of the proximal part of the wound and using fine blunt nosed dissecting scissors, again under direct vision, cut the proximal part of the flexor retinaculum on the ulnar side of the median nerve. Check that all fibres of the retinaculum have been divided, because any residual uncut fibres can cause persistent median nerve compression. Again

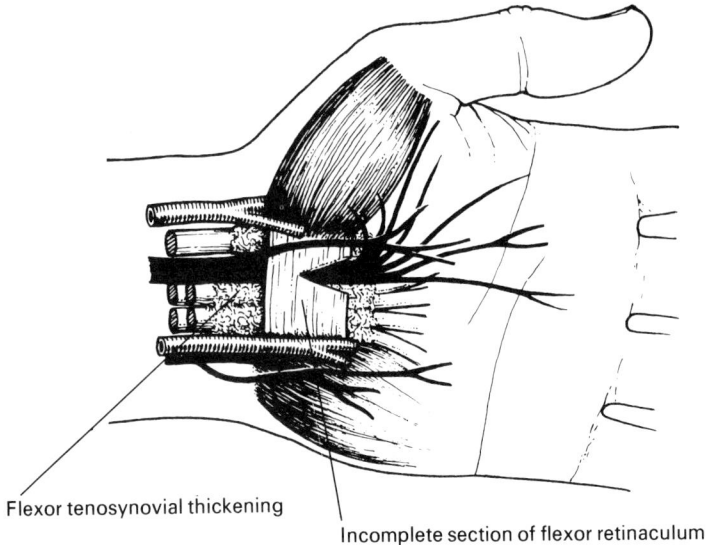

Flexor tenosynovial thickening

Incomplete section of flexor retinaculum

Fig. 5.30 Causes of persistent or recurrent carpal tunnel syndrome

under direct vision, cut the volar carpal ligament and deep fascia of the forearm proximal to the retinaculum.

Now expose the median nerve and decide whether any further surgery is required, e.g. external neurolysis, epineurotomy, or internal neurolysis. External median neurolysis is indicated if the nerve is obscured or compressed by thick fascia. This is not a routine procedure. An epineurotomy, division of the epineurium, is indicated if there is constriction of the median nerve. Internal neurolysis is required if there is interfascicular scarring, manifested by palpable induration of the nerve or obliteration of the median artery. Internal median neurolysis may also be indicated where there is persistent pain and para-aesthesia or where there has been recurrent carpal tunnel syndrome (Curtis 1973, Gassmann et al 1977). Exposure of the terminal branches of the median nerve is not a necessary routine unless there has been selective impairment of a sensory digital branch or branches, or the recurrent thenar branch.

Flexor tenosynovectomy is rarely indicated during operations for carpal tunnel decompression. Removal of synovium can create raw bleeding surfaces which heal by excessive scar, forcing adhesions around the flexor tendons and limiting tendon glide and grip strength. The indications of flexor tenosynovectomy include:

(a) Gross hypertrophy and compression of the median nerve.
(b) Interference with flexor tendon glide.
(c) Invasion of the flexor tendons.

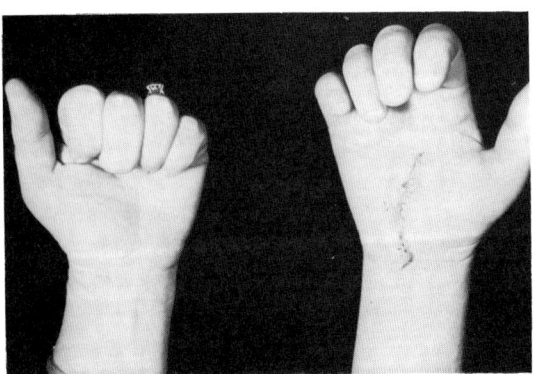

Fig. 5.31 Post-operative swelling, stiffness and palmar fasciitis. Three days after operation this 40 year old secretary developed pain which persisted for three months. She developed a sympathetic dystrophy. There were no pre-operative or operative problems

Suture only the skin and apply a compression bandage and plaster splint for the wrist. Encourage

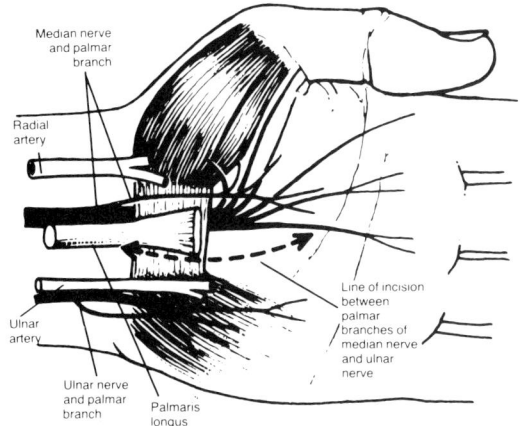

Fig. 5.32 Skin incision. This is made on the ulnar side of the thenar crease, between the palmar branches of the median and ulnar nerves. A vertical line bisecting the ring finger approximates the boundary between these two nerves. This incision avoids all but a few terminal branches of these nerves. The palmar branch of the median nerve lies between the palmaris longus and flexor carpi radialis tendons at the wrist. Accidental division of the palmar branch of the median nerve can lead to a sensitive neuroma in the scar. Caution—'Blind' carpal tunnel decompression through a transverse incision is dangerous and may result in: 1. Cutting the median nerve or its branches. 2. Incomplete division of the flexor retinaculum with persisting symptoms and signs. Blind section makes inspection of the carpal tunnel impossible

gentle finger movements, but maintain hand and arm elevation. Remove the dressing and splint at two weeks and remove the sutures.

Ulnar nerve compression at the wrist

At the wrist the ulnar nerve passes through Guyon's space (Fig. 5.27). The floor of this triangular space is the flexor retinaculum and some muscle fibres of the hypothenar eminence. The multilayered oblique roof consists of the volar carpal ligament that blends distally with the hypothenar fascia, radially with the palmar aponeurosis and proximally with the deep fascia of the forearm. The palmaris brevis also contributes to the roof. The vertical ulnar wall comprises flexor carpi ulnaris, the pisiform bone and the abductor digiti minimi. The space contains the ulnar artery and nerve.

Compression of the ulnar nerve in this space is rare. A ganglion is the most common cause. Other possible causes include proliferative flexor tenosynovitis extending in from the forearm, true or false aneurysms of the ulnar artery, thrombosis of the ulnar artery, fracture of the hook of the hamate with haemorrhage, lipoma or aberrant muscles pressing on the ulnar nerve. Compression of the ulnar nerve in Guyon's space can be caused by repeated blunt trauma.

Preoperative

Assess the patency of the ulnar artery by Allen's test. This may detect thrombosis or aneurysm of the ulnar artery or one of its branches, so causing ulnar neuropathy.

Operation

This space can be decompressed as part of a carpal tunnel decompression procedure. As an independent procedure one can incise on the radial border of the tendon of flexor carpi ulnaris, beginning 2 to 3 cm proximal to the wrist crease and extending in a zigzag fashion across the crease, along the line of the ring finger. It is safer to dissect the ulnar nerve proximal to the wrist and trace it distally through Guyon's space, reflecting in an ulnar direction the tendon of the flexor carpi ulnaris. Dissect and preserve those branches of the ulnar nerve to the hypothenar muscles and palmaris brevis muscle, as well as both superficial and deep branches of the ulnar nerve itself. The palmar branch of the ulnar nerve will probably not be seen but it should be kept in mind.

Postoperative care

As for carpal tunnel decompression.

Complications

As with carpal tunnel decompression these complications may be intra- or postoperative, and are very similar to those complications listed under carpal tunnel decompression.

REFERENCES

Angelides A C 1982 Ganglions of the hand and wrist. In Green D P (ed) Operative hand surgery, Volume 2. Churchill Livingstone, New York. ch 50, p 1635

Conolly W B 1978 Pitfalls in carpal tunnel decompression. Australian and New Zealand Journal of Surgery 48:421–425

Conolly W B 1980 A colour atlas of hand conditions. Wolfe Medical Publications Limited, London

Conolly W B 1984 A colour atlas of treatment for carpal tunnel syndrome. Wolfe Medical Publications Limited, London

Curtis R M, Eversmann W W 1973 Internal neurolysis as an adjunct to the treatment of the carpal-tunnel syndrome. Journal of Bone and Joint Surgery 55 A:733–740

Das S K, Brown H G 1976 In search of complications in carpal tunnel decompression. Hand 8:243–249

Gassmann N, Segmuller G, Stanisic M 1977 Carpal tunnel syndrome. Indication, technique and results following epineural and interfascicular neurolysis. Handchirurgie 9:137–142

Hybbinette C-H, Mannerfelt L 1975 The carpal tunnel syndrome—a retrospective study of 400 operated patients. Acta Orthopaedica Scandinavica 46:610–620

Kilgore Eugene S Jr, Brown L G, Newmeyer W L, Graham W P, Davis T S 1975 Treatment of felons. American Journal of Surgery 130:194–198

Langloh N D, Linscheid R L 1972 Recurrent and unrelieved carpal-tunnel syndrome. Clinical Orthopaedics 83:41–47

Lanz U 1977 Anatomical variations of the median nerve in the carpal tunnel. Journal of Hand Surgery 2:44–53

Lister G D, Smith R R 1978 Protection of the radial artery in the resection of adherent ganglions of the wrist. Plastic and Reconstructive Surgery 61:127–129

McCormack R M 1960 Carpal tunnel syndrome. Surgical Clinics of North America 40:517–520

Macdonald R I, Lichtman D M, Hanlon J J, Wilson J N 1978 Complications of surgical release for carpal tunnel syndrome. Journal of Hand Surgery 3:70–76

McEvedy B V 1962 Simple ganglia. British Journal of Surgery 49:585–594

Neviaser R J 1978 Closed tendon sheath irrigation for pyogenic flexor tenosynovitis. Journal of Hand Surgery 3:462–466

Scott J C, Jones B V 1952 Results of treatment of infections of the hand. Journal of Bone Joint Surgery 34B:581–587

H. G. Thomson

6

Syndactyly

The individualisation of 'simple syndactyly' requires fastidious attention to detail and considerable patience. Even when every effort is made to achieve the best possible correction, the result may be unsatisfactory. As several reviews show, the incidence of unsatisfactory results is often higher than expected (Kettelkamp & Flatt 1961, Emmett 1963, Skoog 1965, Buck-Gramcko 1975, Marumo et al 1976, Bauer et al 1980, Blauth 1980, Micali 1982).

This chapter examines ways of preventing a disappointing outcome. It also provides methods for correcting problems resulting from surgery that has been judged unsatisfactory from either an aesthetic or functional perspective by parents, patients, and hand surgeons.

CLASSIFICATION

Syndactyly is the most common significant congenital anomaly of the hand (Flatt 1977). It may occur in isolation but is also the most common anomaly associated with other congenital hand and foot conditions and more generalised syndromes of minor and major importance. These facts must be kept in mind when attempting to classify it (Kelikian 1974, Entin 1976, Castilla et al 1980). A random group of 196 syndactyly patients seen at The Hospital for Sick Children in Toronto fits well into a broad classification (Table 6.1). The patients with symphalangism (51) were isolated from a contracture evaluation because of their lack of clinical PIP joints, although their DIP joints can have a degree of congenital flexion deformity (Fig. 6.1).

FACTORS LEADING TO UNSATISFACTORY RESULTS

A number of factors may contribute to an unsatisfactory result in syndactyly surgery. Although complications rarely occur in isolation, they are considered individually in this chapter for the sake of clarity.

Preparation of the parent(s)

The difference between what parents may expect and what the actual results of surgery are may be the first source of discontent. For this reason it is extremely important to explain to the parents how

Table 6.1 Classification of syndactyly

	No. of patients	%	No. of web spaces	%
1. (a) Soft tissue syndactyly extending up to PIP	10	6.9	11	3.3
(b) Soft tissue syndactyly extending up to DIP	1	4.8	10	3.0
(c) Soft tissue syndactyly extending up to tip with or without involvement of cuticle	30	20.7	52	15.6
(d) Syndactyly soft tissue contracture	5	3.4	11	3.3
2. Syndactyly with bony fusion or abnormal position	20	13.9	45	13.5
3. Brachysyndactyly	37	25.5	117	35.1
4. Partial ectrosyndactyly	17	11.7	44	13.3
5. True ectrosyndactyly	15	10.3	21	6.3
6. Acrocephalosyndactyly	4	2.8	22	6.6
Total	145	100.0	333	100.0
7. Syndactyly with symphalangism*	51			

*Commonly associated with Poland's syndrome and not included in figures due to clinically fused joints.

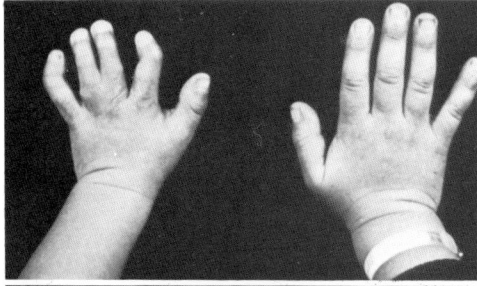
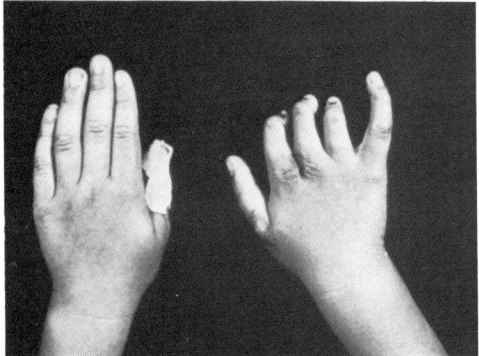
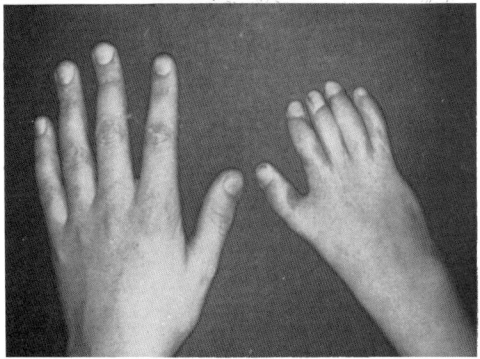

Fig. 6.1 Various types of PIP symphalangism, showing degrees of individualisation, DIP flexion contractures, and angulations

dressing changes, periods of immobilisation, splinting (if used), and subsequent care should also be discussed in detail with the parents.

Contractures

Any passive or active limitation to full extension and flexion is considered a longitudinal axial contracture in this chapter. Although the problem may be very subtle, it should be recognised. Factors which may be responsible for contractures include age and surgical design.

Age

If the syndactyly is complex and involves multiple extremities, there is significant parent pressure to initiate the surgical programme as early as possible, which is understandable. A definite schedule of area combinations, relative to surgical timing, must be planned; for example, left, middle, and ring fingers; left second and third toe. However, errors and complications are more likely when the fingers are very small. At The Hospital for Sick Children, we have found that the incidence of postoperative contracture is much higher if the initial surgery is done before the patient's second birthday than if it is done later (Table 6.2). As much functional and/or aesthetic surgery as possible should be completed by age 6 (grade 1) as this is the initial stage of peer pressure. To accomplish this goal, surgery may be required every six to eight months beginning at age two years.

There are always exceptions to rules and this commonly applies to syndactylies that have a tethering effect. If soft tissue tethering with or

the surgery will be done and what the outcome will be for their child. The explanation should include schematic drawings, drawings on the patient, and a statement of the reasons for choosing the donor site being used. Although this preparation is time consuming and demands patience, it is extremely helpful in creating realistic expectations and eliminating dissatisfaction with results.

In addition to explaining the procedure and outcome it is important to tell the parents how long the surgery will take. We currently allow 2½ hours for one web-space individualisation. The initial

Table 6.2 Surgical contractures related to initial age at operation

Age	No. of operated webspaces	No. of contractures
<6 months	21	*18*
6 months to 1 year	63	*38*
1 to 2 years	84	37
2 to 3 years	69	28
3 to 4 years	25	14
4 to 5 years	17	5
5 to 6 years	16	4
6 to 10 years	24	10
>10 years	14	2
Total	333	156

SYNDACTYLY

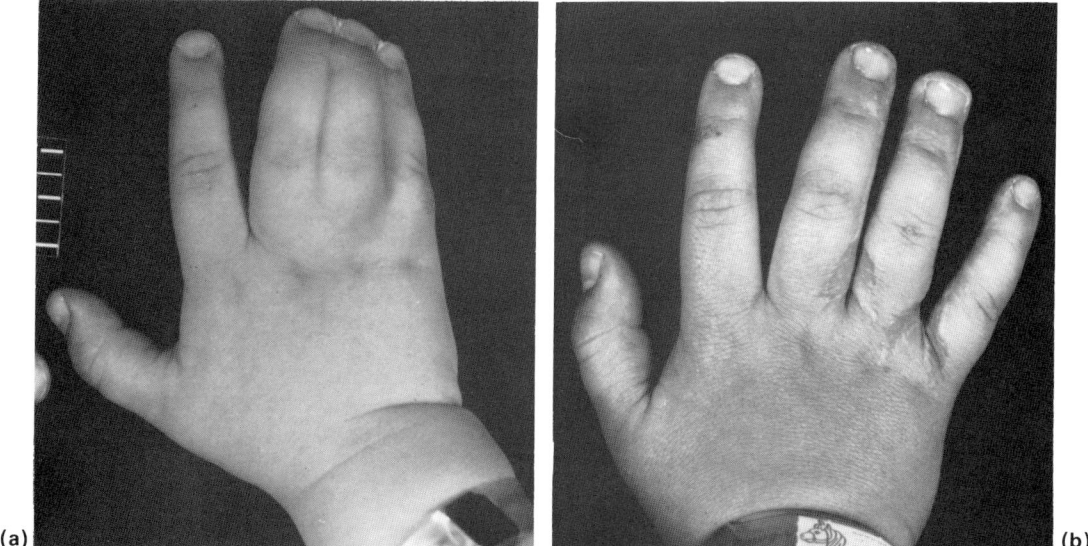

Fig. 6.2 (a) Ulnar soft tissue tethering acrosyndactyly. (b) Postoperative corrrection demonstrating no persistent ulnar angulation due to early correction

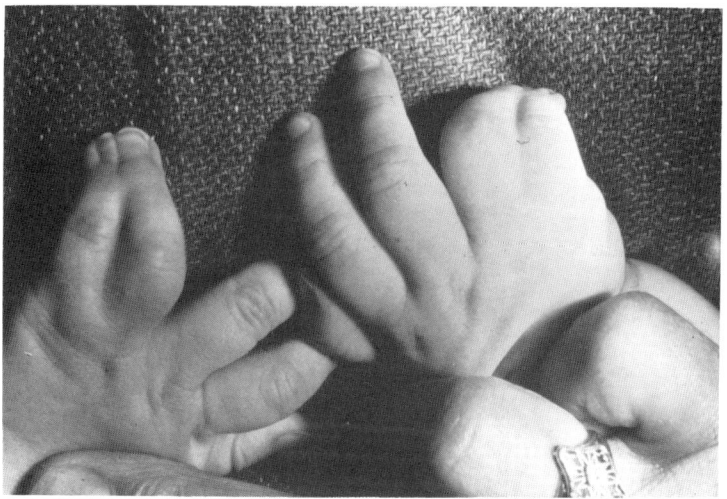

Fig. 6.3 More severe bony and cartilaginous tethering with significant early angulation and almost certain growth distortion

without bony attachments is allowed to persist, long-term secondary growth and soft tissue changes can result in some patients (Figs 6.2 and 6.3). Therefore, initial surgery before age two may be justified. Tethering may be single or multiple and is usually on the ulnar aspect, but it may also be radial (Fig. 6.4).

Surgical design

In many facets of life, design is the foundation for success and this is certainly true for syndactyly repair. If a haphazard approach is used, the surgical result will be unsatisfactory. The actual operative design must be outlined in ink on the patient's

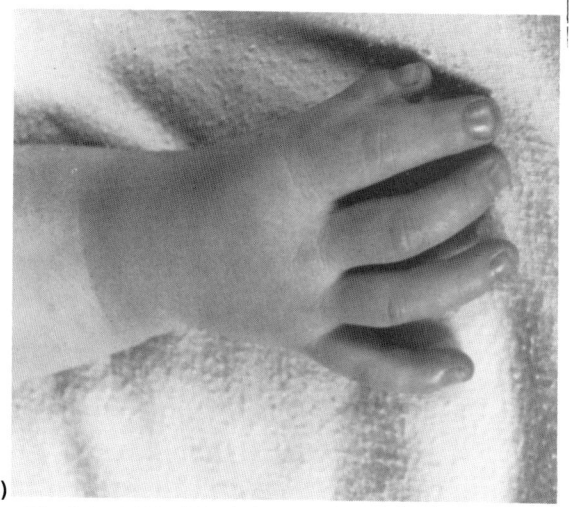 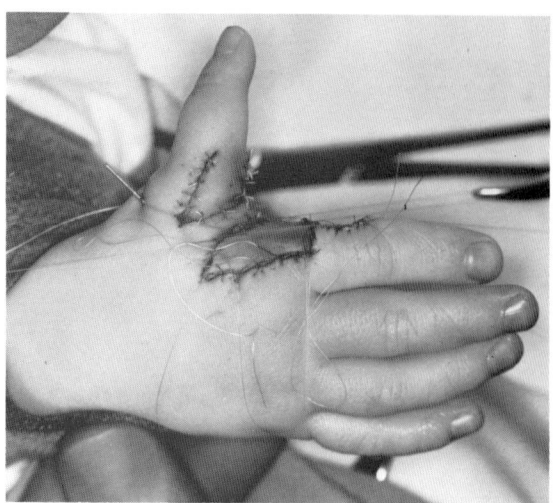

Fig. 6.4 (a) Radial soft tissue syndactyly having a potential tethering effect. (b) Postoperative individualisation with local flap and skin graft with Compère wire as abduction fixator

syndactyly web. This can be done in various ways. I use a sterile drafting pen nib combined with Bonney's blue. However, several available prefabricated pen and ink units which are gas resterilisable are almost as satisfactory.

The location of various critical dorsal or volar points on the geometric design can be determined using a through and through no. 25–27 syringe needle, dividers, and/or the eye. The types of geometric design are well established (Bauer et al 1956, Cronin 1956, Flatt 1962, Blauth & Schneider-Sichert 1981). All of them involve a zigzag volar incision line. The dorsal incision can be either staggered or linear. Rarely, if ever, does an extensor surface linear incision cause a scar contracture after an individualisation (Fig. 6.5). Usually no attempt is made to design skin flaps that completely clothe the separated surfaces. Almost always there is a skin shortage and thus skin grafts must be added to one or both opposing surfaces. However,

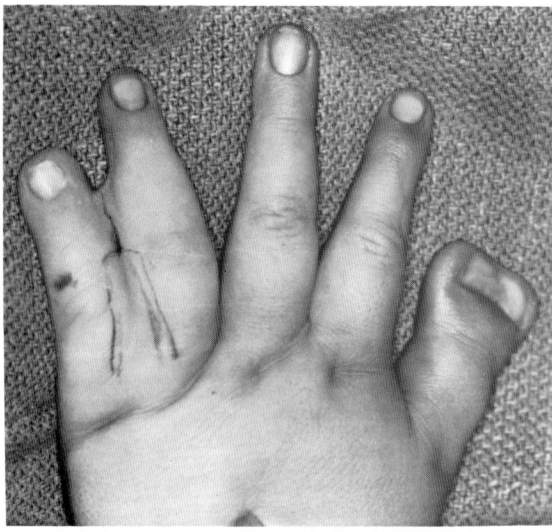 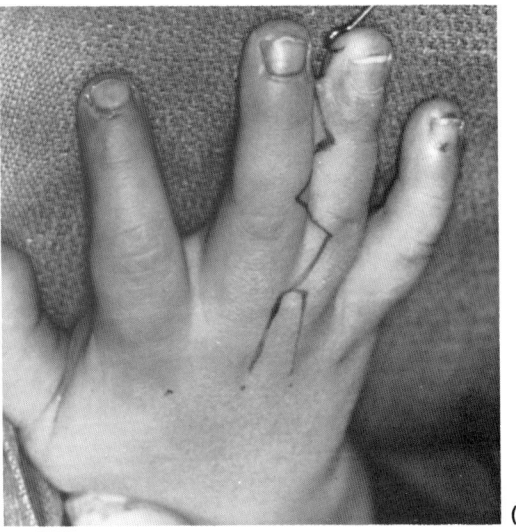

Fig. 6.5 (a) Linear dorsal incision with a jog at the juncture with dorsal web flap; associated radial Type A polydactyly. (b) Zigzag dorsal incision where unusually wide soft tissue web will permit some volar and dorsal interdigitation of gusset plus skin graft

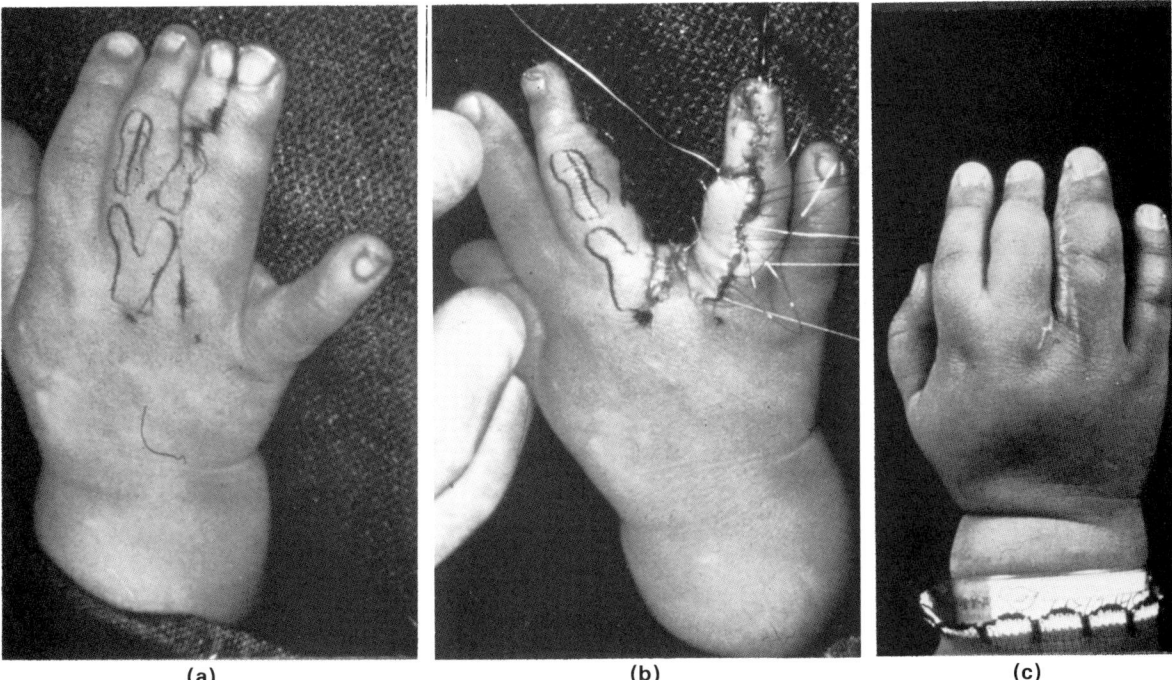

Fig. 6.6 (a) Median polysyndactyly in which the central ray is to be filleted. This provides enough skin for closure of the middle finger and a skin graft insert to the ring finger (b), (c)

in a median polysyndactyly enough skin flap may be salvaged to clothe one finger and skin graft the other (Fig. 6.6).

The volar triangular flap or gusset of the zigzag should be in the region of the joint creases, particularly the proximal phalangeal crease, and should be isosceles in shape. If the flaps are short and broad based, the design is similar to a straight

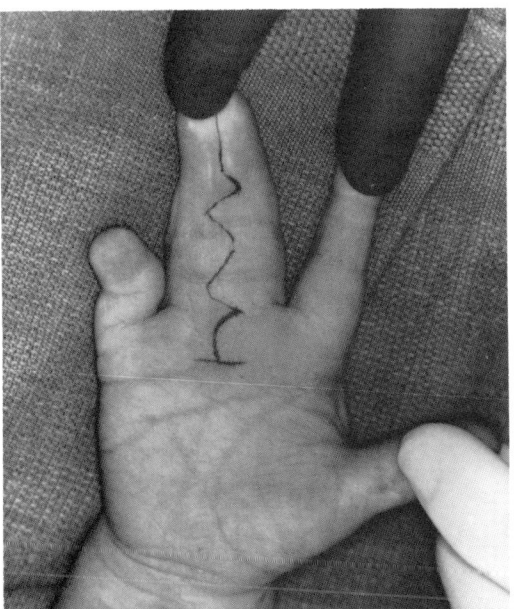 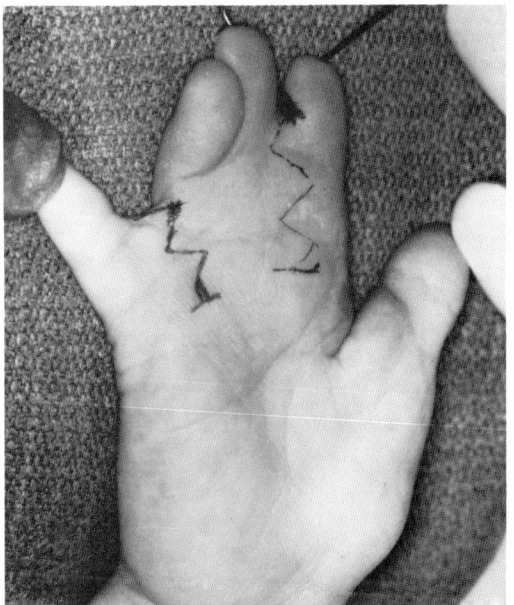

Fig. 6.7 (a) Soft tissue acrosyndactyly with broad-based triangular gusset and proximal 'T' to receive the dorsal flap. (b) Similar design in two syndactylies but with middle and ring web interposed for neurovascular safety

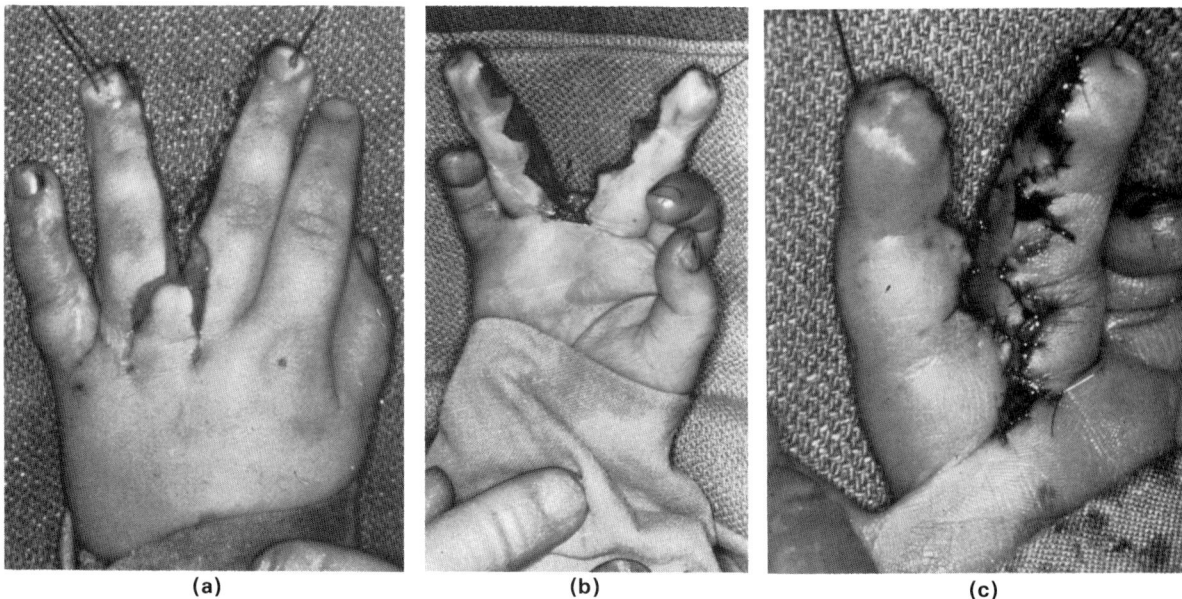

Fig. 6.8 (a) Linear dorsal incision with quadrilateral web flap. (b) Volar triangular gusset formed in region of IP joints. (c) Skin graft inserted with resultant zigzag closure

line which predisposes to contractures (Fig. 6.7). If the flaps are too long, they will reach the extensor surface, dividing the skin graft into two or more parts per finger. Although some surgeons find this acceptable I disagree. It is technically much easier to achieve appropriate tension and survival by inserting a single graft than by using two or three small grafts.

Additional surgical details

Before the incisions are made, the geometric design must be re-evaluated by viewing it from the volar and extensor surfaces. This can be done easily if a sturdy skin hook is passed through the terminal touch pad and nail at the same time. This technique makes the three dimensional operation accessible and thus easier. It is necessary to double check the volar incisions to be sure that they do not cross longitudinally at right angles to a flexion crease, which would automatically result in hypertrophic scar (Fig. 6.8).

So-called 'secondary syndactyly', which presents as a sinus along the congenital web, must be treated with total excision and must not be used as a serendipitous gusset or incision break-up. However, larger sinuses or gaps can be the exception to the rule (Fig. 6.9). Usually the secondary syndactyly phenomenon occurs with the jumbled hand that has small sequestrated parts and is a very depressing picture for the parents. Preparing them to expect a reasonable functional and aesthetic result is a practical and positive approach to an otherwise distressing situation (Fig. 6.10).

After the gusset or triangular flaps are cut and the fingers are individualised, there is a tendency to want to close a proximal triangular flap to the intact margin of the defect because it looks as if that is the way it wants to be placed. However, this will shorten the incision line, resulting in a contracture. When the gusset flaps are outlined, incised, and raised, care must be taken to reduce any possibility of jeopardising the blood supply, which would cause tip necrosis and contracture.

Fastidious care in applying skin grafts, including the preparation of a hemostatic bed with bipolar coagulation, graft immobilisation technique, dressing application, and limb elevation by suspension, all encourage better skin graft survival and maturation (Fig. 6.11).

CONTRACTURE CORRECTION

The frequency of contractures is directly related to the type of syndactyly that originally necessitated

SYNDACTYLY

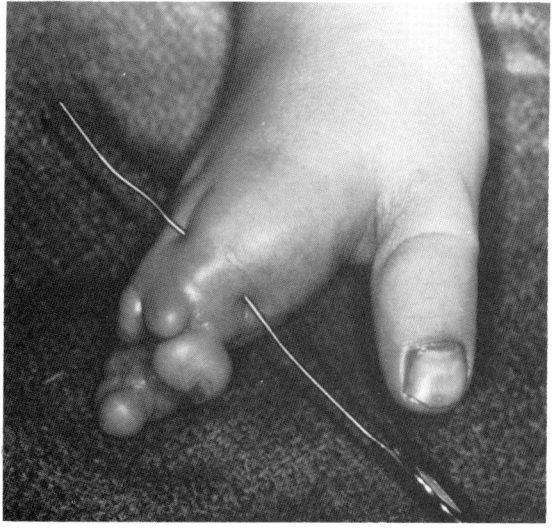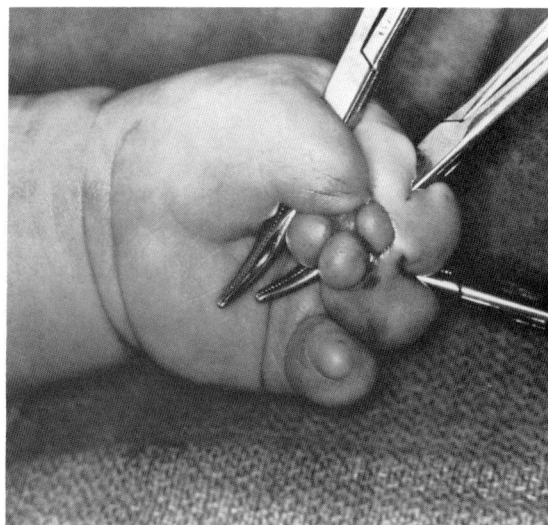

Fig. 6.9 (a) Simple secondary syndactyly in a jumbled hand. (b) Multiple secondary syndactylies which are large and may be used as gussets requiring two skin graft inserts per finger

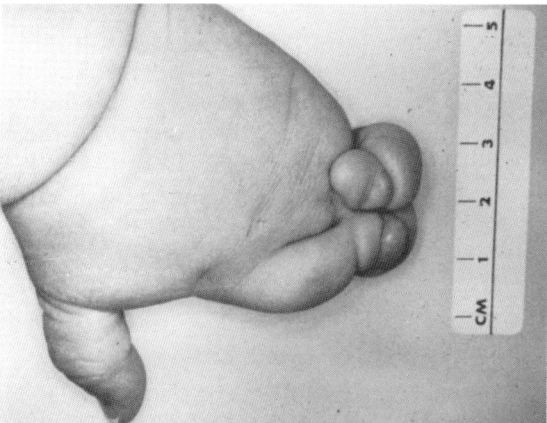

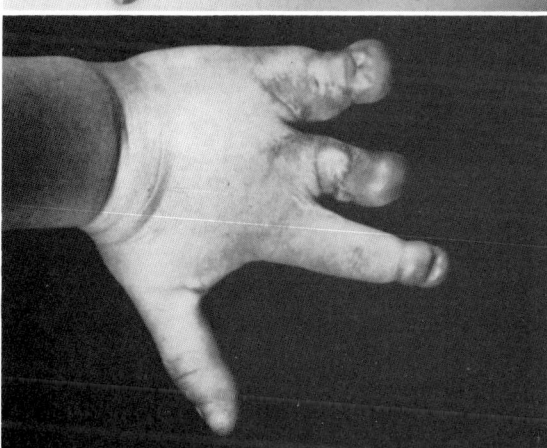

Fig. 6.10 Jumbled hand and functional and cosmetic result after individualisation

surgery (Table 6.3) and is generally greater than expected (Brown 1977, Toledo & Gerr 1979). They can be corrected using either a linear or a diffuse approach, depending on their origin. The least common problem is linear in nature and results from either a lack of or necrosis of the skin gussets. It can be corrected using serial or segmental Z-plasties which must be small distally, but proximally can be progressively larger. Usually there is room for three and possibly four Z-plasties per finger (Fig. 6.12).

The diffuse contracture is a more common problem which in most cases requires early correc-

Table 6.3 Frequency of second operation for contracture relative to type of syndactly

	No. of webspaces operated	Second operation for con- tracture	%
1. (a) Soft tissue syndactyly			
(i) extension to PIP	11	1	
(ii) extension to DIP	10	4	39.7
(iii) extension to tip within cuticle	52	24	
(b) Syndactyly with soft tissue contracture	11	5	45.4
2. Syndactyly with bony fusion	45	38	84.4
3. Brachysyndactyly	117	40	32.2
4. Partial ectrosyndactyly	44	18	40.1
5. True ectrosyndactyly	21	10	47.61
6. Acrocephalosyndactyly	22	16	72.7
Total	333	156	

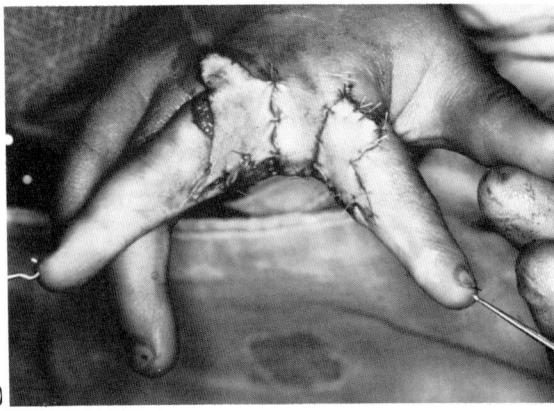
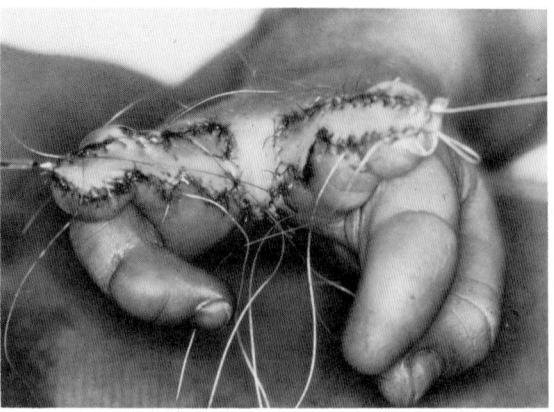

Fig. 6.11 (a) Small skin grafts being tailored with a dorsal web flap interposed. (b) Large skin grafts (acrosyndactyly) with overtie sutures ready to receive bolsters

tion and post-surgical splinting (Fig. 6.13). In the growing child a passive attitude creates a multiplicity of secondary soft and bony tissue changes, including short capsules and collateral ligaments, epiphyseal restriction, and premature closure. The diffuse contracture requires the creation of a volar diamond defect with a skin graft insert. At the time of surgical release, it is important to protect the tethered neurovascular bundles which could be cut inadvertently. The sudden correction of a severe, long-standing contracture of more than 30° can precipitate vascular spasm if full extension and fixed immobilisation by K-wire are achieved (Fig. 6.14).

Distal migration of web-space

The distal migration of the web space after surgical individualisation and thus the reappearance of syndactyly are usually multifactorial in cause and

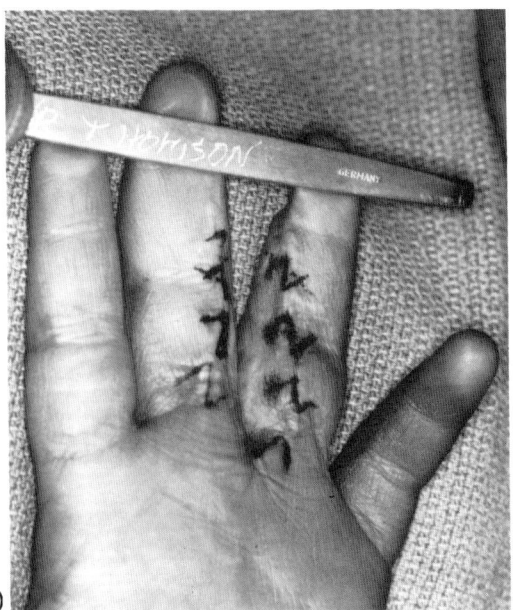
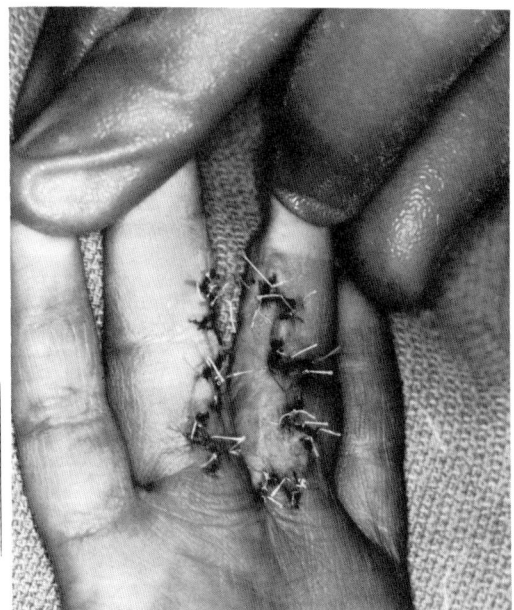

Fig. 6.12 Linear volar contractures (a) lengthened using four serial Z-plasties (b)

SYNDACTYLY

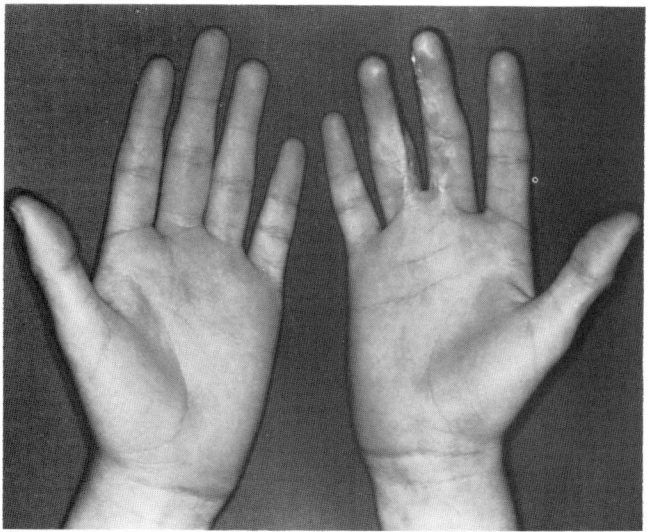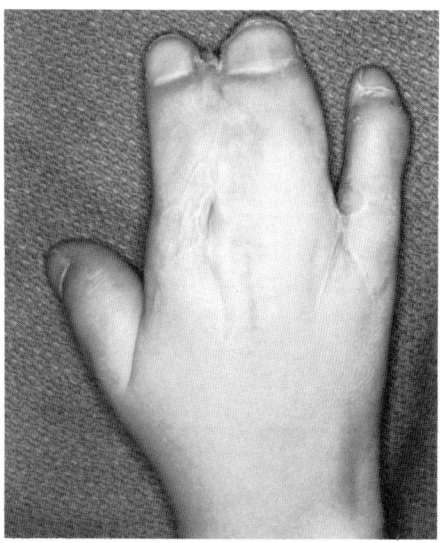

Fig. 6.13 (a) Minor diffuse volar contractures which will require the insertion of a skin graft. (b) Total re-syndactylisation due to loss of web flap and, presumably, necrosis of both skin grafts, and requiring total individualisation

are often associated with some degree of volar contracture. Major factors are web flap design, inadequate initial correction, immobilisation of the flap, or a combination of errors.

Web flap design

The design of the web flap is of paramount importance in web space migration and apparent recurrence of syndactyly. Many flaps have been designed, as discussed in various reviews (Schulstad & Skoglund 1977, Blauth & Schneider-Sichert 1981, Piza & Meissl 1980, Smith & Harrison 1982). Regardless of the choice, however, flap principles must apply, particularly when the flap is random and/or axial in nature. The infringement on flap thickness, width–length ratio, torque, and angu-

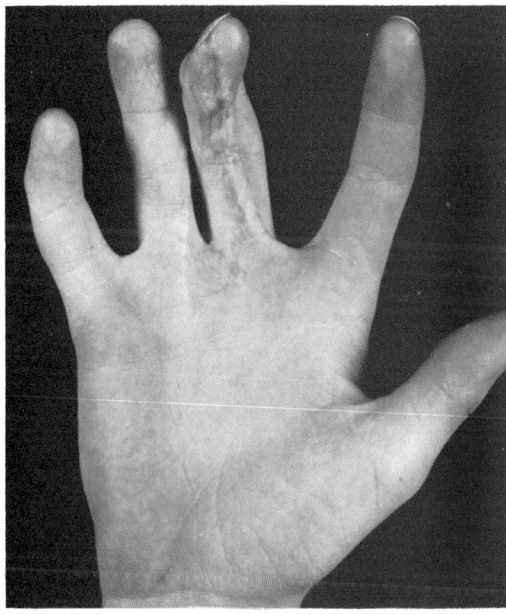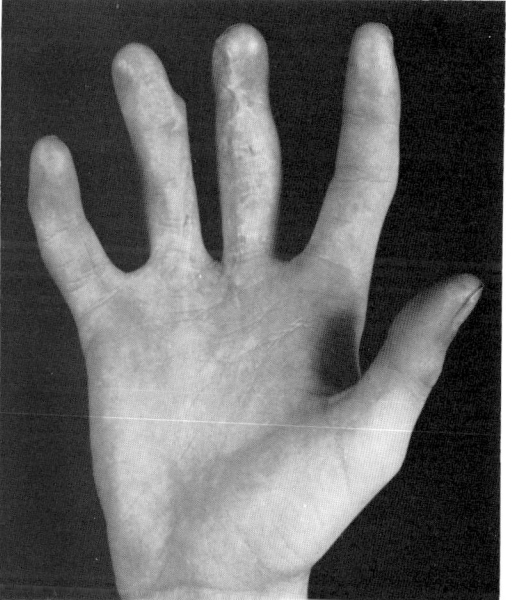

Fig. 6.14 (a) Severe diffuse contracture of middle finger requiring two full thickness skin graft inserts and (b) the late results after prolonged splinting

lation play a negative role in the development of postoperative necrosis and resultant scarring. The flap must have easy dorsal to volar reach without tension. Dragging it means trouble! The reach can be determined by measuring the thickness of the hand through the MCP joint region, relative to the length of the flap, or by using a syringe needle in a through and through fashion to identify the exact location. Usually the flap almost reaches to the dorsal PIP joint before the incision. I prefer to use a dorsal quadrilateral flap (Fig. 6.15).

Inadequate initial correction

When the web space flap is designed, it must be positioned in such a way that it overcorrects or proximally positions the web space. To achieve this it is necessary to bring the base(s) of the flap proximal to the metacarpal heads. The intermetacarpal ligament may have to be transected to permit the flap to sit in this exaggerated position. If a single dorsal flap is planned, the base must be proximally positioned, as must the volar 'T' cut which will receive the flap (Fig. 6.8). If the dorsal base and volar insert 'T' cut are distally positioned, late distal web migration is assured.

Immobilisation of the flap

The immobilisation of the flap with sutures and the type of dressing are important. The dressing should hold the fingers in an abducted position so that there is no pressure on the flap tip from torquing or compression.

Combination errors

If any degree of necrosis affects the web flap(s), gusset flaps, and/or skin graft it will result in distal migration of the web space.

The need for correction of a secondary distal migration of the web is based on functional and aesthetical limitations. If the migration is very mild, there may be no need for correction. However, if it is mild to moderate, significant improvement can be achieved by one or more Z-plasties (Fig. 6.16). These may be in or out of series.

If the resyndactylisation or distal migration is severe and thus aesthetically and functionally undesirable, a more radical method of correction is necessary. Either local or free graft soft tissue must be added. In some instances, particularly when the first web space is involved, an index interposition flap with direct closure or additional skin graft coverage can correct the problem (Fig. 6.17). Severe interdigital/distal web space contracture may require a new dorsal flap with skin graft inserts, i.e. a total recorrection of the syndactyly. In most cases the associated finger contractures have to be corrected at the same time (Fig. 6.18).

Skin coverage

There is some controversy over the type of skin graft or flap that should be used to cover the surface of the defects created after surgical individualisation.

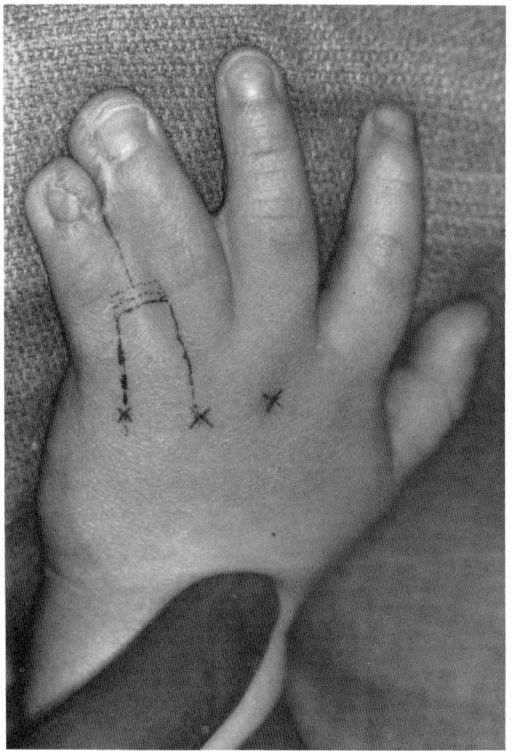

Fig. 6.15 Dorsal MCP dimples (×), web flap outlined with various length possibilities to PIP joint; pedicle flap inserts on distal phalanges

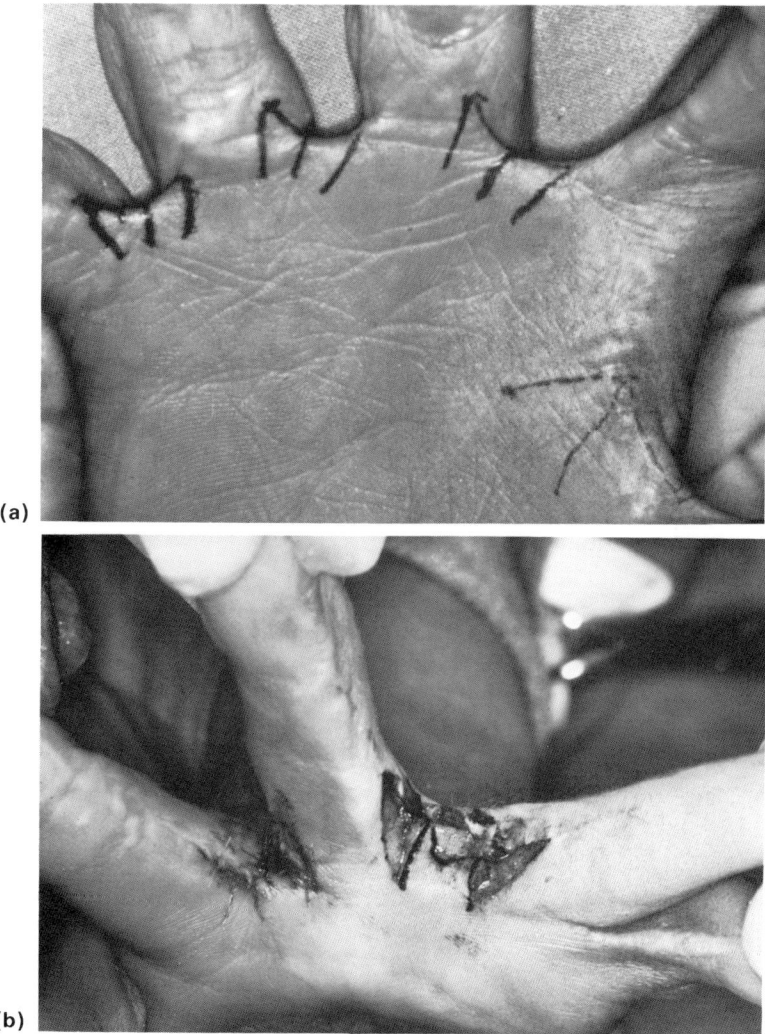

Fig. 6.16 (a) Mild distal migration of webs corrected with out-of-series Z-plasties and (b) double right-angled Z-plasty in the first interosseous web

Partial thickness skin graft

The technique requiring the least experience is the free split or partial thickness skin graft. Large areas of skin can be harvested from the same donor site and can, therefore, cover several individual sites. A mechanical assist such as a Humby knife or a Reese, electric, or pneumatic dermatome is necessary to provide the skin graft. Graft removal, particularly if one is unaccustomed to the equipment, requires careful selection of donor site, e.g. high posterior thigh or buttock, and a test pass of the blade to sample the skin graft thickness. The purpose of this manoeuvre is to reduce the likelihood of taking a thick or full thickness skin graft which would result in scars at the donor site (Fig. 6.19). This phenomenon can occur even in experienced hands and leads to a very unsatisfactory result.

The main advantage of the split thickness skin graft is its ability to survive under adverse recipient site conditions, e.g. seroma, cancellous bone, fat, or interface shearing due to poor dressing. The disadvantages of partial thickness skin grafts lead to some of the common undesirable results in syndactyly repair, such as excessive graft contrac-

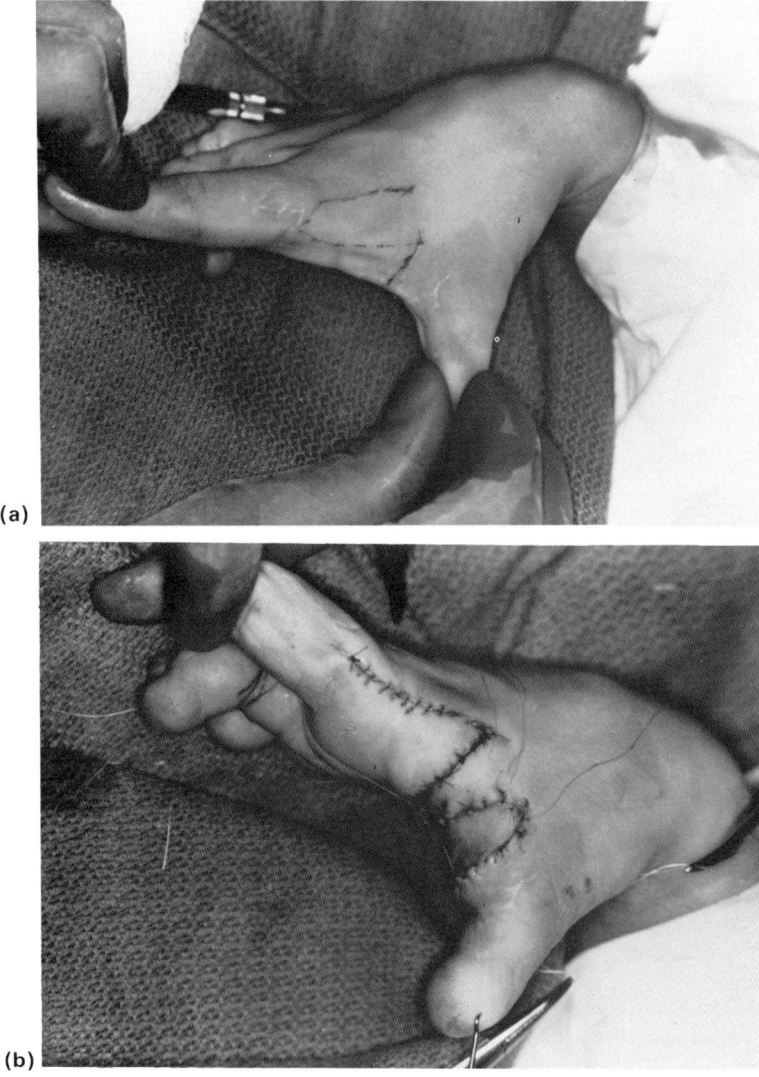

Fig. 6.17 (a) Previously under-corrected mild syndactyly of thumb–index finger with double right-angled Z-plasty. (b) Additional correction with interposition index flap and full-thickness skin graft

tion which causes finger contracture, hyperpigmentation, and poor skin quality match. Nevertheless, some surgeons feel that split thickness skin grafts are the most appropriate method of dealing with the acrosyndactyly of Apert's syndrome where a relatively large graft area is required. The use of free full thickness skin graft donor sites in this circumstance would cause excessive scarring (Fig. 6.20). A review of the clinical results of partial thickness skin graft individualisation of Apert's syndrome patients at The Hospital for Sick Children showed that patients achieved 60% normal finger function compared to their peers in appropriate age and sex groups. Therefore, encouraging parents to anticipate significant benefit with the resultant poker fingers is appropriate.

Full-thickness skin graft

The most desirable method of adding skin is the free full-thickness skin graft because it has better

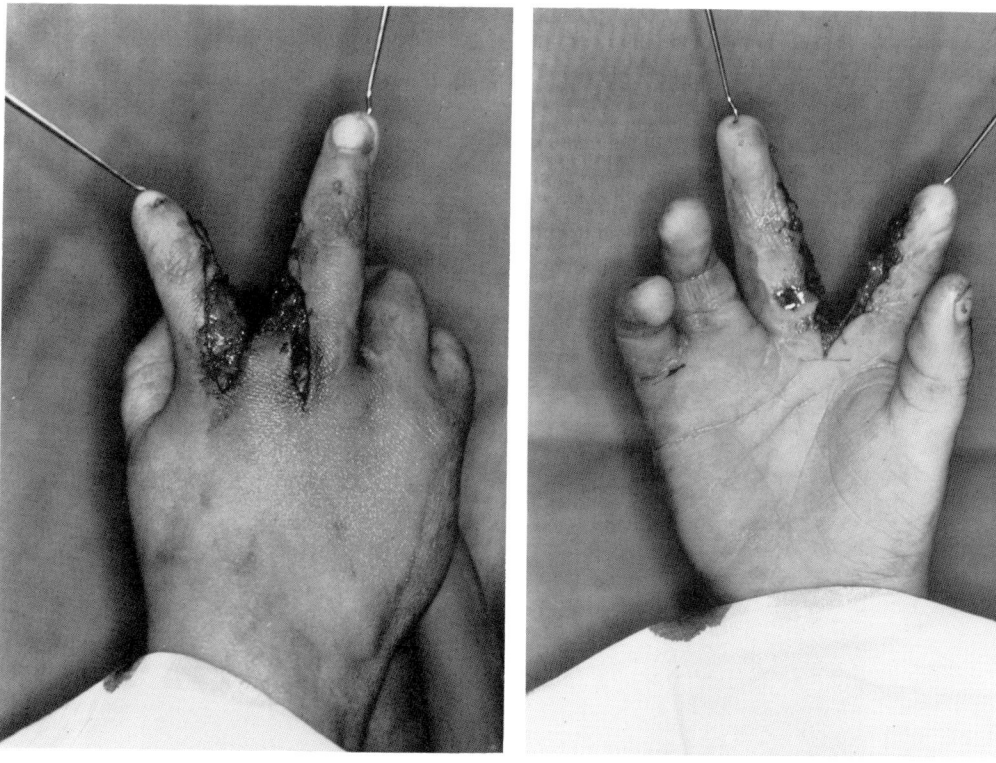

Fig. 6.18 (a) Severe distal migration of web between index and middle fingers is over corrected with recreated dorsal flap. (b) Volar incision with inked 'T' is over corrected

texture, colour, resilience, and sensation and less pigmentation and contraction than partial thickness grafts. The graft must be harvested from selected areas such as the left lower quadrant (bikini area) or inner arm. Using the lower abdominal quadrants as donor sites allows grafts to be harvested from the same donor site at three different times providing they are separated by periods of at least eight months. The groin is a popular area but it can be used only once and is approaching a high melanocyte zone which would encourage late hyperpigmentation. The apparent shortage of donor site availability in bilateral total syndactylisation might suggest the use of a tissue expander. This would require operating on both hands at once and would require longer surgical periods. Probably the concept is not practical in most institutions. After one or two surgical harvestings the standard donor site should appear as a single line, the final result of an intracuticular closure.

Full thickness skin grafts require more attention to tension than partial thickness grafts. The recipient sites always look larger and the skin graft smaller than they are. The use of a moist pattern of silence cloth or any non-stretchy material pressed onto the inked defect margins can be helpful in maintaining the appropriate size of skin graft, and hence the proper tension (Fig. 6.21). Before they are removed, the skin grafts must be marked using either ink or intradermal scratching with the back of the scalpel. This is necessary since a full thickness skin graft loses its shape because of its elastic nature once it is removed from its bed.

A one piece skin graft for each finger defect is better than several skin grafts. All grafts must be tailored to receive the gusset or triangular flaps that have been made in the recipient area (Fig. 6.11).

Occasionally it is possible to use filleted polydactyly units as a reservoir for full thickness replacement skin; this procedure is very imaginative and fulfills the need for similar skin at the graft donor site (Rowsell & Godfrey 1984). A frequently

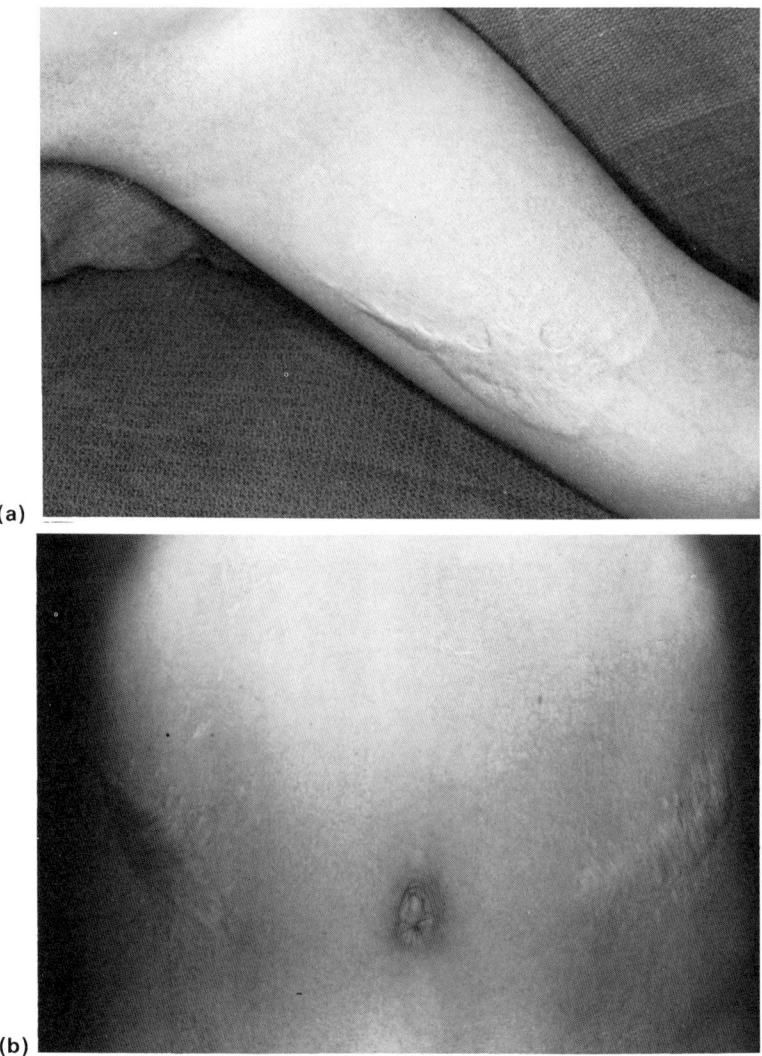

Fig. 6.19 (a) Hypertrophic partial thickness skin graft donor site on forearm. (b) Spread, hypertrophic full thickness skin graft donor sites in a non-selected area

requested donor site is the foreskin, but this particular tissue is very inappropriate because of its unusual texture and great tendency to hyperpigment; it would not give a satisfactory result.

Flaps

Occasionally, both skin and subcutaneous tissues are necessary to avoid an unsatisfactory result. This is particularly true in the first interosseous web space between the thumb and index finger where tightness and restricted mobility are common. A jump flap may be necessary to overcome these problems (Fig. 6.22).

Hyperpigmentation

Hyperpigmentation is rare in Caucasians, particularly if selectivity has been observed, but it sometimes occurs in the darker races. If hyperpigmentation develops within a split thickness skin graft, replacement with a full thickness graft is appropriate (Fig. 6.23). The use of depigmenting topical agents rarely provides permanent changes.

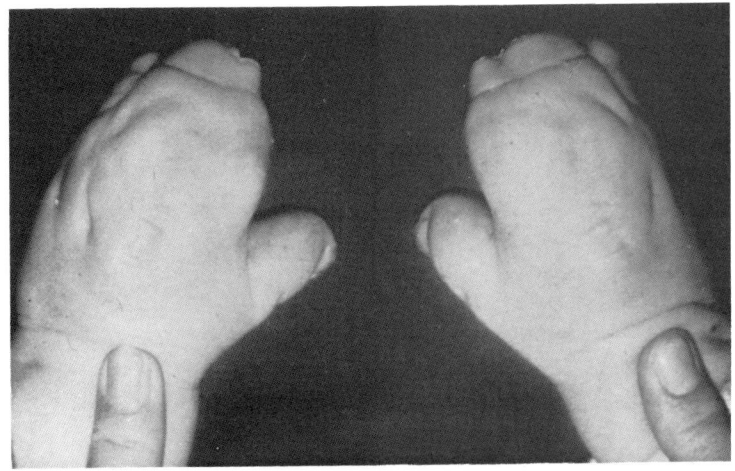

(a)

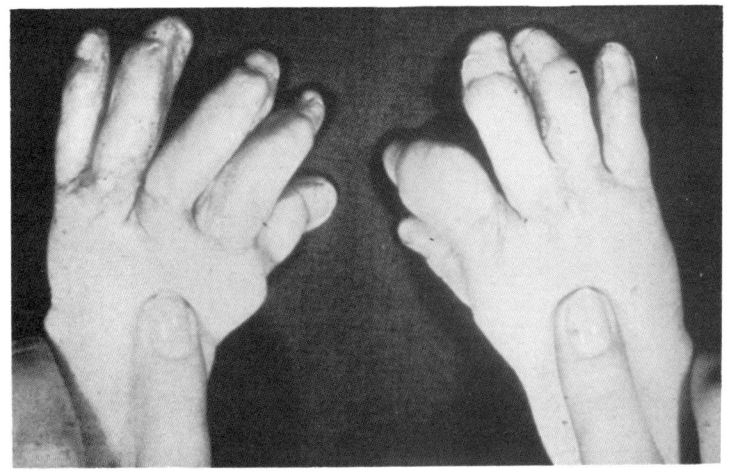

(b)

Fig. 6.20 (a) Acrosyndactyly of Apert's syndrome with (b) post-individualisation 'poker fingers' (split thickness skin grafts used in this particular patient)

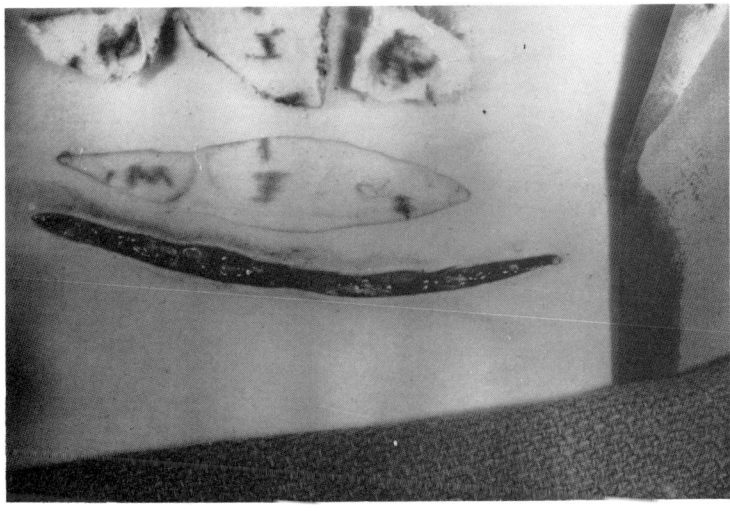

Fig. 6.21 Donor site, left lower quadrant (bikini area) lateral sector just over anterior superior spine, wound subcutaneous layer closed, full thickness skin graft; three silence cloth patterns above

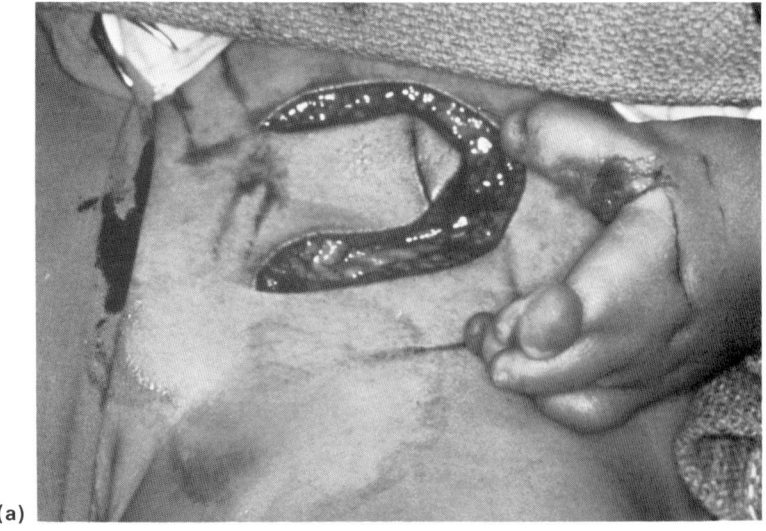

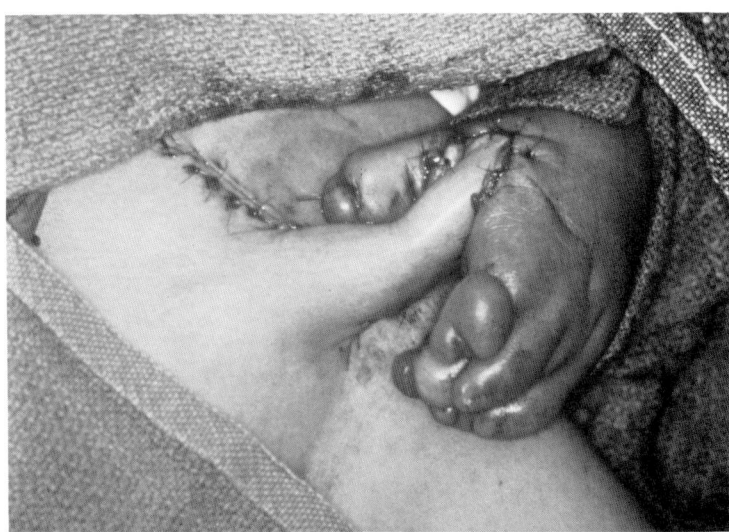

Fig. 6.22 (a) Jumbled hand with adducted thumb space opened with adductor oblique head. (b) Recessed and an abdominal jump flap inserted into defect

Dermabrasion of split and/or full thickness grafts can be attempted but with a guarded potential for success.

Ectopic hair

The survival of hair follicles after a thick partial or full thickness skin graft is possible but not common. This phenomenon may make its appearance at puberty. If the parents are particularly hairy, additional consideration should be given to donor site selectivity and an area such as the inner arm might be selected. Hair follicle survival is more likely with full thickness than with intermediate or partial skin grafts. Replacement surgery is the only means of eliminating this problem. Although professional electrolysis may be used it is not likely to give a permanent result.

Neurovascular bundles

Our patients are very young at individualisation and therefore do not complain of insensitivity or a cold finger if a neurovascular bundle is inadvert-

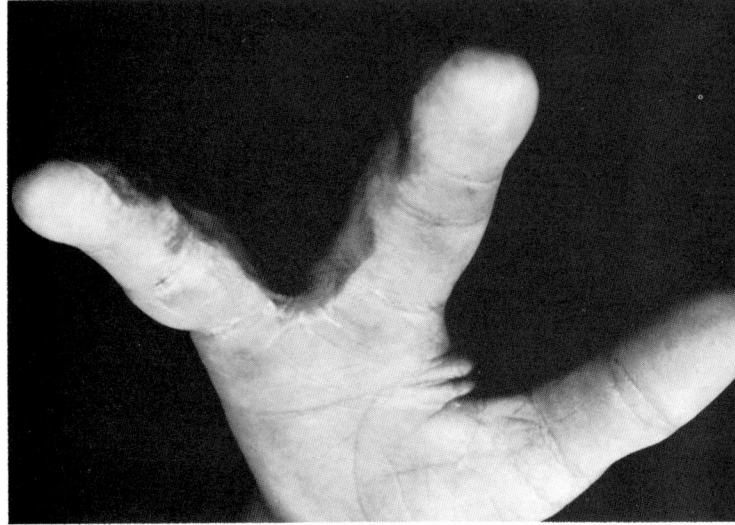 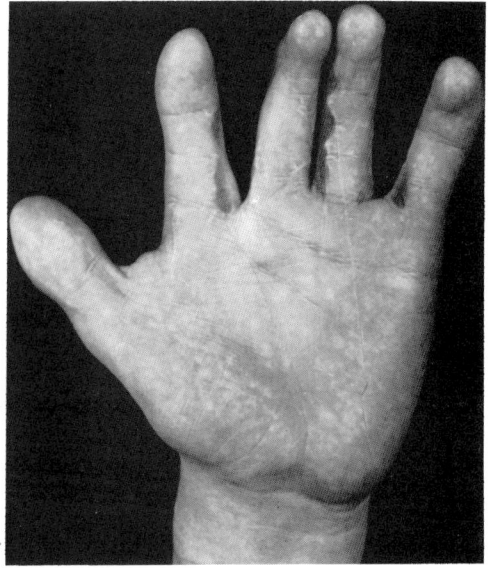

Fig. 6.23 (a) Two-fingered hand with isolated hyperpigmentation of graft. (b) Multiple individualised webs all demonstrating hyperpigmentation

ently transected. Special care must be taken with the neurovascular structures during separation. The most common error is failing to look for them during blunt or sharp dissection. Once they are recognised distally and traced proximally, the distally branching digital artery may have to be ligated. If this is done, it must be carefully documented in the operative notes, particularly if several web spaces are involved, as it may be necessary to make a similar decision relative to adjacent fingers in the future. It would be very unsatisfactory if both digital arteries to a single finger were ligated. Probably the most common application of the ligation principle is the radial aspect of the little finger if conjoint with the ring finger, especially if there are multiple syndactylies.

Similarly, the digital nerve is more frequently a problem because the epineurium has not separated and is joined more distally than the artery bifurcation. If this is the case, the epineurium can be split atraumatically with the back of the scalpel blade to the proximal point where the new web space flap can be comfortably interposed (Fig. 6.24).

A compression dressing can be applied to ensure the survival of the skin graft and may also act as a tourniquet. The finger tips should always extend beyond the dressing so that capillary bed return can be seen and so that Dopler or thermocouple monitoring is possible. This can be accomplished easily if the large hooks already mentioned are left in place during dressing applications.

Neuroma

Secondary neuroma has never been recognised as a problem at our hospital. Secondary neurotrophic changes have not been identified and yet there must have been transected digital nerves over the years. The fact that we have not observed a digital neuroma in an individualised syndactyly patient does not mean that the problem might not occur in an adolescent or adult who has been individualised. However, it raises the interesting general question of whether digital neuromata ever occur in children.

Suture material

The more inert the suture material, the more likelihood there is that the incision scar will be satisfactory. Unquestionably, the time-consuming part of the operation is the insertion of sutures, be they interrupted or continuous. This being the case, both the needle and the suture material itself should be easy to handle. For all well behaved children over three years of age, I use 6–0 monofilament both as interrupted tie-over sutures and as interrupted and continuous skin graft

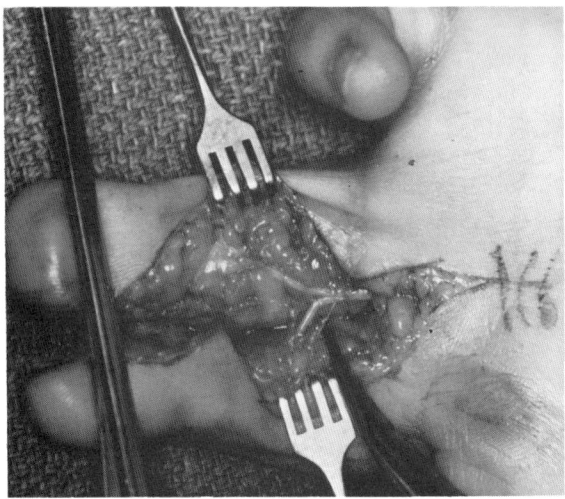 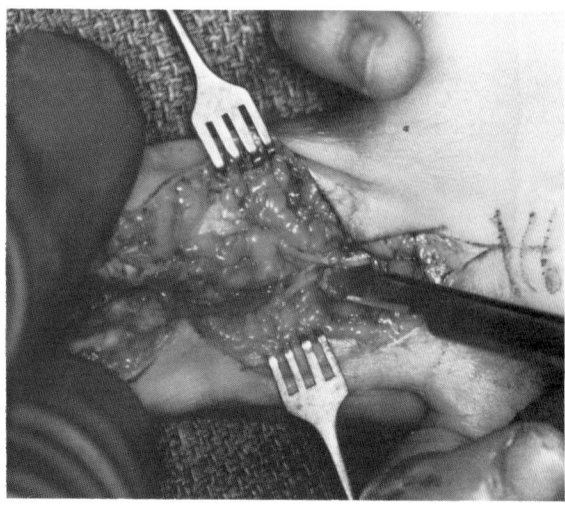

Fig. 6.24 (a) Distal position of digital nerve bifurcation. (b) Epineureum easily split, releasing the two nerves by using back of scalpel blade

fixation sutures. These inert sutures ensure as fine a juncture scar as possible and are easy to remove. However, for all patients under 3 years of age and those who are somewhat older but misbehave, the use of 6–0 polyglycollic acid sutures makes life much easier for the parents, patient, and surgeon. Unfortunately, these sutures appear to be more reactive. Furthermore, they must be left in place for 6 weeks, which necessitates suture line hygiene with soap and water and some form of greasy application such as Vaseline.

Nail-cuticle distortion

Nail-cuticle distortion occurs only when the initial condition is a type of acrosyndactyly, primarily of a bony-cartilaginous nature; it is less likely with a minor soft tissue join. The distortion results from the application of a skin graft on bone, cartilage, and/or joint at the time of primary separation and closure, causing skin graft disruption with residual scar contraction. The literature contains many postoperative pictures of acrosyndactyly fingers showing angulation as well as nail and cuticle distortion.

If the defect to be grafted is in continuity with the remainder of the finger defect and has a very small bony bed of 1 mm or so, it can probably be covered with a small piece of local tissue and the defect can be skin grafted. A simple preoperative test is to grasp each conjoint digit between the index finger and thumb and determine whether there is any movement between them. This gives a good indication of whether there is a cartilaginous or non-radiological bony union. If there is going to be more significant bony exposure and particularly if full thickness skin graft is to be used, the graft will probably become necrotic, leading to angulation and nail bed distortion.

This unsatisfactory result can be prevented by using pedicle tissue to cover the exposed bone and two to three months later a skin graft to cover the remainder of the individualisation (Figs 6.25 and 6.26) (Thomson 1971).

Epiphyseal closure and angulations

Epiphyseal closure and angulations are not a primary problem but are manifested at a much later postoperative date. They may be due to several factors. Partial or complete epiphyseal closure may be secondary to a surgically created scar or may result from the fingers being kinetically tethered due to a congenital finger length irregularity (Figs 6.2 and 6.3). These problems must be anticipated for parents so that they will not be dissatisfied with the results.

Epiphyseal closure and angulations secondary to surgery may result from direct epiphyseal transections during the separation, the most common

SYNDACTYLY 83

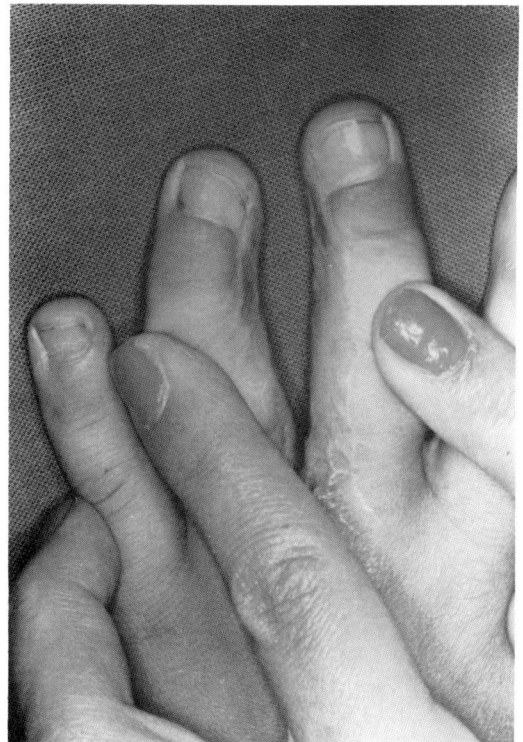

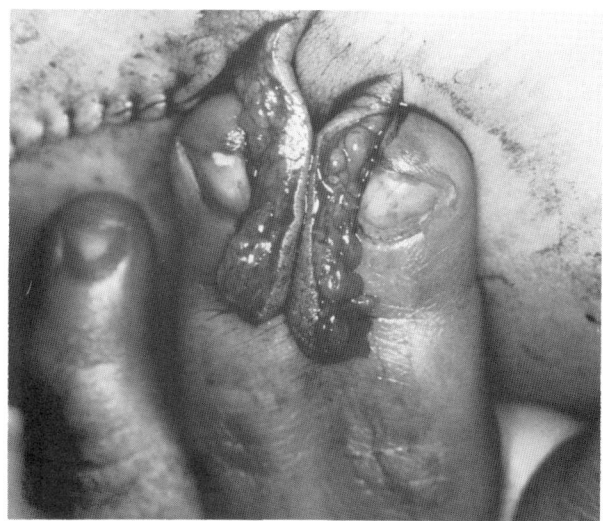

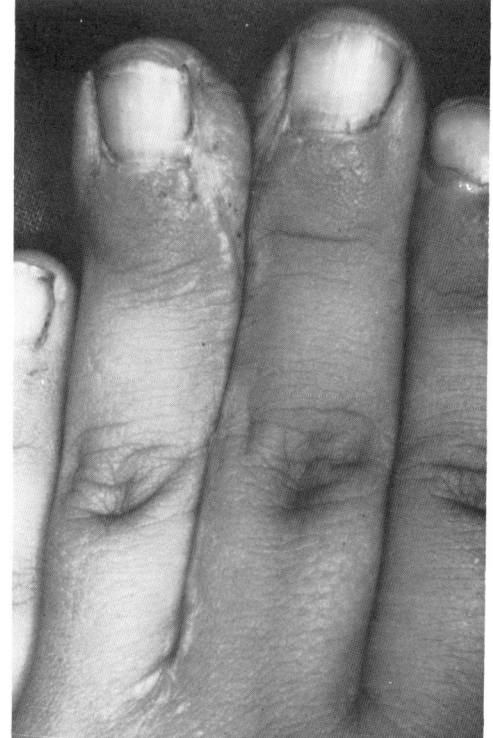

Fig. 6.25 (a) Usual cuticle distortion and digital angulation associated with scar contracture. (b) Double butterfly flaps raised to clothe bare bone. (c) Appearance after maturation of individualisation

example being acrosyndactyly. However, I do not believe this alone causes epiphyseal closure but rather that poor wound healing due to skin graft necrosis and resulting scar formation are contributing factors. Epiphyseal closure or growth delay may also result from prolonged scar contracture. This can be a combination of flexion, radial, and ulnar angulation force (Fig. 6.27) which is directly related to the location, direction, and severity of the scar itself. Anticipation of both these potential consequences of surgery and early surgical release reduce the retardation in epiphyseal growth but

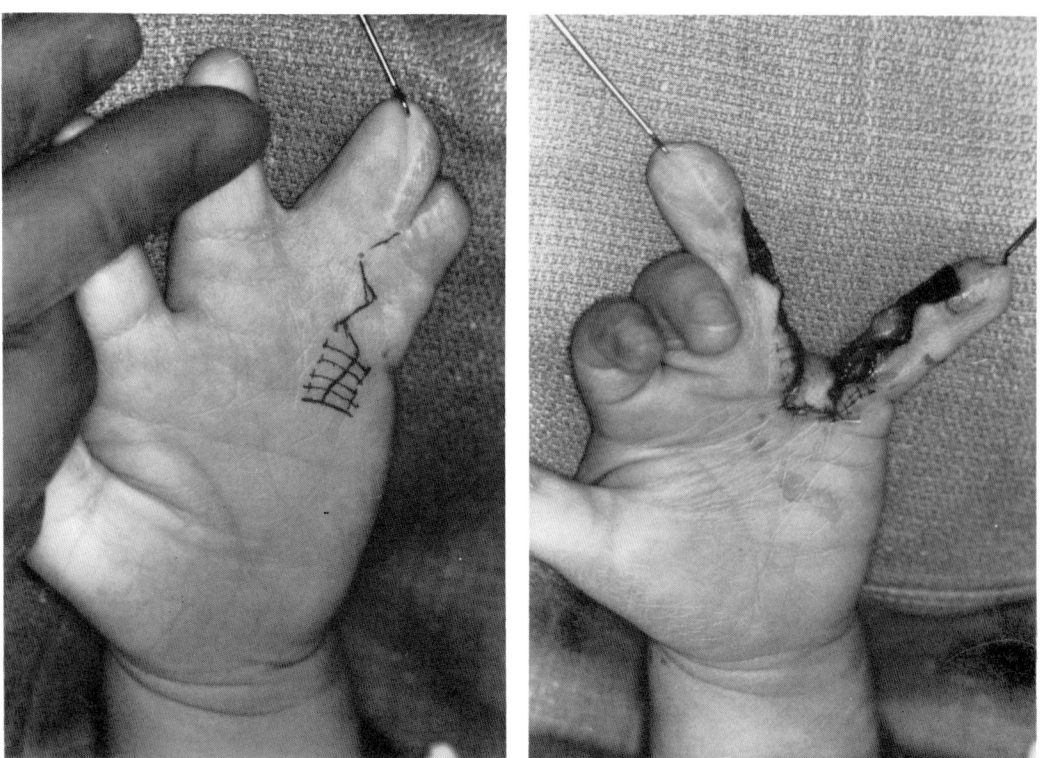

Fig. 6.26 (a) Volar appearance of distal pedicle flaps prior to individualisation demonstrating optimal positions of 'T' incision. (b) Separation completed and ready to receive skin graft inserts

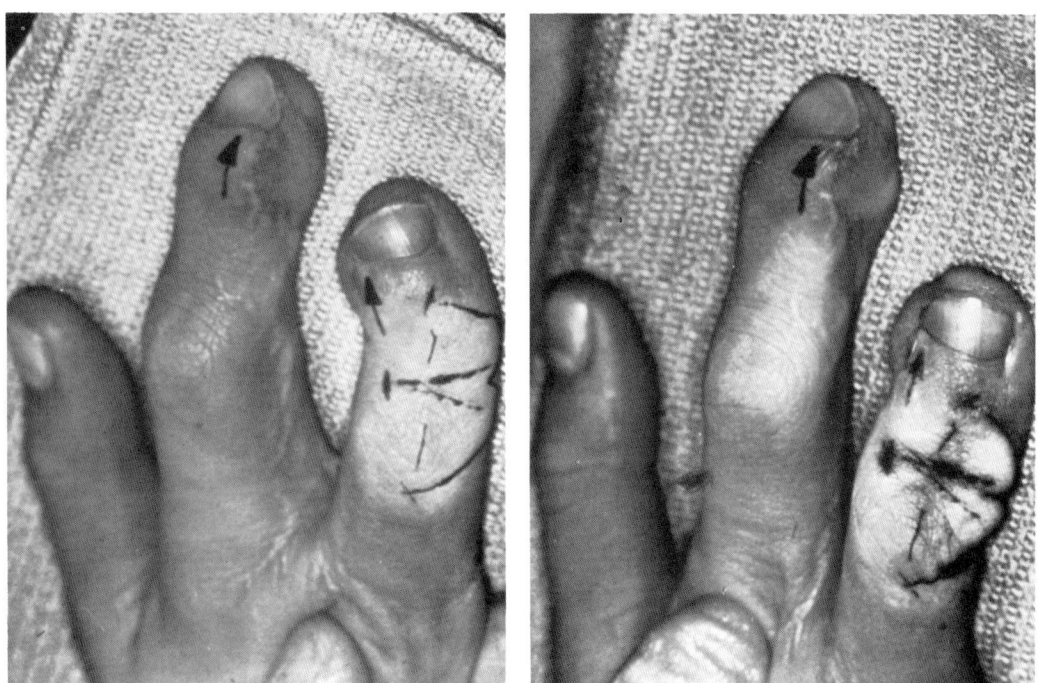

Fig. 6.27 (a) Combination clinodactyly due to scar contracture and delta phalanx. (b) Appearance after corrective ostectomy

SYNDACTYLY 85

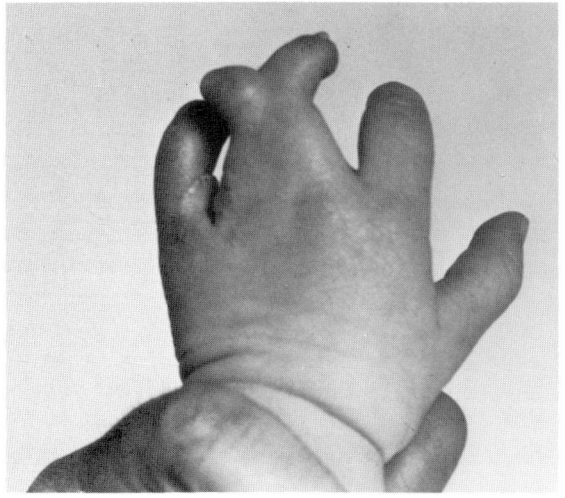
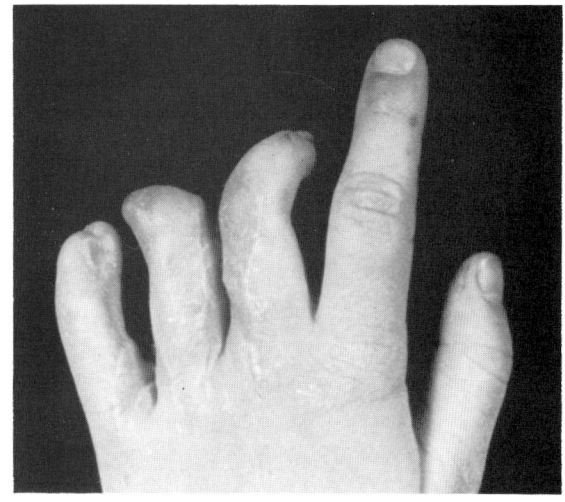
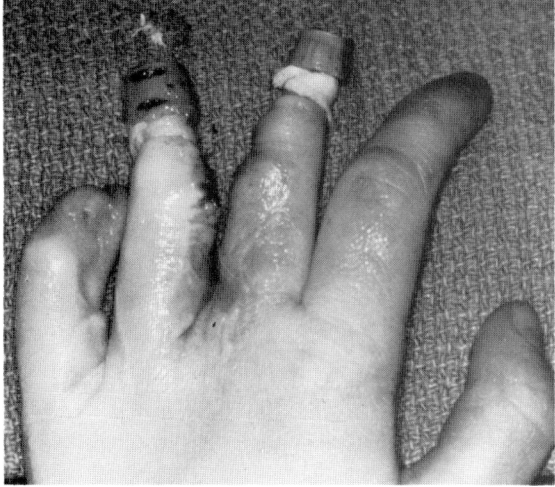

Fig. 6.28 (a) Congenital clinodactyly persisting after individualisation (b). (c) After ostectomies and K-wire inserts, covered with protective corks

cannot reverse a closed epiphysis. There is also an additional variable, the delta middle phalanx which can cause clinodactyly and may or may not be obvious at the time of separation (Fig. 6.28). This angulation, which mimics epiphyseal compression, can be deceiving in the presence of surgical scarring (i.e. a co-existing problem).

Dressings and splints

After an embroidery type operation, it is an insult to both the patient and the surgeon to apply a non-functioning, non-aesthetic dressing and/or splint. Regardless of the high esteem in which the surgeon is held by both parents and peers, a sloppy dressing usually indicates sloppy underlying surgery.

Splints are rarely needed initially. I use them only when there has been some skin graft necrosis and there is the potential of scar contracture. In this case an extension-abduction splint which permits light dressings should be used. The thermoplastic qualities of the splint allow it to be reformed subsequently to fit more snugly when the dressings are discontinued. A two piece (dorsal and volar) splint is preferred; it not only holds the finger in extension, but also applies pressure on the early scar. For two months the splint should be kept in place except during meals, baths, and swimming. Then it should be used only at night for a further month. A similar dressing augmented by initial splinting is used for a secondary postoperative, diffuse contracture or migration of the web.

86 UNSATISFACTORY RESULTS IN HAND SURGERY

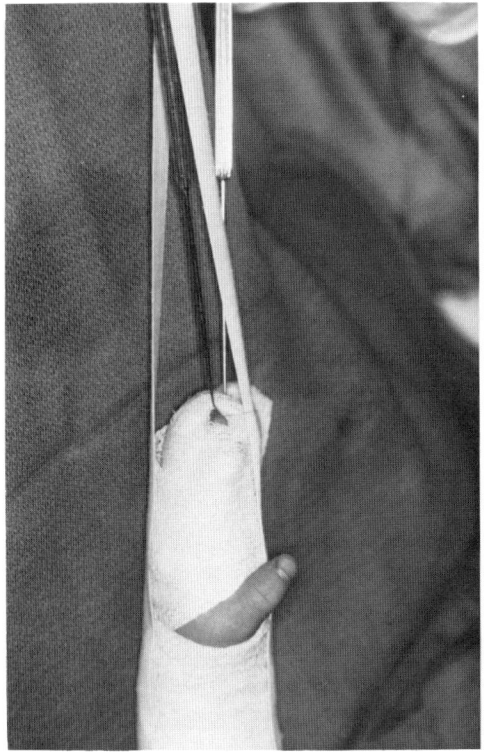

Fig. 6.29 Non-tourniquet suspension dressing; using hypoallergenic skin glue and the 'stove pipe' plaster bandage principle substituting Kling bandage. This is facilitated by the retention of skin hooks through the nails

Overzealous individualisation

Overzealous individualisation may produce undesirable results. Postoperatively, some patients have excellent function with some persistent polysyndactyly, which is usually partial in nature, for example, in the much wider digit with a single broad nail. There may be patient, parent, or general practitioner pressure to individualise rather than leave the ray as it is. However, in this situation it is important to consider the case carefully and not to individualise just because it is possible to do so. Individualisation may not be in the patient's best interests because it may create irregular finger lengths, will mean not having a nail, will not be stable, will not have IP or MCP flexion or extension, and so forth.

The overall rule of thumb, is never to individualise more than one adjacent web space at the same operative session in the same hand. The incidence of undesirable results rises precipitously when this rule is not followed. However, there can be exceptions. For example, if a patient has acrosyndactyly and significant heart disease, comes from 600 miles away, and has only one parent, breaking the rule may be justified and the possibilities should be discussed carefully with the parent.

It is important to adopt a plan with the parents to accomplish as much as possible with each operative session, but never to over commit oneself or the patient. If there are upper and lower extremity syndactyly problems with or without associated deformities, the ipsilateral upper and lower individualisations could be done at one time. Thus, it is important to outline the operative plans for the parents; any of these plans can be altered before, during, or after surgery.

It is worthwhile to alert the parents to the possibility that a single individualisation could be done if other types of minor surgery are being undertaken, such as T & A or hernia. This requires pre-arrangement with surgeons, anesthetists, the family doctor, and the parents.

FINAL PHILOSOPHY

This syndactyly chapter began by considering parent preparation and, because it is so important, will end with the same subject. As surgeons, we may lose sight of the fact that the parents and, where applicable, the patient have no idea what to expect from the newly separated fingers in terms of either function or aesthetics. The parent must be given home therapy exercises for the hand and in the case of a child with Poland's syndrome, arm adduction exercises to build up the usually hypoplastic latissimus dorsi, which may be used for breast–chest contour reconstruction at a later date (Ireland et al 1976, Haller et al 1984). They must also be told what to expect from the hands after surgery when the anomaly is complex as in the unstable joints of ectrosyndactyly, the lack of IP flexion in symphalangism, and the secondary angulation of the delta middle phalanges. The surgeon knows that the quality of the end result will be limited by such anomalies and must not fail to communicate this fact to the parents. Failure to adequately inform the parents leads to unsatisfactory results in their broadest sense. The surgeon's personal explanation of the relevant information assists the parents in their ultimate decision to overcome their natural reticence to let him operate on their child. After the surgery the poker finger of symphalangism is an obstruction and is always getting injured. If parents have been inadequately prepared they will ask why they were not told of this problem before. If they have been well prepared they are likely to have a positive response and often note that the results are better than they expected.

REFERENCES

Bauer T B, Tondra J M, Trusler H M 1956 Technical modification in repair of syndactylism. Plastic and Reconstructive Surgery 17:385–392

Bauer T B, Cronin T R D, Smoot W H 1980 Long-term results in plastic and reconstructive surgery. In: Goldwyn R H (ed) Treatment of Syndactyly. Little Brown & Co, Boston. ch 45, p 812–834

Blauth W 1980 Kongenitale Syndaktylien der Finger. Zeitschrift für Kinderchirurgie und Grenzgebiete Suppl 30:42–53

Blauth W, Helbig B 1981 [So-called recurring syndactyly and its management] Das sogenannte Syndaktylierezidiv und seine Behandlung. Zeitschrift für Kinderchirurgie und Grenzgebiete Suppl 30:53–57

Blauth W, Schneider-Sichert F 1981 Congential Deformities of the Hand: An Atlas of Their Surgical Treatment. Springer-Verlag, New York. ch 2, p 10–71

Brown P A 1977 Syndactyly—a review and long term results. Hand 9:16–27

Buck-Gramcko D 1975 Congenital malformations of the hand: indications, operative treatment and results. Erik Moberg Lecture 1975. Scandinavian Journal of Plastic and Reconstructive Surgery 9:190–198

Castilla E E, Paz J E, Orioli-Parreiras I M 1980 Syndactyly: frequency of specific types. American Journal of Medical Genetics 5:357–364

Cronin T D 1956 Syndactylism: results of zigzag incision to prevent postoperative contracture. Plastic and Reconstructive Surgery 18:460–468

Emmett A J 1963 Syndactylism of the hand: a review of sixty cases. British Journal of Plastic Surgery 16:357–375

Entin M A 1976 Syndactyly of the upper limb. Morphogenesis, classification, and management. Clinical Plastic Surgery 3:129–140

Flatt A E 1962 Treatment of syndactylism. Plastic and Reconstructive Surgery 29:336–341

Flatt A E 1977 The Care of Congenital Hand Anomalies. Webbed Fingers. C V Mosby Co, St Louis. p 170–212

Haller J A, Colombani P M, Miller D, Manson P 1984 Early reconstruction of Poland's syndrome using autologous rib grafts combined with a latissimus muscle flap. Journal of Pediatric Surgery 19:423–429

Ireland D C R, Takayama N, Flatt A E 1976 Poland's syndrome: a review of forty-three cases. Journal of Bone and Joint Surgery 58A:52–58

Kelikian H 1974 Congenital Deformities of the Hand and Forearm. W B Saunders Co, Philadelphia. ch 12, p 333–407

Kettelkamp A B, Flatt A E 1961 An evaluation of syndactylia repair. Surgery, Gynecology and Obstetrics 113:471–478

Marumo E, Kojima T, Suzuki, S 1976 An operation for syndactyly, and its results. Plastic and Reconstructive Surgery 58:561–567

Micali G 1982 Experience treating syndactyly. Annals of Plastic Surgery 9:65–71

Piza H, Meissl G 1980 Spätergebnisse nach operativer Korrektur der Syndaktylie. Zeitschrift für Kinderchirurgie und Grenzgebiete Suppl 30:57–60

Rowsell A R, Godfrey A M 1984 A fortuitous donor site for full-thickness skin grafts in the correction of syndactyly. British Journal of Plastic Surgery 37:31–34

Schulstad I, Skoglund K 1977 Surgical treatment of simple syndactyly. Scandinavian Journal of Plastic and Reconstructive Surgery 11:235–237

Skoog T 1965 Syndactyly. A clinical report on repair. Acta Chirurgica Scandinavica 130:537–549

Smith P J, Harrison S H 1982 The 'seagull' flap for syndactyly. British Journal of Plastic Surgery 35:390–393

Thomson H G 1971 Isolated acrosyndactyly: avoiding postoperative contracture. British Journal of Plastic Surgery 24:357–360

Toledo L G, Ger E 1979 Evaluation of the operative treatment of syndactyly. Journal of Hand Surgery 4:556–564

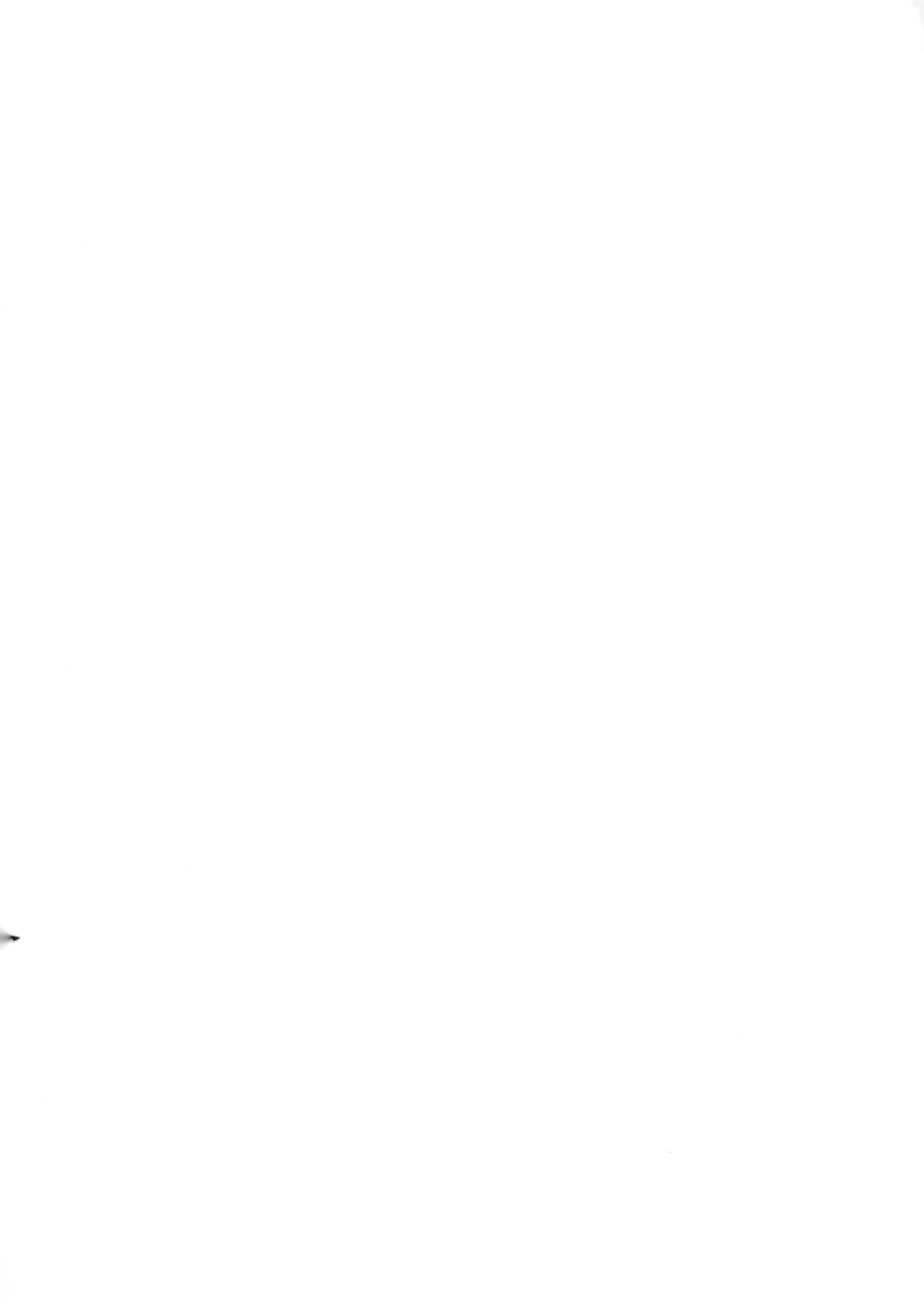

D. W. Lamb

7 Club hand

POTENTIAL COMPLICATIONS OF TREATMENT FOR ABSENCE OF THE RADIUS

Radial absence is such a complex deformity of the forearm, wrist and hand (Fig. 7.1) that it is not surprising that it is notoriously difficult to treat and that complications will be not infrequent. It is essential to have some knowledge of the deficiencies of development which are found in order to try and minimise complications in management. It is not just the bone which fails to develop but also muscles, joints, nerves and vessels (Heikel 1959). It is important for surgeons to be aware of these developmental failures before embarking on any surgery.

The muscles arising from the extensor origin at the lateral condyle are often absent whereas the medial humeral condyle and the flexor muscle origin are usually normal. A flexion deformity of the wrist and weakness of dorsiflexion of the wrist is therefore common (Fig. 7.2). The muscles normally arising from the radius are absent but as the thumb is usually missing or a 'rudimentary' thumb (Fig. 7.3) the absence of flexor pollicis longus and the thenar muscles does not much matter. However, the absence of the radial half of flexor digitorum profundus may be significant as loss of terminal joint flexion of the index finger would effect 'thumb' function if the index is subsequently pollicised (Lamb 1972).

The radius may be totally absent, partially absent, or hypoplastic (Fig. 7.4). The radial carpal bones are usually missing. Absence of scaphoid and trapezium may make the operation of centralisation of the ulna less secure. The elbow joint is often stiff

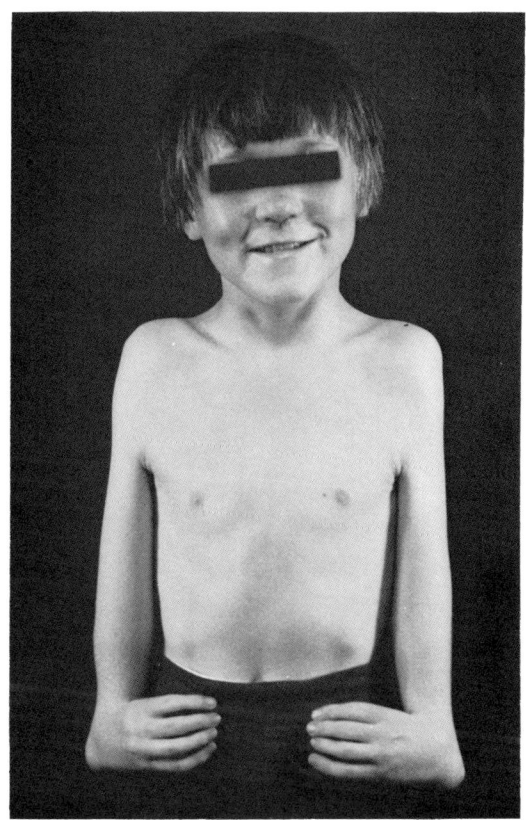

Fig. 7.1 Typical deformity in untreated total absence of the radius. Note the prominence of the lower ulna. There are minor contractures of the proximal interphalangeal joints. There is complete absence of the thumb. This boy was one of twins both of whom had this deformity. This boy had stiff elbows in extension. His brother had full active movement of the elbows

in extension in early life and may develop abnormally due to defects in the capitellum and lateral condyle. Unless elbow movement is restored and there is active flexion to at least 90° it is unwise to

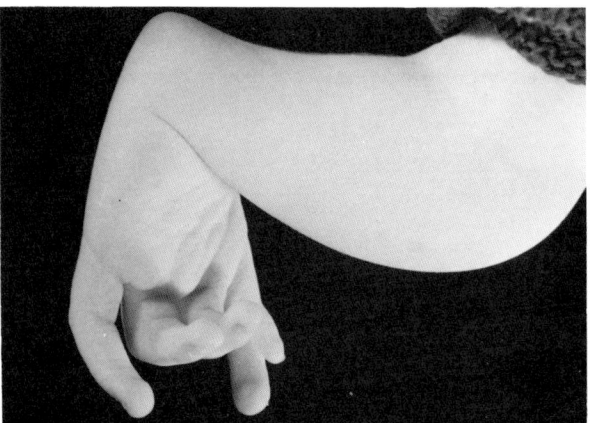

Fig. 7.2 Flexion deformity that may occur in complete absence of the radius rather than the more common radial deviation. It is due to the weakness or absence of the extensor group of muscles arising from the lateral condyle as compared with those on the flexor aspect

correct the wrist deformity. In addition to the joint deformity the elbow flexors are usually poorer than the triceps. The function of the hand is often severely limited by stiffness of the joints and the poor function of the long flexors and extensors and the intrinsic muscles.

Any operative procedure to correct the ugly radial club hand deformity will be disappointing to patient, parents and surgeon unless it is made clear that the hand, even if it has been corrected into a better cosmetic positioning, may function no better. This only applies when the metacarpophalangeal joints are very stiff, usually in an extended position, and the proximal interphalangeal joints have flexion contractures. This lack of function may not matter in the unilateral case and the cosmetic improvement from operation may outweigh this. When the hand joints are less affected, however, we have found no child where correction of a bilateral deformity has led to any functional impairment—in fact usually the reverse is true. It must be remembered that the function of the index and middle fingers are usually much less than the ulnar two digits due to the greater stiffness of the related joints. An ulnar pattern of prehension (Fig. 7.3) is encouraged by both the deformity and the greater dexterity of the ulnar fingers. The surgeon must beware of correcting the wrist deformity when there is a well established ulnar prehension and this is one of the cogent reasons for surgical correction of the wrist deformity early before prehensile patterns become too fixed. The superficial radial nerve is usually missing in the lower forearm and its sensory territory taken over by the median nerve. Not infrequently (between a quarter and one-third of patients at operation) the median nerve divides in the forearm

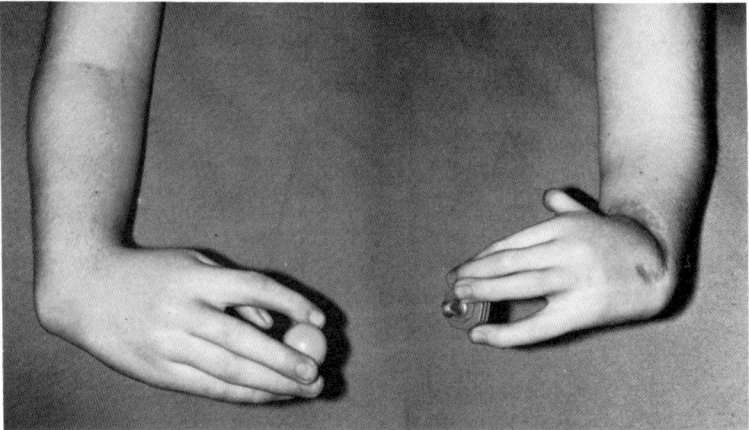

Fig. 7.3 Bilateral absence of the radius. Operation has been carried out on the left side in which centralisation was carried out. There has been some recurrence of deformity. Note the ulnar pattern of prehension on the left side. There is a useless maldeveloped thumb on the left side. On the right side no operation has been carried out. Note that despite a more normal looking thumb the pattern of prehension is a sideways pinch between the index and long fingers. The thumb was in fact of very little functional value

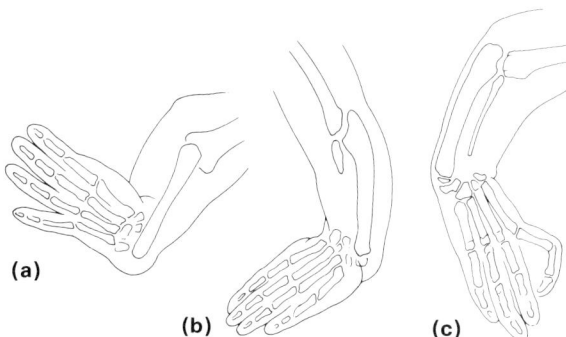

Fig. 7.4 The three types of radial dysplasia (a) total, (b) partial, (c) hypoplasia (reproduced from *The Practice of Hand Surgery*, Lamb & Kuczynski (eds) with the permission of the publishers—Blackwells Medical Publications)

and the more radial division takes over the sensory function of the radial nerve (Lamb 1972).

The radial artery is often small or absent and it is quite common for the radial digital neurovascular bundle to the index finger to be absent. This is obviously of great importance if pollicisation of the index finger is to be performed and knowledge of this may prevent serious ischaemic complications after operation.

Another over-riding thought in the management of radial absence is that this is a deformity which will tend to increase during growth if uncorrected and will tend to recur even after correction (Bora et al 1970, Lamb 1970, Riordan 1955).

The deformity is often correctible passively at or soon after birth but soft tissue contracture will soon develop and lead to an increasing incorrectible deformity. An attempt to prevent or minimise this by splintage at night is advisable and will make the development of postoperative complications less likely. When the radius is absent growth of the ulna is usually completed by the age of 12. The lower ulnar epiphysis, at which most growth takes place, closes prematurely and the forearm is usually anything from one-half to one-third of normal length. Any operation which might lead to even more premature closure of the epiphysis must be approached with great care.

It is important to be sure of the goals to be obtained by any operation before embarking on surgery. Each child must be considered very carefully as an individual problem. There is a wide difference in the clinical presentation. Various principles can be used as guide-lines to try and assess if surgery is justified and to minimise complications.

1. Corrective splinting of the wrist at night.
2. Leave free by day to encourage function.
3. Encourage mobility of a stiff elbow. Never correct the wrist while the elbow is stiff or the hand will not reach the face.
4. Check hand function and joint mobility. Is this good enough to justify correction of the wrist?
5. Never operate to improve appearance alone. Function is all important. If this is always a guiding rule disappointing results and the development of complications will be less common.

Straightening the wrist leads to some loss of wrist movement, which compensates to some extent for the absence of normal pronation/supination. However the increased stability and the improvement in the strength and range of finger movement resulting from the increased mechanical advantage of the long tendons more than compensate for this loss of wrist movement.

OPERATIVE TREATMENT

This can be divided into two stages—correction of wrist deformity and improvement of prehension by pollicisation.

Correction of wrist deformity

Many procedures have been described over the past 100 years. Various types of osteotomy through the ulna may give initial correction but the deformity readily recurs. Replacement of the missing fibula by bone graft (Albee 1928, Starr 1945, Riordan 1955) have been disappointing. The bone graft fails to grow. More recent attempts to transfer the fibula with its epiphysis on a vascular pedicle have been described but the long term effect is not known. The most frequent procedure is centralisation of the carpus over the lower ulna. As already stressed the elbow must be mobile before this operation is done and an appreciation that this is not just absence of bone but severe soft tissue derangement as well. Unless an attempt is made to balance the muscles working at the wrist recurrence of deformity will be frequent. Soft tissue and skin contracture should be prevented by early splintage (Fig. 7.5), corrected by positive splintage (Lamb 1970) or corrected by initial operation if severe.

Various surgical approaches have been described and as long as good exposure of the lower half of forearm and its muscles, the carpus, the lower ulna and bases of metacarpals is obtained the exact approach does not matter. More than one incision can be used. The author has found an incision extending down the volar forearm, curving round the radial side of the wrist onto the dorsum of the hand to be most effective. The median nerve should be immediately displayed as it usually lies displaced to the radial side immediately under deep fascia. It is easily damaged. The division of the nerve into two components should be looked for before any further dissection.

The aim of the operation is to stabilise the lower ulna into central carpus by excising sufficient of the carpus to accommodate the lower ulna with a neat fit. The ulna should be inserted to a depth equal to its transverse diameter (McCon 1974). The flexor and extensor tendons are now lying more centrally. Sometimes the flexor superficialis tendons appear tight and the fingers flex too much at the proximal interphalangeal joints which are already often the site of flexion contractures. The tendons should be lengthened at their musculotendinous junction.

The flexor carpi radialis is transferred to the dorsum of the wrist. The extensor carpi ulnaris is often slack after correction of the wrist deformity and may be shortened. The corrected position is partially maintained by careful closure of periosteum and capsule over lower ulna and carpus and usually reinforced by passing a Kirschner wire up the medullary cavity of the ulna from the 3rd or 4th metacarpal shaft.

The *complications* of this operation may be early and late.

Early complications

1. *Oedema and swelling* is common and often severe. It is unwise to apply a complete circular plaster cast around the forearm and hand. The hand should be elevated for several days. The stiff fingers and poor muscle development prevents the active movement so helpful in dispersing oedema in the normal hand. The tourniquet should always be released before closure of the wound and careful haemostatis achieved. The development of a haematoma will greatly increase the postoperative swelling.

2. *Skin necrosis*. This is unusual although considerable tension on the radial side of the wound occurs after correction of the wrist. The skin has healed well in our cases.

3. *Infection*. This has not been a problem but is a possibility as with any Kirschner wire penetrating skin. We leave the wire cut subcutaneously.

4. Ideally the wire should be passed retrograde down 3rd or 4th metacarpal shaft out through the

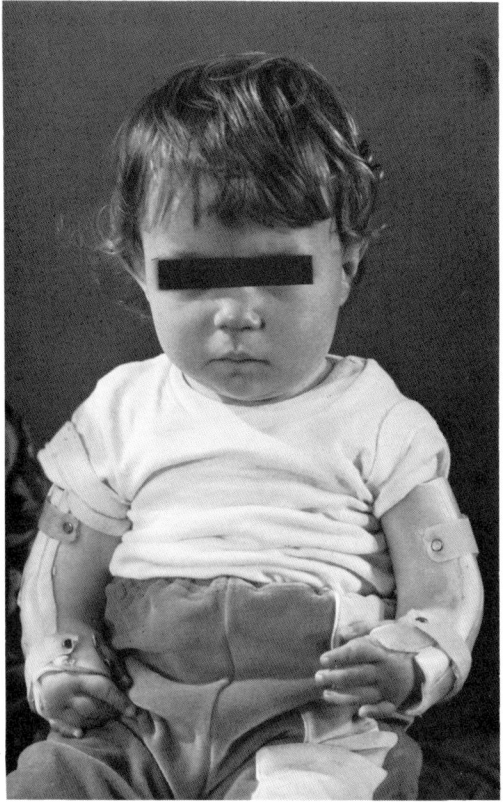

Fig. 7.5 The use of plastic splints in an attempt to prevent progressive radial deviation at the wrist. There is complete absence of the radius on both sides. Note that there is almost normal appearance of the thumb which is nearly always indicative of the absence of radius associated with thrombocytopenia as was the case here

skin and then back across the middle of the corrected carpus and across the centre of the lower ulnar epiphysis. It should pass up the ulna and out at the olecranon. This is seldom possible. If the ulna is curved a corrective osteotomy can be done at one or more sites. A check radiograph of the passage of the K-wire is advisable during operation. Careless passing of the wire might damage other structures. The lower ulna should be dissected extraperiostially. Stripping the periosteum, shaping the lower ulna to facilitate insertion into the carpus or passing the K-wire across the periphery of the epiphysis may all be responsible for later development of premature fusion of the epiphysis.

Late complications

1. *Recurrence of deformity* (Fig. 7.6). Unfortunately this is not uncommon. Care at the original operation is the main prevention of this happening. Inadequate carpal bony remnants on the radial side of the notch, poor closure of the osteo-periostial flap over the ulna and carpus, lack of balancing of the muscles at operation, or lack of postoperative immobilisation may all contribute to recurrence. The K-wire should be left in as long as possible. The longest in my personal series has been 7 years without any sign of affecting ulnar epiphyseal growth. Usually the wire extrudes spontaneously sooner than that. If this extrusion occurs in less than 6 months from operation then external fixation with a closely fitting plaster with the wrist fully corrected and the elbow incorporated at 90° of flexion is required. Continuous external fixation for 6 months postoperatively in plaster and with a readily applied and removable plastic splint for use at night while growth is occurring is recommended.

Deformity may also recur due to breakage of the K-wire. This is usually at the carpal level (Fig. 7.7) and indicates the tremendous deforming forces present. A new K-wire should be inserted. This would also be required if during growth the K-wire no longer controlled the wrist. It must be realised that centralisation is *not* an arthrodesis. It simply stabilises the wrist and will allow some flexion/extension movement.

If during growth the radial or volar or combined deformity is recurring further operation may be indicated. If the carpal area is stable a corrective ulnar osteotomy may be all that is required. If the deformity is recurring at the carpus then repetition of the centralisation with muscle transfers to balance the deforming forces may be needed.

2. *Premature fusion of lower ulnar epiphysis.* This may occur if the lower ulna is stripped subperiosteally, handled roughly, the K-wire inserted carelessly or an osteotomy performed through the ulna too near to the epiphysis. While we have had

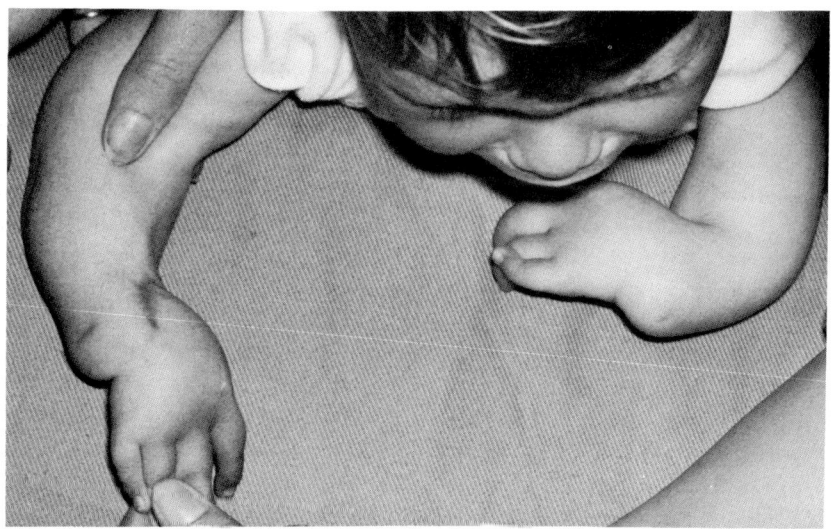

Fig. 7.6 Centralisation has been carried out on the right side for absence of the radius a year previously. An unsatisfactory placement of the lower end of the ulna in the carpus has resulted in some early recurrence of deformity

94 UNSATISFACTORY RESULTS IN HAND SURGERY

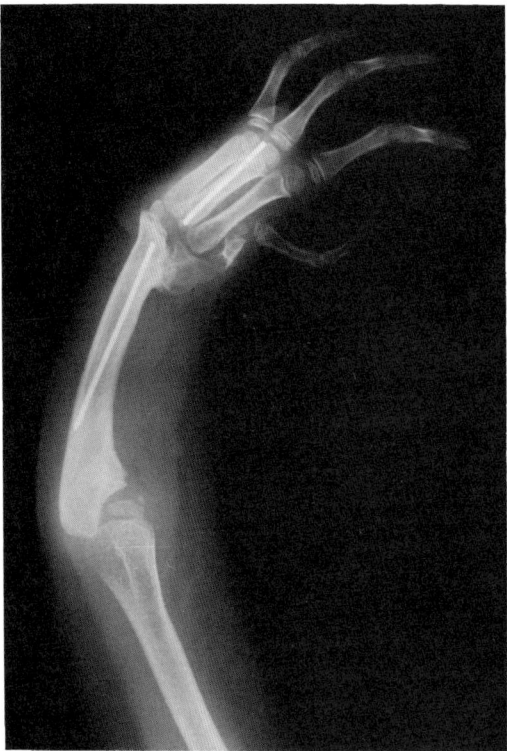

Fig. 7.7 Radiograph showing centralisation of the ulna in the carpus controlled by a Kirschner wire passed up the medullary cavity and across the metacarpal. The pin has broken at the carpal level. Note the hyperextension deformity of the thumb

no personal examples of this complication we have seen some cases in which severe stunting of the ulna has occurred (Fig. 7.8). This is a very serious occurrence as the forearm will be so short.

3. In one girl where satisfactory centralisation had controlled a unilateral deformity for several years during growth she began to develop pain in the wrist while working as a children's nurse. Arthritic changes had developed (Fig. 7.9) and now at the age of 21 arthrodesis has been carried out. No doubt this is a complication which may occur in others.

Ulnar lengthening

Because the forearm is normally short attempts to lengthen the ulna have been described (Dick et al 1977). This is not so straightforward as in a normal forearm or when bone lengthening is carried out in a paralytic limb because the soft tissues are tight and contracted. Few successful examples have been described and there is always the danger of non-union occurring, as following simple osteotomy, although we have not seen this. The advantages gained with 4–5 cm of lengthening and the potential dangers involved suggest this is not a procedure often required. It may have more place in the hypoplastic radius to try and equalise the lengths of the two forearm bones.

Pollicisation

Once the wrist deformity has been corrected the hand approaches objects in a more normal fashion and the ulnar type of prehension is no longer appropriate. Changing the prehension pattern to the radial side of the hand is an important readjustment and best done early—about the age of one year. Consideration must be given to pollicisation and the index is the most appropriate digit although its structure is often very poor. The M–P joint often has an extension contracture but this does not matter as it will become the new carpo-metacarpal joint of thumb but some stabilisation is required to prevent development of an ugly complication mentioned later.

There is often a flexion contracture of the proximal interphalangeal joint but again this does not matter too much as it will be the new metacarpophalangeal joint of the thumb. If the flexion contracture is too great for satisfactory appearance and function then the joint can be arthrodesed. As already mentioned the index profundus may be absent or poor. Without active flexion of the interphalangeal joint of the new thumb its function will be much poorer. In none of our children who have had an index pollicisation in radial absence has the appearance or function of the thumb been nearly as good as where this is done with a normal index (e.g. four-fingered hand, five-fingered hand). Children and parents, however, feel it has been an improvement both in function and appearance. The operative procedure used by the author is an amalgam of the incision described by Barksy (1958) with a dorsal digital extension (Buck-Gramcko 1971), rotation of the digit 150° on its longitudinal axis and on its neurovascular bundle (Littler 1953), reattachment of

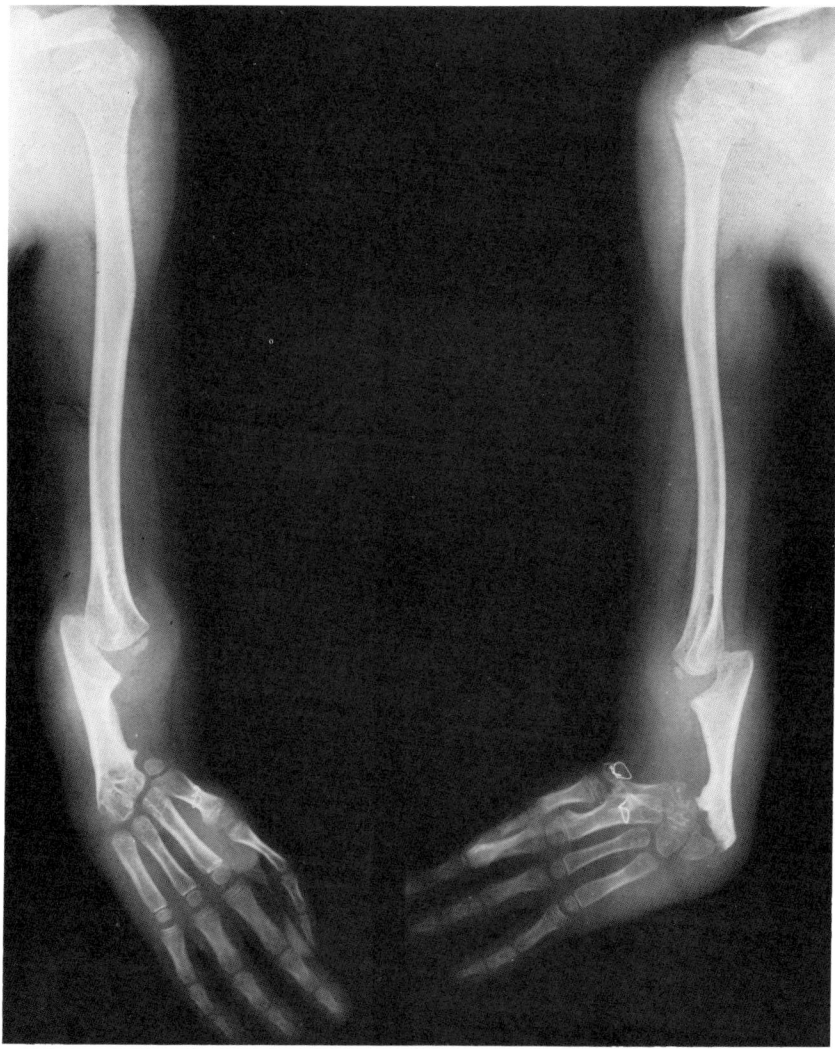

Fig. 7.8 Early osteotomy of the lower ulna near the epiphysis which has resulted in premature fusion of the epiphyses and very short forearms

the 1st dorsal and 1st volar interossei to the extensor tendon at the new M–P joint level (Riordan 1955), and rotation of the metacarpal head as described by Buck-Gramcko (1971) to prevent the ugly hyperextension deformity at the base of the new thumb. Attention to all of these important details will prevent many of the possible complications.

Again the complications may be early and late.

Early

1. *Vascular.* The most serious complication is loss of the 'thumb' due to ischaemia. This may result from damage to the ulnar digital vessels during the operation. As the radial vessels are often absent great care is required in the dissection of the ulnar vessels and in their separation from the branch to the radial side of the middle finger. Even after successful separation the vessels may become 'kinked' as the digit is being rotated on its longitudinal axis. This may occur when the proximal three-quarters of the metacarpal shaft is being removed but this kinking is unlikely unless the artery is trapped by a loop of the nerve which sometimes surrounds the vessel. The presence of pulsation in the vessel and the absence of any

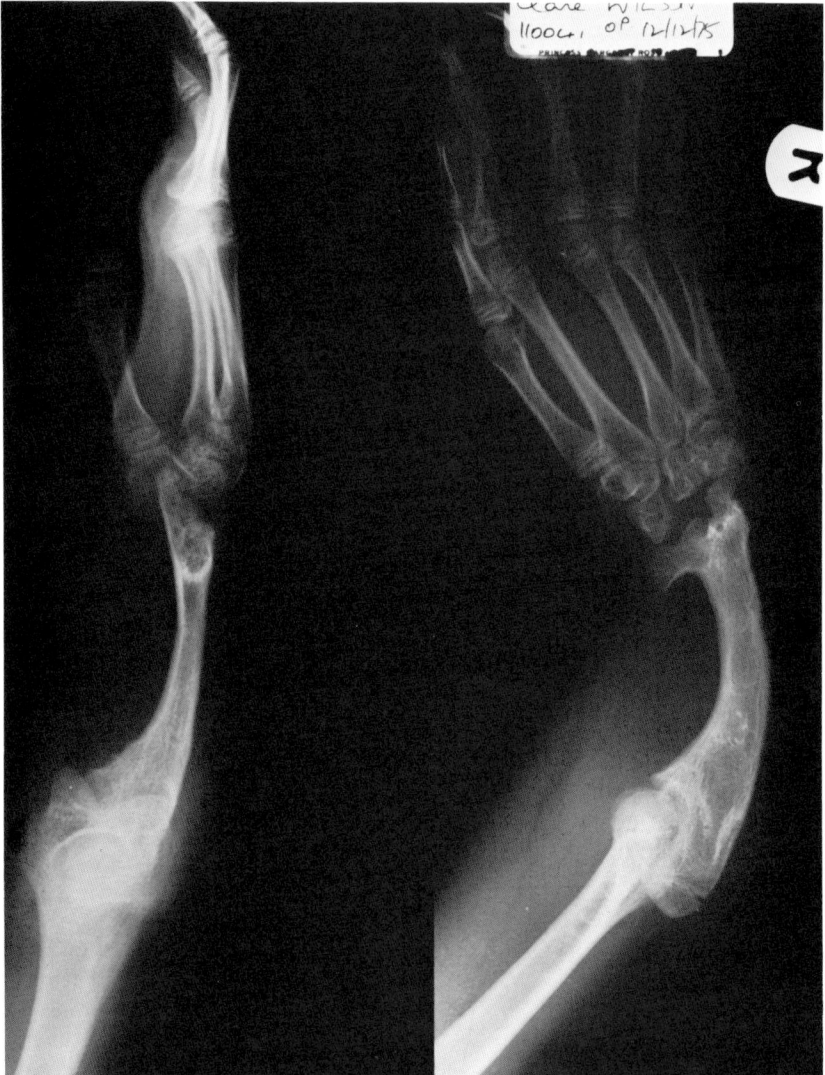

Fig. 7.9 Centralisation at an early age for absence of the radius. Good correction was maintained during adolescence. Note that a thumb is present. This was an example of absent radius in thrombocytopenia. At the age of 20 the patient began to complain of increasing pain in the wrist and she required an arthrodesis

kinking must be checked carefully when the tourniquet is released. Fortunately total ischaemia is a most rare complication but it is a disaster when starting with only four and sometimes only three digits. Much more likely is a failure of adequate venous drainage. The venous drainage is mainly on the dorsum and great care is required to protect the veins on the dorsum of the index finger and on the hand when separating the second and third metacarpals. Some blueness of the transposed digit is not infrequent two or three hours after operation but it usually corrects spontaneously. If not, the dressings are removed and if this does not improve the colour the skin is released by removing some of the stitches. Haematoma is infrequent if careful haemostasis has been achieved at operation but if it is a factor in compressing the circulation then it should be evacuated.

2. *Neurological.* Separation of the components of the nerve in the second metacarpal interspace into

the branches of the adjacent sides of index and middle finger is part of the operative procedure. This is done gently by the back of a 15 blade scalpel or Watson–Cheyne dissector. It is important that the nerve be dissected back to the base of the palm so that the ulnar digital nerve to index is not kinked as the digit is rotated. Temporary numbness may be noted in the pollicised index after operation but unless the nerve has been damaged by clumsy dissection this soon recovers.

3. *Skin healing.* This is seldom any problem. Even if the skin flaps cannot be closed completely at operation this is unimportant in the young child and healing takes place readily in two to three weeks with a minimum of scarring. If the new thumb is not shortened by removal of sufficient metacarpal the skin flaps will be tight, will cause more swelling, may obstruct venous return and the skin edges necrose. If a 'dangle' thumb has previously been removed the skin flap to form the new thumb web may have had its blood supply damaged. In one such case this was obvious on release of the tourniquet and the ischaemic skin was replaced by a skin graft.

Late complications

1. *Length of thumb.* This is a matter of judgement at operation. The thumb normally reaches the prox-imal interphalangeal joint of the index. The pollicised index should reach that of the middle finger. This usually means removal of all of the second metacarpal but the head. Removal of this amount of bone relaxes skin, blood vessels and nerves and reduces the incidence of the early complications.

In the early development of pollicisation for congenital abnormalities there was a tendency to make the thumb too long in case growth subsequent to operation was not as much as in the intact fingers. This has not been the case. An overlong thumb can be unsightly (Fig. 7.10) but this can easily be rectified at a later date by shortening.

Much more difficult to correct is the thumb that has been made too short. This is only likely to happen if one of the phalangeal epiphyses undergoes premature closure. This could result from damage to the epiphysis during operation or possibly as a result of some ischaemia. This complication must be rare and I have only seen one example (Fig. 7.11).

2. *Appearance of the thumb.* The index which has been put in a thumb position without rearrangement of the intrinsics looks like a finger in the wrong position (Fig. 7.12). Where the interossei have been released and reattached (Riordan 1955) the digit looks and works like a thumb (Fig. 7.13). If the thumb has not been rotated on its longitu-

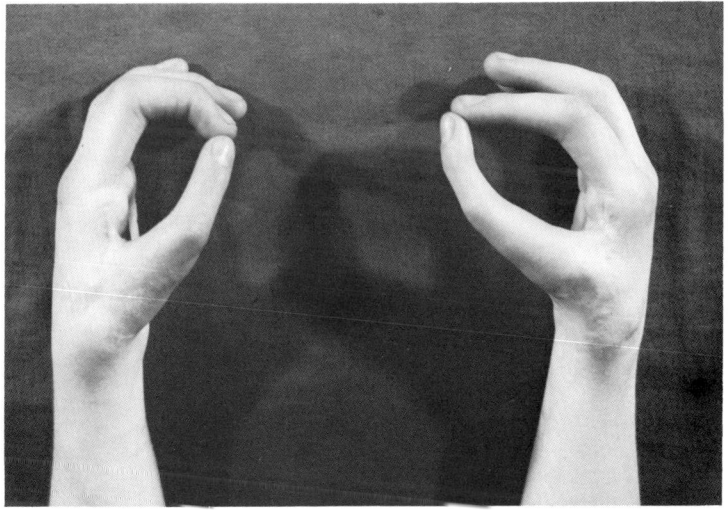

Fig. 7.10 Good functional bilateral pollicisation of the radial digit on both sides but, particularly on the right side, the thumb has been made unduly long which is a little unsightly

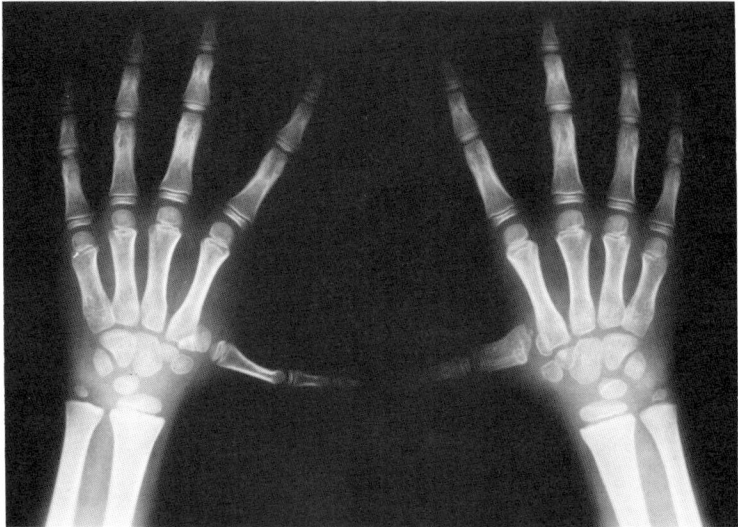

Fig. 7.11 This boy with a bilateral 5-fingered hand has had pollicisation of both radial digits. X-ray shows that premature fusion of the basal epiphysis of the proximal phalanx of the radial digit on the right has occurred leading to shortening of the new 'thumb' and functional impairment

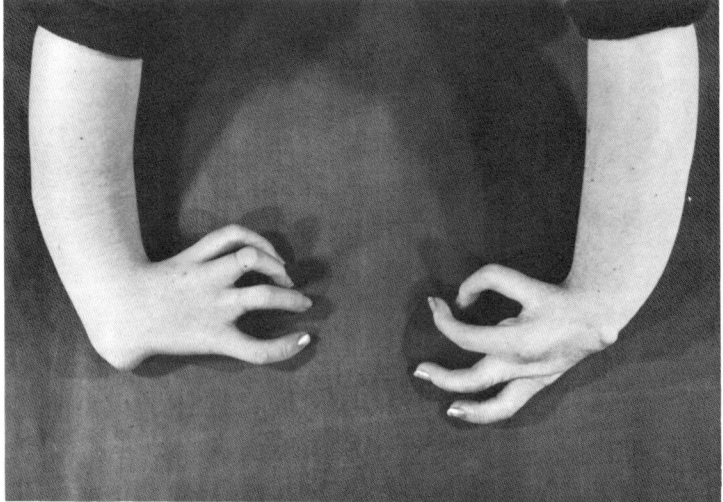

Fig. 7.12 Bilateral absent radius and severe bilateral radial deformity. Elbow flexion was severely restricted. On the left side a posterior release of the elbow and transfer of the triceps to biceps provided over 90° of active flexion at the elbow following which centralisation was carried out. A subsequent transfer of the radial digit into the thumb position was carried out. This operation was performed before the importance of the rearrangement of intrinsic muscles was appreciated and although there is some reasonable function the appearance is that of a finger in a thumb position

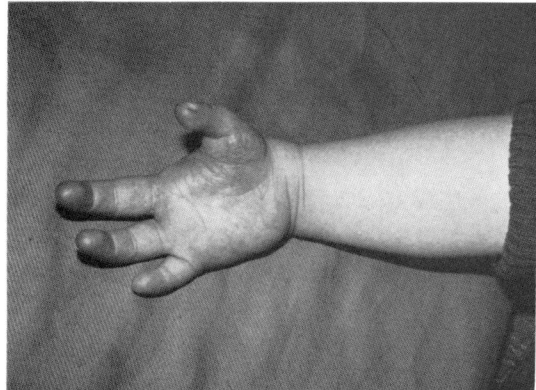

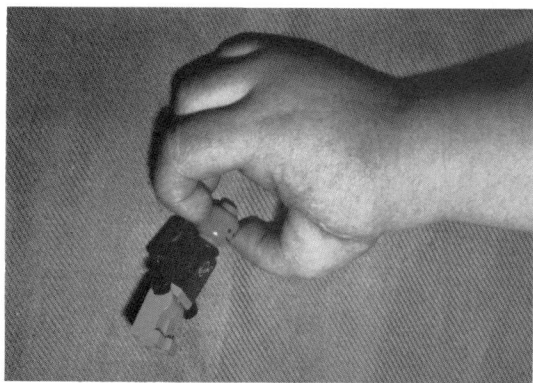

Fig. 7.13 This child with a four-fingered hand has had a good cosmetic and functional pollicisation of the radial digit. Note the appearance of thenar muscles by the rearrangement of the first dorsal interosseous

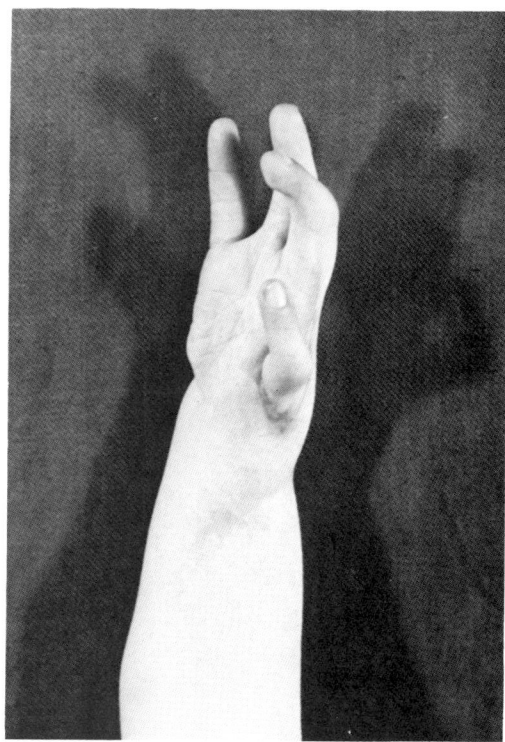

Fig. 7.14 Pollicisation has been carried out here after centralisation of the carpus in absent radius. Good control of the wrist has been obtained. An unsatisfactory degree of rotation of the thumb has resulted in the thumb lying inadequately placed and allowing a web contracture

dinal axis through about 150° there will be insufficient rotation to get pulp to pulp pinch and a thumb web contracture may develop (Fig. 7.14). A hyperextension deformity at the base of the thumb is very ugly and readily develops if rotation of the second metacarpal head to tighten up the volar plate and capsule (Buck-Gramcko 1971) is not carried out (Fig. 7.15). This will increase if there is also a flexion contracture at the new metacarpophalangeal joint (Fig. 7.16) and it will affect function also.

3. *Bony fusion at the base of the thumb*. In early attempts at pollicisation it was advocated that bony stability at the base of the thumb was the aim. This is easily obtained by removing the central portion of the second metacarpal and fixing the head to the base by K-wires. However much better function is obtained if there is mobility at the base of the thumb. By the rearrangement of the interossei as already advocated some useful control and movement of the thumb is obtained. If bony fusion occurs then this function is lost and this should be considered to be a complication and justifies reoperation.

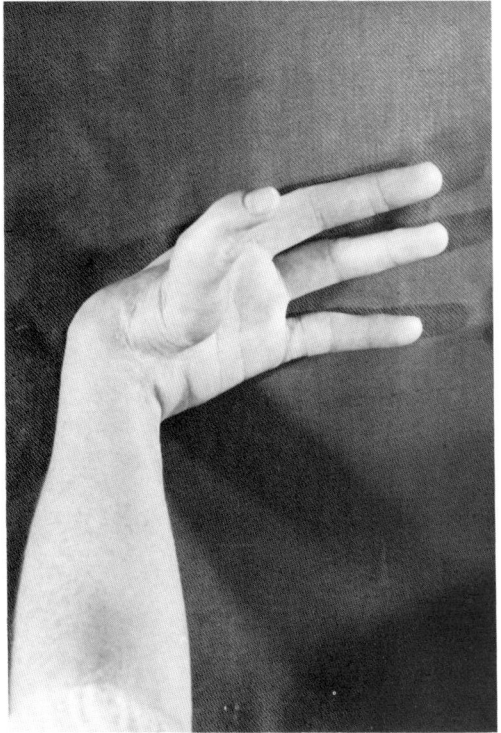

Fig. 7.15 Absent radius and pollicisation of the radial digit. A hyperextension deformity at the base of the thumb has been allowed to develop due to lack of rotation of the metacarpal head described by Buck-Gramcko. This is a very ugly deformity which also affects function

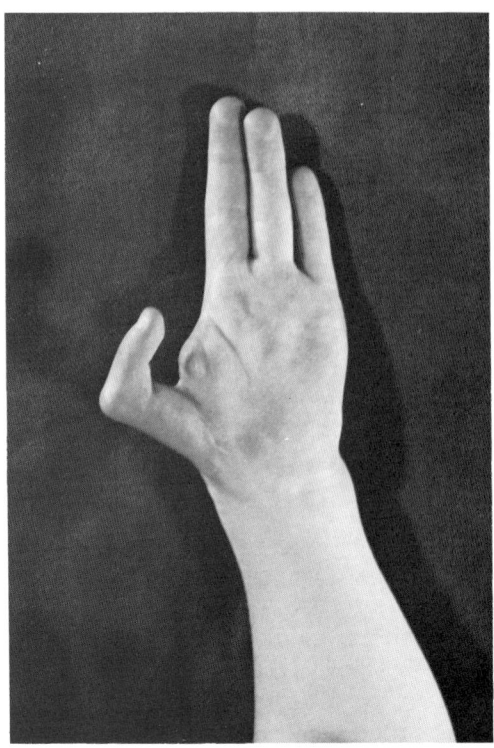

Fig. 7.16 Pollicisation of the radial digit. The digit had a flexion contracture of the proximal interphalangeal joint which has become more marked following transposition

REFERENCES

Albee F H 1928 Formation of radius congenitally absent condition seven years after implantation of bone graft. Annals of Surgery 87 : 105–110

Barsky A J 1958 Congenital anomalies of the hand and their surgical treatment. Charles C Thomas, Springfield, Illinois

Bora F W Jr, Nicholson J T, Cheema H M 1970 Radial meromelia. The deformity and its treatment. Journal of Bone and Joint Surgery 52-A : 966–979

Buck-Gramcko D 1971 Pollicisation of the index finger. Method and results in aplasia and hypoplasia of the thumb. Journal of Bone and Joint Surgery 53-A : 1605–1617

Dick H M, Petzolot R L, Bowers L R, Rennie W R 1977 Lengthening of the ulna in radial agenesis—a preliminary report. Journal of Hand Surgery 2 : 175

Heikel H V A 1959 Aplasia and hypoplasia of the radius. Studies on 64 cases and on epiphyseal transplantation in rabbits with the imitated defect. Acta Orthopaedica, Scandinavica, Suppl. 39.

Lamb D W 1970 Club hand : absent radius. In Charles R, Smith R eds. Operative Surgery, 2nd edn, Vol. II, The Hand (Pulvertaft R G ed). Butterworth, London. p 12–16

Lamb D W 1972 The treatment of radial club hand. Absent radius aplasia of the radius, hypoplasia of the radius, radial paraxial hemimelia. Hand 4 : 22–30

Littler J W 1953 The neurovascular pedicle method of digital transposition for reconstruction of the thumb. Plastic and Reconstructive Surgery 12 : 303–319

MacCon M B 1974 Radial club hand. A review of 106 cases. Thesis for Ch.M. (Orth.), Liverpool, England

Riordan D C 1955 Congenital absence of radius. Journal of Bone and Joint Surgery 37-A : 1129–1140

Starr D E 1945 Congenital absence of the radius. A method of surgical correction. Journal of Bone and Joint Surgery 27 : 572–577

L. G. Bayne

8

Thumb duplication

Unsatisfactory results following treatment of thumb duplications frequently are due to poor preoperative analysis and planning. The surgeon who simply ablates the accessory digit will frequently end up with a poor functional and cosmetic result. Reconstructive surgery of the duplicated thumb requires a basic knowledge of the abnormal anatomy present. If correction is inadequate then a deformity can become accentuated by abnormal dynamic structural forces. The ultimate goal of treatment is restoration of the anatomical relationships of the remaining structures and to align the growth plates perpendicular to the long axis of the digit. This will ensure, as growth continues, that the correction will be maintained.

CLASSIFICATION

There is a wide spectrum of degrees of duplication of the thumb. Thus a classification is necessary to image which type of duplication a specific discussion concerns. Numerous classifications have been devised by various authors. The classification favoured by most is the one proposed by Wassel (1969). This classification is based on the degree of skeletal union involved in the duplication and includes seven separate classes. The classification proposed by Marks & Bayne (1978) (Fig. 8.1) is much more simple and is based on the level of duplication, that is, 1. the distal phalangeal level, 2. the proximal phalangeal level, and 3. the metacarpal level. The triphalangeal thumb and the thumb with the delta phalanx are not included. They represent a different problem altogether and, therefore, should be considered separately. There is a wide variation in the degree of duplication at each level. Therefore, it is most appropriate to consider the level of the duplication and the degree of duplication at each level when considering a surgical correction. There are certain basic abnormalities to anticipate at each level, and ingenuity at the time of operation must be applied to deal with the various degrees of duplication.

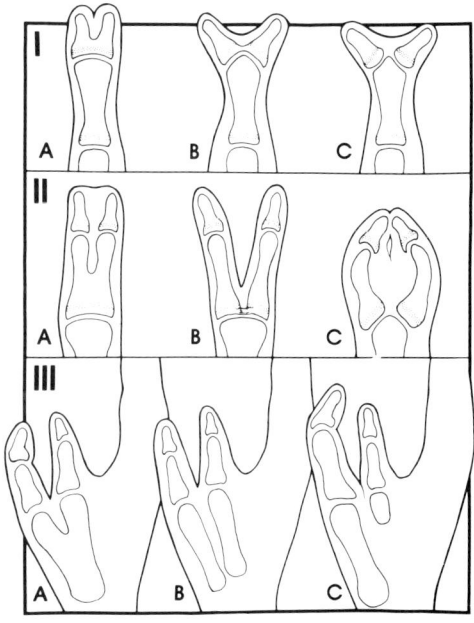

Fig. 8.1 Classification (Marks & Bayne 1978). Duplication is classified according to level of occurrence. Type I— Duplication at the distal phalangeal level (A) Incomplete, separation. (B) Complete duplication, bases joined by cartilage plate or fibrous septum. (C) Complete duplication. Type II— Duplication at the proximal phalangeal level. (A) Incomplete separation. (B) Complete duplication, joined at base. (C) Complete duplication. Type III—Duplication at the metacarpal level. (A) Incomplete. (B) Complete. (C) Mixed.

SURGICAL CONSIDERATIONS

Surgical procedures to correct congenital defects are now being performed earlier in the child's life than previously thought necessary. This is especially true in the preaxial type, as the thumb plays such an essential role in the function of the hand. Delay is necessary in some cases where there is a need to determine which thumb is most functional. Other factors such as size, progression of deformity and nail development need to be considered when deciding which thumb is to be salvaged. It may, in some instances, be necessary to transfer distal portions of one thumb to the proximal portions of the second thumb to make the most pleasing and functional digit. Thus correction may be delayed to 1–2 years of age. It is also essential for the surgeon to point out to the parent what they can expect from the surgery. The duplicated thumb is an abnormal thumb and will not appear the same as the opposite thumb. It will usually be smaller, thinner, and may not be as functional due to the restricted motion or due to a lax joint (Fig. 8.2). Show the parent the difference in the two thumbs. It will also be helpful to point out to the parent that a second procedure may be necessary to correct any residual angulation that may develop with later growth, or to correct hypermobility of the joints.

SURGICAL TECHNIQUES

Type I deformities

There is no one technique that will suffice for all deformities. Basically all corrective procedures can be placed into two categories. The first type of correction is typified by the Bilhaut–Cloquet (1890) procedure which involves excision of a central wedge of tissue from the adjacent parts of both duplicated structures, and then joining of the remaining lateral portions (Fig. 8.3). This procedure has the advantage of reconstructing a more normal sized thumb but is more difficult than it appears. The physis have to be accurately approximated or unequal growth will occur. The nail matrix and bed has to be approximated accurately to obtain a satisfactory appearing nail. A divisional line, however, will always be present. If the bases

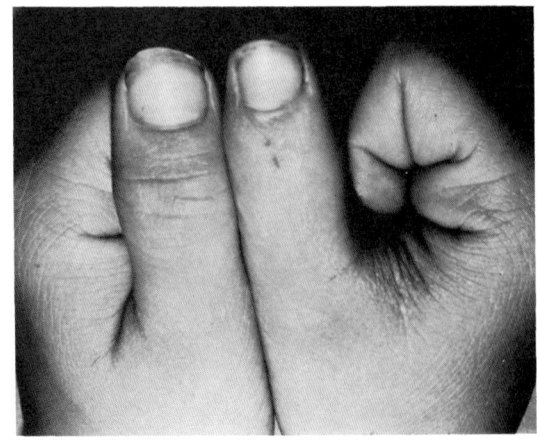

Fig. 8.2 Comparison of reconstructed duplicate thumb with patient's normal opposite thumb

of the two phalanges are not united centrally but are divergent, then getting them together will be difficult without releasing the collateral ligaments, and thus jeopardising the joint stability and function (Fig. 8.4). This procedure, in my opinion, is only useful in Type 1A patients who have a partial duplication of the distal phalanx.

The second type of corrective procedure involves ablating one of the parts but salvaging various structures to augment the remaining part. It has the disadvantage of not being able to make the digit as large as the opposite thumb. However, the distal segment can be made larger by augmenting it with tissue from the ablated part.

Variations in surgical treatment depend on the level of duplication and the degree of involvement. In Type 1B and 1C deformities, where there is

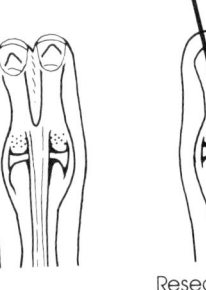 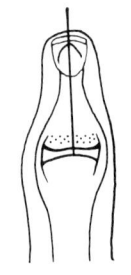

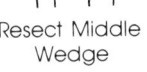

Resect Middle Wedge   Pull Two Halves Together

Fig. 8.3 Schematic drawing of the Bilhaut–Cloquet procedure. Type 1A reconstruction

THUMB DUPLICATION 103

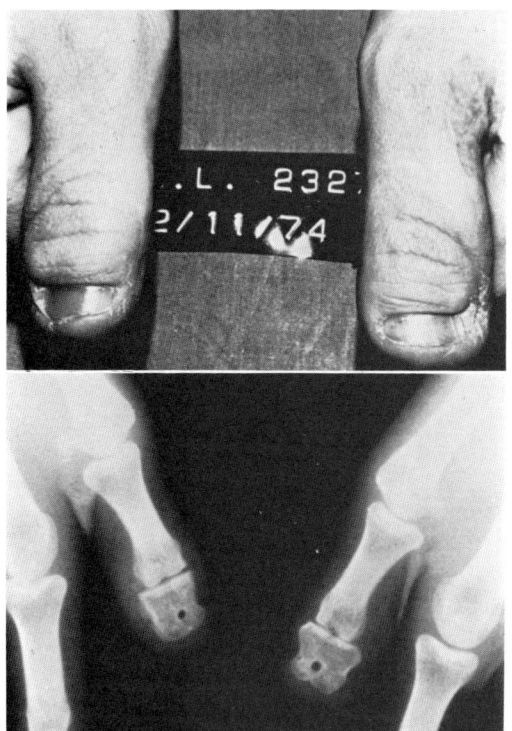

Fig. 8.4 Type IA duplication reconstructed by the Bilhaut–Cloquet method. Note the irregularity of the soft tissue and the nail, and the excessive width of the distal phalanx

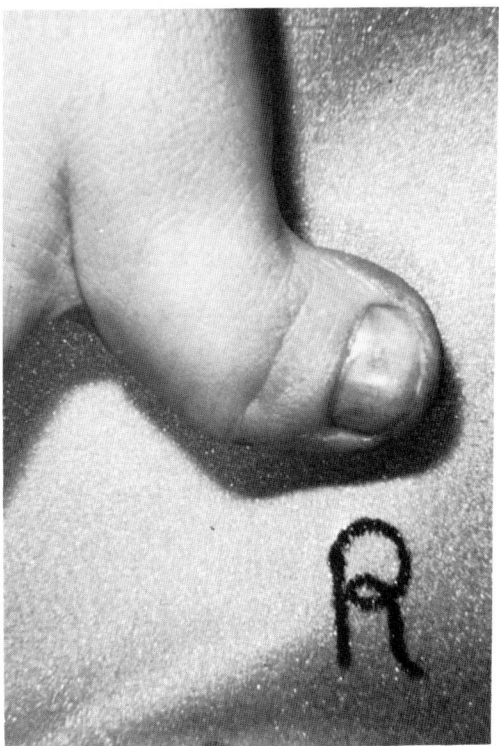

Fig. 8.5 Thumb with residual angulation due to skin deficit

complete duplication of the distal phalanx, it is best to pick the most functional and pleasing part and ablate the other. In most instances the ulnar part is the part that is salvaged.

Unsatisfactory results are usually due to failure to recognise abnormal anatomical structures and to properly reconstruct the remaining part.

Skin contractures should not occur (Fig. 8.5). There is usually sufficient skin from the ablated part to cover any defect. Incisions should be made along the lateral aspect of the thumb. Z-plasties may be necessary to break up any type of contracting incisional lines, or if necessary a rotational flap can be fashioned from the excess skin.

In asymmetrical duplications of the distal phalanx there are two separate distal phalanges which diverge from a common proximal phalanx (Fig. 8.6). The abnormal anatomical structures are:

1. The flexor and extensor tendons will be bifurcated.

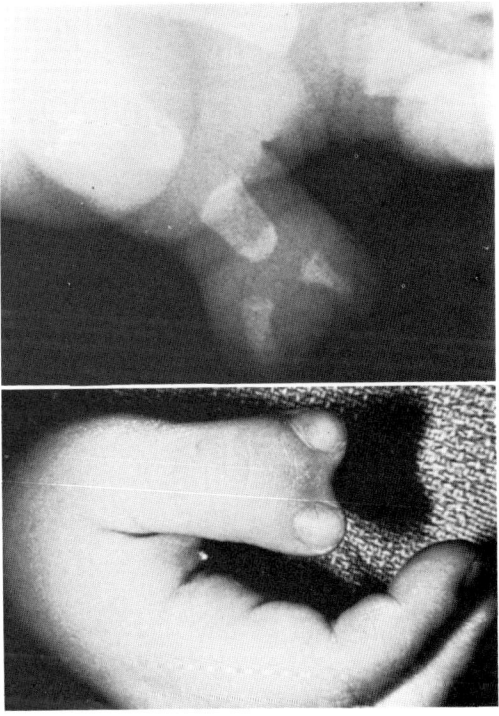

Fig. 8.6 Type IC duplication

2. The head of the proximal phalanx is enlarged to accommodate the two phalanges, often having two separate facets which are congruent with the articular surface of the respective phalanx.

3. Each distal phalanx has but one collateral ligament.

Reconstruction of this type of duplication (Fig. 8.7), will require reconstruction of the distal joint, centralisation of the tendons, and correction of the alignment so the joints and the physis are perpendicular to the longitudinal axis of the thumb.

Joint reconstruction begins with excising one of the distal phalanges, saving the slip of the extensor tendon and as much of the lateral capsule and collateral ligament as possible. The bifurcated slip of the flexor tendon is cut off smooth so as not to become entrapped by the flexor pulleys and prevent flexion of the distal joint. To reconstruct the radial or vacant side of the distal joint the capsule and collateral ligament salvaged from the amputated part is used. If the distal phalanx is displaced laterally then it will tighten the remaining collateral ligament and displace the distal phalanx from its congruent articular groove. Both of these factors will impede motion of the distal joint. A wedge resection of the head of the proximal phalanx will sufficiently narrow the head so that the capsular and collateral ligament reconstruction can be accomplished without disrupting the normal articular arc of the remaining phalanx (Fig. 8.7).

Correction of the angulation of the distal joint is usually necessary so as to align the joint surface and the physis perpendicular to the long axis of the thumb. This is accomplished by a closing wedge osteotomy. The osteotomy and joint reconstruction can then be protected by an intermedullary K-wire placed from the tip of the phalanx to the base of the proximal phalanx.

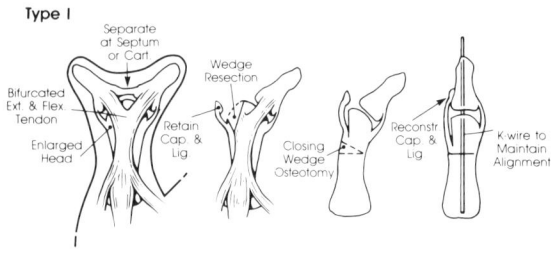

Fig. 8.7 Type IC reconstruction

Realignment of the extensor tendons is necessary to ensure adequate motion and prevent angulation. The bifurcated slip can be used as a transverse retinacular ligament to maintain the extensor tendon centralised over the distal joint.

Occasionally in Type I deformities it will be necessary to augment the lateral nail fold with a portion of skin saved from the lateral surface of the ablated part, thus creating a lateral skin flap. This will give a more pleasing appearance (Fig. 8.8).

The factors producing unsatisfactory results in distal duplications are:

1. Failure to adequately reconstruct the collateral ligament.
2. Failure to trim the bifurcated flexor tendon to prevent triggering.
3. Failure to realign the extensor tendons.
4. Failure to correct angulation.

Type II deformities

Duplications that occur at the proximal phalangeal level will usually present additional abnormal anatomy (Fig. 8.9).

1. There can be double angulation. The distal joint is angulated in one direction and the proximal joint in the opposite direction.
2. The intrinsic muscles are attached to the radial most part which is usually the most deformed and less functional.
3. The extensor tendons are duplicated with a common hood. The flexor tendons are duplicated and both the extensor and flexor tendons will be subluxed across the distal joint.

Reconstruction of Type II deformities is much more complicated. It involves the correction of a double angulation and the salvaging and reconstruction of the intrinsic muscles of the thumb (Fig. 8.10).

The metacarpophalangeal joint is reconstructed in a similar manner as the distal joint in Type I deformities, i.e. wedge resection of the metacarpal head—collateral ligament and capsular repair—corrective osteotomy.

The proximal phalanx is osteotomised to correct the distal joint alignment when necessary.

The extensor and flexor mechanisms, because of

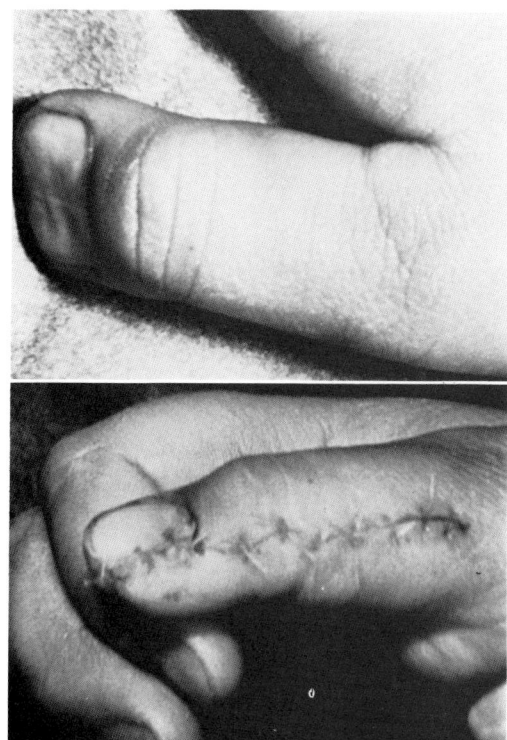

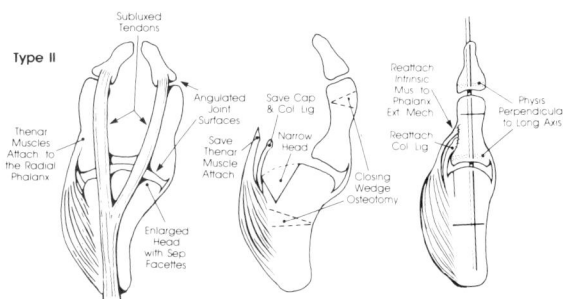

Fig. 8.10 Type IIC reconstruction requires transferring the thenar muscle attached to the radial part and correction of double angulation

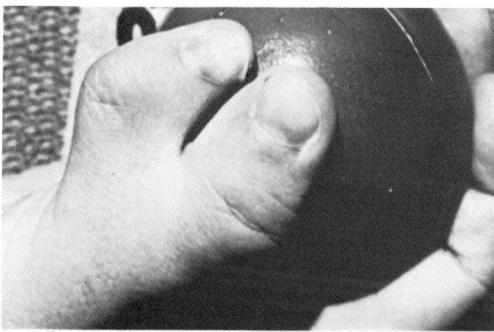

Fig. 8.8 Type IA duplication showing reconstruction of lateral nail fold

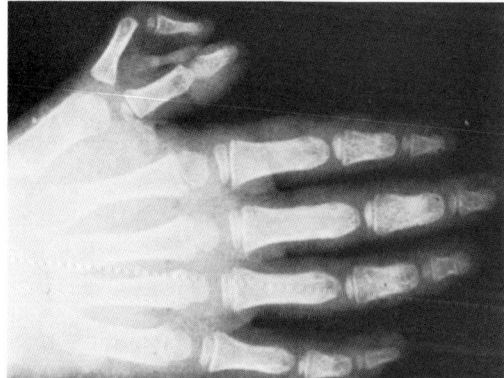

Fig. 8.9 Type IIC duplication

their more proximal bifurcation and broad septal connections, are subluxed across the distal joint. The extensor tendon is centralised by utilising a portion of the septum as a transverse retinacular ligament. The flexor tendons may require reconstruction of the A-3 pulley after careful excision of the bifurcated portion.

The thenar muscles are usually attached to the radial duplicated part. This is the part most often removed. Thus thenar muscles will have to be transferred to the proximal phalanx and extensor hood to prevent instability of the MP joint and loss of the extensor and abduction function of the thumb (Fig. 8.11).

Unsatisfactory results thus result from:

1. Failure to correct the double angulation.
2. Failure to realign the extensor and flexor tendons.
3. Failure to stabilise the MP joint either by reconstruction of the joint or failure to reattach the thenar muscles.
4. Failure to reattach the thenar muscles with resultant loss of abduction function of the thumb.

Type III deformities

Duplications that occur at the metacarpal level vary greatly in degree of deficiency and duplication (Fig. 8.12). Reconstruction will require much more ingenuity by the surgeon. Because Type III deformities vary so greatly, certain examples will be discussed.

When the thumbs are completely reduplicated they are usually similar in size and shape, and

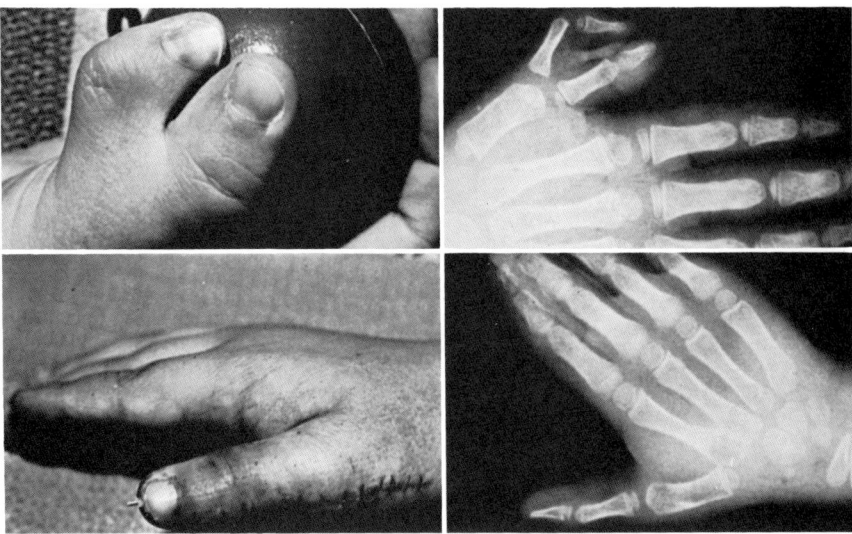

Fig. 8.11 Type IIC—Before and after reconstruction

frequently syndactylised (Fig. 8.12b). Reconstruction will require:

1. Carpometacarpal joint reconstruction.
2. Transfer of the intrinsic muscles to the remaining part.
3. Frequently reattachment of the abductor pollicis longus tendon.
4. Reconstruction of the thumb index web space, either by widening the web space and deepening the web space with double Z-plasty, or by utilising a sliding skin flap with a skin graft as described by Brand (1963) (Fig. 8.13).

When the duplication is incomplete, that is, the metacarpal sharing a common base, the reconstructive procedures are carried out similarly as to a complete duplication with the exception of not having to reconstruct the carpometacarpal joint (Fig. 8.14).

In a mixed quality of duplication the best appearing thumb metacarpal is deficient proximally and is unstable (Fig. 8.15). The radially more complete thumb is thin, angulated, and the distal joints are stiff. The ulnar part has flexion and extension but no stability. The radial part has intrinsic function and a mobile carpometacarpal joint. In order to obtain the best appearing thumb with good function, parts of each thumb will have to be used. Reconstruction requires removal of the radial thumb at the mid-metacarpal level, and transposing the ulnar placed thumb to the radial metacarpal. The extensor pollicis brevis, abductor pollicis brevis and the adductor pollicis are transferred to the transposed part. The flexor and extensor tendons are transferred intact with the ulnar component. This gives a thumb utilising the distal portion of the ulnar thumb and the proximal portion of the radial thumb (Fig. 8.16).

DISCUSSION

Muira (1977, 1983) reported 49 patients with duplications of the thumb, all of which showed some impairment following ablation. Twenty-two

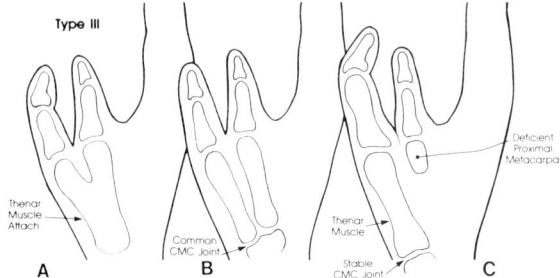

Fig. 8.12 Type III—Duplications vary greatly. (A) Incomplete separation. (B) Complete duplication. (C) Mixed

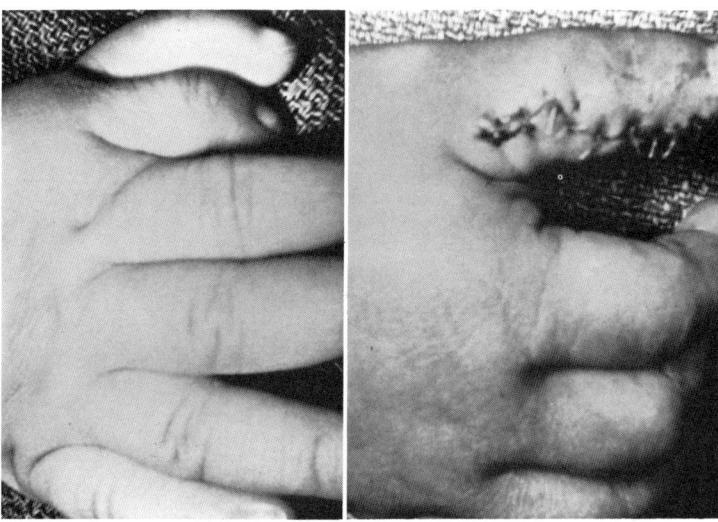

Fig. 8.13 Type IIIB—Before and after reconstruction

of the patients had insufficient abduction or had an ulnar deviation deformity of the metacarpophalangeal joint. Twenty of these patients were improved with reinsertion of the abductor pollicis brevis or thenar muscles. Fourteen patients had zigzag deformities with ulnar deviation of the metacarpophalangeal joint and radial deviation of the interphalangeal joints, primarily due to failure of correction of the angulation at the initial operation. Some of the patients had poor aesthetic

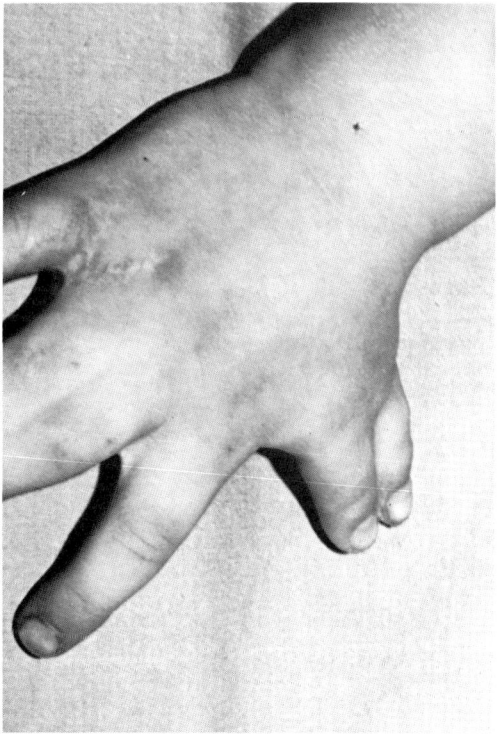

Fig. 8.14 Type IIIA duplication

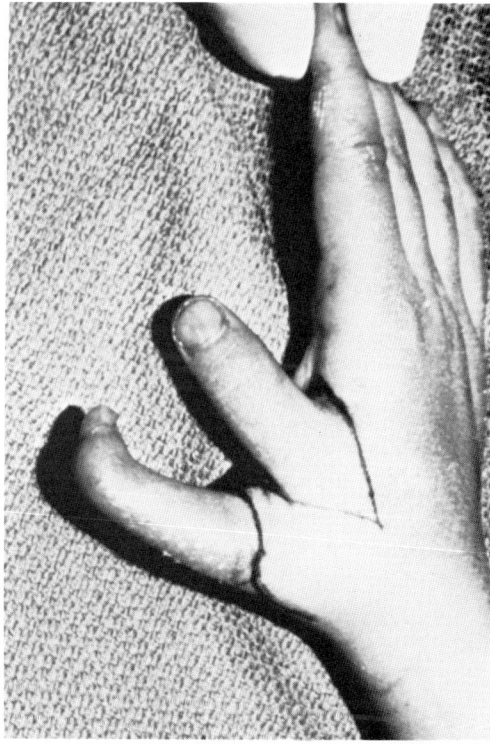

Fig. 8.15 Type IIIB duplication

108 UNSATISFACTORY RESULTS IN HAND SURGERY

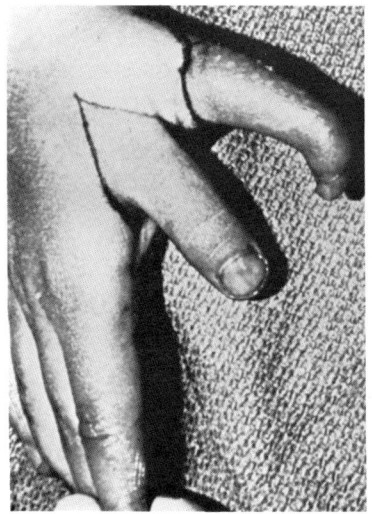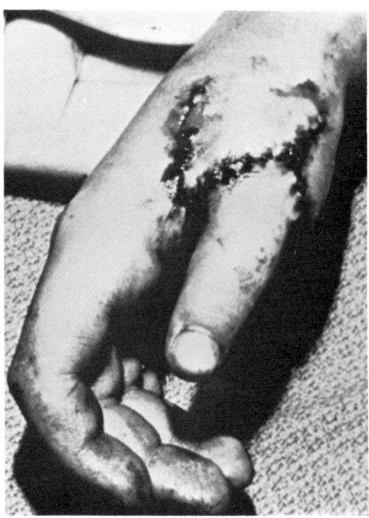

Fig. 8.16 Type IIIC—before and after correction

results following the Bilhaut–Cloquet procedure. This is similar to my experience.

Unsatisfactory results can be reduced with proper preoperative analysis of the abnormal anatomy and planned reconstruction. The key to reconstruction is to:

1. Reconstruct a joint that is stable and mobile.
2. Centralise the flexor and extensor tendons.
3. Transfer intrinsic muscles.
4. Align the joint surfaces and physis perpendicular to the long axis of the thumb.

REFERENCES

Brand P W 1963 The hand, by Milford L. In: Crenshaw A H (ed) Campbell's Operative Orthopaedics, 4th edn. C V Mosby, St Louis, p 229

Bilhaut M 1890 Gerison d'um pouce bifide per un nouveau procede operatoire. Congres Francaise de Chirurgie, 4:576, 1890

Marks T W, Bayne L G 1978 Polydactyly of the thumb: Abnormal anatomy and treatment. Journal of Hand Surgery 3:107

Miura T 1977 An appropriate treatment for postoperative Z-formed deformity of the duplicated thumb. Journal of Hand Surgery 2:380

Miura T 1983 Polydactyly in Japan. Hand 15(1):22

Wassel H D 1969 The results of surgery for polydactyly of the thumb. Clinical Orthopaedics 64:175–93

J. W. Littler, V. R. Hentz and V. D. Pellegrini

9

Thumb reconstruction

Following significant injury to the thumb, either through trauma or developmental mishap, restitution of normal function and appearance is seldom accomplished. Given this limitation of surgical reconstruction, the definition of 'unsatisfactory' varies widely. For the surgeon, the origin of an unsatisfactory result is either an error of omission (poor preoperative planning or failure to anticipate potential problems) or commission (faulty technique or misguided postoperative management). Alternatively, 'success' is primarily dependent upon achieving the potential improvement for the patient and the patient's family. It is therefore imperative that all parties involved have realistic expectations of the outcome from surgical or non-surgical treatment alternatives. An appropriate plan is formulated only after consideration of the patient's occupation and functional demands, psyche, motivation and committment to post-operative therapy. Each individual case must be evaluated on its own merits and shortcomings because in the final analysis, as Gaul (1969) has suggested, 'the owner of the hand is the only one who really knows how to evaluate the results'.

Function is of the utmost importance, however aesthetic considerations may occasionally be of equal concern. Requisites for satisfactory thumb reconstruction can be categorised into three primary areas. Pollex is derived from the Latin term polleo and implies strength. The importance of length, strength, stability and free lateral movement of the thumb has been eloquently stated by Sir Charles Bell (1832) in the frequently quoted Fourth Bridgewater Treatise. These considerations may well be viewed as comprising the *structure* of the thumb. Secondly, skin *sensibility* is of utmost importance in protecting the digit and allowing manipulation and assessment of objects independent of visual guidance. Finally, the *posture* of the thumb concerns its attitude and mobility with respect to the remaining four fingers. These three areas of consideration assume variable importance depending upon the level and magnitude of the thumb deficit. Accordingly, efforts at surgical reconstruction must focus on the particular areas of deficiency peculiar to the individual case.

In discussing the origin, avoidance, and treatment of complications in surgical reconstruction of the thumb, we will consider both conventional and microsurgical approaches to problems of post traumatic loss and congenital deficiency.

COMPLICATIONS IN CONVENTIONAL RECONSTRUCTION FOR TRAUMATIC LOSS

Just as the priorities in post-traumatic thumb reconstruction vary with the level of amputation, the potential causes of an unsatisfactory result differ according to the particular level of deficit. We will discuss the most commonly accepted advantages and shortcomings of specific reconstructive procedures as they relate to the five levels of injury to the thumb illustrated in Fig. 9.1.

Level I

This zone includes the distal two-thirds of the terminal phalanx, the nail structures, and the volar tactile surface to the interphalangeal joint flexion crease. Functional priorities for injury at this level

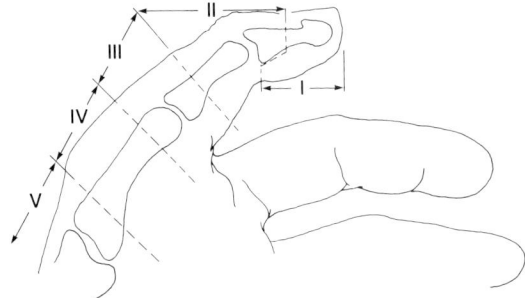

Fig. 9.1 Levels of traumatic loss of the thumb. I: Distal half of terminal phalanx, nail plate and matrix, and volar soft tissue of entire terminal segment. II: Through proximal phalanx leaving intact MCP joint. III: Proximal to or through MCPJ with nearly entire metacarpal and intrinsic musculature with preservation of trapeziometacarpal joint. V. Loss through or proximal to trapeziometacarpal joint

focus on stable and sensate skin coverage and preservation of the nail, both for cosmetic reasons and its functional contribution to dorsal skin fixation. Because terminal hypesthesia presents less of a problem than an irritable tender neuroma or unstable skin coverage, the time honoured commandment that the thumb should never be shortened solely to facilitate skin closure would seem to be overemphasised (Bruner 1954). Sacrifice of several millimeters of bone to gain a well-padded sensate tip is a profitable exchange. However, the functional importance of the nail structure should not be underestimated and preservation of bony length to support the nail plate is justified. Shortening of the skeleton mandates comparable shortening of the nail mechanism to avoid an unsupported nail matrix sloping in a volar direction and resulting in a clawed nail. Similarly, meticulous repair of the nailbed and a smooth dorsal bony surface are necessary to avoid a split or thickened nail. The decision to sacrifice length at the expense of the fingernail is most difficult with bone injury at the middle of the distal phalanx where further shortening often leaves the little remaining nail structure unsupported (by bone). Should shortening be elected, deliberate ablation of the germinal matrix will avoid later problems with an unsatisfactory nail remnant.

A detailed discussion of the numerous methods for management of the thumb tip injury is not within the scope of this text. However, application of general principles will help avoid the specific complications and minimise the shortcomings peculiar to each technique. Digital nerves should be shortened proximal to the level of existing skin to avoid formation of an irritable neuroma in an area vulnerable to unbuffered repetitive trauma. Split and full thickness skin graft coverage provide the least additional bulk to the tip and if unstable require later revision. Healing by secondary intention often provides a well contoured tip with adequate bulk, however, some bony shortening is frequently necessary. Lateral or volar V–Y advancement flaps provide sensate skin with satisfactory bulk but are limited to mobilisation of only several millimeters. The more extensive volar advancement flaps require mobilisation to the proximal flexion crease of the thumb and afford an additional 1–2 cm of coverage (Fig. 9.2). Vascular problems are rare provided meticulous dissection is employed (Fig. 9.3). While flexion contracture at the terminal joint is infrequent, loss of normal hyperextension occurs in more than one-third of cases when compared to the contralateral thumb (Posner & Smith 1971, Kelleher 1972). Sensory innervated cross finger flaps are complex procedures requiring surgical assault on an otherwise normal digit (Brailliar & Horner 1969, Gaul 1969, Miura 1973). The distal extent of radial nerve innervation should be tested preoperatively with local anesthetic blockade to avoid performing a complex procedure for transfer of ultimately anesthetic skin. Mobilisation of radial sensory branches risks irritation of those temperamental nerves and may invite a reflex sympathetic dystrophy. The period of immobilisation may jeopardise the integrity of the thumb web in an already injured digit and, as with other flap procedures, contracture following immobilisation is more pronounced in patients of increasing age over 40. A considerably more involved approach is that of the neurovascular island pedicle flap as described by Littler (1952). With nearly normal length and excellent mobility as is present in Level I injuries, traction on the neurovascular pedicle during the extremes of extension–abduction of the thumb can result in a sensitive hyperaesthetic skin island of little functional value (Tubiana & Duparc 1961, Murray et al 1967, McGregor 1969). The greater utility of this sensory island flap rests in reconstruction of the more severely injured thumb as discussed below.

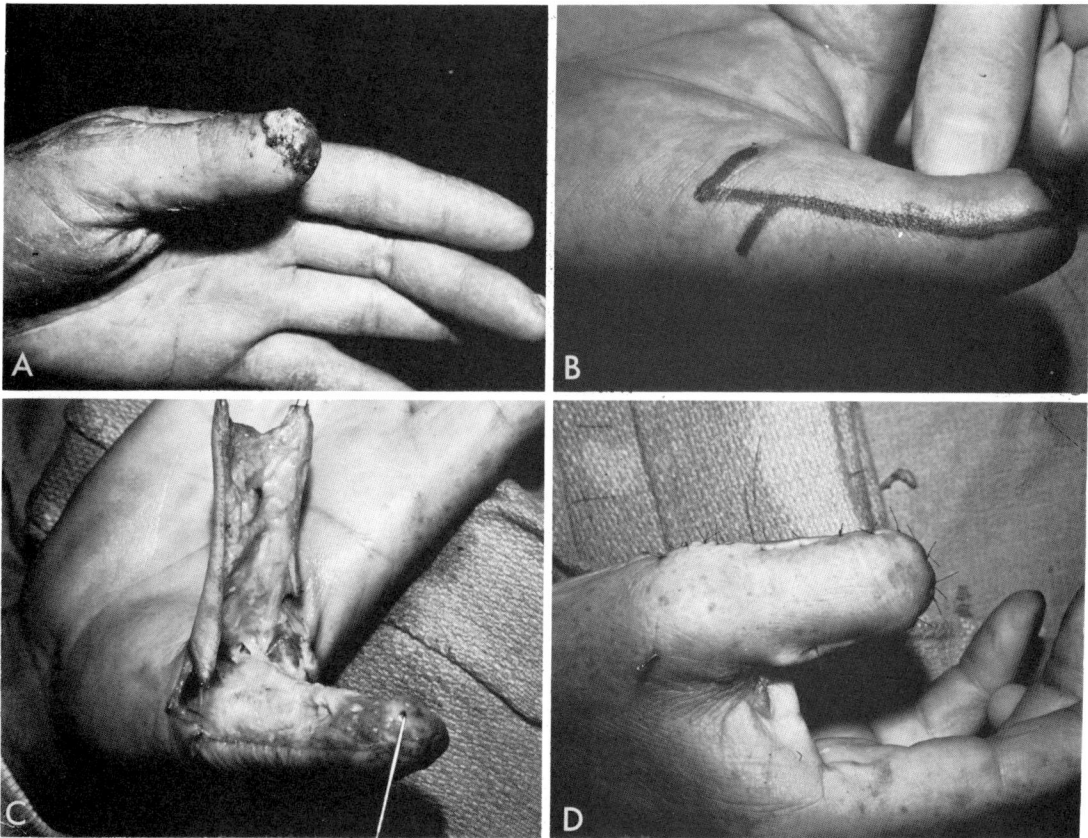

Fig. 9.2 (a)–(d) The volar soft tissue can be advanced distally 1–1.5 cms. A small Z-plasty on either side at the proximal end of the incision provides for additional advancement

All of the many procedures advocated for late reconstruction of the injured nail and supporting matrix are technically complex. Results are often unsatisfactory and residual deformity frequent. Acute repair of the nail matrix continues to be the most efficacious approach to the nailbed injury, while complete ablation of the germinal matrix and remaining nail remains the most reliable procedure for both the irreparably damaged nail structure in the acute setting and the problematic late deformity.

Level II

This includes loss of the terminal joint with shortening of the proximal phalanx to the junction of the proximal and middle thirds. *Sensibility* and stable skin coverage are the primary concerns in reconstruction at this level. Function is surprisingly good following this injury if stable sensate skin coverage is provided along with a mobile MCP joint and a normal commissure. *Structure* is moderately compromised due to the skeletal shortening, however restoration of length at the expense of lesser quality skin coverage is not a profitable trade-off. If local flaps are not available to provide satisfactory coverage of the amputation stump, then more creative and complex soft tissue rearrangement is required with its attendant risks and complications. Radial sensory flaps, whose risks were already discussed, provide a relatively large surface area encompassing nearly the entire dorsum of the proximal segment of the index finger out to each mid lateral line with the functional limitation of 10–15 mm two point discrimination (Brailliar & Horner 1969, Gaul 1969). A dorsal

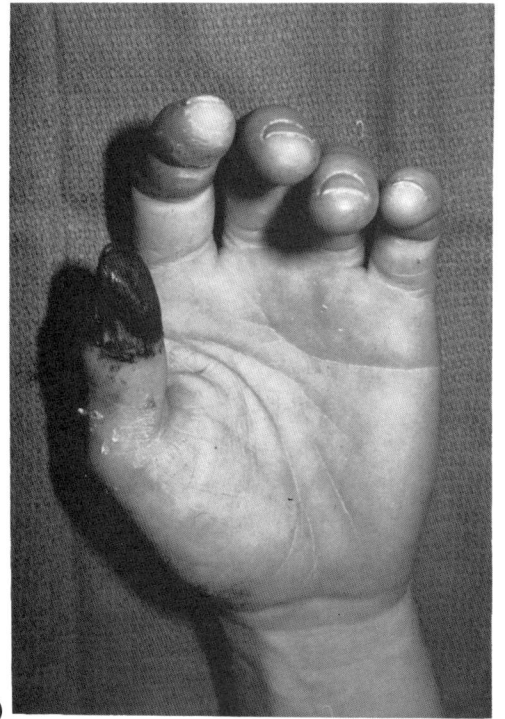
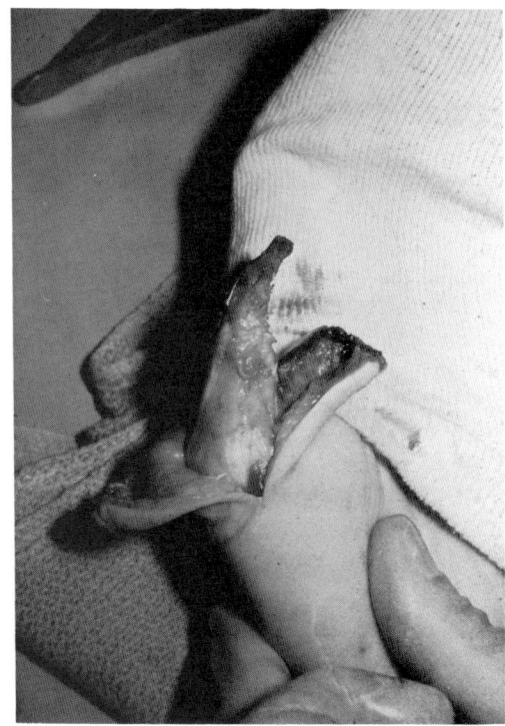

web rotation flap based distally on the palmar skin of the intact commissure has been described by McFarlane (1962) as providing ample skin to resurface areas distal to the metacarpophalangeal joint. The thin subcutaneous layer provides for good quality coverage with satisfactory fixation of the skin and usually allows for preservation of the web space during immobilisation. As with other local flaps, sensory reinnervation of the transposed skin is usually minimal and results in a relatively analgesic working surface.

The neurovascular island pedicle when utilised for reconstruction of Level II injury is less likely to be complicated by traction hyperaesthesias. The incidence of hyperaesthesias has approached 50% in some series with the least satisfactory results consistently occurring in the less severely injured thumbs with relatively normal length and good

Fig. 9.3 (a)–(c) The volar soft tissues remain well nourished when advanced on the neurovascular bundles. It is not feasible to combine a volar advancement with a similar advancement of dorsal soft tissues without risk of necrosis of the dorsal flap

range of motion (Murray et al 1967). As the dissection is complex and extensive, it should not be routinely employed as a primary or emergency procedure. Preferably the flap can be harvested from an already extensively injured digit scheduled for amputation. Murray (1974) recommends harvesting skin from the proximal and middle segments thereby preserving skin and sensibility in the donor fingertip. This approach provides a larger skin paddle for coverage of more extensive defects, however it has a shorter pedicle and limited mobility for transfer with greater risk of traction hyperaesthesias. Additionally, proximal and middle phalanx skin is less well innervated and transection of terminal nerves may lead to dysaesthesias in the donor fingertip. Lack of cortical reorientation of the donor digit to the thumb is a frequent problem and occurs to at least a partial degree in only 50% of patients. Little improvement occurs beyond 2 years and poorer results are obtained in individuals beyond the third decade of life. Alternatively, the digital nerve to the skin pedicle may be divided and sutured to the proximal segment in the thumb stump to alleviate the need for corticosensory reorientation (Fig. 9.4). Ultimate pedicle sensibility is then dependent on the results of microsurgical neurosuture with an anticipated diminution in two-point discrimination when compared with that of the intact skin

before transfer (Morrison et al 1980, Schlenker et al 1980, Poppen et al 1983). This may be an acceptable compromise in light of follow-up studies demonstrating absent two-point discrimination in up to 80% of island pedicle flaps transposed on intact nerves despite preservation of sharp–dull discrimination (Murray et al 1967). Even without this high level sensibility, the skin islands have reliably produced a functional durable surface with callus formation attesting to use and absence of trophic changes. An important caveat concerns the use of this procedure in thumbs afflicted with causalgic pain, especially resulting from avulsion injuries (Tubiana & Duparc 1961). The procedure has not alleviated symptoms in this situation nor has the theoretical advantage of providing additional circulation to the injured thumb provided any improvement in cold intolerance. Therefore, while neurovascular island pedicle skin transfer from an adjacent digit provides very functional and durable skin coverage, many of the anticipated benefits from preserving the integrity of artery and nerve have not been realised in subtotal thumb reconstruction.

Another alternative for skin coverage is that of the distant pedicle flap with its attendant risks and complications. The traditional groin flap offers satisfactory skin coverage at the expense of a bulky and mobile subcutaneous layer, poor sensibility, and dependency leading to edema and significant stiffness of the hand. The infraclavicular pedicle flap eliminates the significant disadvantage of dependency and stiffness when it can be employed in the male, however, a visible unsightly scar usually precludes its use in women.

Functional and aesthetic remedies for a modest deficit in thumb length include creating an illusion of increased length through deepening of the thumb web space or phalangisation. This may augment the breadth of the hand allowing firm grasp of larger objects. Web deepening is limited by necessary preservation of most of the adductor to ensure a strong pinch and grip (Brown et al 1970). Littler (1974) has emphasised the tetrahedral configuration of the thumb web in contrast to a simple cleft or commissure. In the absence of soft tissue contracture and with preservation of pliable web space musculature, a traditional Z-plasty will often suffice to broaden the web space. While a

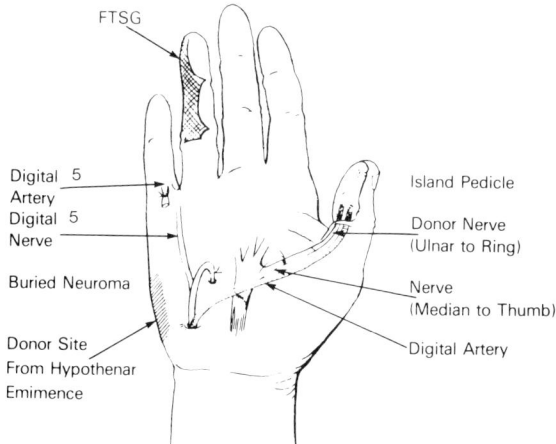

Fig. 9.4 The need for cortical reorientation can be avoided by suture of the proper digital nerve of the neurovascular island to the stump of one of the digital nerves to the thumb. However, sensibility is then dependent on the quality of the neural repair and axonal regeneration

standard 60 degree Z-plasty produces somewhat of a cleft, this effect may be minimised by using a four flap Z-plasty with better distribution of tension in the tissues.

Frequently with severe contracture of the first web provision for additional skin is necessary, usually from local flaps, analagous to the syndactyly release (Fig. 9.5). The subcutaneous tissue of distant flaps retains the phenotypic characteristics of the site of origin and may all too well reflect changes in body weight (Fig. 9.6). Systematic division of the first dorsal interosseous muscle followed by the leading edge of the adductor is usually sufficient, however, extreme contracture requiring complete release of the adductor may be fraught with significant flexion-adduction weakness. This situation may be avoided by recession of the adductor with more proximal reattachment to the shaft of the metacarpal (Tubiana & Roux 1974). Proximal adductor origin release as described by Matev (1970) maintains functional continuity but does not allow for significant deepening and contributes little to the phalangisation of an already shortened thumb amputation. The web space may be further enlarged by resection of a useless index ray (Brown et al 1970).

Skin sufficient to resurface the web provides a marked increase in functional breadth. More efficient conservation of tissues might include pollicisation of the damaged index finger onto the

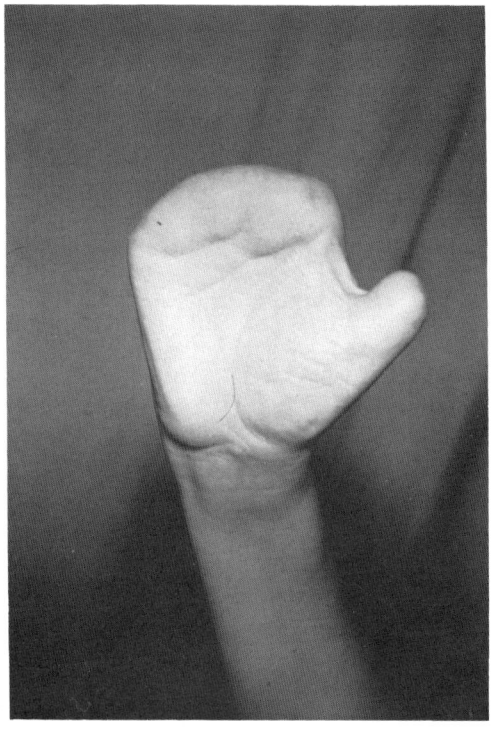

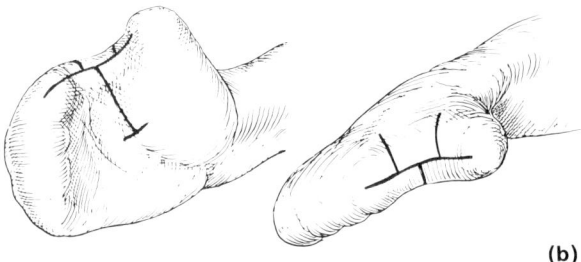

(b)

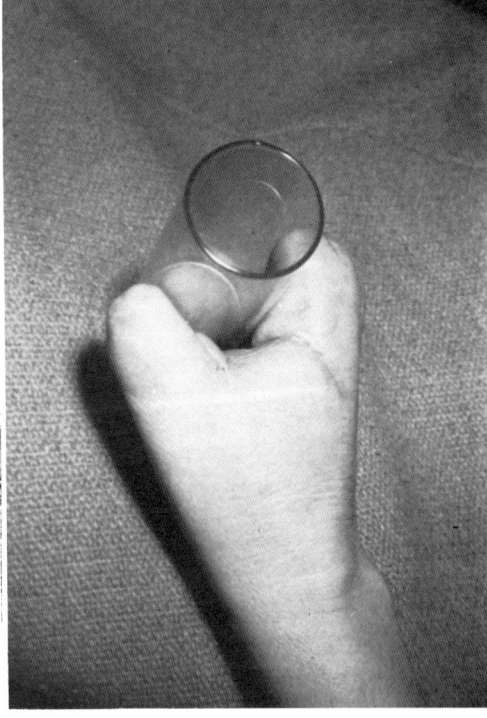

(c)

Fig. 9.5 (a)–(c) The remaining thumb skeleton can be provided an appearance of greater length by deepening the first web space. A rearrangement of the soft tissue much like that for release of syndactyly, rather than a standard Z-plasty, is advocated. This results in an increased ability to grasp objects of greater diameter

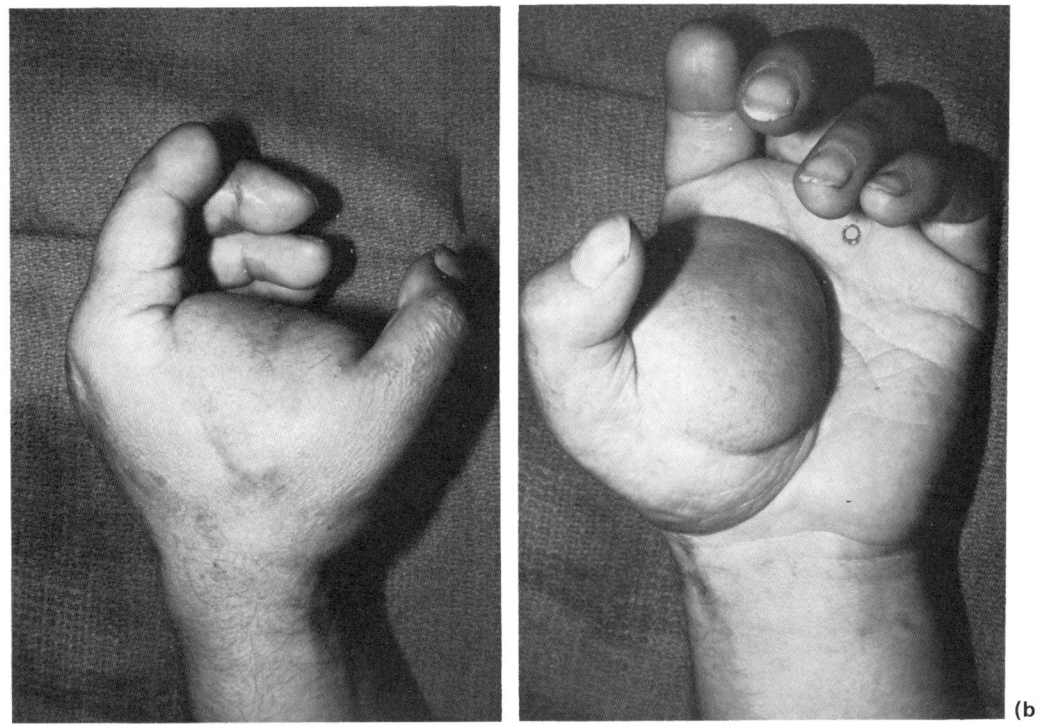

Fig. 9.6 (a) and (b) The choice of distant flaps for coverage of defects or as an element in osteoplastic pollicisation must take into account future changes in patient body weight. The abdominal flap retains the fat storage capabilities of the donor site. In this case, marked weight gain is reflected in the development of a bulky flap that interferes with function

thumb stump thereby gaining thumb length in conjunction with web space restoration. In extreme cases trapeziometacarpal capsulotomy or even trapezium excision may be required to ensure sufficient thumb metacarpal abduction to provide a functional web space. During proximal dissection in the web, care must be taken to avoid injury to the perforating radial artery and its princeps pollicis branch so as not to jeopardise thumb circulation. Additionally, recurrence of web space contracture may require prolonged splinting of the thumb in palmar abduction for up to 6 months postoperatively, along with tendon transfer to augment poorly functioning thenar musculature.

Level III

This is the most common level of traumatic amputation and is associated with some of the most difficult decisions in thumb reconstruction. This zone extends from the base of the proximal phalanx to the metacarpal neck, sparing most of the thenar and antithenar musculature and the trapeziometacarpal articulation. Stable skin coverage with adequate tip *sensibility* is of utmost importance. In addition, injury to the web space frequently requires a large amount of flap skin for resurfacing. Shortening of skeletal *structure* to this degree results in a significant loss of function, especially with concommitant web injury and ensuing contracture. Without injury to the soft tissues of the web and preservation of good thumb-index breadth, satisfactory function may be retained (Fig. 9.7) and even augmented by phalangisation as previously discussed. More commonly this degree of skeletal shortening combined with significant injury to the web space necessitates the addition of 'real' length to the thumb skeleton in addition to resurfacing of the web. Where reconstruction is necessary, restoration of skeletal length assumes importance equal to provision of stable sensate coverage.

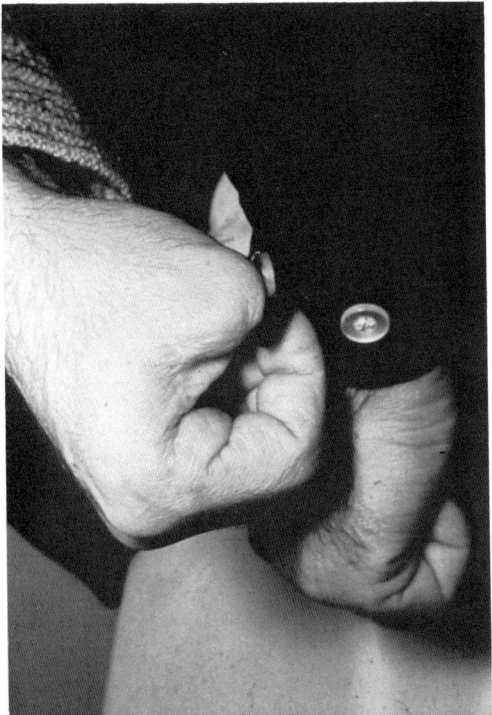

Fig. 9.7 The loss of some portion of the thumb is, in itself, insufficient indication for reconstruction. If the remaining digits have normal function, and the web remains soft, the residual thumb stump may possess substantial thumb-like function

Mechanisms for skin coverage have been discussed. When extensive web space injury or contracture exists, pedicle skin flaps such as dorsal rotation flaps or distant flaps are most frequently employed (Brown 1972). The 'Chinese' or radial forearm flap provides a large area of well vascularised skin at the expense of sacrificing the radial artery. With injury to the thumb, patency of the palmar arch through the ulnar artery must be ensured so as not to add the further insult of vascular insufficiency. Additionally, a sizeable split skin graft may be required to close the donor site frequently resulting in an unsightly donor defect.

Relative lengthening of the skeleton by phalangisation has already been discussed. Further web deepening with destruction of the adductor musculature makes this a less satisfactory procedure than for more distal levels of thumb injury. Real lengthening of the skeleton is required and may be accomplished by a number of operative approaches.

The 'cocked hat' flap or 'thumb stall' of Gillies is one of the older operations for this problem (Gillies & Millard 1957). A major shortcoming of this approach is the requisite for pre-existing stable skin coverage of the amputation stump, a significant problem with injury at this level. Placement of a bone graft beneath tenuous skin cover which is to be circumferentially incised and advanced distally may result in wound breakdown, bone resorption, and a sensitive non-functional tip. With attainable lengthening of only 1–1.5 cm in the face of these attendant risks, it is not surprising that this procedure is only infrequently employed.

Matev (1970, 1979) has pioneered metacarpal lengthening through gradual distraction and this method now enjoys renewed enthusiasm as evidenced by the manufacture of a host of new mini-external fixator frames. A cooperative patient and a near full length metacarpal shaft are required. Gradual distraction of approximately 1 mm per day has resulted in an 80–100% lengthening of the metacarpal shaft over 2–4 months time. Benign pin track infection is the most common complication and responds well to meticulous pin site care and minimising skin tension and motion around the pins. Vascular compromise represents a significant potential complication, particularly in the adult, and can be avoided by proceeding slowly with distraction both initially and after a 50% gain in metacarpal length. Slough of the distal skin is a difficult problem requiring creative skin flap gymnastics and is best treated by avoidance of ischemia during distraction lengthening. Distal sensibility transiently diminishes during the lengthening but returns to normal preoperative levels at the conclusion of the distraction process. Children frequently do not require bone grafting to consolidate the gap produced during lengthening; however, adults do require autogenous bone grafting with significant risk of fracture if protection is not provided during the process of incorporation and maturation of the graft. Finally, as with any other long bone lengthening procedure, the stability of proximal and distal joints must be carefully assessed. Abnormal soft tissues frequently represent the greatest resistance to lengthening and may result in a flexion deformity of the proximal phalanx remnant at the metacarpophalangeal joint or, less commonly, progressive dorso-radial subluxation of the trapeziometacarpal joint. Metacarpal lengthening represents a very satisfactory method of thumb reconstruction in the child with active periosteal new bone formation provided there is careful parental monitoring of the procedure. With meticulous attention to detail in avoiding ischemia during distraction, successful lengthening may also be achieved in the injured adult thumb without a mobile proximal phalangeal remnant.

Osteoplastic reconstruction was previously characterised by anesthetic mobile skin covering a rigid skeleton prone to resorption and had fallen into disfavour prior to the introduction of the neurovascular island pedicle flap. Improvements in both strategy and technique have enhanced the results; however, significant problems remain. The reconstruction consists of multiple stages requiring construction and attachment of a tubed pedicle flap, takedown of the pedicle, insertion of a corticocancellous bone graft, and provision of sensation through a neurovascular island pedicle flap. With increased experience the reconstruction may be accomplished in two stages with provision of a tubed skin pedicle and insertion of a bone graft at the first stage followed by takedown of the pedicle and a neurosensory island flap as the second stage, or some similar combination thereof. The tubed groin flap has been the traditional donor for skin coverage; however, the need for prolonged immobilisation in a dependent position, a thick subcutaneous tissue layer resulting in a mobile skin envelope, and a frequent need to 'delay' division of the pedicle have fueled the search for an alternative means of skin coverage (Fig. 9.8). The infraclavicular region serves as an excellent site for pedicle skin coverage in the male and avoids the problems of dependency and a thick subcutaneous layer (Chase 1969). An unsightly prominent donor scar discourages its use in a young woman. Loss of the skin tube to vascular insufficiency may be avoided by 'delay' of pedicle division, however, this adds another procedure. The optimal time for placement of the graft remains a matter of individual surgeon preference. In an effort to optimise vascular ingrowth into the bone graft by providing a double-ended flow through circulation, Gillies has advocated insertion of the graft at a time between that of attachment of the tube and division of its pedicle (Gillies & Millard 1957). This approach has theoretical appeal but adds another operative stage. Others have advocated insertion of the graft at the time of the tube construction to expedite the process. The graft itself should be 1–2 cm shorter than required to restore normal length to the injured thumb to compensate for the loss of dexterity with the equivalent of fused metacarpophalangeal and interphalangeal joints. Normal length without normal flexibility and control frequently results in less than optimal function (Flatt 1964). The anteromedial region of the tibia and iliac crest have been the most popular donor sites for corticocancellous graft. Osteogenic potential of the iliac crest and the need for cast protection of the leg following tibial graft harvest to avoid pathologic stress fracture would appear to make the pelvis a more favourable graft donor (Fig. 9.9). However, the inherent curvature of the ilium and accessibility of the tibial cortex have perpetuated the use of the leg as donor site. Proper graft position should restore the normal flexion arc to the thumb and may be accomplished either by proper orientation of the natural curvature of the graft or creating a greenstick fracture at an appropriate level (Fig. 9.10). Chase (1969) has further elaborated on the details of graft placement at the same time a neurovascular island pedicle flap is added to the thumb. He has described an elegant technique for fixation of the dorsal skin of the tube to the periosteum of the bone graft and then uniting the skin of the neurosensory pedicle to this dermalperiosteal unit to enhance fixation of the sensate skin on the volar working surface of the thumb. However, debulking of dorsal subcutaneous tissue and additional fixation of the volar soft tissues to the tip of the bone graft may still be necessary to minimise excessive skin mobility. Bone disappearance from the terminal segment of the graft has been a troublesome problem without a clearly identified cause. Since bone resorption is an active process requiring a blood supply, relative avascularity would not appear to be an explanation for this phenomenon. Resorption may well be a manifestation of disuse atrophy of the part secondary to suboptimal sensibility in the overlying skin or hypersensitivity at the very tip of the bone graft.

In spite of shortcomings in restoration of sensibility and the limited cortical reorientation of

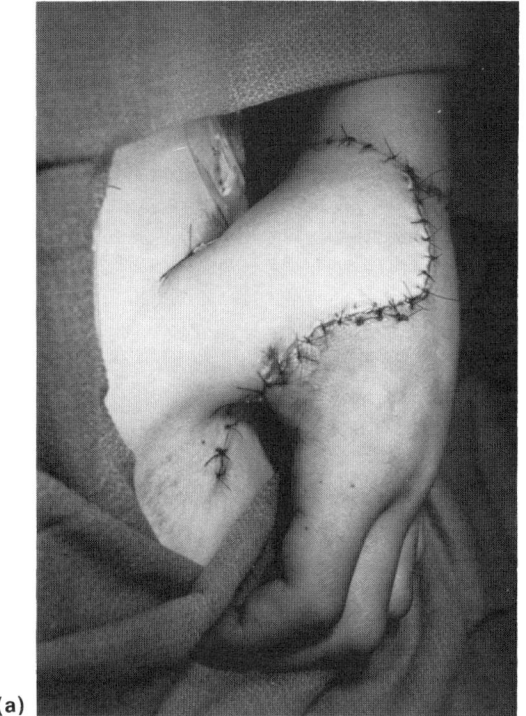
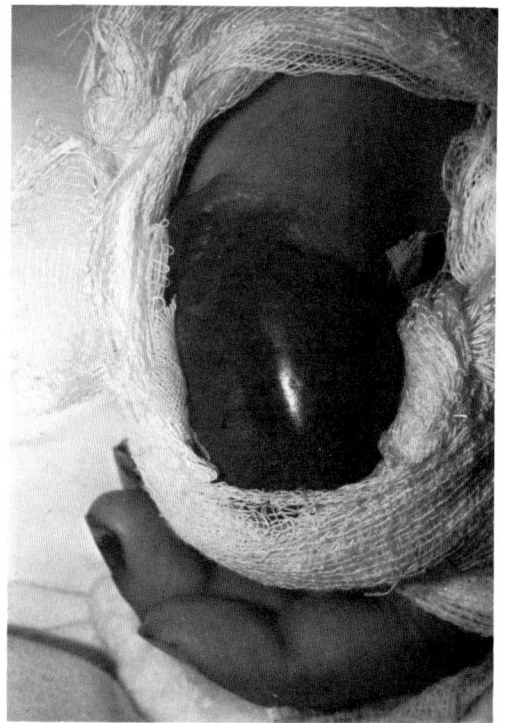
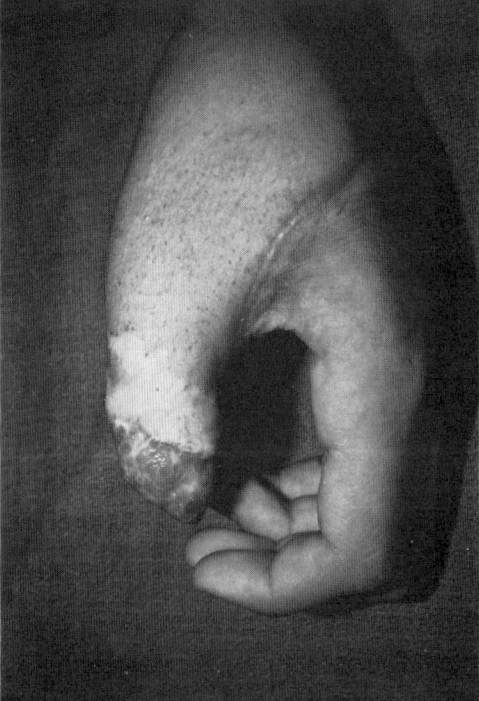

Fig. 9.8 (a)–(c) Osteoplastic pollicisation, because of the multiple stages offers numerous opportunities for the development of complications leading to an unfavourable result. In this case, a very long groin flap was used to cover the remaining skeleton after an avulsion injury. There was no way to temporarily occlude the pedicle to determine if revascularisation of the flap via newly formed recipient site vessel was adequate to nourish all the flap. Following division of the flap, the distal soft tissue suffered from ischemia with subsequent loss of some length of the flap

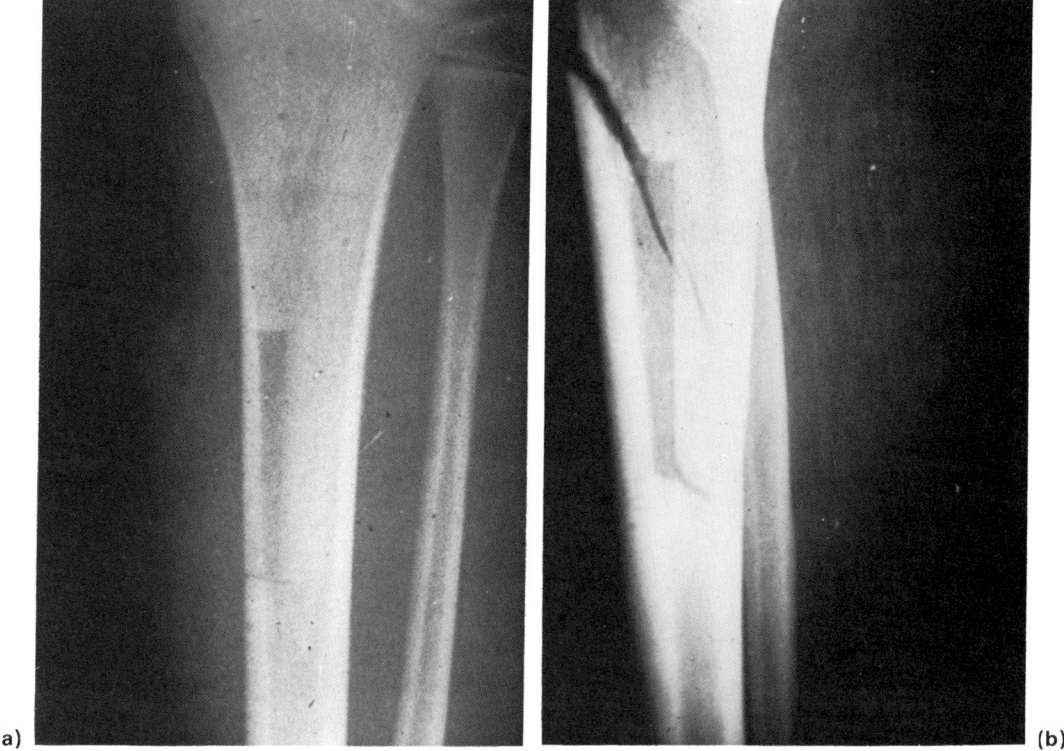

Fig. 9.9 (a) and (b) Attention to detail must extend to the postoperative period. The harvesting of a bone graft, e.g. om the anterior surface of the tibia focuses stresses transmitted through the tibia upon weight bearing (stress risers). A period of 6 weeks of non-weight bearing, or protected ambulation in an orthosis is necessary to avoid a potential pathologic tibial fracture

the innervation of this transferred skin, the neurovascular island pedicle flap remains a major improvement in osteoplastic thumb reconstruction. Best results with this approach are obtained with nearly complete preservation of the metacarpal and the surrounding intrinsic musculature to control the critical trapeziometacarpal articulation (Fig. 9.11). With less than one-half to one-third of the normal length of the metacarpal intact, the abnormal proportions of the reconstructed thumb and a loss of intrinsic control of the basal joint result in less than satisfactory results from osteoplastic thumb reconstruction.

Pollicisation of a normal digit from a full complement of four normal fingers represents an alternative approach to thumb reconstruction with the significant advantage of providing normal sensibility (Tanzer & Littler 1948, Littler 1953, 1966, 1974, 1976, Reid 1969). The development of microsurgical free transfer of toe to thumb has intensified the controversy surrounding sacrifice of a normal finger for reconstruction of Level III injury (Cobbett 1969, Lister et al 1983). Much less controversial is the pollicisation of an injured digit, seen frequently with traumatic damage to the thumb (Sallis 1963, Littler 1977). This represents the ultimate in 'conservation of tissues'; adding length, sensibility, and function to the thumb position while affording an opportunity for web reconstruction if the index or long fingers are transferred. Any of the four fingers may be utilised depending on the degree of injury; however, the proximity and functional independence of the index finger provides for the easiest and most successful transfer (Littler 1977, Burton & Littler 1983). For the three ulnar digits more complex incisions and skin flaps are required and the vascular pedicle is more susceptible to mechanical

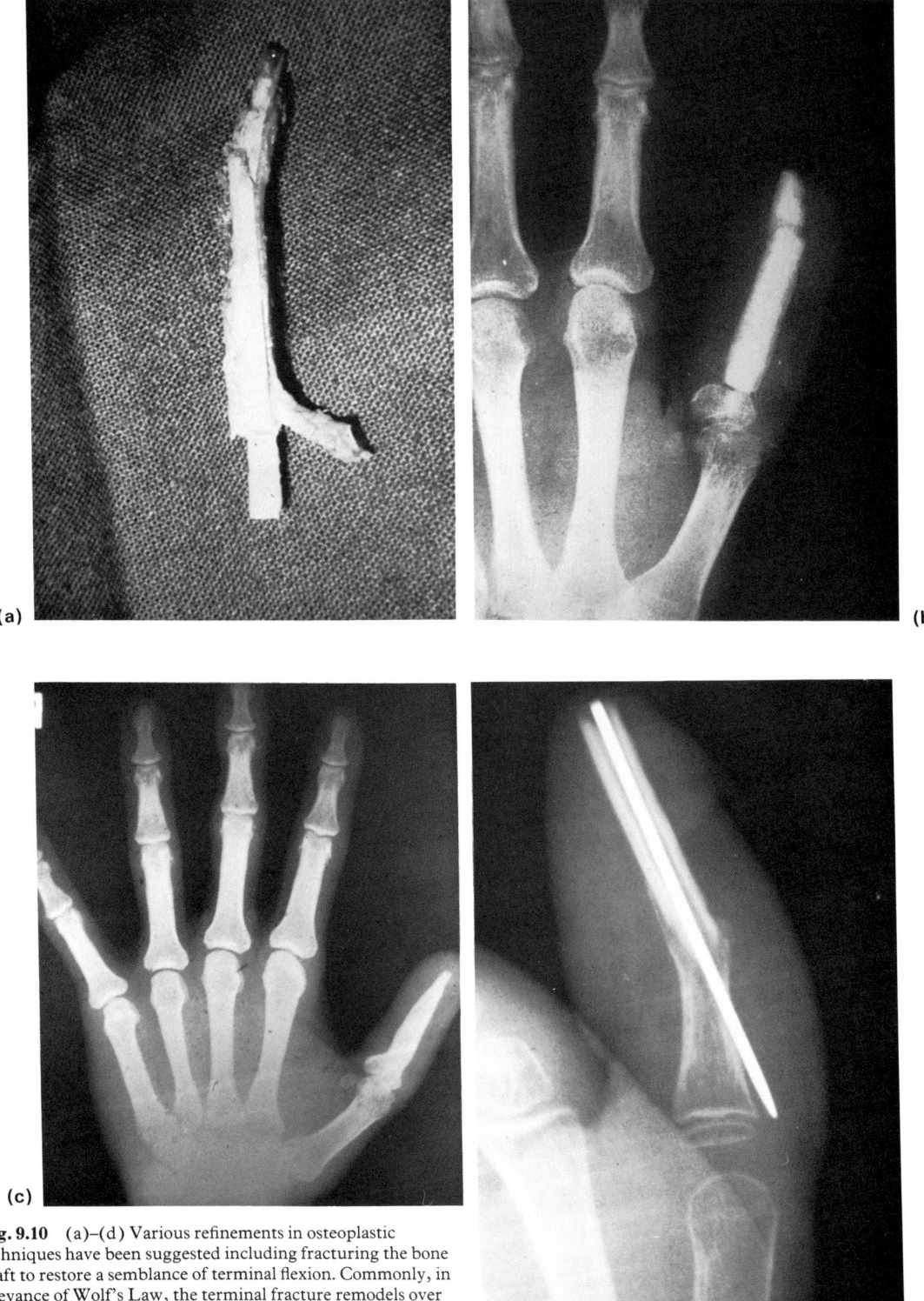

Fig. 9.10 (a)–(d) Various refinements in osteoplastic techniques have been suggested including fracturing the bone graft to restore a semblance of terminal flexion. Commonly, in obeyance of Wolf's Law, the terminal fracture remodels over time. This occurs to a lesser degree when the bone graft itself is fixed to the recipient site in some flexion

THUMB RECONSTRUCTION

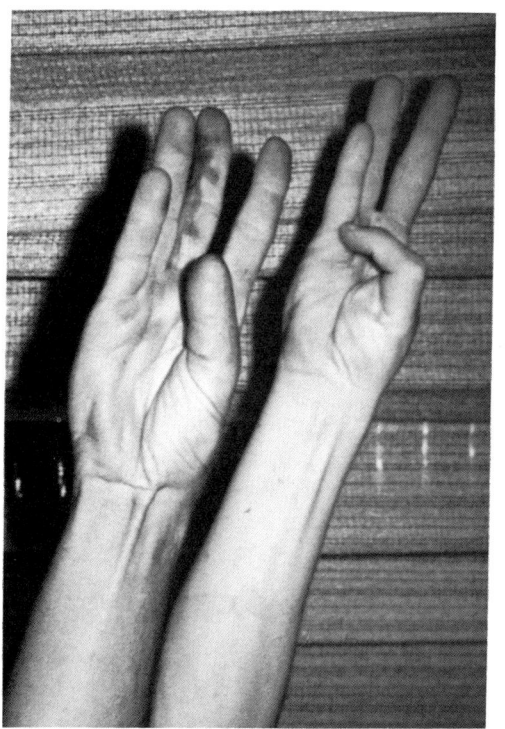
(a)

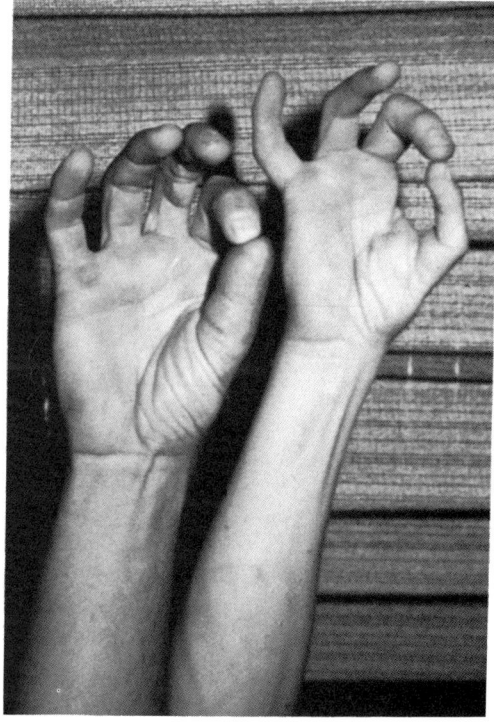
(b)

(c)

kinking or compression beneath intact skin bridges. Preservation of a dorsal vein is extremely difficult when transposing the long finger and impossible when pollicising the ring or little fingers. Abnormal vascular anatomy resulting from the original injury should be delineated by preoperative arteriography. Severely damaged and scarred skin covering the web space and thumb should be excised and replaced by either local flaps during the pollicisation or a distant flap in a separate preliminary procedure. The technical details of pollicisation will be discussed in a subsequent section.

Level IV

Injuries involving the proximal and middle thirds of the thumb metacarpal are associated with significant loss of intrinsic muscle control of the basal joint and represent a major challenge for thumb reconstruction. Priorities include restoration of length, stability of the trapeziometacarpal

Fig. 9.11 (a)–(c) The appearance of an osteoplastic reconstruction is compared to the result following index pollicisation

joint, and a sensate working surface. As the available length of metacarpal diminishes, the likelihood of osteoplastic thumb reconstruction providing a satisfactory result also dwindles. This leaves pollicisation, of an uninjured or preferably an injured digit as is available in greater than two-thirds of cases, as the preferred method (White 1970, Kelleher 1972, Stern & Lister 1981, Hentz 1985). No single individual has contributed more to the refinement and mastery of surgical detail of this operation than Littler (Fig. 9.12). Problems and complications contributing to an unsatisfactory result following pollicisation can be divided into three general categories: skin incision and web reconstruction, vascular compromise, and management of the skeleton.

Skin incision and web reconstruction

The design of skin incisions and local flaps is guided by the need to excise unsatisfactory skin over the thumb and web space, interrupt constricting scar at the base of the new thumb, and provide for satisfactory configuration and coverage of the reconstructed web space. The complex design of the skin incisions is only a small reflection of the requisite preoperative planning. Inadequate skin coverage must be recognised and most frequently is replaced by local flaps. Occasionally distant flap coverage is necessary as a preliminary procedure to pollicisation. Transfer of the index finger contributes significantly to restoration of an adequate web space. Littler has perfected the use of interdigitating dorsal and volar web flaps while others have relied on varying combinations of Z-plasties to achieve the same end (Littler 1974, 1977, Burton & Littler 1983). The leading distal edge of the newly constructed web should remain at the level of the metacarpophalangeal joint of the reconstructed thumb which corresponds to the PIP joint of the transposed index finger. This necessitates longitudinal incisions to that level on the index ray to allow for positioning of the web and added skin for coverage of the reconstructed intrinsic musculature. The tendency towards more proximal placement of the web results in a grotesque thumb substitute with an overly slender profile and illusion of excessive length.

Vascular compromise

Vascular compromise of the transposed digit remains the most devastating complication; however, it is extremely infrequent and can be avoided through adequate preparation and meticulous surgical technique. Vascular injury following trauma should be thoroughly evaluated with preoperative arteriography to determine the feasibility of digital transposition on an intact, and possibly solitary, vascular pedicle. Dissection is begun in the palm to verify neurovascular integrity. Inclusion of perivascular fat in the pedicle preserves small venous channels accompanying the digital arteries. The pedicle is routed through a plane superficial to the flexor tendons with particular care to avoid kinking, constriction secondary to previous scar formation, tunnelling beneath tight skin bridges, and excessive rotation which might serve to compromise vascular flow to the digit. Brisk return of satisfactory circulation to the pollicised digit following release of the tourniquet is essential and anything less than suitable vascularity should be immediately investigated until a cause is discovered and rectified. Surgical delay of the transfer is possible as a salvage manoeuvre but is seldom necessary (Bowe 1963). Postoperative vascular insufficiency is avoided by elevating the operated part to promote satisfactory venous drainage, release of constricting dressings, and the use of sympathetic blockade to reduce vasospasm. Adequate venous drainage is ensured through preservation of a dorsal vein. As previously mentioned, this luxury is not permitted when transposing a more ulnar digit and maintenance of a small palmar skin bridge may provide an additional margin of safety.

Management of the skeleton

Skeletal management encompasses both posture and stability of the reconstructed thumb. Posture implies both length and attitude of the thumb relative to the remaining digits. Because the true thumb metacarpophalangeal joint is a condyloid articulation, it normally allows 15–20 degrees of pronation on the long axis of the ray. This articulation is inadequately replaced by the ginglymoid proximal interphalangeal joint of the index

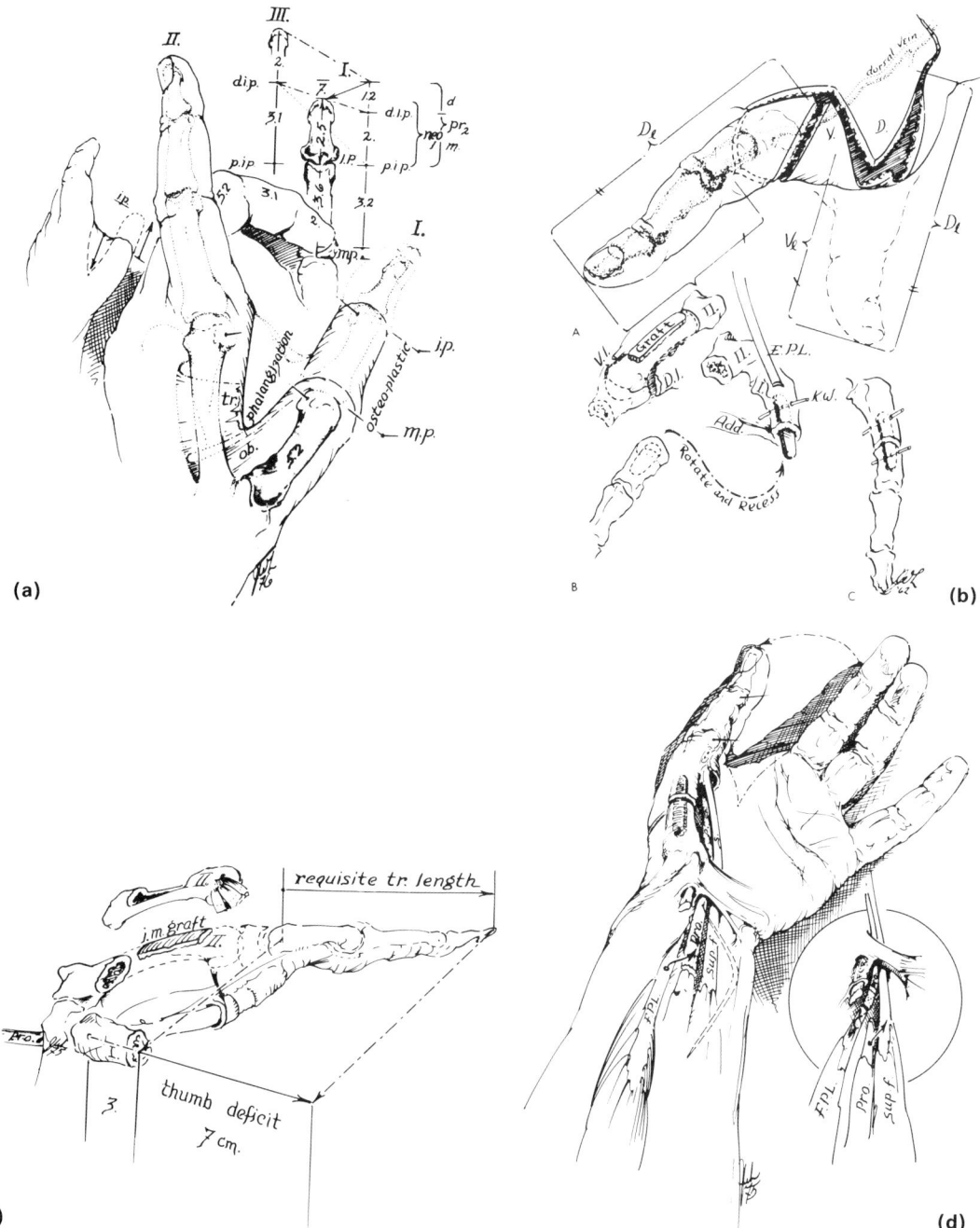

Fig. 9.12 (a)–(d) Littler's depiction of thumb reconstruction with emphasis on pollicisation. Phalangisation achieves 'relative' lengthening, osteoplastic reconstruction ideally restores thumb length to the IPJ level, and pollicisation most closely restores a mobile thumb of nearly normal size (a). Sequential skeletal dimensions are best approximated by long finger pollicisation but overall thumb length is equally well replaced by proper deployment of the index digit. Preoperative measurement of volar and dorsal skin lengths adds precision in thumb reconstruction (b). Interdigital dorsal and volar web flaps and recession–abduction–pronation of the transposed part are critical steps in technique. An intramedullary bone graft fixed by transverse wires is used to restore an average skeletal length of 10–11 cm (c). Secondary suture of the FPL to the profundus tendon of the neothumb enhances independence of function and affords an opportunity to increase flexor tone (d)

finger and therefore the pollicised segment should be rotated an additional 15–20 degrees relative to the thumb metacarpal. Likewise, the thumb interphalangeal joint, which pronates 10–15 degrees during flexion, is replaced by the index terminal joint which rotates into supination. Thus, the pollicised segment requires 120–140 degrees of rotation (pronation) relative to its original position (Burton & Littler 1983). The elasticity of the soft tissues neutralises the surgeon's attempted rotation so that it is rare to have overrotation of the pollicised segment. A good intraoperative guide is to align the reconstructed thumb tip to oppose the ring finger. Functional rotation of the basal joint may be further enhanced by an opposition transfer, and the superficial flexor of the pollicised digit is a readily available motor. When at least half the metacarpal length and the accompanying intrinsic musculature are intact such a transfer is usually unnecessary and is best performed as a secondary procedure after demonstration of a functional deficit. Secondary adjustment of flexor tendon tone or transfer of flexor pollicis longus to the reconstructed thumb may be desired for enhanced functional independence and active flexion. Appropriate length of the transposed segment may be calculated from comparative radiographs of the injured and normal thumbs. From both cosmetic and functional standpoints, it is far better to err on the side of a shorter reconstructed thumb than one endowed with excess length.

Instability of the bony juncture between thumb metacarpal and transferred segment is an infrequent occurrence. Union can be achieved through use of either a free intramedullary graft or a spike from the proximal phalanx of the transposed digit fixed to the thumb metacarpal remnant with K-wires. Unfortunately, hyperextension instability of one or both of the transposed interphalangeal joints is a frequent reminder of the complexity and delicate balance of the intrinsic and extrinsic musculature (Figs 9.11c and 9.13). Powerful metacarpophalangeal joint flexion is lost through amputation of the sesamoids and detachment of the proximal phalangeal insertion of the flexor pollicis brevis, adductor pollicis, and abductor pollicis brevis. The loss of extrinsic flexor tone following recession of the pollicised digit along with transfer and readjustment of the extensor tendons aggravates the tendency towards interphalangeal joint hyperextension. The two slips of the superficial flexor insertion on the middle phalanx of the pollicised index finger can be used to reinsert the adductor pollicis and flexor pollicis brevis on their respective ulnar and radial sides, respectively, to restore strong metacarpophalangeal flexion though at the expense of intrinsic extensor tone to the terminal joint (Kelleher 1972). Alternatively, Littler has suggested shortening and transfer of the index superficial flexor to the pollicised proximal or middle phalangeal segments of the reconstructed thumb to enhance pinch. Finally, fusion of the new metacarpophalangeal joint (formerly PIP joint) serves to simplify and stabilise the system (Littler 1952). Index finger pollicisation offers a potentially excellent functional reconstruction for injuries at the mid-metacarpal level. In addition to restoration of length it provides normal sensibility, independence of motion, and potential for stability that characterise the normally functioning thumb. However, because of the complexity of the digit being imitated, satisfactory functional restitution will not be achieved by a single operative procedure in all cases. Secondary procedures directed at specific functional deficits may occasionally be necessary, and were indicated in 80% of cases in one series of thumb reconstruction by pollicisation of a previously injured digit (Harkins & Rafferty 1972).

Level V

These injuries involve loss of the unique trapeziometacarpal joint along with its associated governing intrinsic musculature. This degree of anatomic loss makes osteoplastic thumb reconstruction a fruitless undertaking. Pollicisation of another digit is the only viable conventional alternative to restore thumb function. The trapeziometacarpal articulation of the thumb is extremely difficult to reproduce in the adult and is best replaced by fusion of the base of the transposed proximal phalanx to the remaining carpus in the strategic fist projection rather than attempt transfer of the index metacarpophalangeal joint. This leaves a situation not unlike that with congenital deficiency of the thumb where the first dorsal and first volar interosseous muscles may be reattached to the lateral bands of

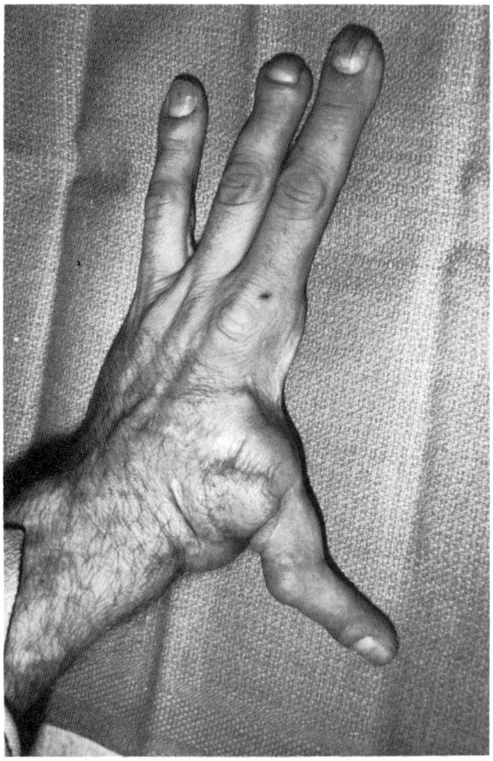

THUMB RECONSTRUCTION 125

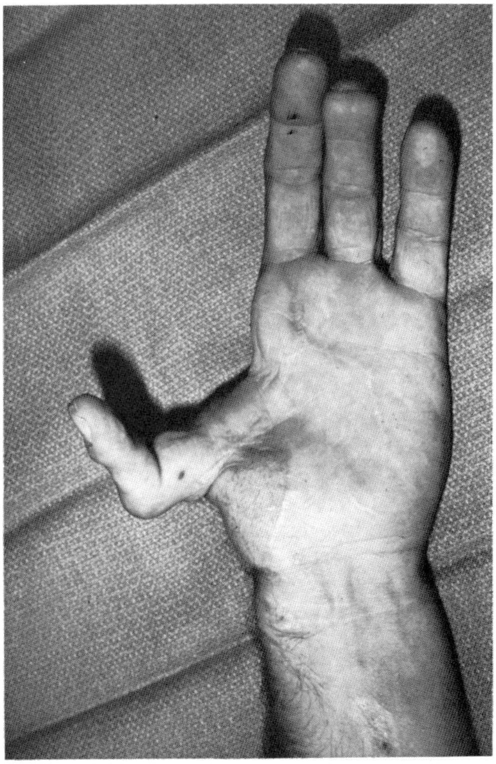

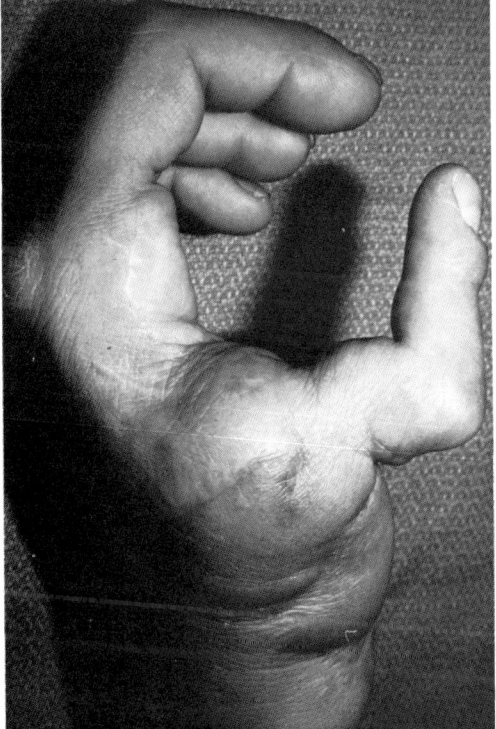

Fig. 9.13 (a)–(c) Dynamic stabilisation of the transferred metacarpophalangeal joint into the carpometacarpal joint position is very difficult to achieve. When the basal joint has been destroyed and the index digit is to be transferred, it seems best to fuse the base of the proximal phalanx to the remaining radial carpal element or base of 2nd metacarpal

the transposed digit at the level of the former proximal interphalangeal joint to function primarily in extension of the terminal two segments. Alternatively, one of the interosseous muscles may be attached to the former superficialis insertion on the middle phalanx to provide for strong flexion of the newly created metacarpophalangeal joint. In any event, the more essential functional attribute of the basal joint system of the thumb is stability rather than mobility. The only caveat is that in fusing the proximal phalanx to the carpus a modest degree of extension in the plane of the palm must be provided so that the fingers are free to close unobstructed by the newly created thumb.

COMPLICATIONS IN CONVENTIONAL RECONSTRUCTION FOR CONGENITAL DEFICIENCY

A great variety of thumb malformations exist on the basis of abnormal intrauterine development. In general, digits in the preaxial opposable position may be amenable to reconstruction by addition or deletion of particular components or may require total reconstruction. Problems complicating management of the salvageable thumb are not within the scope of this discussion.

Although many of the principles in total thumb reconstruction by index finger pollicisation for congenital absence are similar to those employed following traumatic loss of the thumb, three areas of special consideration deserve attention.

It is frequently difficult to decide when a structurally deficient thumb with less than a normal complement of skeletal components is salvageable by staged reconstruction. If the abnormal thumb significantly varies from normal size, it is best to ablate that member and proceed with pollicisation of the next most radial digit. Conservation of tissues may still be employed to a limited extent in creating the illusion of a thenar eminence by subcutaneous burial of these non-functional remnants. A much more diminutive part such as a pouce floutant should be ablated in the nursery before emotional and psychological attachment make this rational treatment difficult.

A second area of controversy concerns the timing of pollicisation. Recommendations vary from under one year of age to the third or fourth year of life. A reasonable compromise of between one and two years of age recognises the time during which the child is beginning to develop and incorporate more complex patterns of thumb function.

Finally, associated anomalies must be considered prior to the selection and performance of a surgical procedure. This includes systemic disorders like thrombocytopenia accompanying radial aplasia with intact thumb and concomitant developmental problems such as with the longitudinal deficiency syndromes.

In pollicisation for the congenitally absent thumb, surgical principles are identical to those as discussed previously for post-traumatic thumb reconstruction with several notable exceptions. Design of the skin incisions and web reconstruction remain complex but are somewhat simplified by the absence of scarred tissue in need of excision. Skin flap design should provide for interruption of the circumferential incision at the base of the pollicised digit and aim to place the volar incision such that it simulates a thenar crease. Sufficient skin is available to provide for excellent web reconstruction such that the lines of incision are dictated more by their anticipated position following pollicisation than by a need to create large strategic flaps to reconstruct the web. Absence of a true thenar cone frequently gives the false impression of excessive length because of the slender appearance of the pollicised digit. This can be avoided by adequate distal advancement of the abductor indicis and first volar interosseous muscles to the level of the proximal interphalangeal joint by attachment to the respective lateral bands, correct placement of the leading edge of web skin at this same level, and preservation of tissues from a non-functional thumb to provide bulk in simulation of a thenar eminence. Vascular compromise may be related to unanticipated anomalous structures. Malformation of the vascular arches are most frequent on the preaxial side of the extremity with anomalous intermingling of the digital artery and nerve at a frequency of 15–20% and an absent radial digital vessel to the index ray in the four-fingered hand in up to 25% of cases. Because of the relative predictability of anomalous structures and increased risk of the use of contrast media in young children, arteriography is seldom indicated. Dissection is begun in the palm to ascertain the blood supply of the pertinent digit with the usual meticulous care taken in identifying and isolating these structures.

With absence of the trapezium as the radial member of the proximal transverse carpal arch, strategic positioning of the pollicised digit volar to the base of its former metacarpal is essential in providing the foundation from which satisfactory opposition to the remaining fingers can take place. Palmar projection of 40 degrees from the plane of the hand is recommended and Buck-Gramcko (1971) has introduced the valuable concept of palmar rotation of the pollicised metacarpal head as it simulates the trapezium to prevent hyperextension at the new basal joint. Although the plasticity and growth potential of the infant skeleton allows the metacarpophalangeal joint of the index finger to be deployed as a trapeziometacarpal joint, the unique articular relationship of the latter is never fully realised and accordingly, the pollicised digit must be rotated 150 degrees into pronation. Both Littler (Hentz & Littler 1977) and Buck-Gramcko (1971) have emphasised the need for complete epiphyseal arrest of the transposed index metacarpal head to avoid late overgrowth of the new 'trapezium' and subsequent deformity (Fig. 9.14). Differing opinions exist regarding the advisability of primary opponensplasty, most frequently employing the flexor superficialis tendon from the pollicised digit when available (Kelleher 1972, Harrison 1973, Manske & McCarroll 1985).

With full knowledge that secondary procedures are frequently necessary, it would seem prudent to delay opponensplasty until such time as a specific functional deficit is identified. This allows the tendon transfer to be conducted in a more attentive manner rather than at the conclusion of an already long and arduous pollicisation, avoids additional surgery in those patients where it is unnecessary, and affords the additional benefit of increased cooperation during postoperative retraining in the older child. When the superficial flexor tendon is not available for transfer from the pollicised digit, shift of the abductor digiti minimi can provide augmentation of opposition while adding bulk to the thenar eminence.

Accepting the fact that a normal thumb can never be created from a finger due to clear anatomical differences, excellent functional and cosmetic results can be achieved by index pollicisation for congenital pollical deficiency. Best results have been obtained in the hand with a skeletally deficient hypoplastic thumb where functional intrinsic thenar musculature can be salvaged and in the five-fingered hand with a normally sized radial digit available for pollicisation. There remains a need for secondary procedures to enhance functional performance in up to 50% of hands, with the most frequently performed procedure directed at improving opposition and palmar abduction. Handling of large objects is significantly improved by pollicisation, however, there is evidence to suggest that fine manipulative skills persist in the preoperative pattern of side to side prehension when this activity is carried out in the third or fourth interspaces (Manske & McCarroll 1985).

Alternatives to complete digital pollicisation should be considered in longitudinal radial deficiency syndromes. Longitudinal deficiency of preaxial development resulting in radial aplasia should initially be treated by wrist stabilisation if elbow flexion is sufficient to allow the centralised wrist continued access to the head and mouth. Should wrist stabilisation not be indicated or abnormal joint motion and motor-tendon units be present in the radial most digits less than optimal function will result from formal radial digit pollicisation. Absence of the first dorsal interosseus muscle identifies a group of hands that will likely need formal opponensplasty to restore this function. Buck-Gramcko (1971) has emphasised the importance of an independent extrinsic profundus flexor to the radial most digit in predicting the success of pollicisation in the radial club hand. Flexion deformity in the interphalangeal joints of the pollicised digit may necessitate arthrodesis in a more functional position if passive correction is not possible or this is not overcome by muscle rebalancing at the time of pollicisation. The hand with radial aplasia is more likely to require secondary reconstructive procedures than the otherwise well-developed extremity in need of a normally functioning thumb. Because of the suboptimal results in this situation, Hentz & Littler (1977) have recommended abduction–pronation–recession osteotomy of the metacarpal of the most

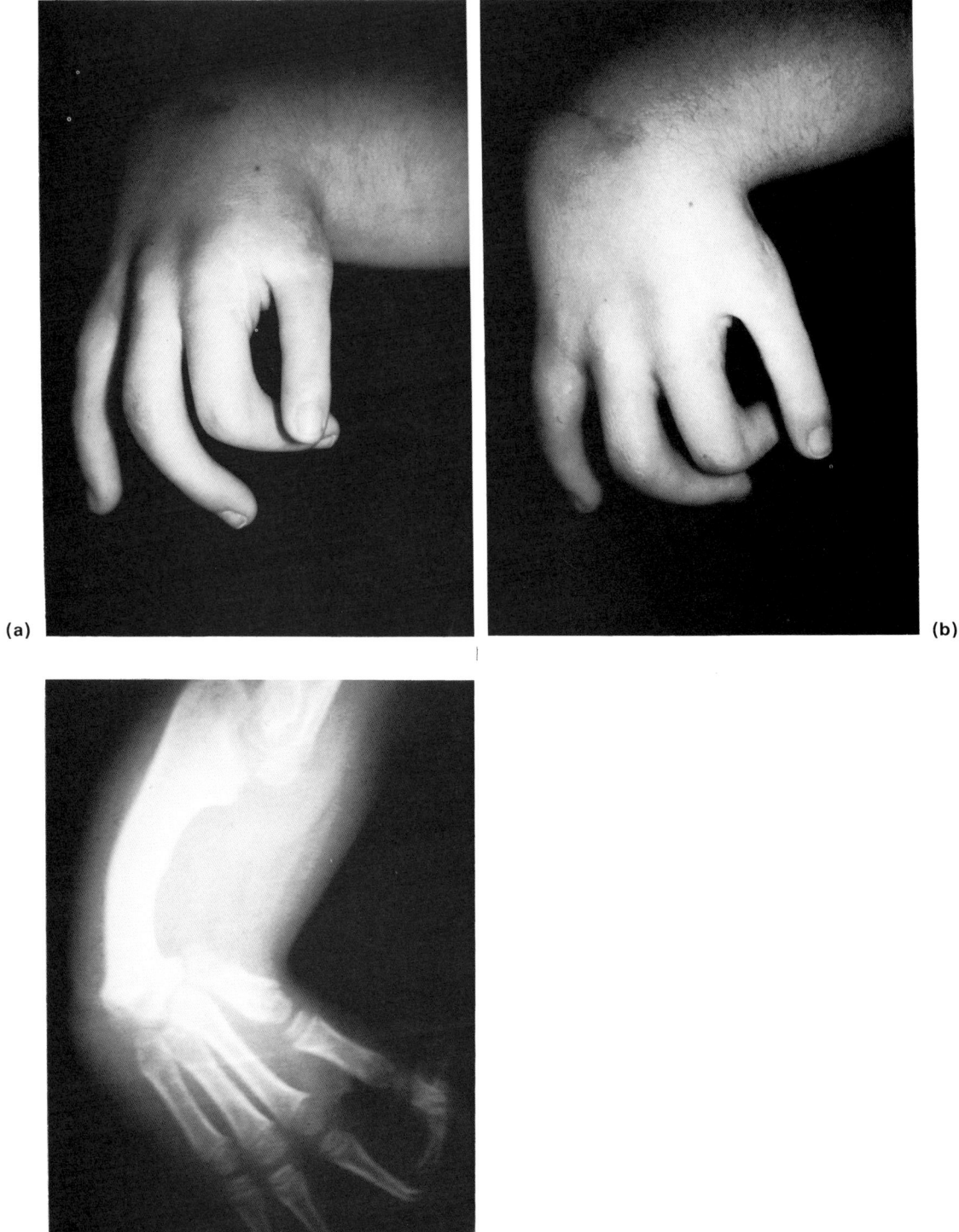

Fig. 9.14 (a)–(c) Insufficient abduction and rotation along with continued epiphyseal growth of the transposed metacarpal head have reduced this pollicised index finger to minimal functional value

radial digit in an effort to capitalise on the natural tendency of this ray towards pronation for prehension with the adjacent fingers (Fig. 9.15). The procedure is carried out through a limited surgical exposure which avoids the need for motor unit rebalancing and extensive dissection of the neurovascular bundles. It provides a more functional hand unit without significantly changing its appearance or risking the viability of the operated finger. Most importantly, the procedure does not preclude later formal pollicisation should the parents or patient elect this more complex procedure for optimal functional restoration.

COMPLICATIONS IN MICROSURGICAL RECONSTRUCTION FOR TRAUMATIC THUMB DEFECTS

In 1966, Buncke demonstrated the technical feasibility of free toe to thumb transplantation in rhesus monkeys. Cobbett (1969) was the first to achieve this clinically. His success was soon followed by many others who demonstrated the practicality of this method in providing an additional reconstructive alternative in creating a thumb substitute. In some centres, microvascular free toe to thumb transfer has become the procedure of choice for reconstruction of the thumb following its loss by trauma. Its place in the reconstructive surgical armamentarium has not been achieved smoothly. Indeed, many early reports demonstrating truly inferior results were proudly published indicating that, as in digital replantation, mere survival of the transferred part was not synonymous with satisfactory function. Functional success requires more than heterotopic survival of a composite part or proficiency with the operating microscope. Success requires attention to the many details of preoperative planning, surgical execution and postoperative management. From these unfavourable results have come changes in surgical philosophy, design, and technique that, when properly employed, have made toe to thumb transfer a dependable reconstructive alternative.

Free toe to thumb transfers have been employed

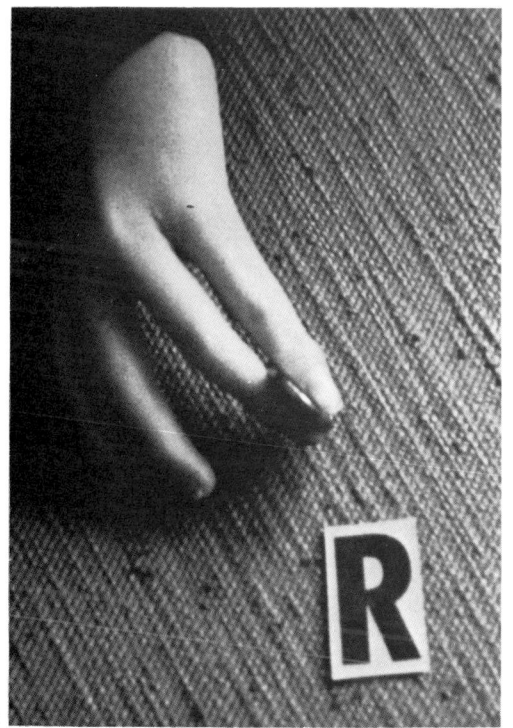 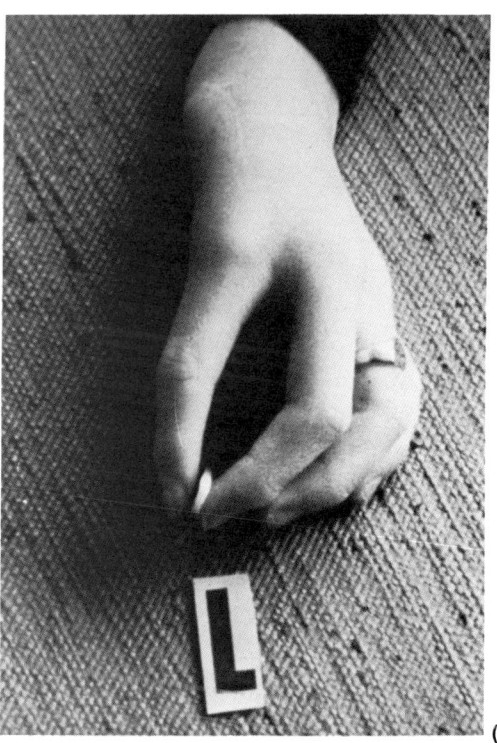

Fig. 9.15 (a) and (b) Abduction–pronation–recession osteotomy of the radial digit in radial longitudinal deficiency enhances the natural tendency to opposition as demonstrated by the left hand compared with the unoperated right side

for traumatic amputations at Levels II through V and rarely for Level I injuries. There are three, and perhaps four, principal procedures that have been useful, including all or part of the great or second toe or some type of combination of great toe and second toe parts (Foucher et al 1980). This plethora of reconstructive methods can be confusing to the surgeon trying to match the patient's needs with the correct surgical procedure. Many unfavourable results can be traced to inattention to detail in this crucial analytic process.

Preoperative planning

I. *Analysis of recipient site requirements*

The functional requirements of the thumb have been outlined above. The choice of procedure must be governed by the functional demands of the patient and the remaining skeletal length, functioning joints, soft tissues and thenar muscles. In terms of priority, remaining skeletal length and the presence of functioning thenar muscles are the most important prerequisites in guiding the choice of a microvascular reconstructive procedure. In contrast to many of the conventional reconstructive procedures such as osteoplastic pollicisation, transfer of a toe or toe part is more akin to replacing 'like with like'; and the operation can be potentially tailored to the recipient site requirements far more readily than with conventional reconstructive techniques. Therefore, choosing the correct procedure is paramount in avoiding an unsatisfactory result. Rather than discuss in detail various procedures for amputations at various sites, we will discuss some of the constraints that guide the choice of various procedure (Fig. 9.16).

A. Great toe transfer. Transfer of the entire length of the great toe to the thumb appears most indicated in amputations at or somewhat proximal to the metacarpophalangeal joint (Stern & Lister 1981). Typically, the base of the proximal phalanx of the toe is fused to the remaining thumb metacarpal; flexor and extensor tendons, vessels and digital nerves are repaired to corresponding members. The additional length of the toe phalanges will provide a thumb substitute of potentially near normal length. Only one joint, the

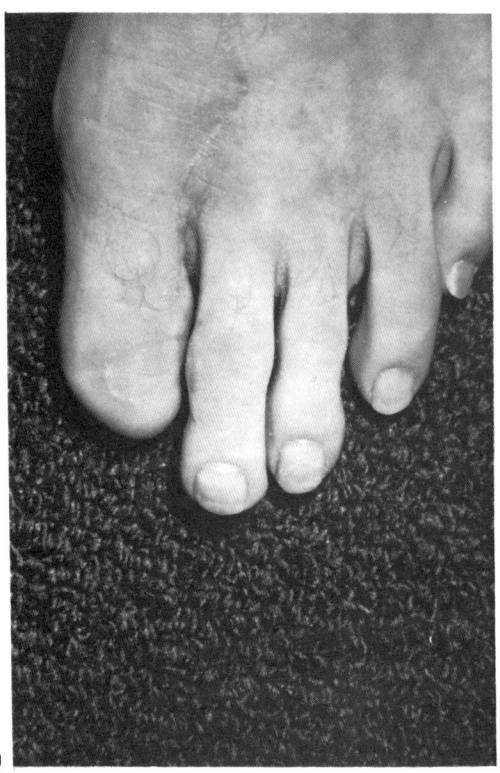

(a)

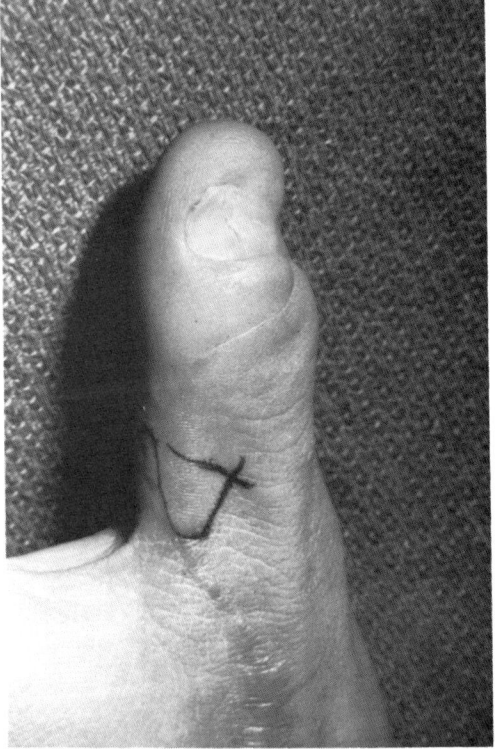

(b)

THUMB RECONSTRUCTION 131

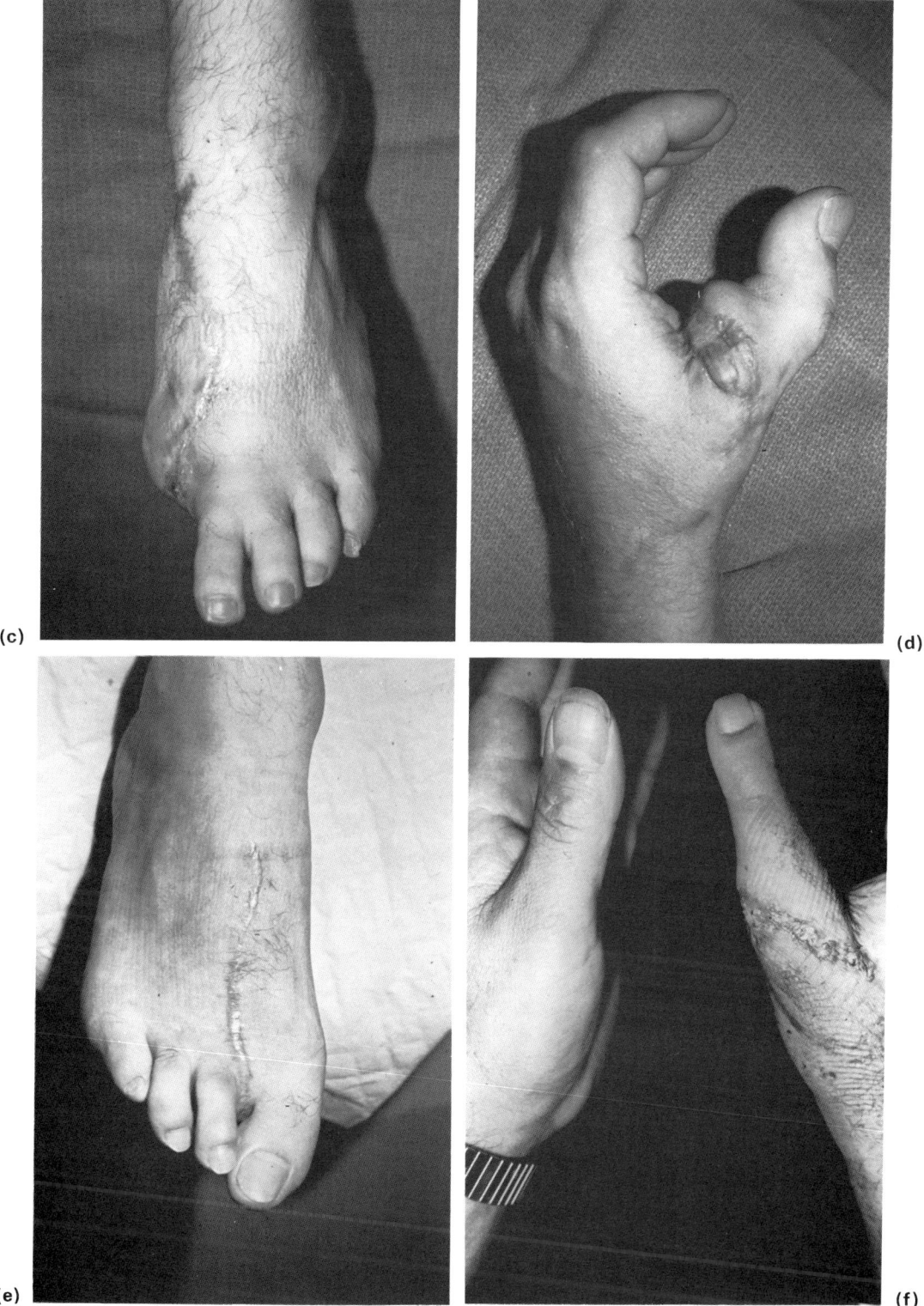

(c) (d)
(e) (f)

Fig. 9.16 (a)–(f) The aesthetic result for the recipient as well as the donor site following the several common methods of thumb reconstruction by microvascular transfer of all or part of the first or second toe. Pictured are the results following partial great toe transfer (a, b), transfer of the complete great toe (c, d), and second toe transfer (e, f)

interphalangeal joint, requires muscle-tendon control. One can anticipate recovery of protective sensation and the result is typically a thumb somewhat broader than normal with the nail plate somewhat larger than normal but with potentially great strength and stability for grasp (Poppen et al 1983). The addition of a fingernail is an important adjunct and the presence of even a small amount of terminal joint flexion and extension makes this reconstruction extremely functional and aesthetic. The principal complaints relate to the abnormally large size and configuration of the pulp and nail. As time passes, the pulp atrophies somewhat and the part achieves a more thumb-like appearance (Fig. 9.16). Secondary surgery to improve the overall appearance includes narrowing of the nail plate and recreating the nail fold and removing a wedge of pulp to diminish its bulk. Only fair recovery of 2-point discrimination, averaging between 10–15 mm, may be related to the technical limitations of microsurgical neurorrhaphy and the pre-existing population of sensory end organs in the toe.

B. *Second toe to thumb transfer.* The second toe can be transferred in place of the great toe for defects at the levels mentioned above (Lister et al 1983). It can also be utilised to restore a thumb-like appendage for more proximal amputations such as through the proximal metacarpal or basal joint area. When the second toe plus metatarsal is to be transferred, there is insufficient foot skin to cover the transferred metatarsal. Therefore, provisions for additional skin must be made either prior to or at the time of toe transfer. In contrast to the great toe, the second toe is long and spindly, the distal phalanx bulbous, and primate-like (Fig. 9.16e & f). Stability of pinch is not as great as with great toe transfer. This probably relates less to the diminutive size of the tip than the difficulty in stabilising interphalangeal joints. Control of these joints has proved exceedingly difficult, particularly following transfer for more proximal amputations where sufficient numbers of thumb intrinsic muscles no longer exist. To simplify the system, one may choose to fuse one or another of the interphalangeal joints or utilise the tendon of the short toe extensor as an intrinsic transfer to provide better extensor tone to the interphalangeal joints. The intrinsic muscles of the toe metatarsophalangeal joint may then be attached to the flexor contribution of the intrinsic cone of muscles at the thumb recipient site.

C. *Partial toe transfers.* A very elegant method to reconstruct more distal missing portions of the thumb utilises a portion of the great toe. This so-called 'wrap-around' procedure described by Morrison et al (1980) is best reserved for amputations distal to the metacarpophalangeal joint. Because no additional joint motion is added, the potential for dexterity is somewhat reduced in those cases lacking a functional metacarpophalangeal joint. However, the presence of a nail of near normal size and shape adds tremendously to the functional and aesthetic result (Fig. 9.16a & b).

II. *Analysis of donor site morbidity*

The choice between a great toe and second toe transfer is frequently based on surgeon's preference. There are, however, instances where great toe transfer is relatively contraindicated for aesthetic or functional reasons. The apparent deficit at the donor site following second toe transfer is less obvious than that following transfer of the great toe (Fig. 9.16c & e). Following great toe transfer, provided that a first metatarsal head is present, gait appears relatively unaffected. On careful analysis, however, many patients report a feeling of imbalance on uneven surfaces especially when walking barefooted, difficulty in 'pushing off', and weakness in 'cutting' while running (Poppen et al 1983).

III. *Planning of the procedure*

Careful preoperative planning will be reflected in the smooth uneventful progression of the operation. Technical options are best considered beforehand rather than at surgery. Among frequently neglected details are the following:

1. Reviewing anatomic variations of the vascular system.

2. Making a preoperative clay or alginate model of the part of the foot to be transplanted and matching it with the recipient site in order to avoid harvesting a toe that doesn't precisely fit the defect or with vessels that ultimately lie on the wrong side.

3. Studying X-rays of the foot and hand to determine the proper skeletal-soft tissue relationships.
4. Arteriography of the recipient site especially if the initial injury is one of avulsion of the thumb.
5. Precisely locating the traumatic neuromas of the thumb. This is very important when the injury has been avulsive in nature.

IV. *Errors in surgical execution*

Attention to detail in all phases of the operative procedure minimise the opportunities for untoward results. There should be an unhurried progression of the operation from beginning to end. Many small details are important, including a well-hydrated patient and a warm operating room. The method of preoperative planning as described by Lister et al (1983) should be read by anyone contemplating this procedure.

A. Donor site dissection. While doppler examination of the dorsal arterial anatomy has been helpful, it is not totally reliable. Few authors recommend arteriography of the donor foot in every occasion. What is necessary is the avoidance of inflexibility; the desire to make the transfer 'work' off the dorsal vasculature when the first dorsal intermetatarsal artery is diminutive is but one example. The surgeon must be prepared to dissect the volar arch if this is clearly the dominant arterial supply to the toe (Morrison et al 1978). Other donor site errors include failure to maintain the peritenon over extensor tendon that are not to be harvested and failure to remove a sufficient length of the remaining second metatarsal to allow narrowing of the foot if the second toe is to be transferred (Fig. 9.17).

B. Recipient site errors. Many problems at the recipient site follow failure to heed basic microvascular principles e.g. resecting back to normal vessels, avoiding tension, and meticulous microvascular repair. The sequelae of errors of judgement are vascular thrombosis, emergency surgery and the high likelihood of partial or total loss of the transfer. Obviously, survival of the part must be paramount. However, unfavourable results follow inattention to the details of adequate functional restoration and survival of the transfer does not constitute success. The sequence of reconstructive steps must provide for:

1. An adequately stabilised skeleton best accomplished by some method of rigid internal fixation as opposed to percutaneous K-wires.
2. Properly balanced dorsal and volar tendons.
3. Nerve repairs performed as accurately as the vascular anastomosis.
4. Meticulous microvascular anastomoses.

The basis for elegant reconstruction has long been atraumatic technique carried out in a bloodless field. The urge to rapidly restore circulation at the expense of the other steps should be resisted. However, once embarked, the surgeon should never leave the Operating Room until adequate arterial and venous flow are established. Occasionally the transferred part will not be perfused via the anastomosed artery. If anastomotic patency can be confirmed, a search for a poorly ligated side branch should be carried out. Failing to discover an obvious source of inadequate perfusion, the surgeon is best advised to adopt a nihilistic attitude, apply local vasodilators making certain that the part stays warm and then waiting for relief of spasm. A tensionless skin closure using full thickness or split thickness skin grafts is preferable to a tight skin closure.

V. *Donor site morbidity*

The donor site is a significant source of patient dissatisfaction. Typically, closure of the donor site is delegated to the least experienced member of the surgical team. Closure of the donor site requires the same attention to detail as in designing the operation or performing the microvascular repairs (Fig. 9.18). This is especially true in closing defects following the 'wrap-around' procedure where skill and ingenuity in closure pay large dividends in terms of patient satisfaction. Opportunity for errors abound and include:

1. Breakdown of the wound secondary to primary closure under excessive tension.
2. Improper choice and position of skin grafts (Fig. 9.18).
3. Improper resection of remaining digital nerves causing painful neuromas.

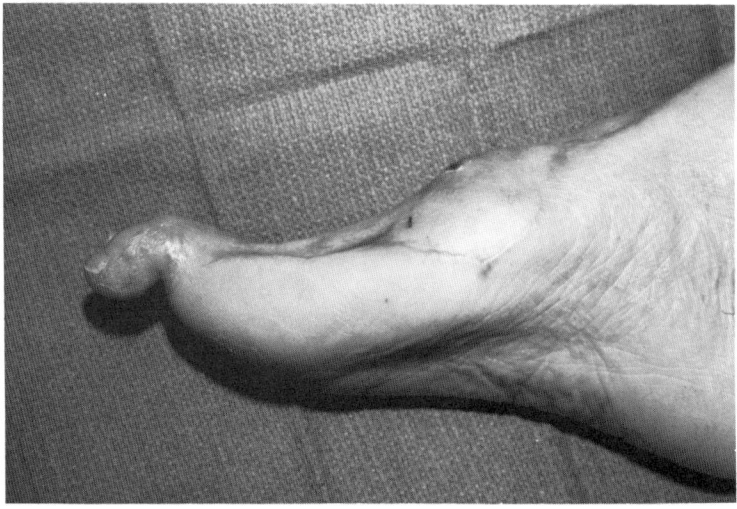

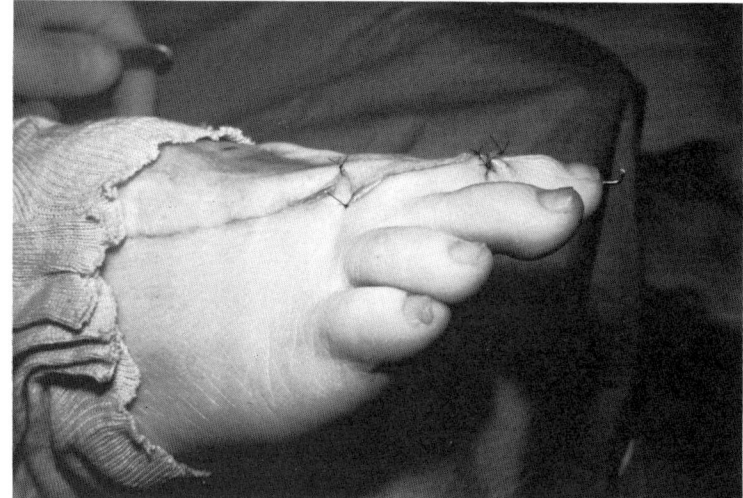

Fig. 9.17 (a) and (b) Attention to detail extends to precisely locating incisions so that with healing and scar contraction, a pathological contracture does not develop. In (a), following transfer of the great toe including a paddle of dorsal foot skin, the patient developed a hammer toe deformity secondary to contraction of the scar at the interface of foot skin and skin graft. This could have been avoided by breaking up this linear scar with several half Z-plasties at the time of closure. Instead, the patient required a formal hammer toe procedure including phalanx resection to allow comfortable shoe wear (b)

4. Inadequate resection of the second metatarsal following second toe transfer with development of hallux valgus.

VI. *Specific technical problems*

Some technical aspects of the various procedures bear emphasising in the quest to prevent complications and untoward results.

A. Great toe transfer. If the metatarsal head is to be transferred, it should be fixed to the recipient metacarpal in a slightly flexed position to avoid hyperextension instability at the reconstructed metacarpophalangeal joint.

B. Second toe transfer. The arc of motion of the second toe metatarsophalangeal joint is also one of extension. To avoid instability in extension at this joint, great care is required in rebalancing the extensor and intrinsic muscle system. It may be useful to fix the second metatarsal head into some flexion to prevent problematic hyperextension instability.

C. 'Wrap-around' flap. Retaining some portion of the distal phalanx as a part of the flap means that the bone graft employed to provide additional length can be placed as an interpositional graft. Bone graft resorption is minimised over that of a terminal graft.

VII. *Postoperative care*

The cause of unfavourable results may occur at any stage of the planning and execution. However, the most disastrous problems typically become evident in the early postoperative period. The management of a failed microvascular anastomosis will not be discussed here. Early recognition of an impending failure is of paramount importance in preventing the ultimate unfavourable result, that is total loss of the transfer. Some system of continuous postoperative monitoring utilising temperature probes, pulse oximeters, or pulse photoplethysmography, are more reliable than intermittent observation of the transferred part. An activist attitude toward anything other than normal or near normal circulatory status is necessary. The transferred part should appear hyperperfused secondary to denervation when compared to its fellow digits.

VIII. *Management of complications*

Complications may occur early, for example occlusion of the anastomosis, or late, for example instability of the transfer, or may occur at either the recipient site or the donor site.

Recipient site problems. Sources of dissatisfaction following survival of all or part of the transferred first or second toe include failure to achieve both functional and aesthetic goals.

Function. 1. lack of motion at the transferred joints; 2. instability of transferred joints during forceful activities; and 3. improper position compromising pinch and grip.

Aesthetics—1. the great toe is too large; 2. the second toe tip too bulbous and the nail too small.

The management of these sources of dissatisfaction do not differ appreciably from similar problems with other methods of thumb reconstruction save a proper level of concern for avoiding injury to the dominant vessel. For many functional problems, secondary surgery can be safely carried out including:

1. Tendolysis of flexor and extensor tendons to provide better motion, carried out when the skeleton is stable.
2. Shortening of the extensor mechanism to improve extension of interphalangeal joints.
3. Muscle-tendon transfers to improve power of movement or stability particularly to provide for missing intrinsic muscles.

For some toe transfer procedures there remain functional problems without ready solutions. The metatarsophalangeal joint of the toe is primarily a joint whose range of motion is into extension while the proximal interphalangeal joint of the toe has primarily flexor functions. Better motion and stability will occur at one or the other of the transferred joint, rarely both.

For many aesthetic sources of dissatisfaction, the passage of time is the best solution. The pulp of the great toe will atrophy over time producing in many people a quite acceptable thumb substitute. If atrophy is insufficient, a central wedge can be removed from the pulp, the nail narrowed by excising nail plate and germinal matrix and the nail fold reconstructed. The second toe typically remains spindly in shape with a foreshortened nail and a round bulbous tip. The appearance can be improved by a V-Y advancement of the pulp to elongate the tip, simultaneously transferring a split thickness skin graft of sterile matrix from another toe to lengthen the nail.

IX. *Toe transfer for congenital absence of the thumb*

The primary application for microvascular toe transfer for congenital absence is in the child born with both absent thumb and absent adjacent digits (O'Brien et al 1978). For such conditions, the second toe has traditionally been transferred to provide sufficient length and numbers of joints. The principal sources of complications associated with the replacement of congenitally absent thumb by microvascular toe transfer is in locating suffi-

136 UNSATISFACTORY RESULTS IN HAND SURGERY

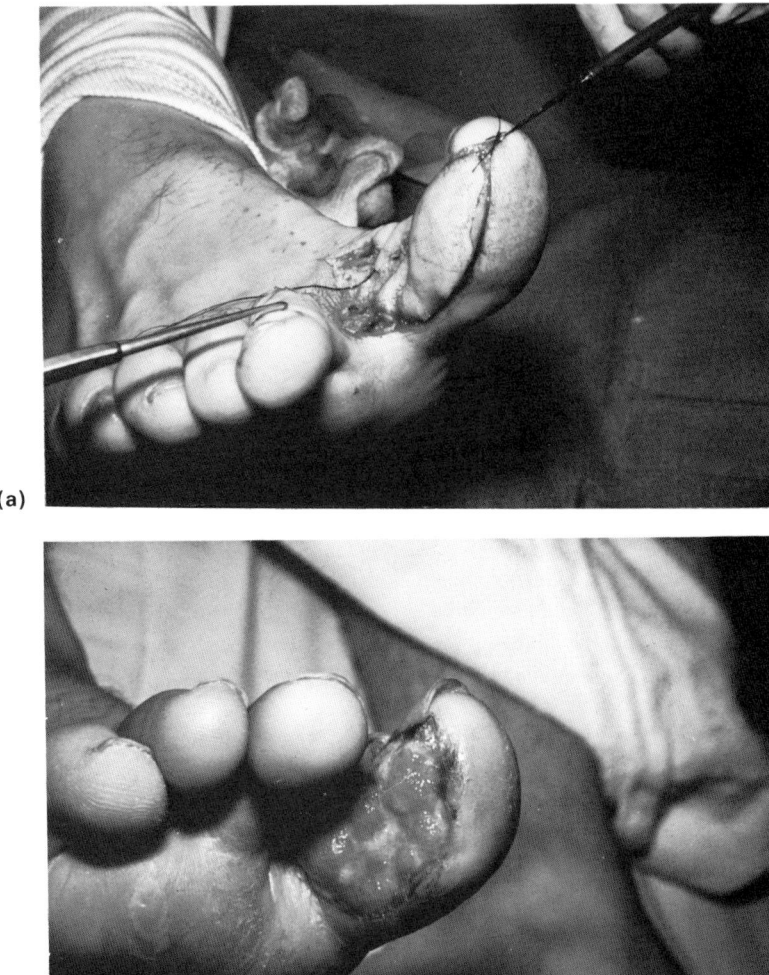

Fig. 9.18 (a)–(d) (loss of graft): A neurovascular island was transferred to the thumb to resurface a defect. The donor site was covered with a full thickness skin graft while the attention of the senior microsurgeons was focused on the microvascular repairs (a). The skin graft was lost (b), and the patient subsequently developed acute osteomyelitis of the proximal phalanx (c), requiring prolonged hospitalisation and debridements that ultimately left him with a stiffened, shortened toe (d)

cient numbers of functional nerves and tendons with which to reinnervate and power the transferred part. Great care must be taken in assessing the hand. The best results have been obtained in those thumb absences thought secondary to intrauterine amputations or ring constriction syndrome. Transverse terminal deficiency states with absence of the digits lends itself poorly to transfer because of absence of more proximal structures with which to reinnervate or power a transferred part. For the more common thumb absences associated with longitudinal deficiency states such as radial ray deficiencies or radial club hands, the benchmark for success remains the index digital transposition and toe transfer in this situation seems a poor choice.

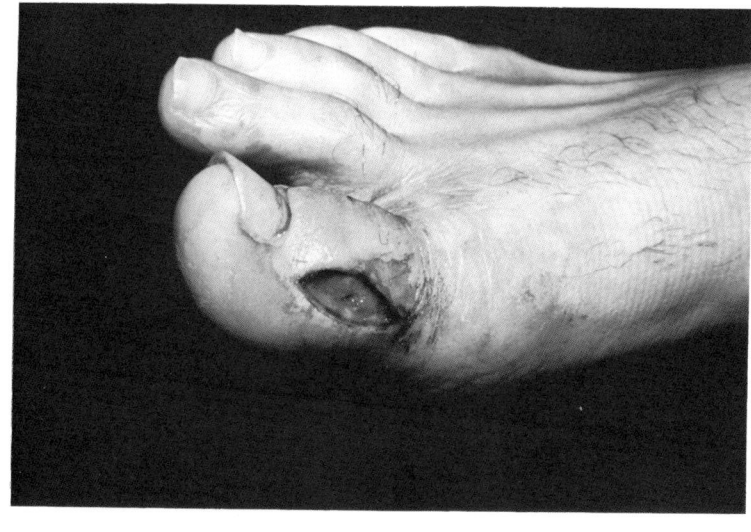
(c)

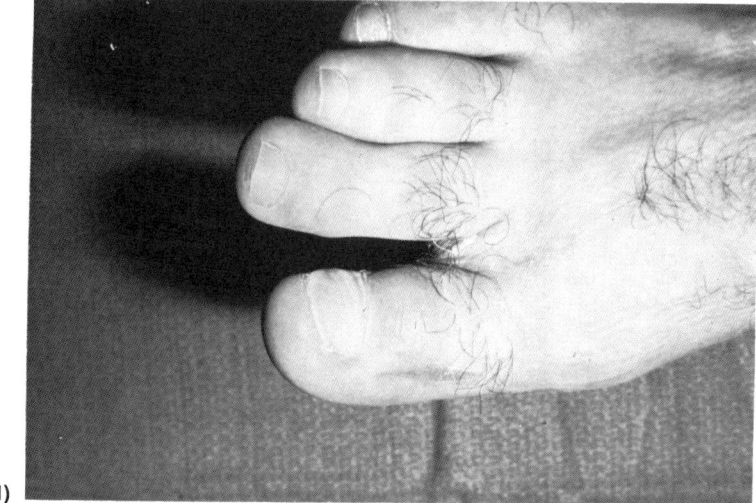
(d)

SUMMARY

Restoration of function to the most important digit of the hand occupies a significant portion of the energies of the hand surgeon. The evolution of the contemporary approach to this problem has progressed through sequential waves of enthusiasm for local tissue salvage and rearrangement, staged distant pedicle reconstruction, adjacent digital transposition, and, most recently, microsurgical reattachment of amputated digits and transfer of composite parts. Given a set of functional needs, the choice of method for thumb reconstruction is largely determined by the ease and reliability of performance; that is, primum non nocere, in other words, the ability to avoid the problems and complications implicit in any technique ultimately determines its utility. Accordingly, we have attempted to discuss the value of these techniques in the context of their complications and their avoidance. The development of free tissue transfer has been surrounded by controversy over its indications and functional results. Additional experience with this procedure will more clearly define its final place in the surgical armamentarium for thumb reconstruction. Undoubtedly, this will occur at a time when other new methods with their own complications, such as allograft replacement of the injured thumb, will start the process all over again.

REFERENCES

Bell C 1832 The hand. Its mechanics and vital endowment as envincing design, 3rd edn. W. B. Pickering, London. p 162
Bowe J J 1963 Thumb construction by index transposition. Plastic and Reconstructive Surgery 32:414–424
Bralliar F, Horner R 1969 Sensory cross finger pedicle graft. Journal of Joint and Bone Surgery 51A:1264–1268
Brown H, Welling R, Sigman R, Flynn W, Flynn J E 1970 Phalangising the first metacarpal. Plastic and Reconstructive Surgery 45:294–297
Brown P 1972 Adduction-flexion contracture of the thumb. Correction with dorsal rotation flap and release of contracture. Clinical Orthopaedics and Related Research 88:161–168
Bruner J 1954 Salvage of the 'all but amputated' thumb. Plastic and Reconstructive Surgery 14:244–248
Buck-Gramcko D 1971 Pollicisation of the index finger. Method and results in aplasia and hypoplasia of the thumb. Journal of Bone and Joint Surgery 53A:1605–1617
Buncke H J, Buncke C M, Schultz W P 1966 Immediate Nicoladani procedure in rhesus monkey or hallux to hand transplantation utilising micro-miniature vascular anastomoses. British Journal of Plastic Surgery 19:332
Burton R I, Littler J W 1983 Thumb reconstruction. In: Evart's C M (ed) Surgery of the musculoskeletal system, 1st edn. Churchill Livingstone, New York. Vol 1, sec. 2, ch 19, p 501–519
Chase R A 1969 An alternate to pollicisation in subtotal thumb reconstruction. Plastic and Reconstructive Surgery 44:421–430
Cobbett R R 1969 Free digital transfer. Journal of Bone and Joint Surgery 51B:677
Flatt A E 1964 An indication for shortening of the thumb. Description of technique and brief report of five cases. Journal of Bone and Joint Surgery 46A:1534–1539
Foucher G, Merle M, Maneraud M, Michon J 1980 Microsurgical free partial toe transfer in hand reconstruction. Plastic and Reconstructive Surgery 65:616
Gaul J S 1969 Radial innervated cross finger flap from index to provide sensory pulp to injured thumb. Journal of Bone and Joint Surgery 51A:1257–1263
Gillies H, Millard D R 1957 In: The principles and art of plastic surgery. Little, Brown Co, Boston. Vol 2, p 484–488
Harkins P, Rafferty J 1972 Digital transposition in the injured hand. Journal of Bone and Joint Surgery 54A:1064–1069
Harrison S 1973 Pollicisation for congenital deformities of the hand. Proceedings of the Royal Society of Medicine 66:1–4
Hentz V R 1985 Conventional techniques for thumb reconstruction. Clinical Orthopaedics and Related Research 195:129–143
Hentz V R, Littler J W 1977 The surgical management of congenital hand anomalies. In: Converse J (ed) Reconstructive Plastic Surgery, vol 6, 2nd edn. W B Saunders, Philadelphia. Ch 79, p 3306–3349
Hentz V R, Littler J W 1977 Abduction-pronation and recession of (2nd) metacarpal in thumb agenesis. Journal of Hand Surgery 2:113–117
Kelleher J C 1972 Pollicisation. In: Goldwyn R M (ed). The unfavourable result in plastic surgery. Avoidance and treatment. Little, Brown and Co, Boston. Ch 33, p 475–488
Lister G D, Kalisman M, Tsai T M 1983 Microvascular toe to hand transfers. Plastic and Reconstructive Surgery 71:372
Littler J W 1952 Subtotal reconstruction of the thumb. Plastic and Reconstructive Surgery 10:215–226
Littler J W 1953 The neurovascular pedicle method of digital transposition for reconstruction of the thumb. Plastic and Reconstructive Surgery 12:303–319
Littler J W 1966 Digital transposition. In: Adams J P (ed) Current Practice in Orthopaedic Surgery, Vol 3. C V Mosby, St Louis. Ch 8, p 157–172
Littler J W 1974 Restoration of the amputated thumb. In: Symposium on frequent hand problems in plastic and reconstructive surgery, Vol 9. C V Mosby, St Louis. Ch 20, p 202–213
Littler J W 1976 On making a thumb: 100 years of surgical effort. Journal of Hand Surgery 1:35–51
Littler J W 1977 Reconstruction of the thumb in traumatic loss. In: Converse J M (ed), Reconstructive Plastic Surgery, 2nd edn. W B Saunders, Philadelphia. Ch 80, p 3350–3367
Manske P R, McCarroll H R 1985 Index finger pollicisation for a congenitally absent or non-functioning thumb. Journal of Hand Surgery 10A:606–613
Matev I B 1970 Thumb reconstruction after amputation at the metacarpophalangeal joint by bone lengthening. Journal of Bone and Joint Surgery 52A:957–965
Matev I B 1979 Thumb reconstruction in children through metacarpal lengthening. Plastic and Reconstructive Surgery 64:665–669
McFarlane R M, Stromberg W B 1962 Resurfacing of the thumb following major skin loss. Journal of Bone and Joint Surgery 44A:1365–1374
McGregor I A 1969 Less than satisfactory experiences with neurovascular island flaps. Hand 1:21–22
Miura T 1973 Thumb reconstruction using radial-innervated cross finger pedicle graft. Journal of Bone and Joint Surgery 55A:563–569
Morrison W A, O'Brien B M, MacLeod A M 1980 Thumb reconstruction with free neurovascular wrap-around flap from the big toe. Journal of Hand Surgery 5:575–583
Morrison W A, O'Brien B M, MacLeod A M, Gilbert A 1978 Neurovascular free flaps from the foot for innervation of the hand. Journal of Hand Surgery 3:235–242
Murray J F 1974 The missing thumb. In: Symposium on frequent hand problems in plastic and reconstructive surgery, vol 9. C V Mosby, St Louis. Ch 21, p 214–222
Murray J F, Ord J V, Gavelin G E 1967 The neurovascular island pedicle flap. An assessment of late results in sixteen cases. Journal of Bone and Joint Surgery 49A:1285–1297
O'Brien B, MacLeod A M, Black M M, Morrison W A 1978 Microvascular great toe transfer for congenital absence of the thumb. Hand 10:113
Poppen N K, Norris T R, Buncke H J 1983 Evaluation of sensibility and function with microsurgical free tissue transfer of the great toe to the hand for thumb reconstruction. Journal of Hand Surgery 8:516–531
Posner M A, Smith R J 1971 The advancement pedicle flap for

thumb injuries. Journal of Bone and Joint Surgery 53A:1618–1621

Reid D A C 1969 Pollicisation—an appraisal. Hand 1:27–31

Sallis J G 1963 Primary pollicisation of an injured middle finger. Journal of Bone and Joint Surgery 45B:503–505

Schlenker J D, Kleinert H E, Tsai T M 1980 Methods and results of replantation following traumatic amputation of the thumb in sixty-four patients. Journal of Hand Surgery 5:63–70

Stern P J, Lister G D 1981 Pollicisation after traumatic amputation of the thumb. Clinical Orthopaedics and Related Research 155:85

Tanzer R C, Littler J W 1948 Reconstruction of the thumb by transposition of an adjacent digit. Plastic and Reconstructive Surgery 3:533–547

Tubiana R, Duparc J 1961 Restoration of sensibility in the hand by neurovascular skin island transfer. Journal of Bone and Joint Surgery 43B:474–480

Tubiana R, Roux J P 1974 Phalangisation of the first and fifth metacarpals. Indications, operative technique and results. Journal of Bone and Joint Surgery 56A:447–457

White W F 1970 Fundamental priorities in pollicisation. Journal of Bone and Joint Surgery 52B:438–443

J. F. Murray

10 Amputations

Amputation of one or more digits of the hand is a common operation. While a few are done for vascular problems and malignant tumours, the vast majority are the result of trauma or its sequelae. It is one of the most frequent causes of permanent disability in patients with industrial hand injuries. There is an obvious physical impairment of function but there are also varying degress of less obvious psychological pathology in the form of depression, introversion, phobias, and nightmares as a result of the anatomical loss of an exposed part of the body. How severe this is depends more on the patient's personality, emotional stability, cultural background and home environment than on the extent of the loss in the hand.

Ratliff (1974) confirmed the observation of Rank et al (1968) that 'complications of finger amputations are distressing and common place'. In his series, one-third of 61 digit amputations performed by casualty officers and registrars developed complications. Thompson (1963) stressed the importance of primary care and showed that healing time was prolonged fourfold when amputations of fingers were done by untrained and unsupervised personnel. The operation requires the facilities, planning, and technical expertise of any hand operation if infection, haematoma, and ischemic or tight skin flaps are to be avoided. These are the forerunners of delayed healing, joint stiffness, and unsatisfactory stumps that in some cases prolong rehabilitation interminably.

THE PAINFUL STUMP

An amputation results in the loss of all or part of the involved digit or digits but a single chronically painful stump impairs the function of the whole hand and also ignites the debilitating problems associated with chronic pain. There are many causes for a painful stump and often more than one is present but, from the point of view of treatment, we can recognise two main groups. Pain and tenderness that emanates from the transsected sensory nerves, that is, neuroma pain, and pain and tenderness from other causes.

Neuroma pain

The clinical manifestations of neuroma pain reflect the events that occur around all the transsected sensory nerves in the stump. Within 24 hours axone sprouting takes place and for about 2 weeks they randomly invade the adjacent traumatised tissue. The neurotrophic effect of denervated skin in the area promotes ingrowth of fibres but most will end up in a disorganised mass enmeshed in connective tissue that we recognise clinically as a neuroma. The histology of a neuroma has been studied in primates and has been shown to vary with its environment (Mackinnon et al 1985). Connective tissue surrounds the disorganised network of nerve fibres. It comprises 80% of the neuroma bulk and contains myofibroblasts that gradually diminish in number (Badalamente et al 1985). Immediately under a scar, nerve filaments grow from the neuroma into the scar and adjacent skin. When the transsected nerve lies in a healthy subcutaneous bed the same sized neuroma develops but there are no sprouting fibres growing into the overlying skin. When the nerve is transplanted into muscle, the fibres are orderly, do not invade and are surrounded by half the amount of connective tissue. Spontaneous and mechanically induced electrical activity originating in the neuroma of a primate has been demonstrated, as well as evidence of re-innervation of denervated skin (Meyer et al 1985). In addition changes occur centrally in the dorsal route ganglion and dorsal horn of the spinal cord (Wall 1983). Sympathetic efferent fibres may stimulate an injured nerve through noradrenaline release and effect a release of chemical pain mediators (Holder & Mackinnon 1984).

Clinical presentations

Although the foregoing takes place around the divided sensory nerves, the majority of patients do not have neuroma pain problems after amputation. When they occur in digit amputations symptoms may be due to the neuroma, the fibres re-innervating denervated skin or both. Neuroma pain (Fig. 10.1 a and b) is localised and emanates from a precise point of tenderness that emits electrical shock sensations with pressure or when gently tapped. Usually it is from a digital nerve incorporated in the stump scar, lies against bone with inadequate padding, or is very superficial under a flexion crease. Branches of the digital nerves or terminal dorsal nerves can cause pinhead sized, tender nodules in the scar. Reinnervated stump skin has altered sensation when it is lightly stroked that varies from an innocuous dysesthesia to disturbing hyperaesthesia. (Fig. 10.1 c) The richly innervated volar skin is primarily involved and the extent of its involvement is evident by a hyperemic blush. If an arm tourniquet is inflated to above systolic pressure the hyperaesthesia gradually diminishes and disappears within 3–5 minutes whereas neuroma tenderness increases. Hyperaesthesia dominates neuroma problems that follow ray amputations (Fig. 10.1d). It was present in over half and significantly interfered with function or virtually disabled 15 of 41 patients with index ray amputations (Murray et al 1978). It is also an annoying complication of a V–Y volar pulp advancement flap for finger tip amputations (Atasoy et al 1970) and neurovascular island flaps when they have been partially denervated by the operation (Fig. 10.1e).

Prevention

Neuroma formation is a constant phenomenon following division of a sensory nerve but 'chronic and disabling pain problems are almost never observed among patients who have experienced rapid primary wound healing followed by early active motion' (Beasley 1981). Primary wound healing ensures healthy environment and minimal scar formation for the terminally divided nerves and a correlation between delayed healing after the initial injury and the severity of the neuroma symptoms has been observed (Laboarde 1982). Early active motion diminishes joint stiffness, promotes the use of the whole hand and is indicative of a well motivated patient.

There are technical details in the operation that help to avoid neuroma problems. In traumatic amputations the neurovascular bundles must be identified on each side and the artery and nerve gently separated. The artery is tied with fine ligature as far distally as possible to ensure a good blood supply to the whole volar flap. It is not known just where branches that innervate a specific area come off the digital nerve but sensation in a volar flap does not seem to be altered if it is resected approximately a centimetre from the wound edge. Dorsal nerves are easily identified in elective amputations and should be cut a few millimetres from the skin margin. If nerves are cauterised with bipolar electrocautery at the level of nerve resection the nerve fibres are destroyed locally, the resulting neuroma is smaller (Gosset 1979, Panagiotis & Defanco 1961) and theoretically the coagulated epineurium seals in the nerve filaments. Hyperaesthesia that complicates ray amputations can be avoided if normal sensation is preserved in the palmar skin involved in wound closure. The digital (and any significant sized nerves) are not resected proximal to the wound edge but rather they are divided about 3 cm within the stump or finger to be amputated (Fig. 10.2a). These 'skeletonised' nerves are transplanted and tacked loosely in a protected area under interosseus muscle of the deleted ray or in some cases into the metacarpal bone (Fig. 10.2b). Gorkisch et al (1983) report prevention of neuroma symptoms in ray amputations by 'centro-central nerve union with autologous transplantation'. The resected nerve ends are

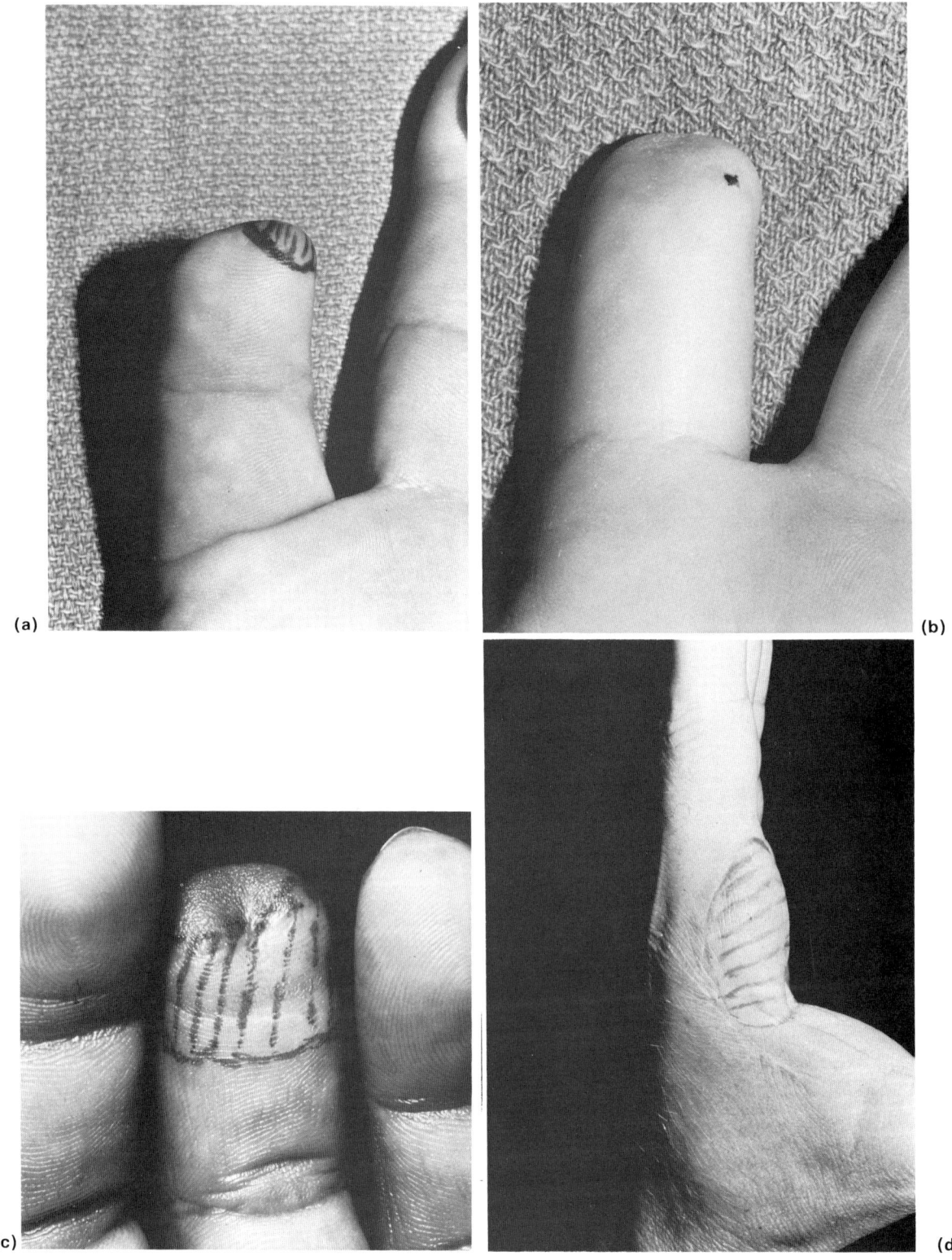

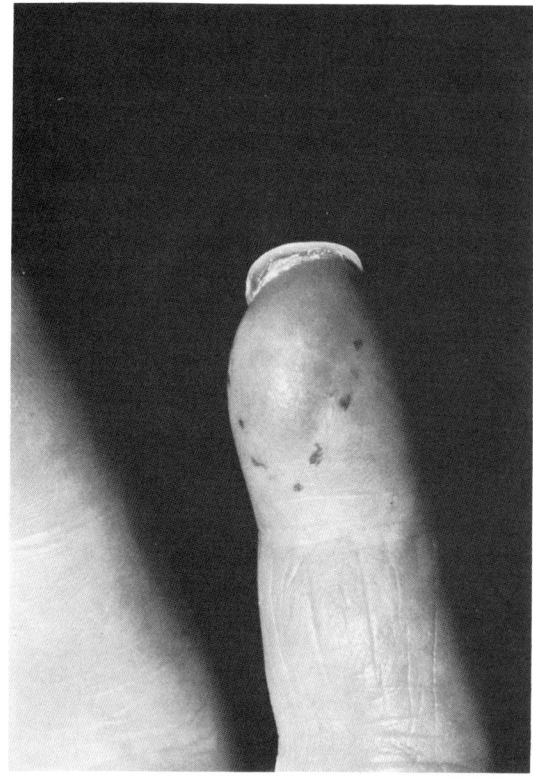

(e)

Fig. 10.1 (a) A localised neuroma in the stump scar of an otherwise healthy amputation stump. (b) Localised neuroma lying immediately under the PIP flexion crease. (c) Hyperaesthetic volar skin associated with neuroma in a digit amputation. The involved area has atrophy of the papillary ridges and is outlined by a faint blush of the skin. (d) The common site of hyperaesthesia involving palmar skin following index ray amputation. (e) Hyperaesthesia of the flap following a 'V–Y' pulp advancement for a finger tip amputation

sutured together, one of them is again divided about 1 cm proximally and sutured at this site. This creates a small nerve graft to trap sprouting axones from each nerve end within an epineurial cuff.

Conservative treatment

The majority of patients with amputation neuroma pain should be given time, at least 3 months, and a trial of non-operative treatment. The guidance and support of a hand therapist using a combination of measures that promote maturation and softening of the tissues, desensitising techniques and getting the patient to use the hand often succeeds in relieving symptoms. It is also an opportunity for the therapist to assess the patient's pain threshold and tolerance and learn of socio-psychological problems that are important when making a decision for surgery.

Operative treatment

The many methods advocated for the surgical management of neuroma pain is evidence of the success of all, some of the time, and of none all of the time. It also suggests that the surgery should be tailored to the clinical presentation of the neuroma pain rather than use a 'routine' operation for all cases. Generally speaking the more complex methods should be reserved for patients who have not benefited from the operation that inflicts the least operative trauma on the painful stump.

Neurectomy. Simple neurectomy is the procedure of choice for all well healed, well vascularised stumps with localised neuroma pain and tenderness. Tupper & Booth (1976) and Tupper (1981) found that it gave results that were comparable to more complex operations. Bipolar cauterisation at the resection site adds nothing to the complexity of the surgery and, as previously noted, has been shown to result in a smaller neuroma. Paradini (1979) had fewer recurrences in patients treated with neurectomy and electrocautery than in a similar series treated by neurectomy alone. Neuromas invading a stump scar are isolated with the scar (Fig. 10.3a), the parent nerve is teased from the subcutaneous fibro-fatty tissue, the scar and neuroma gently drawn distally, resected and

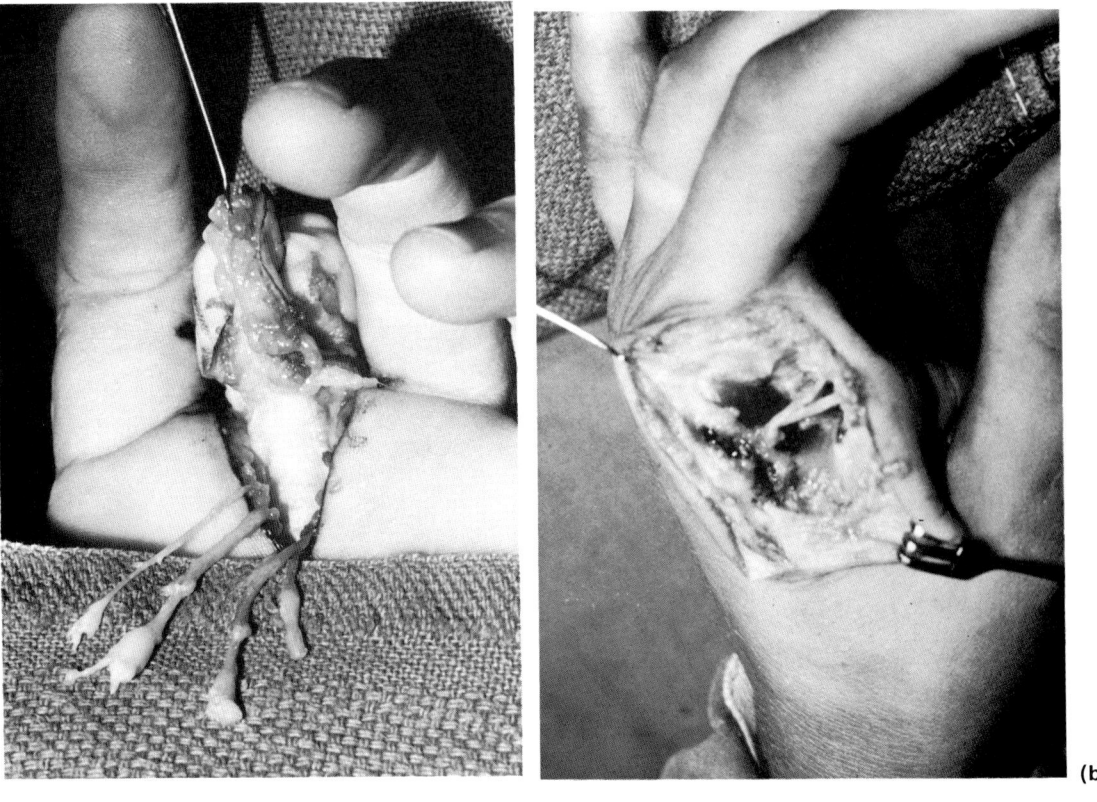

Fig. 10.2 (a) Skeletonising nerves from the stump prior to a fourth ray amputation. (b) Skeletonised nerves from an amputated index finger transplanted dorsally to be covered by first dorsal interosseus muscle. The innervation of palmar skin that is involved in the wound closure is not disturbed

allowed to retract into a scar free bed. Those neuroma not invading scar are isolated after identifying the digital nerve proximal to it and dissecting distally (Fig. 10.3b).

Transplant of neuroma. The intact neuroma is removed from a tender, frequently traumatised site of a stump and when transferred to a healthy well padded protracted environment a hypersensitive neuroma appears to undergo change and lose much of its hypersensitivity (Herndon et al 1976).

The events that occur in terminal resected nerves are avoided by keeping the fibrous capsule of the well formed neuroma intact. A suture of 5-0 catgut is tied to the neuroma capsule. A second knot is made on this suture a few millimetres from the neuroma and the free ends are attached to a straight needle to guide it into the selected, protected site. The needle is passed through the overlying skin and as the suture is withdrawn it is blocked by the second knot at the dermis as the neuroma is kept in the subcutaneous layer. The suture ends are tied at the skin. To avoid traction pain the nerve must not be under tension or transferred into muscle with fibre excursion that could create tension. In hyperaesthetic digital stumps both nerves should be transferred.

In amputations the method is more suited for neuroma problems in short stumps and especially when neuromas lie on the digital palmar crease of a finger or against the proximal phalanx of the thumb where there is little padding and repeated pressure with gripping. In these locations they can be moved to the more sheltered confines of an interdigital cleft or a cushion of muscle (Fig. 10.4). It is not a good method for amputations distal to the proximal interphalangeal joint. Considerable mobilisation of the digital nerve, and therefore denervation of the volar skin is required, and the

AMPUTATIONS 145

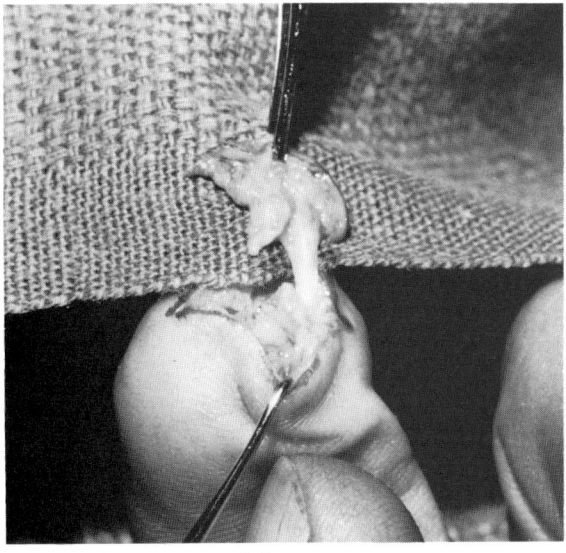

(a)

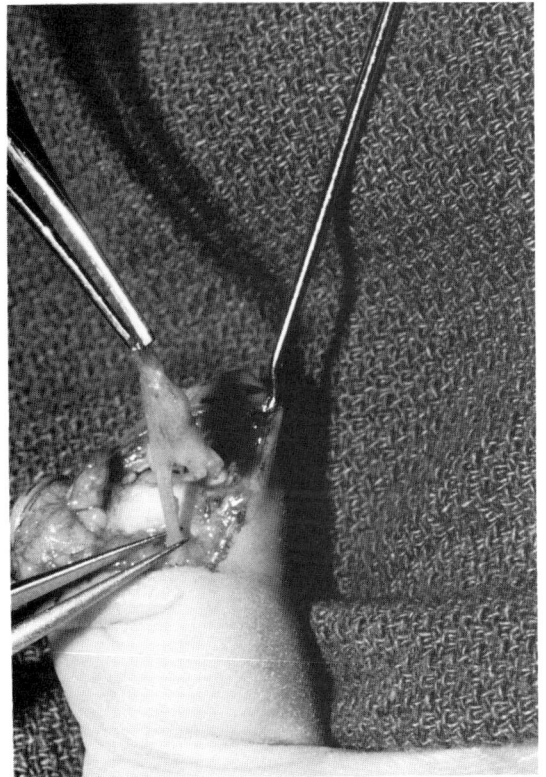

(b)

Fig. 10.3 (a) A neuroma invading stump scar (Fig. 10.1a) is mobilised with segment of scar involved and the nerve traced proximally. (b) Neuroma lying beneath the flexion crease (Fig 10.1b) has been isolated after isolating the digital nerve and dissecting distally. Bipolar cautery is applied at the site of nerve resection and the proximal end allowed to retract

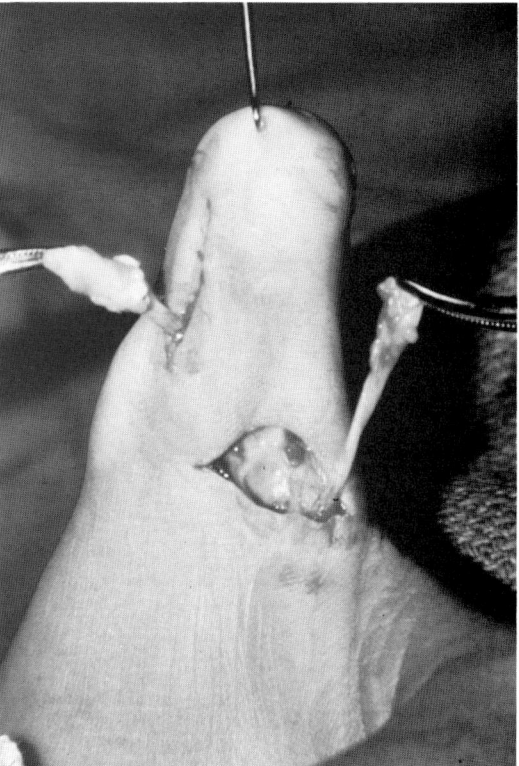

Fig. 10.4 Neuromas at the base of a thumb stump transplanted from area of pressure

only 'protected' site is the lateral or dorsal surface of the stump. It may be less frequently traumatised than on the palmar surface but the neuroma lies on poorly cushioned bone and, at this level of amputation, it is still subject to frequent unexpected trauma.

Revision of amputation stump. The importance of preserving length in a digit, especially the thumb, is one of the commandments of amputation surgery of the hand. Far more important to the function of the hand is comfort! There should be no hesitation about sacrificing length in the interest of comfort at the initial surgery or when certain types of painful stumps are encountered.

When neuroma pain is associated with hyperaesthesia of volar skin of the stump distal to the proximal interphalangeal joint the hyperaesthetic zone should be excised, the neuroma isolated and the bone shortened enough to permit a dorsal flap closure of the wound (Fig. 10.5a). The neuroma is

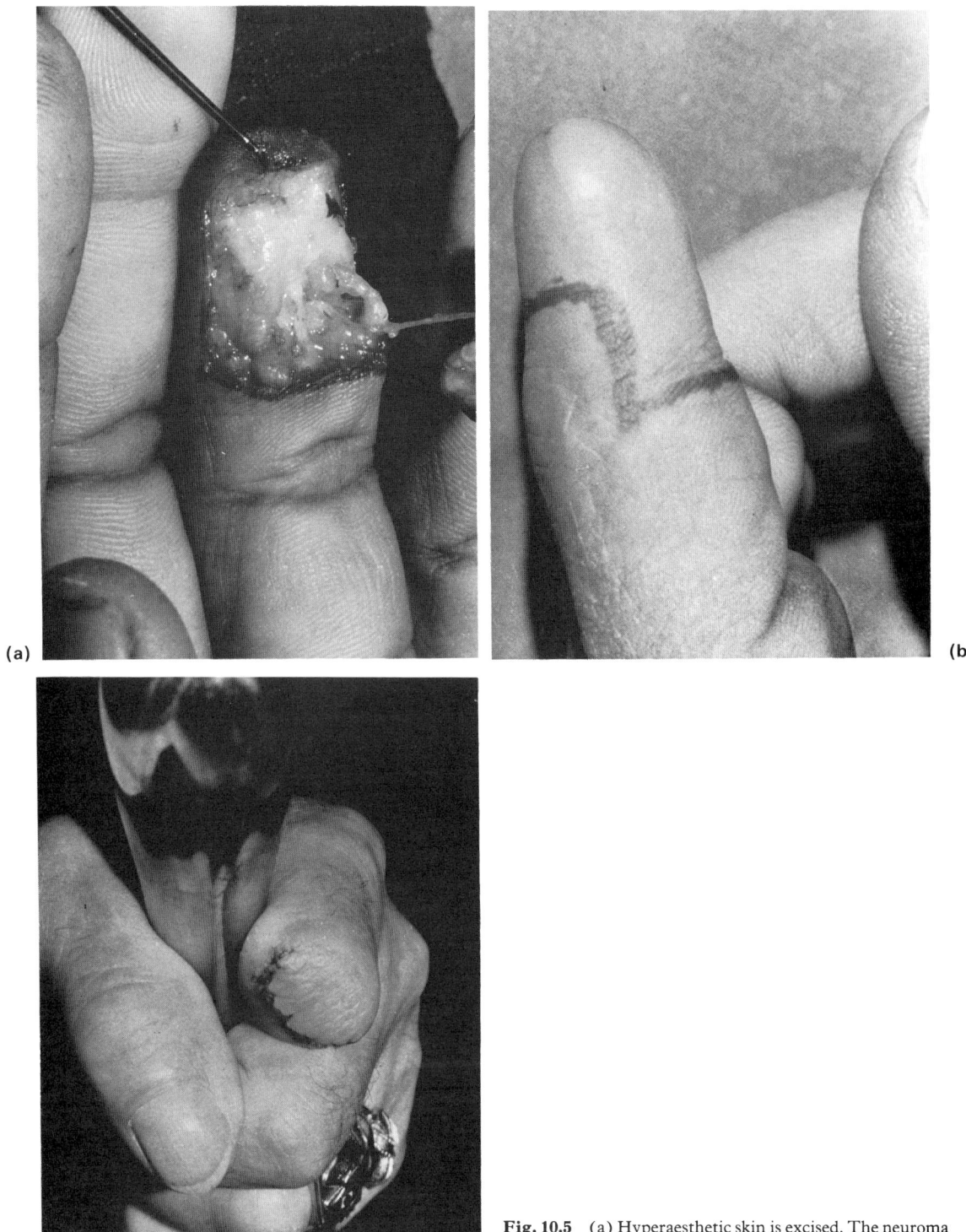

Fig. 10.5 (a) Hyperaesthetic skin is excised. The neuroma cauterised and resected and the stump closed with a dorsal flap following shortening of the phalanx. (b) A diffusely sensitive atrophic stump distal to markings. (c) Following re-amputation

treated by neurectomy and bipolar cauterisation of the nerve.

Re-amputation is required for neuromas encased in tight, atrophic, indurated, sensitive, and often cyanotic flaps (Fig. 10.5b and c). It must be done at the level of soft pliable tissue with normal sensation. There are cases when it might be possible to skeletonise a length of digital nerve from the dystrophic area and transplant it into the bone of the phalanx without tension (Goldstein and Sturim 1985). Laborde et al (1982) noted in a series of 50 patients that the 12 ray amputations that were done for recurrent painful neuroma had the highest reoperation rate and poorest results. One must be particularly cautious about deleting the ray of a digit that has had many operations for neuroma pain. It is particularly important in these people to preserve the normal sensation in the palmar skin as outlined above.

Surgeons tend to identify a single cause for a problem but many factors play a role in the success of failure of operations for pain. In recalcitrant cases, the psyche, pain threshold, monetary gain, job dissatisfaction etc., are more significant causes of failure than the surgery but sometimes this is only appreciated after multiple operations. Patients who demand stump revisions in spite of many previous failures may be examples of mania-operativa, an obsession with pain and disability and seeking relief by repeated surgery (Hunter & Kinnard 1982). We must accept the fact that there are chronic pain problems following amputations in the hand that cannot be 'cured' by peripheral surgery.

Other causes of stump pain

These may be associated with neuroma problems but when there is no clinical evidence of neuroma the 'quiet' neuroma should not be explored or disturbed.

Bony irregularities

All tender stumps must be X-rayed. A bony spur or sequestrated bone fragment can cause localised tenderness similar to a neuroma but without the electric shock quality. Surgical removal gives prompt and lasting relief.

Inadequate padding

These are soft pliable stumps except over the resected bone where there is an inadequate cushion of fat. It may be the result of overstretched dorsal flaps or thin volar flaps that include the flexion crease. Surgical treatment does not involve merely shortening the phalanx but also discarding the thinned covering and resecting enough bone to permit closure with well padded flaps. Inadequate padding also occurs in digit tip amputations through the terminal phalanx that have been covered with a full thickness graft that does not contract and therefore does not draw in the surrounding pulp for padding. Local advancement or local pedicle flaps, sometimes with bone shortening are necessary to provide padding.

Painful nail deformities

1. *Parrot-beak or hooked nail deformity* (Fig. 10.6a). The nail and its matrix are supported by the dorsum of the terminal phalanx with its broad, flat, fan shaped, tuft and the interosseus ligaments that join each end of the tuft to the base of the terminal phalanx. When this support is lost, the nail curves volarly. How much it curves depends on how much support is lost, how much nail bed extends beyond the bone and the degree of scar contracture in the distal pulp. When some of the tuft of the terminal phalanx remains, the interosseus ligaments are intact and the deformity is minimal. This can be relieved by pulp advancement procedures. Operations have been described (Verdan 1981, Atasoy et al 1983) to improve the appearance of more pronounced deformities but probably the best cosmesis is provided by a finger prosthesis (Pillet 1981). In severe cases, the nail covers the end of the digit. It is unsightly, tender and painful where it digs into the volar pulp and should be treated by revision of the amputation and with removal of all nail matrix (Fig. 10.6a).

2. *Nail spurs and cysts* (Fig. 10.6b and c). These seemingly simple problems can, in fact, be very difficult to cure because the germinal matrix that spawns them is not easy to identify. Nail spurs appear a few weeks after the wound is healed and have the discomfort of a chronic hang nail. Cysts may grow slowly over months or even years.

148 UNSATISFACTORY RESULTS IN HAND SURGERY

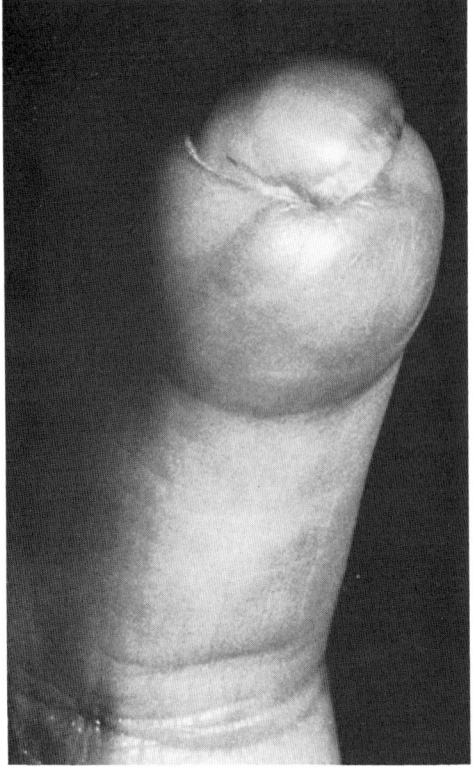

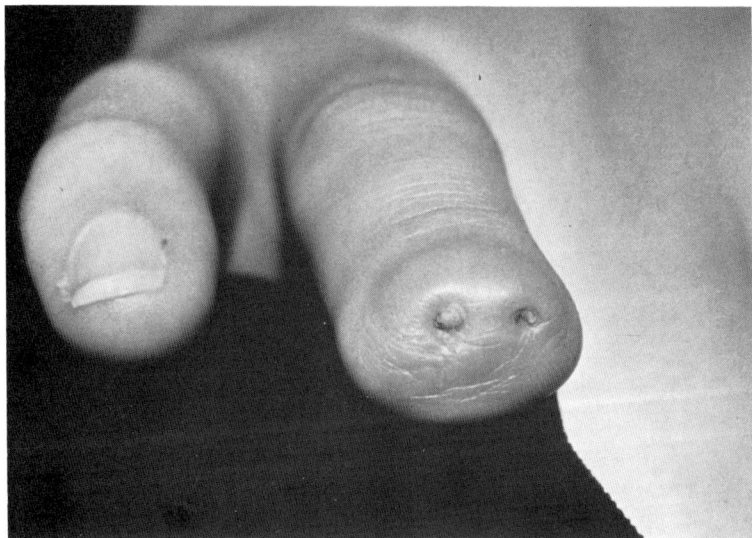

Fig. 10.6 (a) A hooked or parrot-beak deformity of the nail. Note the edge growing into pulp. This degree of hooked nail should be treated by excision of nail matrix and skin graft or re-amputation depending on the quality of the distal pulp. (b) and (c) Nail spurs and nail inclusion cysts that require wide exposure for complete excision of the germinal nail matrix. (d) Exposure for removal of nail cyst and remnants of the germinal nail matrix. Wide exposure is essential to identify all remnants of germinal nail matrix and avoid damage to the extensor tendon insertion

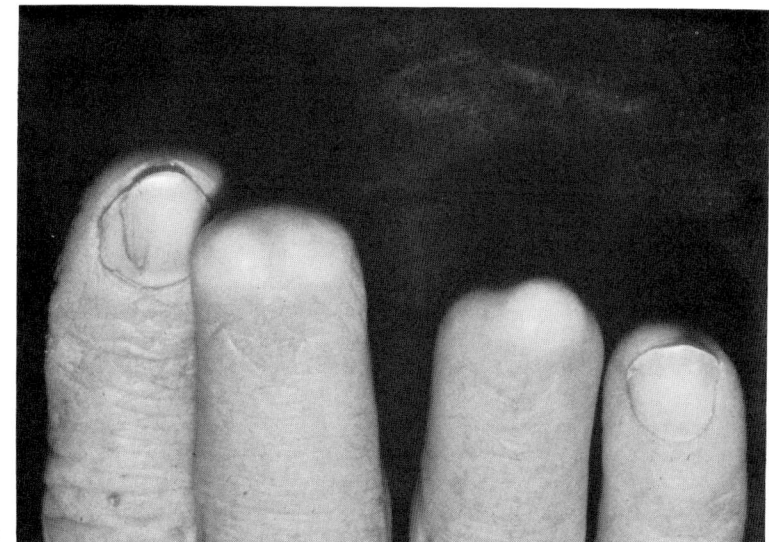

(c)

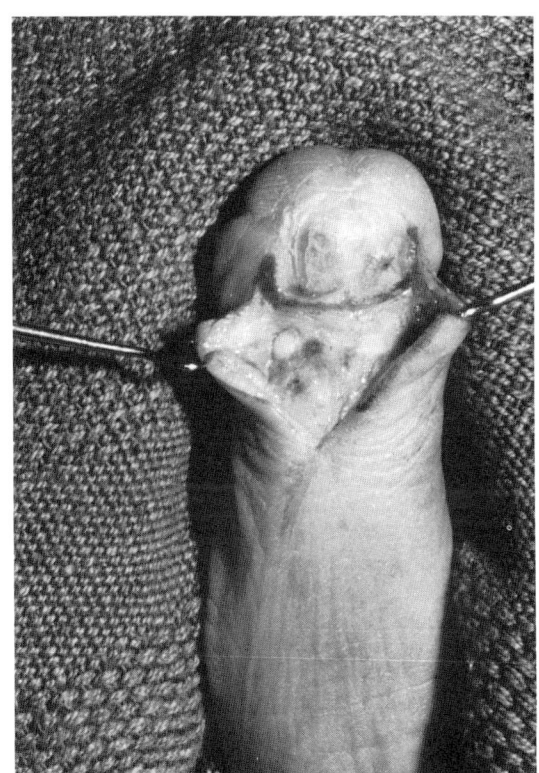

(d)

Generous exposure and loop magnification is essential to remove all remnants of the germinal matrix responsible for all these problems if recurrence is to be avoided (Fig. 10.6d).

TENDON PROBLEMS FOLLOWING FINGER AMPUTATIONS

The tendons of amputated fingers can cause impaired function and symptoms that are often overlooked or not recognised. These include profundus tendon blockage (the quadriga syndrome) the lumbrical plus syndrome, intrinsic plus deformity, weakness of stump flexion, palm tenderness and carpal tunnel syndrome.

Profundus tendon blockage (quadriga syndrome)

The disability involves the *uninjured* fingers. The syndrome of quadriga is a term coined by Verdan (1960) to describe the profundus tendon imbalance that results if this tendon is advanced and sewn over the stump of an amputated finger. The same imbalance occurs if excursion of the resected profundus tendon of an amputated finger is restricted by adhesions that develop spontaneously after a primary traumatic amputation or are present in elective amputations that are done for failed tendon surgery or post-traumatic joint stiffness (Neu et al 1985). Because of the common muscle origin of the profundi, the interconnection of its tendons proximal to the carpal tunnel and the origin of the lumbrical muscles just distal to the carpal tunnel, adhesions of a profundus tendon in the palm or an amputation stump will restrict or 'block' the full excursion of profundi going to the intact fingers (Fig. 10.7a).

Clinical presentation

The patient has weakness of grip for small calibre objects and often inability to make a fully clenched fist. Some patients experience a cramping pain in the wrist and forearm with repetitive gripping. This is thought to be due to stretching of synovium in the carpal tunnel between the adherent and non-adherent tendons and to the shearing stress between muscle fibres going to the fixed and free tendons. There is full flexion and power of the distal interphalangeal joints of the intact fingers when the proximal two joints are held extended but, when the patient makes a fist, there may be no flexion or power in the terminal phalanx (Grade III—Fig. 10.8a) reduced flexion and power (Grade II) or full flexion but reduced power (Grade I). In the small finger, a Grade III blockage will reduce flexion of the proximal interphalangeal joint if the superficialis is weak or absent.

Prevention

Profundus tendon blockage is prevented after primary traumatic amputation by early mobilisation of all the intact fingers and amputation stumps through their full range of movement during the first week after injury. All elective amputations for post-traumatic stiffness or failed tendon surgery should have the profundus tendon to the finger resected in the palm at the time of amputation.

Surgical treatment

Some patients with a Grade II blockage and most with Grade III, in one or more fingers, are candidates for operation. The profundus tendon to the amputated finger or fingers is exposed through an extensile incision in the palm. In most single finger amputations the tendon will be adherent in the stump or near the entrance of its fibrosseus tunnel in the palm. The site of fixation does not need to be exposed. The profundus is divided proximal to it and separated from the overlying superficialis down to the origin of the lumbrical muscle. It must glide freely through the carpal tunnel before it is divided at this level and a segment removed. If the amputated finger has a functioning proximal interphalangeal joint, the lumbrical tendon going to the stump should be resected to prevent a lumbrical plus problem occurring in the amputated finger. Adhesions of the profundus tendon can occur at the palmar entrance of the carpal tunnel and a more extensive exposure and excision of all tethered tendons and tenolysis of the intact ones at this level is required. This occurs occasionally in single finger amputa-

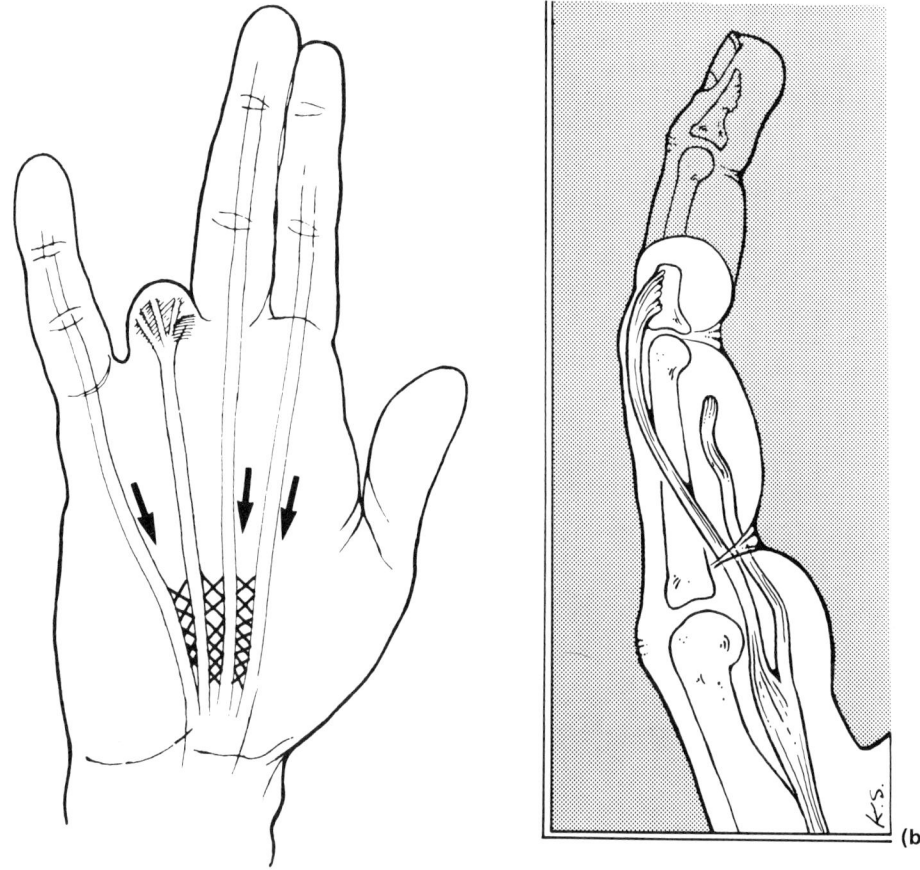

Fig. 10.7 (a) Profundus tendon blockage. The adherent stump of the profundus tendon impedes full proximal excursion of the profundi to intact fingers. (b) The lumbrical plus syndrome. Retraction of the nonadherent resected end of the profundus tendon results in its force being transferred to the lumbrical muscle and extensor expansion. Extension of the mid-phalanx stump occurs as the lumbrical origin moves proximally with attempted flexing of the finger

tions but is more common when more than one has been amputated.

The lumbrical plus finger (Parkes 1970)

Although this condition also involves the profundus tendon, the pathomechanics is totally different from profundus tendon blockage (freely moving verses an adherent tendon) and the disability involves the amputated finger and only those fingers amputated distal to a mobile proximal interphalangeal joint (Fig. 10.7b). The patient appears to be quite uncooperative because attempts to flex the proximal interphalangeal joint of the stump result in active extension. It is due to the proximal migration of the profundus tendon with the lumbrical origin after its insertion is detached from the distal phalanx. 'Paradoxical extension' occurs when the patient attempts to flex and the power of the profundus is diverted to the extensor expansion via the lumbrical insertion.

The problem is corrected surgically by division of the lumbrical tendon just proximal to its insertion into the extensor expansion. This should be done as a prophylactic measure when a finger is amputated through the middle phalanx.

Intrinsic plus deformity

This is an iatrogenic deformity that occurs mainly in the long finger after an index ray amputation. To increase the abduction and flexion power of the

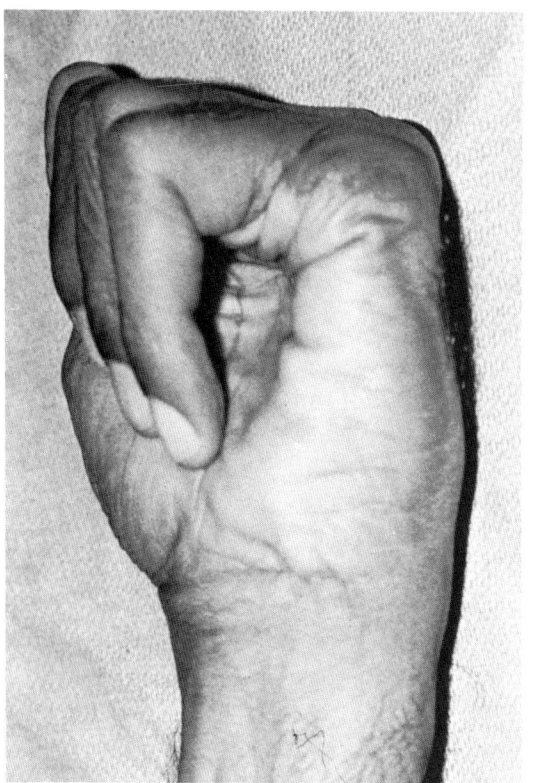
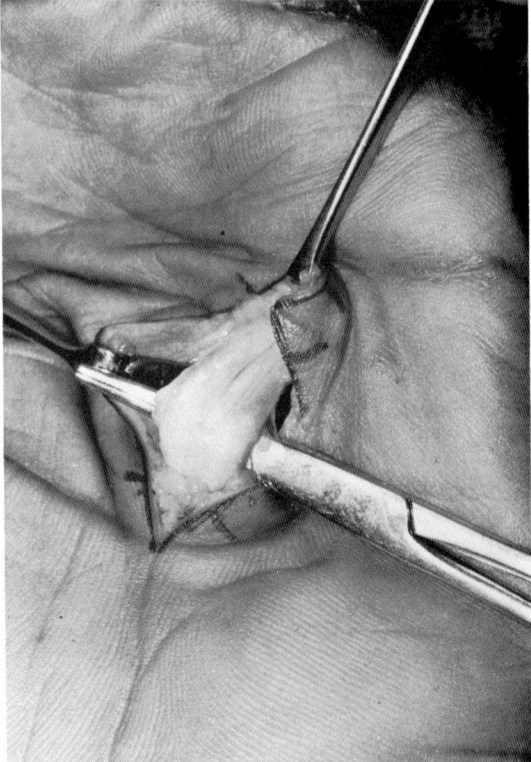
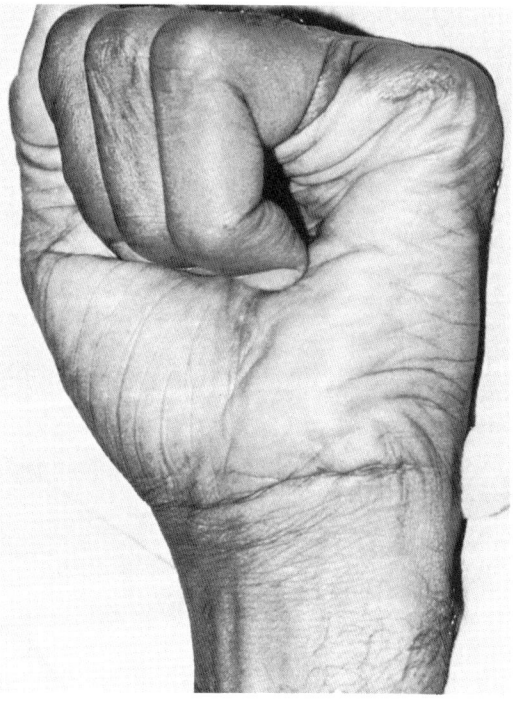

Fig. 10.8 (a) A Grade III profundus tendon blockage of the ring and long fingers following small finger amputation at the MP joint. (b) The profundus tendon is firmly adherent distal to the operative site. (c) Full flexion restored in terminal phalanges of ring and long fingers following release of the adherent profundus in little finger stump

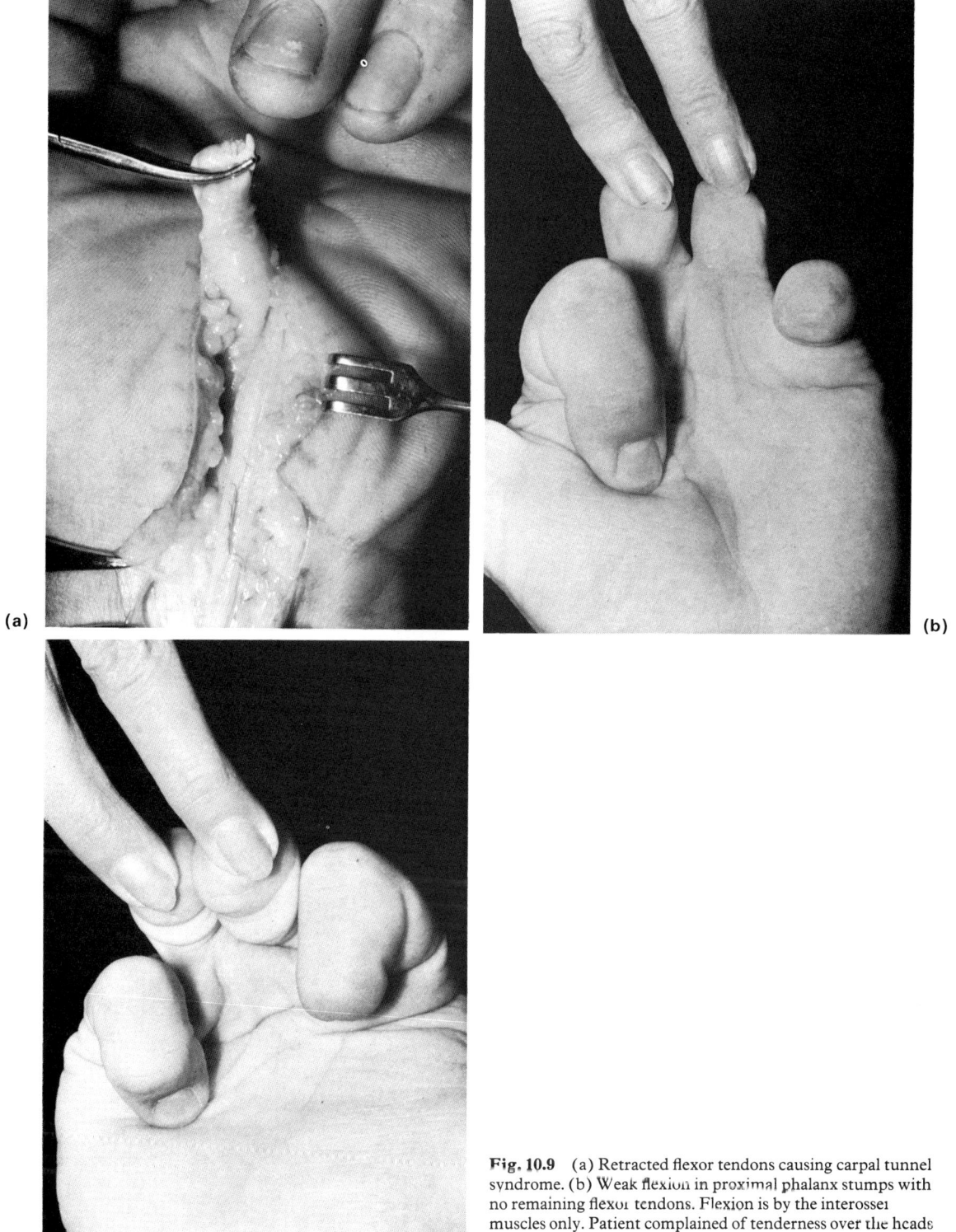

Fig. 10.9 (a) Retracted flexor tendons causing carpal tunnel syndrome. (b) Weak flexion in proximal phalanx stumps with no remaining flexor tendons. Flexion is by the interossei muscles only. Patient complained of tenderness over the heads of the metacarpals. (c) Excellent power in stumps with superficialis tendons intact

154 UNSATISFACTORY RESULTS IN HAND SURGERY

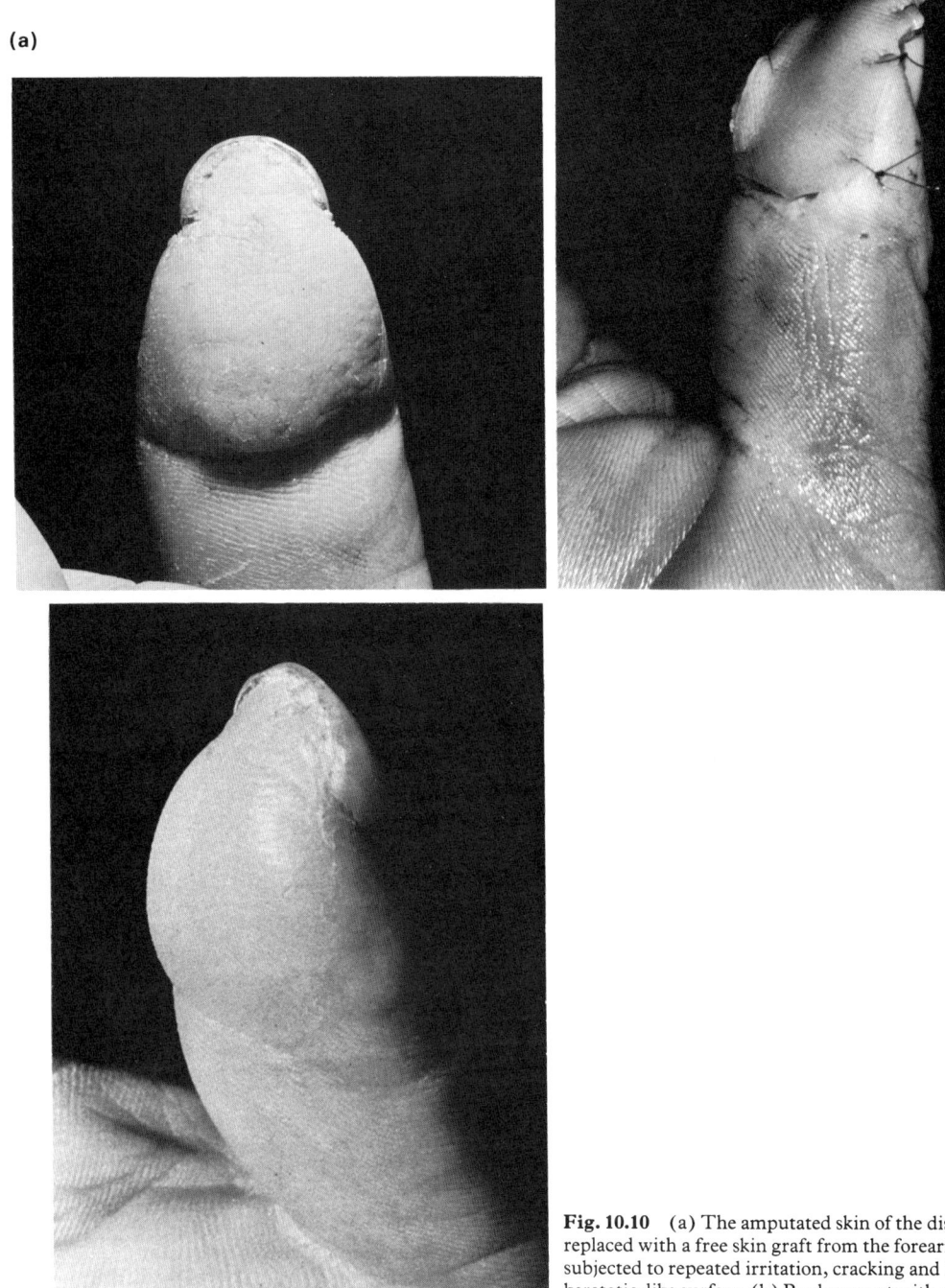

Fig. 10.10 (a) The amputated skin of the distal pulp has been replaced with a free skin graft from the forearm. It has been subjected to repeated irritation, cracking and has developed a keratotic-like surface. (b) Replacement with a free skin graft of a glabrous split skin graft from the hypothenar region. (c) Normal skin surface of pulp restored

long finger that is to assume the role of the deleted index, the tendon of the powerful first dorsal interosseus muscle if often incorporated into the radial side of the extensor hood of the middle finger. If attached with too much tension, it causes an intrinsic plus deformity with flexion of the metacarpophalangeal joint and hyperextension at the proximal interphalangeal joint. The important function of this muscle after index ray amputation is to provide a well padded contour for the thumb, long finger web and the tendon should be sutured without tension over the second dorsal interosseus muscle. When the deformity does occur it is easily corrected by a tenotomy of the tight first dorsal interosseus tendon.

Miscellaneous problems

The management of the flexor tendons in digit amputations has received rather casual attention. It has been mainly a case of pulling them down and cutting them off under tension so they will retract out of the way. Problems can occur with this manoeuvre in amputations through the proximal phalanx. If both tendons are resected under considerable tension they 'snap' back into the palm and form a ball of rolled up yellowish avascular tendon encased in thickened gelatinous synovium. The patient is aware of a fullness at the base of the palm of the hand that often increases in size and causes discomfort with heavy manual work. In addition to profundus tendon blockage, it can cause nerve compression symptoms by impinging on the sensory nerves that exit from the carpal tunnel (Fig. 10.9a). Furthermore the absence of both tendons from a proximal phalanx stump causes a decrease in its bulk, weak flexion and tenderness over the metacarpal head in the palm that no longer has the buffering effect of a tendon. The weakness is more pronounced in the long and

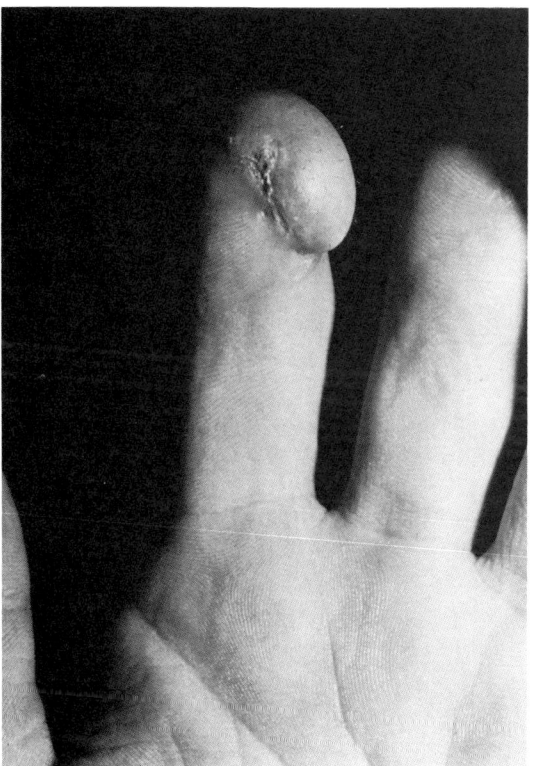
(a)

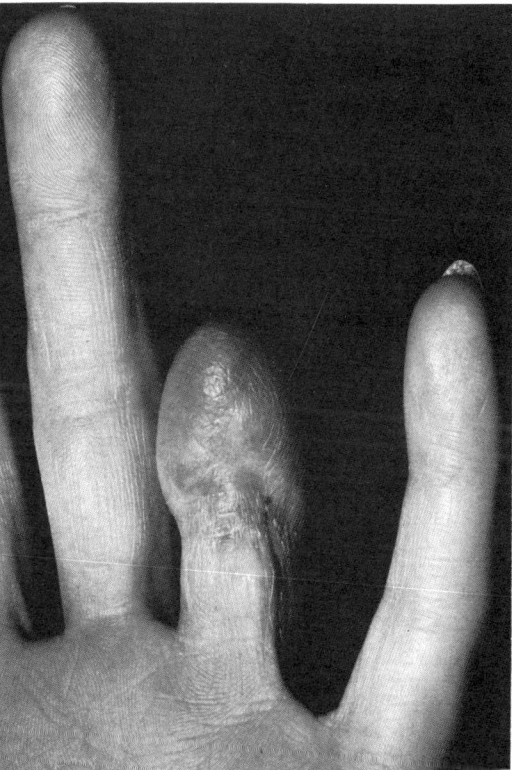
(b)

Fig. 10.11 (a) Distant pedicle flaps are not suitable for covering the ends of digit amputations. (b) Trunk flap to a ring avulsion injury that serves no functional use and is esthetically unacceptable. Treated by ring finger ray deletion

ring finger stumps that have less powerful intrinsic muscles to flex the proximal phalanx.

It is possible to avoid these problems. The profundus tendon is isolated and cut separately under gentle traction and allowed to retract. The superficialis is sutured under normal tension to the fibrosseus tunnel of the proximal phalanx and the independence of superficialis has no detrimental effect on the movement of the intact digits.

UNSATISFACTORY SKIN COVER IN AMPUTATIONS

Free skin grafts

These are the most frequently used grafts in digit tip amputations. The donor site is usually the forearm, inner arm, buttock or thigh. In black skin patients, deep pigmentation on the more lightly pigmented palmar skin is unsightly. The nonglabrous skin from the above donor sites, regardless of thickness, becomes dry, hypertrophic, fissured, and sensitive in patients whose hands are exposed to hard manual work, chemicals, machinery, or cold temperatures (Fig. 10.10a). These should be replaced with free grafts of glabrous skin from the ulnar side of the hypothenar eminence or, for larger areas, from the instep of the foot (Fig. 10.10b and c).

Abdominal pedicle flaps

Abdominal flaps are not suited for covering the end of an amputated digit (Fig. 10.11a). The functional inefficiency of insensitive skin on a blob of mobile abdominal fat is matched by its unsightly appearance and the joint stiffness that follows immobilisation required by the flap transfer. While avulsion injuries that deglove the thumb or multiple fingers may require a trunk flap, the hot dog appearance and function of a single finger avulsion amputation covered in this way is invariably a disappointment to the patient (Fig. 10.11b).

REFERENCES

Atasoy E, Ioakimidis E, Kasdan M L, Kutz J E, Kleinert H E 1970 Reconstruction of the amputated finger tip with a triangular volar flap. Journal of Bone and Joint Surgery (Am) 52:921–926

Atasoy E, Godfrey A, Kalasman M 1983 The 'antenna' procedure for the 'hook nail deformity'. Journal of Hand Surgery 8:55–58

Badalamente M A, Hurst L C, Ellstein J, McDevitt C A 1985 The pathobiology of human neuromas: An electron microscopic and biochemical study. Journal of Hand Surgery 10-b:49–53

Beasley R 1981 Surgery of hand and finger amputations. Orthopedic Clinics of North America 12:763–803

Gosset J Surgical diathermy in the prevention and treatment of amputation neuromata of the fingers. In: Campbell D K, Gosset J (eds) Mutilating Injuries of the Hand. Churchill Livingstone, Edinburgh, p 175–176

Gorkisch K, Boese-Landgraf J, Vaubel E 1983 Treatment and prevention of amputation neuromas in the hand. Plastic and Reconstructive Surgery 73:293–296

Herndon J H, Eaton R G, Littler J W 1976 Management of painful neuromas of the hand. Journal of Bone and Joint Surgery 58A:369–373

Hunter E A, Kennard A B 1982 Mania operativa: an uncommon recognised cause of limb amputation. Canadian Journal of Surgery 25:92–93

Laborde K J, Kalisman M, Tsu-Min Tsai Results of surgical treatment of painful neuromas of the hand. Journal of Hand Surgery 7:190–193

Mackinnon S E, Dellon A L, Hudson A R, Hunter D A 1985 Alteration of neuroma formation by manipulation of its micro environment. Plastic and Reconstructive Surgery 76:345–352

Meyer R A, Srinwasan R, Campbell J N, Mackinnon S E, Dellon A L 1985 Neuro-activity originating from a neuroma in the baboon. Brain Research 325:255–260

Murray J F, Carman W, MacKenzie J K 1977 Transmetacarpal amputation of the index finger: a clinical assessment of hand strength and complications. Journal of Hand Surgery 2:471–481

Neu B R, Murray V F, MacKenzie J K 1985 Profundus tendon blockage: quadriga in finger amputations. Journal of Hand Surgery 10A:878–883

Pardini A G 1979 Treatment of painful amputation neuroma of the digits by cauterisation: a comparative study. In: Campbell D A, Gosset J (eds) Mutilating Injuries of the Hand. Churchill Livingstone, Edinburgh, p 177–179

Parkes A R 1970 The lumbrical plus finger. The Hand 2:164–167

Petropoulos P C, Stefanko S Experimental studies of post-traumatic neuromas under various physiological conditions. Journal of Surgical Research 1:235–248

Pilet J 1981 Prostheses in amputations of the finger tips. In: Pierse M (ed) The Nail. Churchill Livingstone, Edinburgh, p 90–91

Rank B K, Wakefield A R, Hueston J T 1986 Surgery of Repair as Applied to Hand Injuries, 3rd edn. E. S. Livingstone, Edinburgh

Ratliff A H C 1969 Amputation of the fingers and thumb. The Hand 1:137–138

Thompson R V 1963 Essential details in the technique of finger amputations. Medical Journal of Australia 2: 14–18

Tupper J W, Booth D M 1976 Treatment of painful neuromas of sensory nerves in the hand: a comparison of traditional and newer methods. Journal of Hand Surgery 1: 144–151

Tupper J W 1981 Correspondence News Letter 61: American Society for Surgery of the Hand

Verdan C 1960 Syndrome of quadriga. Surgical Clinics of North America 40: 425–426

Verdan C 1981 Plastic surgery of the claw nail. In: Pierre M (ed) The Nail. Churchill Livingstone, Edinburgh, p 93–101

Wall P D 1983 Alterations in the central nervous system after deafferentation: connectivity control. In: Bonica J J, Lindbolm U, Iggo A (eds) Advances in Pain Research Therapy, Vol. 5. Raven Press, New York, p 677–689

D. A. Campbell Reid

11 Skin grafts and pedicle flaps

SKIN GRAFTS

Origin of unsatisfactory results

In order to understand the reasons for unsatisfactory results it is necessary to remind oneself of certain basic principles in the use of skin grafts. It is a remarkable fact that a piece of skin, of either partial or full thickness, when completely detached from one part of the body, will survive transference to another and still remain viable. This obviously depends upon a rapid revascularisation, but before this can take place, the skin must survive through a plasmatic exchange between it and the recipient site during the first 48 hours. The skin's metabolic requirements are met in this way. Anything which interferes with this process, therefore, will lead to graft failure.

Graft failure

May be due to:

(a) Lack of vascularity in the graft bed. Necrotic tissue following inadequate debridement at the time of initial trauma may account for this. This lack of vascularity may also be of relative degree. This is seen where certain viable structures are laid bare in the wound and whose blood supply is insufficient to nourish a free graft. These structures include the bone of metacarpals or phalanges denuded of their periosteum, tendons, flexor or extensor, stripped of their sheaths or paratenon, and bare cartilage or joint capsules (Fig. 11.1). Open joints, too, may be included in this category.

(b) Lack of contact between a skin graft and the bed upon which it is placed. Anything which interferes with the close contact of the graft and its bed will obviously prevent the graft from picking up its new blood supply by ingress of new capillaries from the bed. The most likely cause for this is the accumulation of a haematoma. Progressive bleeding, which may only be a capillary oozing, lifts the graft from its bed and forms a barrier which, uncorrected at an early stage, will result in partial or total necrosis of the graft.

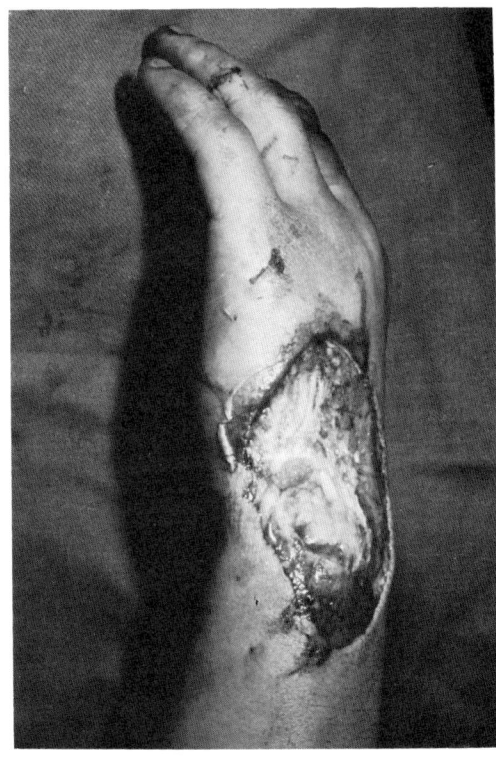

Fig. 11.1 Defect where flap replacement is essential. Note the exposed wrist joint and the extensor carpi ulnaris tendon

Infection is a less frequent cause of graft failure. The accumulation of pus beneath a graft will similarly lift the graft from its bed. This is purely a mechanical effect and is likely to be produced by an organism such as the staphylococcus. A more serious effect of infection upon a graft is seen with the β-haemolytic streptococcus which produces a powerful exotoxin. This has a lytic effect on a skin graft and will destroy even a recently established one.

(c) Mechanical factors may also be responsible for graft failure in the hand. The graft may become displaced due to inadequate fixation and this is particularly important in the early postoperative period. It should be pointed out, that for the successful 'take' of a skin graft, pressure on the graft is not essential. In fact, provided one can prevent a graft from becoming dislodged, the delayed exposed grafting technique may be employed. This operation involves taking a split skin graft at the same time as the wound is cleansed and covered with a non-adherent dressing. The graft is then stored temporarily in the refrigerator and subsequently applied to the defect once the patient has recovered from the anaesthetic. Close nursing supervision is essential and any collection beneath the graft is carefully evacuated as required. There is little place for this technique in hand surgery, however.

Instability

This depends on a number of factors such as the thickness of the graft, the site of the graft and whether or not there is adherence to deep structures. A full thickness graft has a less certain overall 'take' than a split skin graft and, even if it takes fully, it is several weeks more before it has consolidated. The surface layer typically peels off. Once it has matured, however, it provides reasonable cover and is unlikely to break down. Such a graft is unsatisfactory in finger-tip repair for other reasons which will be discussed subsequently. Instability is most likely to be seen where split skin grafts are used, for example, over a joint on the extensor aspect of hand or fingers, or over the volar aspect (especially tactile surfaces) where constant flexion movements and exposure to trauma are liable to cause breakdown in the grafted areas.

Contracture

This is one of the commonest complications causing an unsatisfactory result following a free graft. It is more frequent after a split skin graft than a full thickness one which possesses elastic tissue and can stretch to a certain extent. The contracture is usually a flexion one where a split skin graft has been used to cover a defect over the volar aspect of a digit. Any such graft extending forwards of the midlateral line is almost certain to produce contracture of a digit.

Hypersensitivity

This undesirable result is likely to be seen in a graft which is adherent to underlying tissues such as bone. This is most troublesome where a tactile surface is involved. A graft applied following a digital-tip amputation through the terminal phalanx is most likely to display this complication. One has to distinguish between hypersensitivity caused by an unsatisfactory graft and that due to a

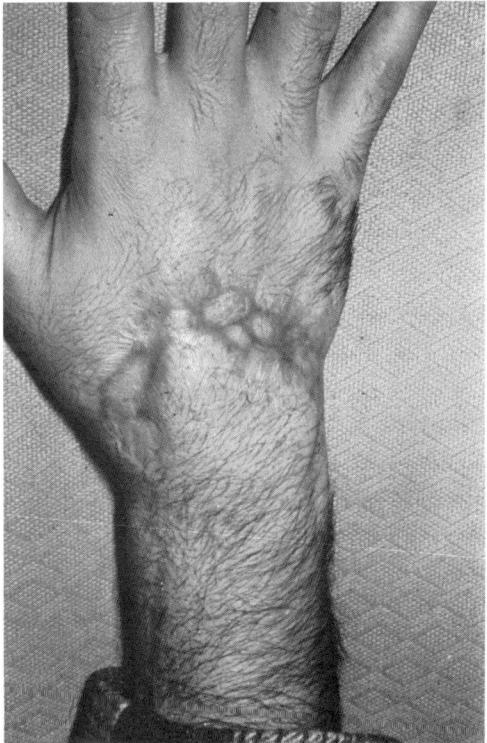

Fig. 11.2 Ugly appearance on the back of the hand due to patch grafts

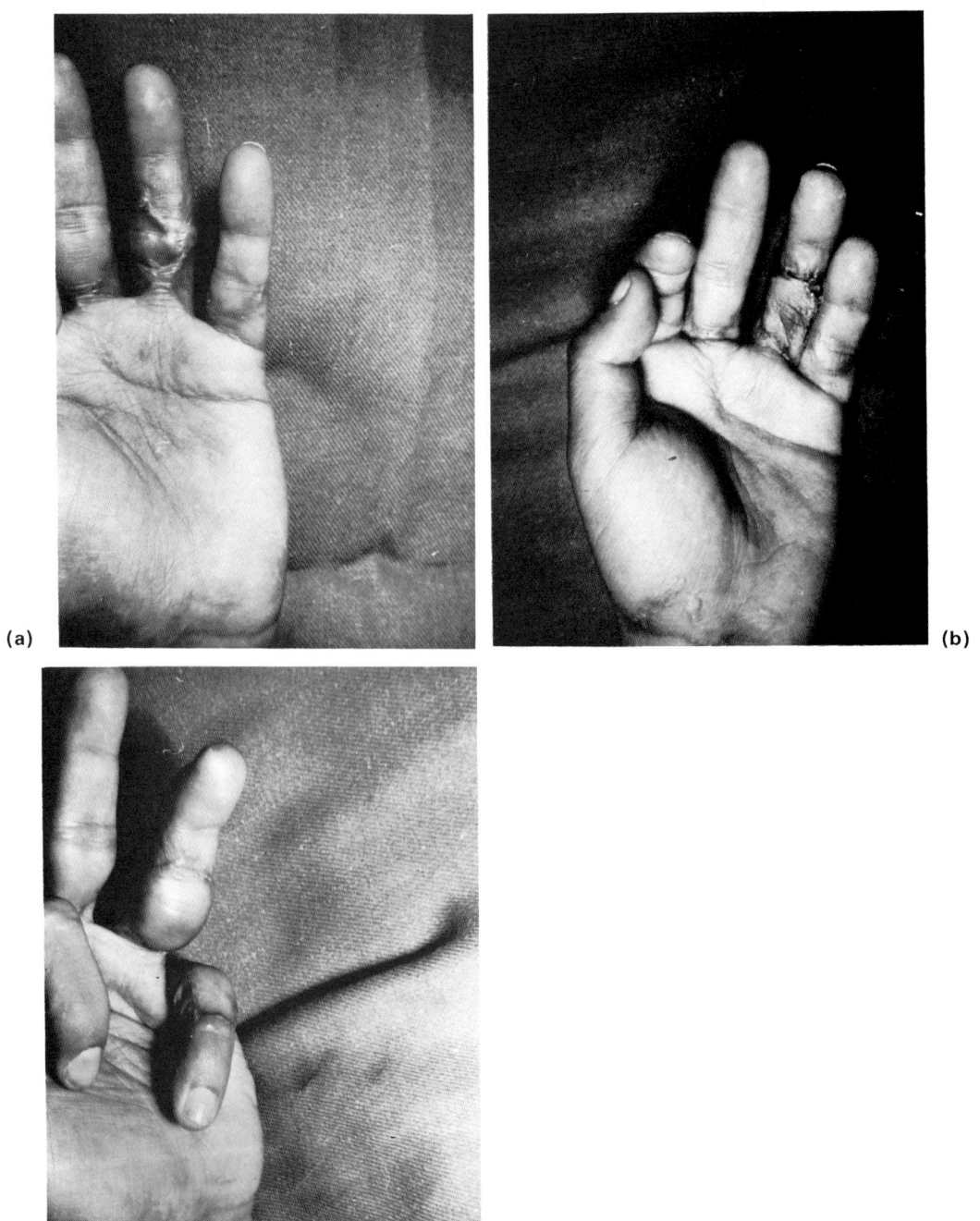

Fig. 11.3 (a) Division of flexor tendons to left middle and ring fingers. Primary skin grafting to defect in ring finger with associated scarring. (b) and (c) Cross-finger flap prior to tendon grafting. (d) and (e) Result of flexor tendon grafts

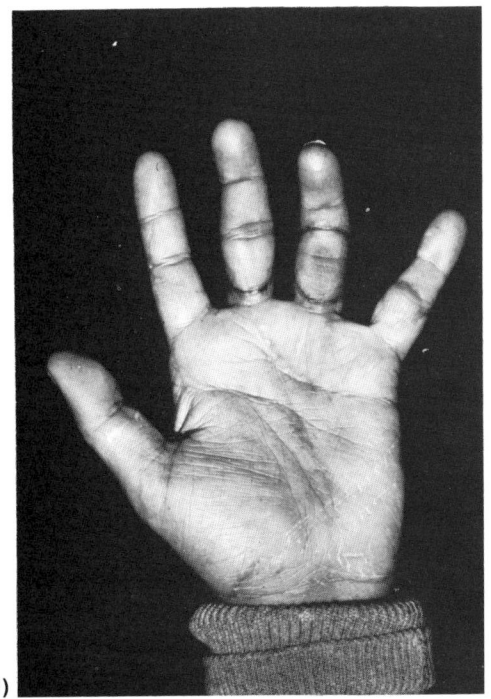
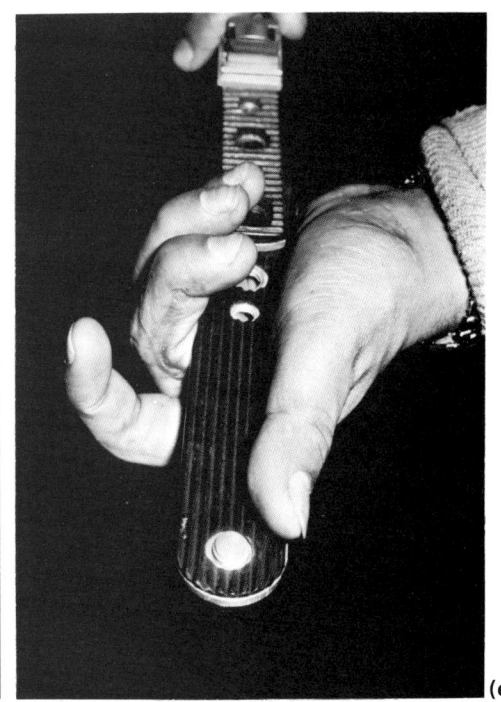

(d) (e)

neuroma. In fact, the two problems may well be combined.

Lack of sensation

Skin grafts, in time, develop protective sensation but this is inadequate on the important tactile surfaces of the digits where gnostic sensation is required for adequate function. Poor results are seen from this point of view where grafts, either split skin or full thickness skin, have been used to repair loss of finger-tip other than a minor defect, or the end of the thumb.

Cosmetically unsatisfactory results

Poor cosmetic results are seen where split skin grafts have been applied in patches, particularly over the back of the hand (Fig. 11.2). This gives an ugly patchwork appearance with scarring between each adjoining piece of skin. This is even uglier if the scarring is hypertrophic. A poor appearance may also result if a graft becomes excessively pigmented. Wide variations of pigmentation abnormalities may be encountered in the dark-skinned races. Excessive pigmentation in grafts may alternate with areas completely lacking pigmentation where grafts have failed, with residual scarring. This gives an extremely ugly mottled appearance and may be the cause of much embarrassment and distress.

Skin grafts give poor cosmetic results when applied to finger-tips following amputation. It is not only the appearance of such grafts but also their failure to buttress the nail resulting in the unsightly parrot beak deformity.

Associated involvement of deep structures

The result of skin grafts in sites where tendons have been divided or avulsed must be considered unsatisfactory as further surgery on the tendons cannot be undertaken, generally speaking, through a scarred skin-grafted area (Fig. 11.3).

Prevention of unsatisfactory results

Graft failure

Prevention of haematoma is the single most important factor. Control of bleeding is absolutely vital before applying the graft and complete haemostasis must be secured. Initial debridement and wound exploration in primary surgery following trauma should be undertaken in a bloodless field but before applying a skin graft the tourniquet must always be removed. Similarly, when using a skin graft in elective surgery, the initial stage of the procedure should be performed under tourniquet control but the tourniquet must always be released and the cuff removed prior to applying the graft. The arm should then be elevated for a few minutes to allow the reactive hyperaemia to settle. Meticulous haemostatis is best achieved by the use of bi-polar coagulation. Once having sutured the graft in place one must then ensure that no further bleeding occurs. The space beneath the graft is syringed out with saline using a dental cavity syringe. A secure dressing is immediately applied. This is an important part of the operation and should not be delegated to others. Where a graft is applied to the back of the hand with its convex surface, a tie-over dressing is not required as is essential when securing a graft over a concavity. A routine hand dressing is applied as follows (Fig. 11.4). A single layer of vaselined gauze covers the graft which is then secured or not, as the case may be, by a tie-over dressing using a bolus of cotton wool wrung out in saline. Fluffed gauze is now applied over the graft and small pieces of gauze between the fingers. A pad of autoclaved steel wool is placed in the palm of the hand. Two rolls of orthopaedic wool (Velband) cover the dressings and extend from hand to upper forearm. Firmly applied crepe or Kling bandages secure the dressing providing even, though not excessive, compression to hand and forearm. The steel wool acts as a springy mesh allowing air to permeate which prevents maceration of the palm. It also helps to splint the hand in a comfortable position of function. A volar plaster cast may be used, in addition, with the wrist in slight extension. Such a routine should prevent displacement of the graft and prevent oozing under it. There is a balance to be maintained in the hand between absolute immobilisation, to allow for take of the graft, and a degree of mobilisation particularly of uninvolved joints to prevent stiffness. Generally, a compromise must be adopted allowing some movement of uninvolved digits. This, combined with elevation of the arm in the first 48 hours, will assist in control of oedema.

The presence of necrotic tissue should be avoided by adequate debridement of the wound under tourniquet control, checked by observing the vascularity of the resulting bed following release of the tourniquet. All foreign material should also be removed.

Failure of graft as a result of its being used to cover exposed bone lacking periosteum, bare tendons, cartilage or open joints may be prevented by the initial use of some form of pedicled flap. This will also prevent such disasters as tendon sloughing due to inadequate blood supply. Only a flap will provide the necessary fresh blood supply in such an instance. A volar defect on a finger leaving intact but exposed flexor tendons denuded of their sheaths is an indication par excellence for an immediate cross-finger flap. This is a highly skilled procedure requiring a meticulous technique. It is also of paramount importance in safeguarding the functional integrity of a finger and for these reasons it is worthwhile emphasising some features of the operation (Fig. 11.5). An accurate pattern of the defect is made and this is applied to the dorsal aspect of the adjoining donor finger making the defect just slightly larger than the pattern and not allowing the base to extend volarwards of the midlateral line. The flap must be designed so as to fit comfortably, with the digits lying in a relaxed semiflexed position free from tension. The defect on the donor finger should be placed between joints as far as possible, though with an extensive longitudinal wound to be covered this will not be possible. However, where the skin over the dorsum of the proximal interphalangeal joint has to be used, no harm will be caused provided the defect is skilfully repaired with either a thick split skin graft or a full thickness one. The author has not experienced restriction of flexion in a donor finger where the defect over a joint has been managed in this way.

The flap is raised at the level of the paratenon covering the extensor apparatus where a well-defined tissue plane will be found. This dissection is performed under tourniquet control. The flap is then hinged on its base through 180 degrees. Having ensured that the flap comfortably covers the whole of the defect, the tourniquet is released and the cuff removed from the arm. Full haemostasis is then secured and either a thick split skin

SKIN GRAFTS AND PEDICLE FLAPS 163

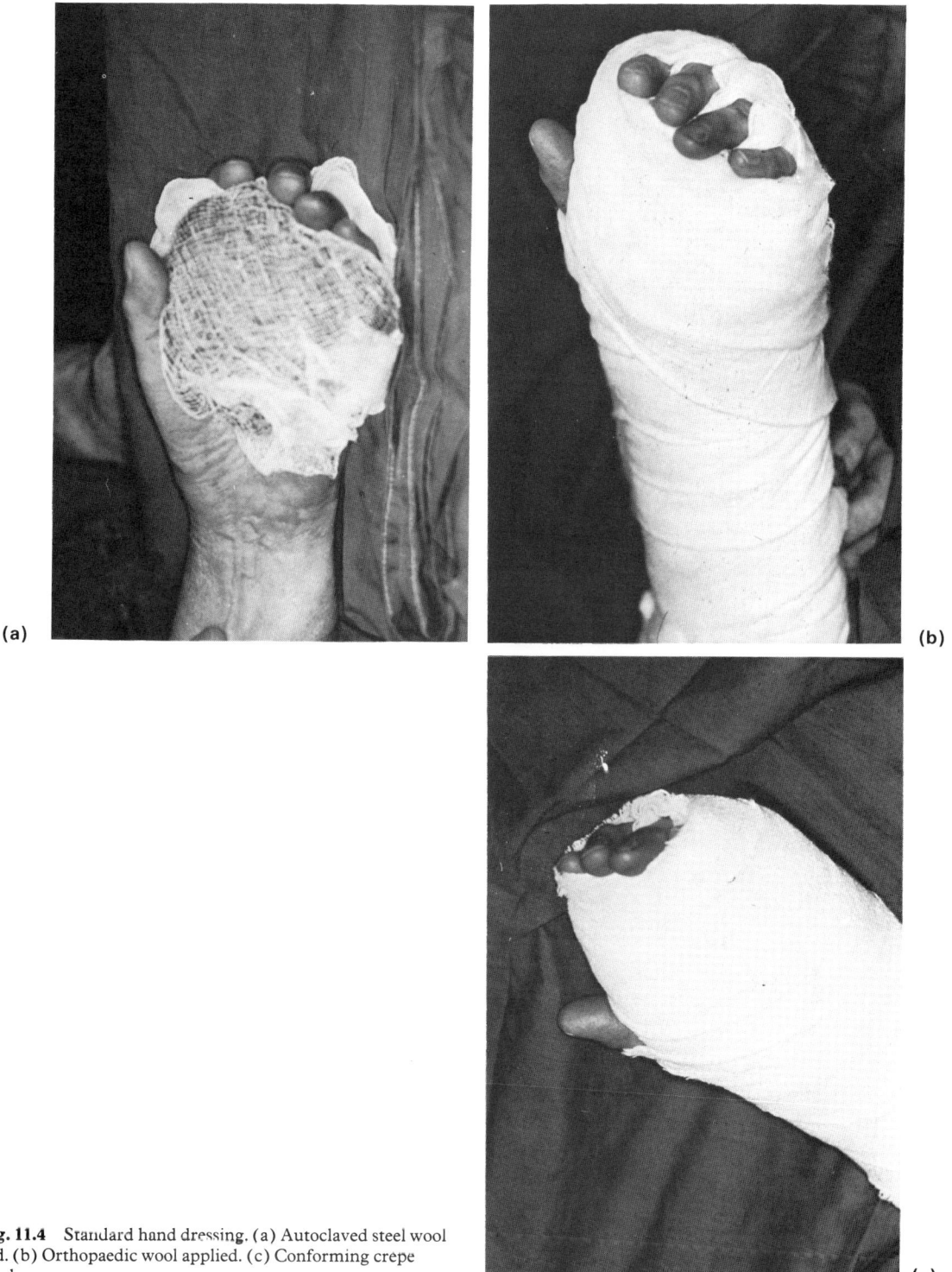

Fig. 11.4 Standard hand dressing. (a) Autoclaved steel wool pad. (b) Orthopaedic wool applied. (c) Conforming crepe bandage

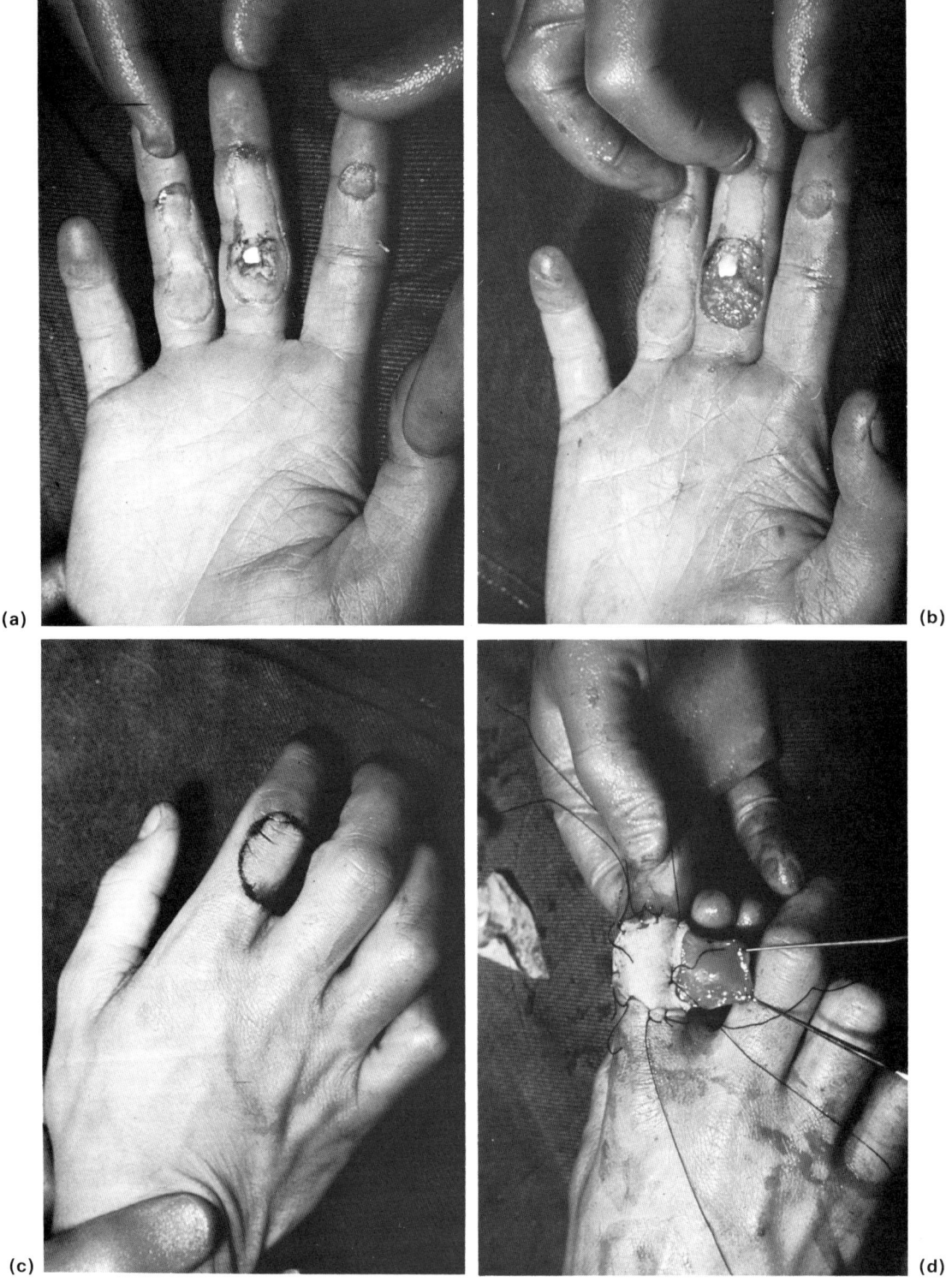

SKIN GRAFTS AND PEDICLE FLAPS 165

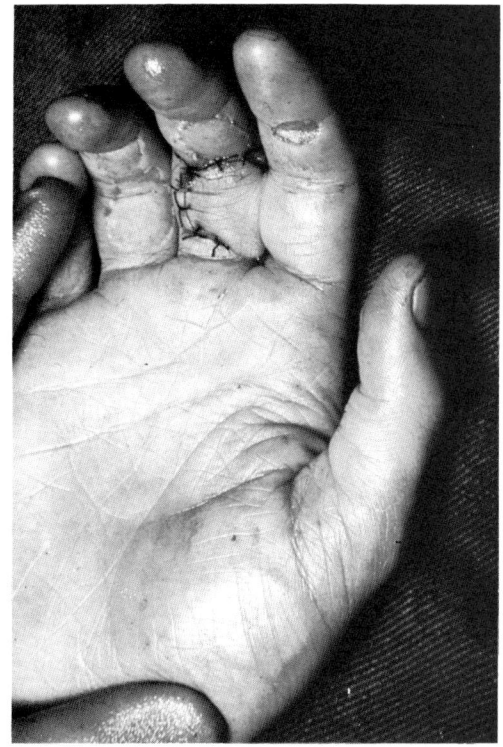

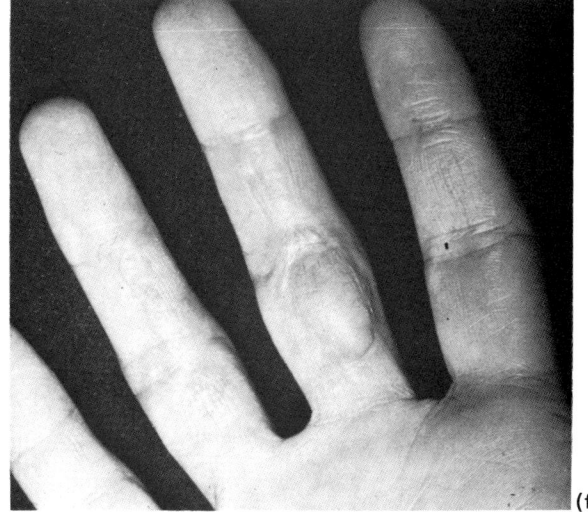

Fig. 11.5 (a) and (b) Initial defect showing exposed flexor tendon. (c) and (d) Cross-finger flap marked out and raised on index finger. Split skin graft applied to the secondary defect. (e) Flap sutured to defect. (f) and (g) Result 6 months later

166 UNSATISFACTORY RESULTS IN HAND SURGERY

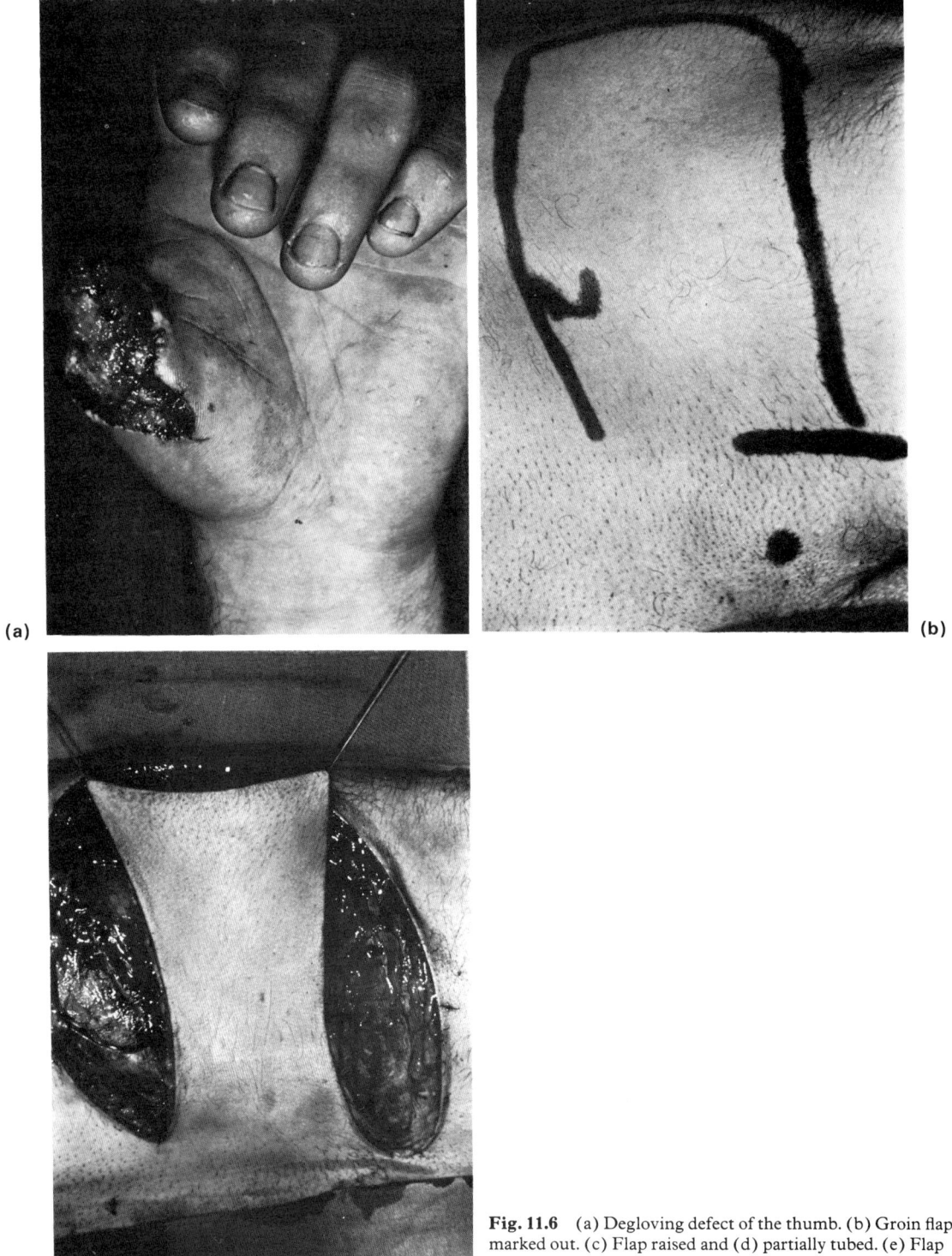

Fig. 11.6 (a) Degloving defect of the thumb. (b) Groin flap marked out. (c) Flap raised and (d) partially tubed. (e) Flap covering the defect. Note that the seam lies along the ulnar border

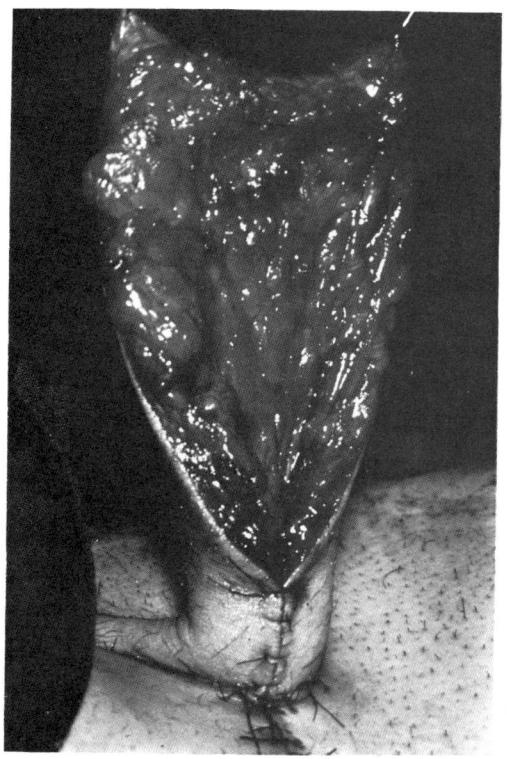
(d)

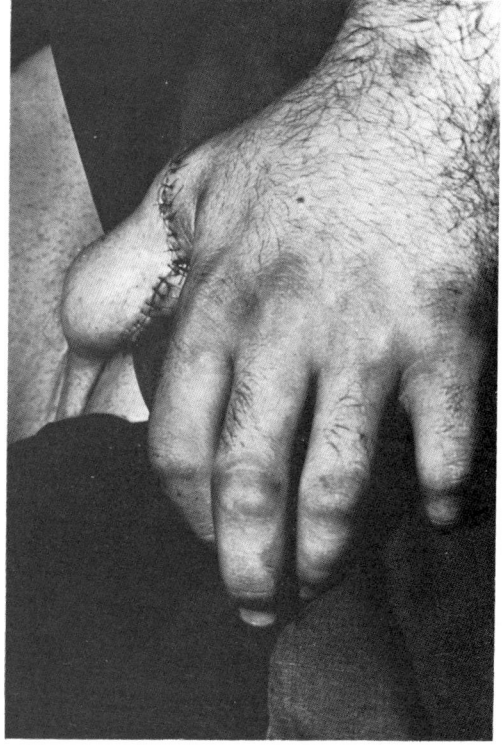
(e)

graft or a full thickness one is sutured into the defect and held firmly in place by a tie-over dressing. This technique is assisted by the insertion of one or two basting sutures through the deep tissues of the bed close to the base of the flap. This enables the bolus dressing to be snugged into position right up to the base of the flap while not interfering with its blood supply. It must be stressed that, on no account should these sutures pick up the base of the flap. Finally, the flap is sutured into the defect on the recipient finger. The backs of the fingers and hand are dressed and padded. The bridge of the flap is covered with a single layer of vaselined gauze. Fixation is achieved by bandaging the fingers over a substantial steel wool pad in the palm and reinforced by strips of 2.5 cm elastoplast applied longitudinally. A plaster cast is unnecessary. Part of the flap should be left sufficiently exposed so that its viability may be checked postoperatively.

The base of the pedicle is divided at 10 to 14 days. Provided the flap initially has been designed so as to cover the whole of the defect, little trimming and insetting should be required.

Larger defects requiring pedicled flap cover are best managed by the use of a groin flap. The groin flap is an axial pattern flap (McGregor & Jackson 1972) depending for its survival on one named vessel, the superficial circumflex iliac. The groin flap offers a number of advantages in the primary cover of a hand defect. As an axial pattern flap, it is possible to raise a flap of considerable dimensions notably as regards its length. A length to base ratio of 3 or 4 to 1 enables one to cover a defect using a long pedicle which may be tubed and which will allow appreciable mobility to the hand. This is an important factor in combating oedema. It is the method of choice in the management of a totally degloved thumb. There are certain features of technique and modifications of design which merit discussion in some detail (Fig. 11.6):

The extremities of the inguinal ligament, pubic tubercle medially and anterior superior iliac spine laterally, are marked out. The position of the femoral artery just below the medial end of the inguinal ligament is then marked. The skin flap is now outlined with its base centred over the medial end of the inguinal ligament and extending outwards over the iliac crest. The superficial circumflex iliac artery arises from the femoral artery about 1.5 cm below the inguinal ligament. The flap must include this vessel and its accompanying vein which drains to the long saphenous vein. The vessels, though they must run the length of the flap, need not necessarily be centrally placed in it, however. The flap is raised from its distal end and at the level of the deep fascia. As one progresses medially, great care must be taken when approaching the medial border of the sartorius muscle where the superficial circumflex iliac artery penetrates the deep fascia. Normally it is not necessary to raise the flap medial to this point but if one requires an even longer pedicle, the deep fascia may be incised here to free the vessels so as to obviate any danger from kinking. The proximal part of the flap is then tubed and the distal part is sutured to the defect on the hand. Another feature of the groin flap is that there is a relatively thin subcutaneous layer. Further, careful reduction of this by thinning may be undertaken at the time of attachment. A flap with a width of up to 10.0 cm will cover most defects and with a flap of such a size it is possible to close the secondary defect by direct approximation after undermining the edges and flexing the hip slightly. Closure by a subcuticular suture will leave a scar lying in the groin crease which should be acceptable to all including female patients. Delaying the division of a groin flap is advisable. Under a local anaesthetic at 3 weeks, a small transverse incision is made over the base of the pedicle to expose the superficial circumflex iliac artery and accompanying vein. These are ligated and divided. Final division of the flap is undertaken 7 to 10 days later. An alternative technique is to loop a prolene thread around the vessels in the base of the flap at the time it is raised and leave the prolene ends emerging from the wound. The prolene loop is then tied off at 3 weeks.

Failure due to mechanical factors

These should be prevented by the expert application of a dressing as already described.

Instability

This may be prevented to a certain extent by avoiding the use of free grafts over exposed bone, e.g. finger-tip amputations through the terminal phalanx. The choice of skin cover in any particular circumstance or situation is a matter of surgical judgement in each case.

Contracture

This may be anticipated as a possible complication in any defect extending on to the volar aspect of a digit, and a split skin graft should be avoided in these circumstances. Grafting a granulating surface is also more likely to produce a contracture. Wherever possible, allowing a wound to granulate should be avoided. In primary trauma, for example, the aim should always be to graft defects at the time to ensure clean healing and prevent the formation of granulation tissue. Where a graft has been placed on the volar aspect of a digit, lively splintage should be instituted as soon as the graft has taken satisfactorily and this should help to prevent, or at least control, flexion contracture. Capener lively splints are most useful for this (Fig. 11.7).

Hypersensitivity

This is a complication which cannot necessarily be avoided but one should not use a free graft on finger or thumb-tip where the terminal phalanx is exposed.

Lack of sensation

This must be anticipated as an initial feature of all forms of skin cover with the exception of the neurovascular flap. Reinnervation occurs in time but the quality of sensation depends upon the type of skin replacement. Cross-finger and thenar flaps develop better sensation than Wolfe grafts which, in turn, are superior in this respect to split skin grafts (Porter 1968). Local flaps should be used for defects over tactile surfaces whenever possible and, in the case of the thumb, one should seriously consider an innervated cross-finger flap as a primary measure if at all feasible. In elective cases, the use of an innervated flap should always be considered for the thumb.

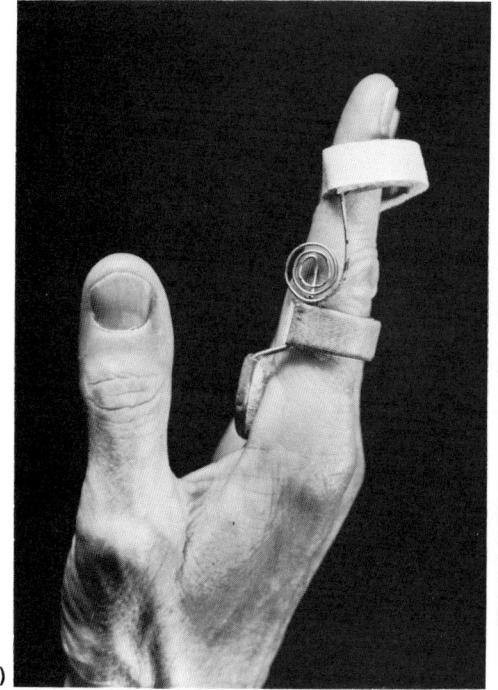 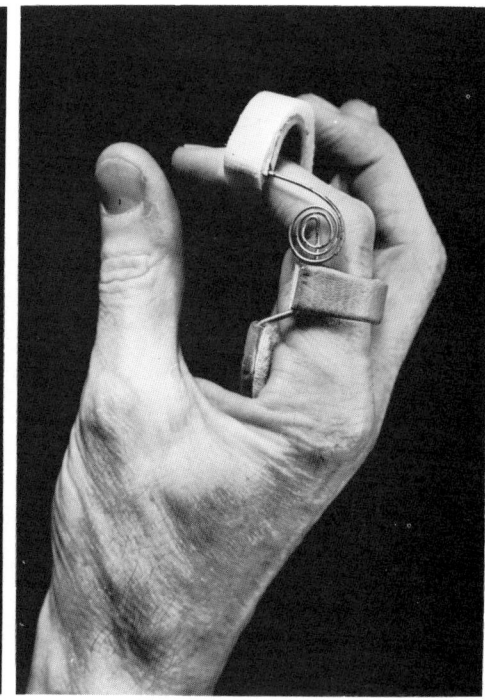

Fig. 11.7 (a) and (b) Capener lively splint to encourage extension

Poor cosmetic results

Grafts for the back of the hand should always be applied in the form of sheets, preferably of thick split skin, and with the fingers flexed at the metacarpophalangeal joints (Fig. 11.8). Skin, too, is best taken from the arm or forearm where the colour match is likely to be better than that using skin from the thigh.

Management of unsatisfactory results

Graft failure

When this is due to the presence of necrotic tissue following inadequate debridement, the area will almost certainly be infected at the time of the first dressing. This should be dealt with by repeated saline dressings to facilitate separation of slough and to encourage formation of healthy granulations. Adherent slough should be trimmed away and as soon as the surface appears healthy a further skin graft should be applied. If tendons and bones are involved, these will have to be dealt with as required. Exposed devitalised tendon should be excised and avascular cortical bone drilled. Once a vascular bed has been established in this way, a further split skin graft should be applied as provisional cover and to achieve healing. Subsequent reconstruction will require definitive flap replacement. In the absence of gross sepsis the immediate application of a flap under full antibiotic cover may be performed. This provides the only chance of saving exposed tendons by the introduction of a fresh blood supply. Failure due to haematoma, provided there is no infection, is treated by re-grafting as soon as possible. If skin has been banked at the first operation, this may be applied without the need for a further anaesthetic after preparing the surface. Should a graft become displaced at an early stage by faulty dressing and fixation, re-grafting should be undertaken without delay.

Instability of graft

Such a complication occurring in a grafted fingertip following amputation is best treated either by the Kutler (1947) technique or the Atasoy (1970)

170   UNSATISFACTORY RESULTS IN HAND SURGERY

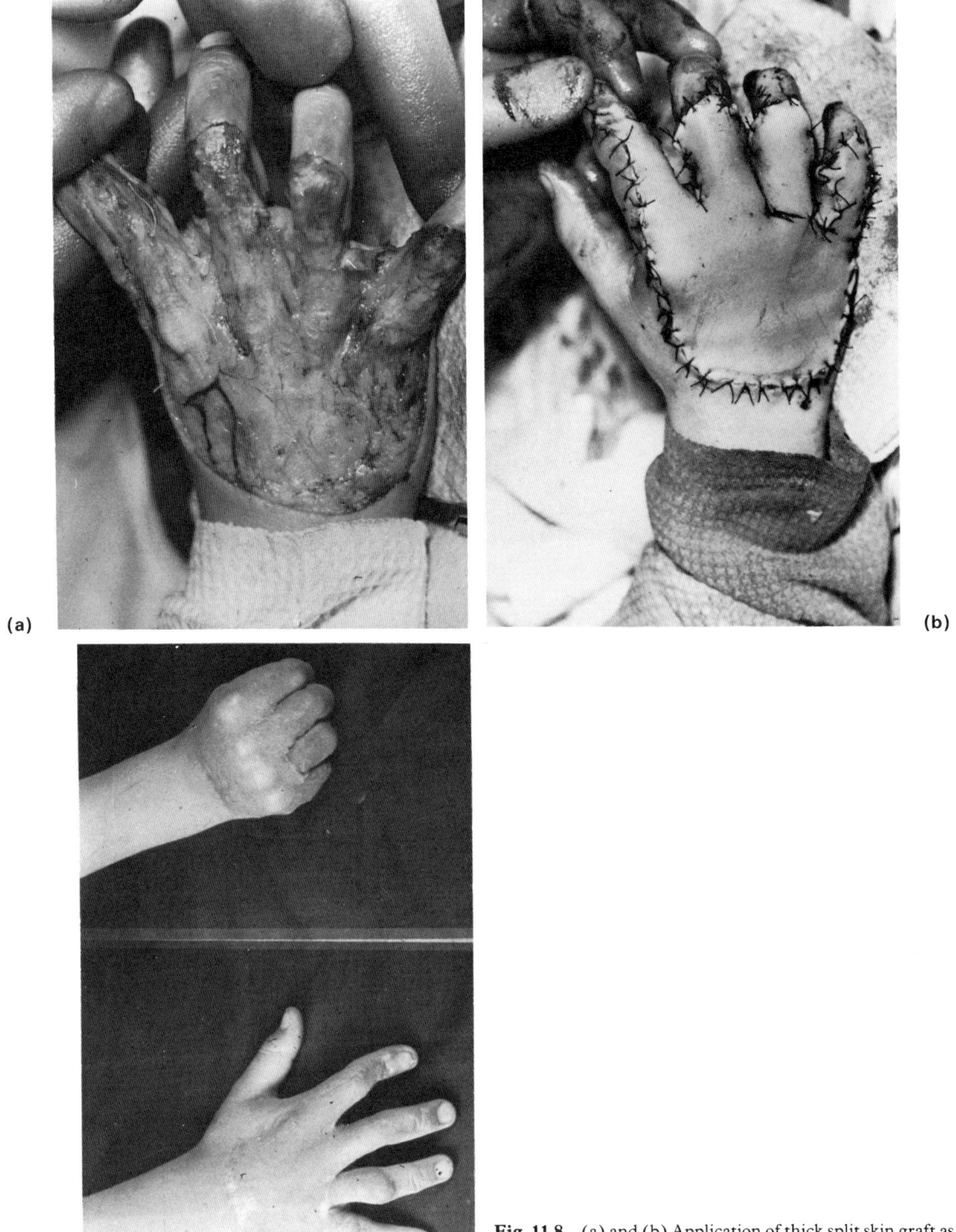

Fig. 11.8 (a) and (b) Application of thick split skin graft as a sheet to defect on the back of the hand. (c) Note satisfactory cosmetic and functional result

method whereby local flaps are shifted on pulp pedicles to replace the defect following excision of the graft. These are, in fact, minute neurovascular flaps and provide good sensitivity. They may only be used to cover small defects. For more extensive defects, either a cross-finger flap or a thenar flap should be used. These flaps develop good sensation within 6 months and result in an extremely acceptable cosmetic result providing the necessary bulk to replace lost pulp and to buttress the nail (Fig. 11.9). This tends to prevent the ugly parrot beak deformity.

Instability in a graft over the dorsum of the hand or digits may be corrected, where this is a relatively minor problem, by simply shaving (tangential excision) the surface and overgrafting with a split skin graft. This reinforces the area and may be adequate to allow the part to resist the trauma of constant movement, pressure and knocks. Failing this, and where breakdown is a more serious matter, the area should be excised and covered with a flap. A local flap such as the sliding transposition one (Smith 1982) may be used on the dorsum for small defects, otherwise a distant flap will be required. A cross-forearm flap is useful to cover a volar defect particularly on the ulnar side. The dorsum of the hand lies comfortably against the forearm enabling a flap to cover the defect completely on the volar aspect. Such a flap also provides skin of good texture with little fat (Fig. 11.10). The alternative is either a chest or groin flap. Instability and/or hypersensitivity of a grafted area over the thumb-tip has an even greater significance because of the vital part played by the thumb in opposition pinch, and grasp generally. The better method is to excise the graft and advance a double pedicle flap as originally described by Moberg (1964). The terminal phalanx should be trimmed minimally. Longitudinal midlateral incisions are made on either side of the thumb to the proximal segment. They are linked by a transverse incision over the interphalangeal joint through which the neurovascular bundles are mobilised having raised the flap containing the bundles to this level. The flap is then advanced to cover the defect over the end of the thumb. The secondary defect is covered with a full thickness skin graft which is secured by a tie-over dressing. A larger defect may be covered by extending this flap proximally to the thenar eminence. A defect up to 3.0 cm in length may be closed in this way (Dellon 1981).

Contractures

Flexion contractures following grafting usually require the addition of skin. Z-plasties are only applicable for linear contractures. The contracture is released by a transverse incision across the site of maximal contracture and then undermining the edges. The incision must be taken out to the midlateral lines and, if the skin on either side is thin and of poor quality, this must be excised back to a healthy bleeding edge. Provided the bed also has an adequate blood supply with no exposed tendon, for example, then a full thickness graft will provide satisfactory skin cover. Such a graft may be taken from the flexion crease of the elbow, though this site is better avoided in a female patient, or from the groin. Once the graft has taken satisfactorily, a lively splint should be used.

Where the bed is not suitable for a free graft, a flap must be used. A cross-finger flap provides the best means of cover over the volar aspect of a finger. If the contracture also involves the joint capsule, a capsulectomy may be performed at the same time. It is also useful to hold the proximal interphalangeal joint in a semi-extended position by driving a Kirschner wire across it. The wire may be removed when the cross-finger flap is divided and a lively splint may then be employed.

This also applies in an elective procedure where scarring has to be replaced by a flap prior to undertaking tendon grafting where the tendons have been destroyed in the original injury (Fig. 11.11).

Lack of sensation

Gnostic sensation over the tactile surface of the thumb is necessary for efficient function. Every effort should be made to achieve this in one of the following ways:

(a) Advancement of a neurovascular flap on its two bundles as already described.

(b) An innervated cross-finger flap from the dorsum of the index finger and adjoining hand.

172 UNSATISFACTORY RESULTS IN HAND SURGERY

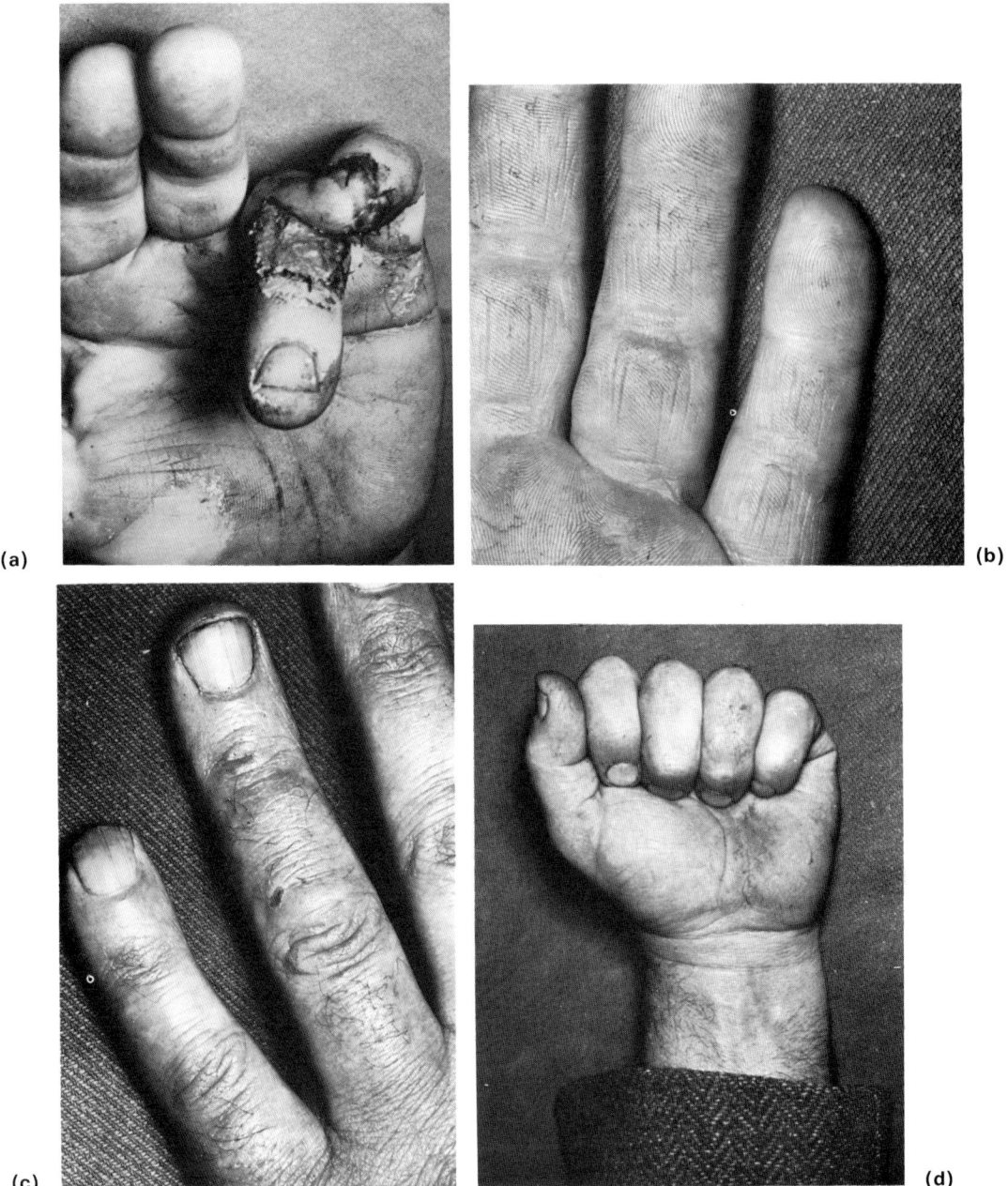

Fig. 11.9 (a)–(d) Cross-finger flap to replace tip of the little finger. Note the excellent contour of the terminal pulp which has been restored with satisfactory buttressing of the finger nail

Such a flap includes the terminal branches of the radial nerve. Some technical details of the use of this flap will be discussed under pedicle flaps.

(c) A neurovascular island from the dorsum of the index finger as described by Foucher & Braun (1979) which is based on the terminal branch of the first dorsal interosseous artery. It is drained by one or two veins and is innervated by the terminal branches of the radial nerve.

(d) A heterodigital neurovascular island flap

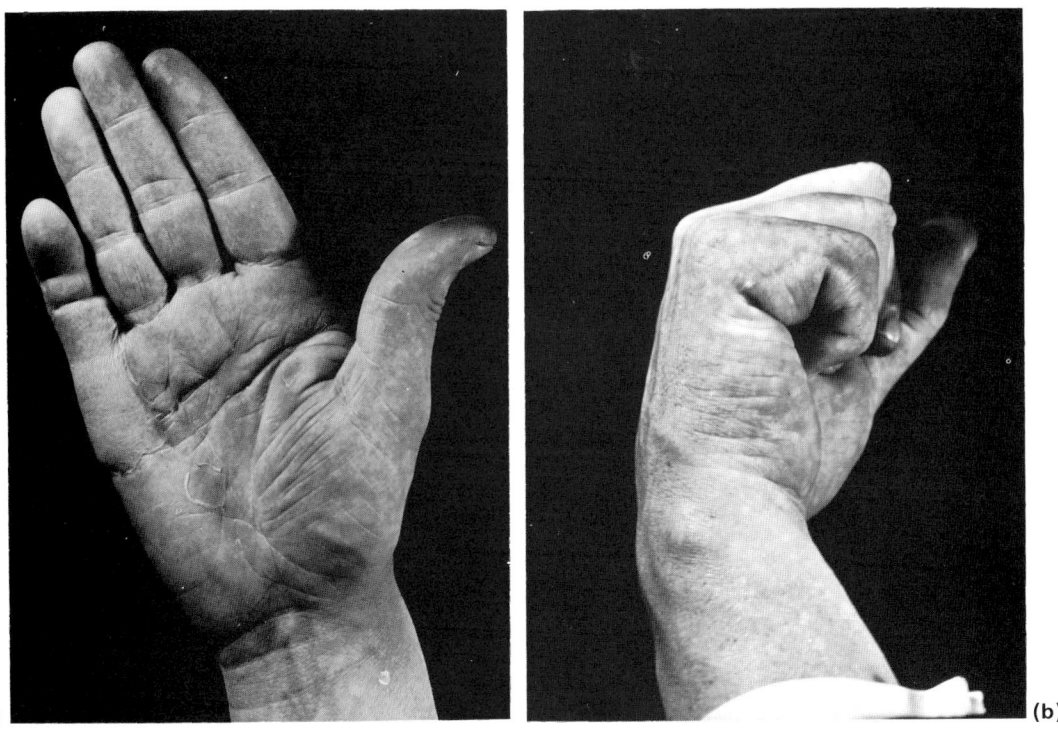

Fig. 11.10 (a) and (b) Cross-forearm flap replacing a skin defect on the palm of the hand. No thinning of this flap has been undertaken

(Littler 1961) taking an island of skin from the middle or ring finger.

(e) The flag flap (Vilain 1952, Vilain & Dupuis 1973, Iselin 1973) which consists of a narrow pedicle (the flag pole) on the dorsum of the index finger over its base incorporating the terminal branch of the dorsal metacarpal artery, terminal filaments of the radial nerve and a superficial vein. The flap expands distally (the flag) taking the skin from the dorsum of the proximal segment of the finger.

Poor cosmetic results

Where the skin is stable but has an ugly appearance due to a patchwork of small grafts and scarring on the back of the hand and, provided function is not limited by the scarring, then shaving off the surface and overgrafting with one single split skin graft may be undertaken. This results in a greatly improved cosmetic appearance. It is advisable for the patient subsequently to wear a pressure glove for 3 to 6 months. Shaving and grafting may also be undertaken for marked mottling due to variations in pigmentation.

PEDICLE FLAPS

Origin of unsatisfactory results

Unlike skin grafts, pedicle flaps have their own blood supply entering by their pedicles (bases). The survival of a flap depends upon the maintenance of this blood supply in sufficient quantity to nourish the whole of the flap. A number of factors must be taken into account when discussing unsatisfactory results. These include design of the flap, its dimensions, site of origin and anything which might interfere with its blood supply including its venous drainage.

Flap failure due to necrosis

The commonest cause of necrosis in a flap is seen after trauma particularly where flaps of skin are

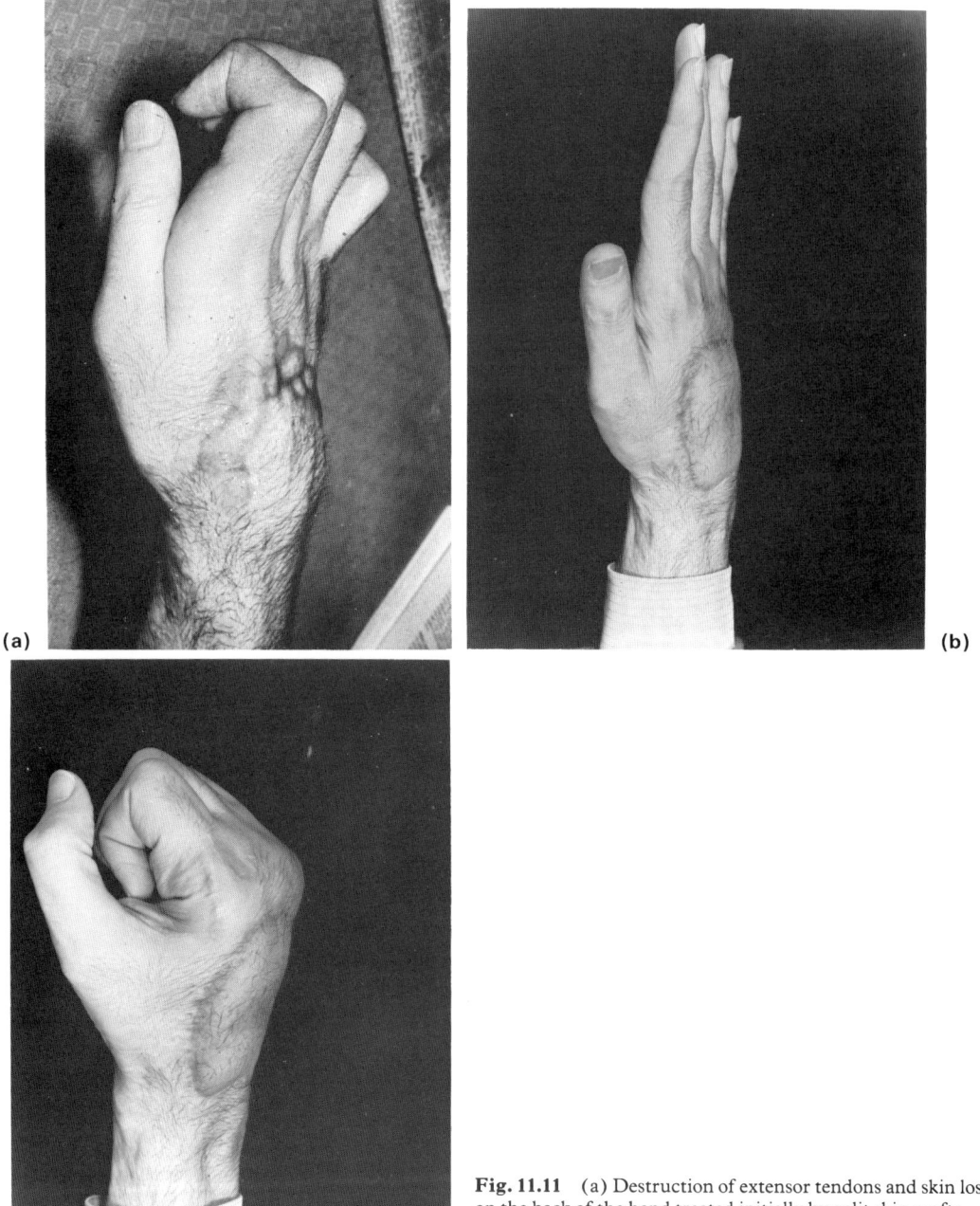

Fig. 11.11 (a) Destruction of extensor tendons and skin loss on the back of the hand treated initially by split skin grafts. Note the tenodesis effect as the patient attempts to make a fist. (b) and (c) Replacement of scarred, skin-grafted area by groin flap and extensor tendon grafts

partially avulsed. There is a temptation to suture back such a flap regardless of the prevailing conditions and this frequently results in necrosis, partial or complete. The chances of this happening are even greater when the flap is based distally. A distally based flap will have an impaired venous drainage. This combined with other factors such as tension following suture, aggravated by oedema due to the trauma and possible faulty positioning of the limb, will result in increasing congestion. The increased back pressure effect on the venous system will eventually lead to an obstruction to the arterial flow comparable to the chain of events seen with a strangulated hernia.

Necrosis may also occur in flaps transferred either locally or from a distance immediately following trauma or as definitive procedures. This may be due to incorrect design of flaps particularly in the case of local flaps such as the Z-plasty and rotation flap. Further important factors in failure are tension from other causes and mechanical obstruction of the pedicle.

Necrosis may also occur at the time a flap is divided and inset.

Infection is usually only a contributory factor in flap necrosis.

Flap failure may also be due to premature detachment, for example, in the immediate postoperative period before the patient has recovered from the anaesthetic.

Prevention of unsatisfactory results

Avulsion flaps

The viability of the flap should be assessed by a simple clinical test described by Climo (1952). The edge of the flap is gently wiped with a gauze swab soaked in saline. A sluggish flow of dark blood from the subdermal plexus indicates a congested flap with impaired venous return whereas a brisk flow of bright red blood means a satisfactory blood supply and a viable flap. Absence of any blood, of course, indicates total ischaemia and an already non-viable flap. If a congested flap is then sutured back in its original place, the added tension in the flap, even if there is no actual skin loss, combined with the inevitable oedema accompanying the injury, will further slow the venous return and lead on to arterial obstruction. The result will be necrosis of the affected flap or at least part of it.

If the viability test indicates an appreciable degree of venous congestion, it is advisable to resect the distal part of the flap particularly if, in addition, there is evidence of crushing of the skin surface (Fig. 11.12). Alternatively, where there is less congestion, having trimmed the skin edge, the rest of the flap may be laid back on its bed without attempting to stretch it in any way. The secondary defect, whether from resection of the damaged part of the flap or left after replacing the flap on its bed so as to take up its own relaxed position, is covered with a split skin graft provided the bed is suitable. Where the bed is not suitable and important structures are exposed then a more radical resection of the involved flap should be undertaken and a primary pedicled flap used to cover the defect.

Proximally based avulsion flaps have a better prognosis but even with these it is advisable simply to lay the flap back if re-suturing it in place is not possible without tension (Fig. 11.13).

Necrosis may also occur in other flaps. Some degree of necrosis is most frequently seen following division and insetting of a flap. One important factor here is whether or not there has been an adequate primary implantation of the flap. The aim should be as near as possible to a complete covering of the defect at the primary operation. Unless this is achieved, it is a mistake to think that one can use part of the bridge, at the time the pedicle is divided, without risking loss of some of the flap particularly if it is further fashioned and inset. In these circumstances, and also when an axial pattern flap is used, a delay operation should be employed before final division is undertaken as already discussed.

Incorrect design of flaps

All flaps must be designed according to recognised principles. If a Z-plasty is considered to correct a linear scar adjoining a graft, then it should only be undertaken in the case of a well established full thickness graft. The optimal 60° angle to the flaps should be used. There must be no tension particu-

176 UNSATISFACTORY RESULTS IN HAND SURGERY

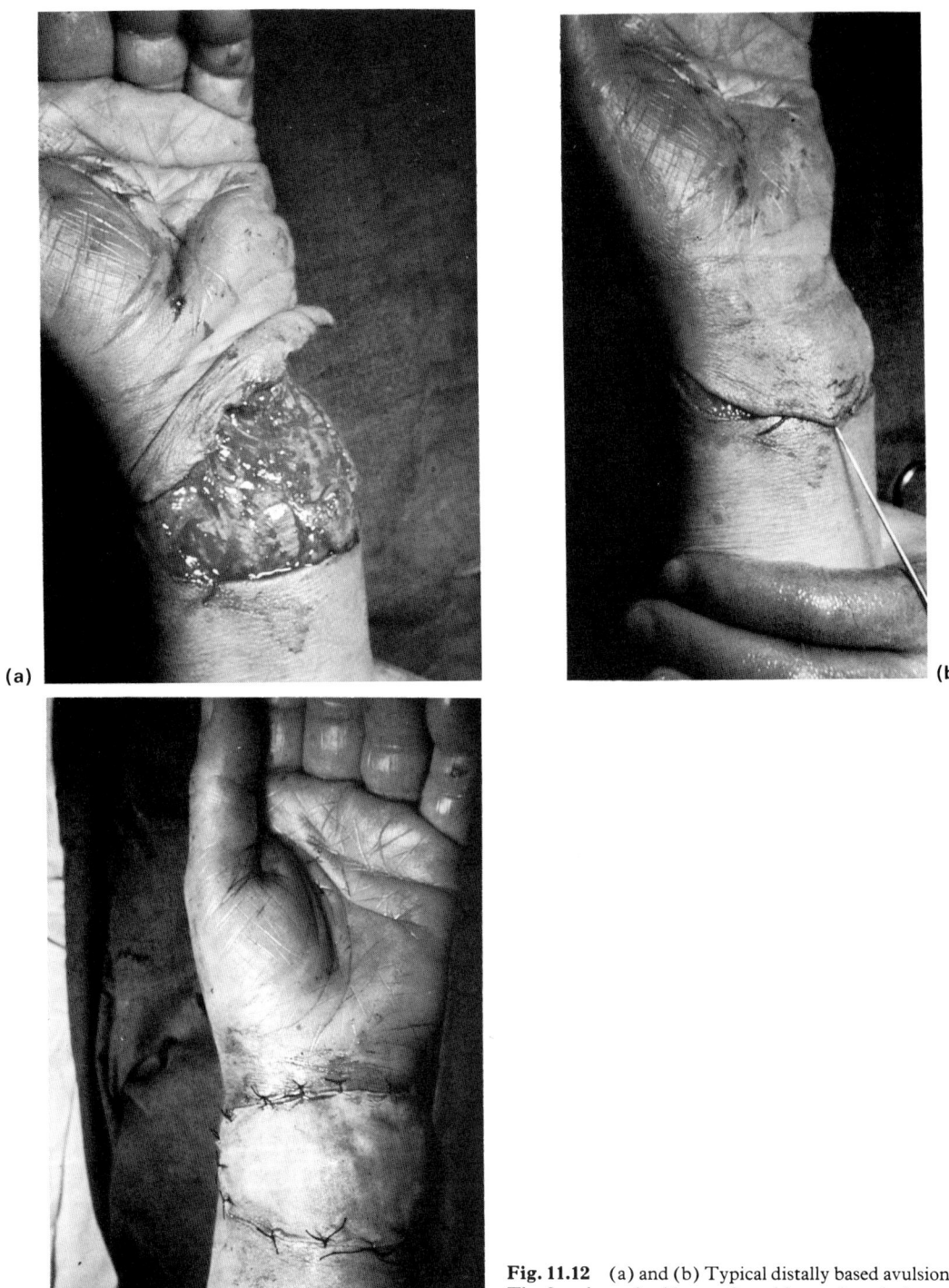

Fig. 11.12 (a) and (b) Typical distally based avulsion flap. The flap showed evidence of crushing and marked congestion. (c) Affected part of flap resected and replaced by split skin graft. (d) and (e) Result seen six months later. Note the shrinkage of the graft and satisfactory hand function

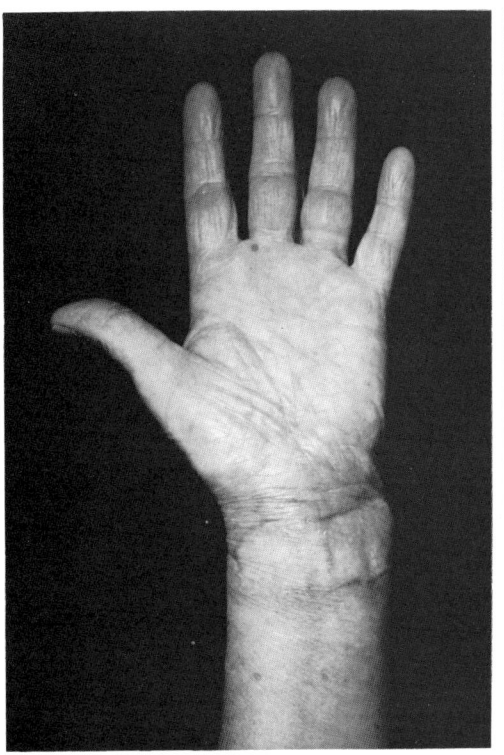
(d)

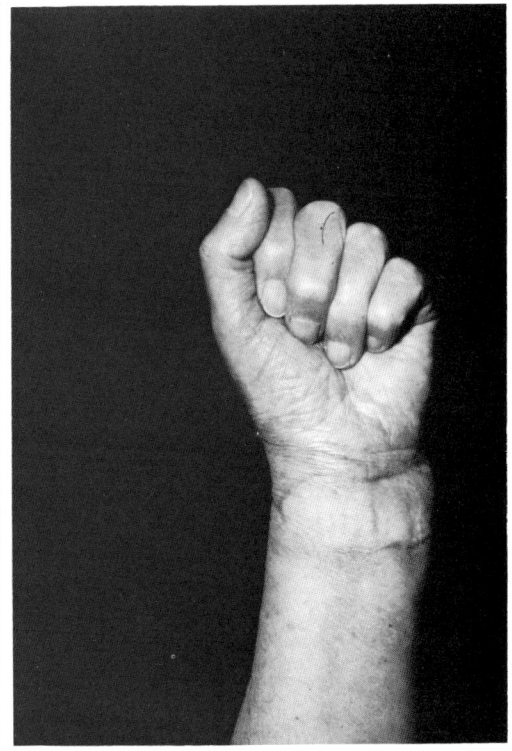
(e)

larly when this technique is used on the flexor aspect of a digit with its convex surface. The flaps must not be based on scars.

Tension

Anything which causes tension on flaps is likely to result in necrosis. Poor design has already been mentioned. Haematoma is an extremely important cause. Meticulous haemostasis is essential for both flap and the bed to which it is to be applied. Excessive pain after an operation on the hand, particularly where flaps are involved, must always be taken seriously. It probably indicates a haematoma and the wound must be taken down and inspected, i.e. where flaps have not been left exposed. One or two sutures should be removed and haematoma evacuated. Infection is a further factor and one which is likely to be associated with haematoma. Appropriate antibiotics should be given.

Flaps which are too thin

The main blood supply to the skin is in the subdermal plexus. Ideally, one should leave some subcutaneous tissue in the flap. It may be difficult to ensure this in the process of a Dupuytren's dissection, for example, when the underlying tissue may be adherent to the overlying skin. Serious consideration should be given to resection of skin and grafting in such circumstances.

Faulty suturing

When suturing a triangular flap (Z-plasty) the apex is the part most at risk. This should be secured in place by a special 3-point suture which only picks up the subcuticular layer of the apex of the flap, and emerges beyond the bay on either side into which the apex is to be fitted (Fig. 11.14). When the stitch is tied the apex is gently snugged into the bay. If interrupted sutures are inserted right up to the apex on either side, carelessly placed sutures may well strangulate the apex of the flap.

178 UNSATISFACTORY RESULTS IN HAND SURGERY

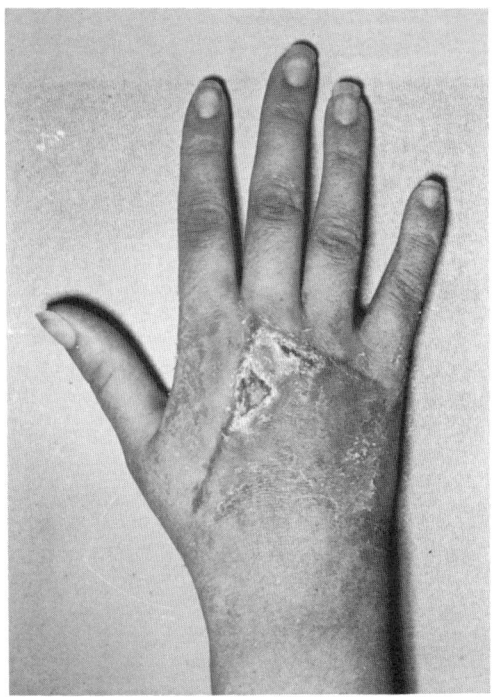
(a)

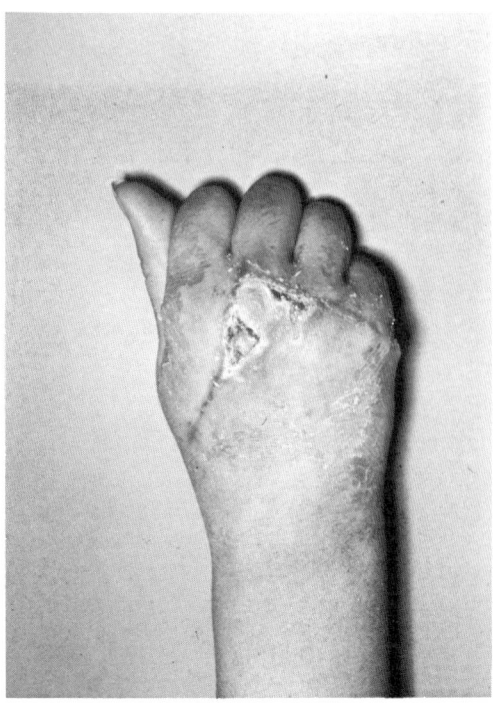
(b)

Fig. 11.13 (a) and (b) Proximally based avulsion flap which has been sutured back. Note the necrosis of the distal part and restricted flexion of the fingers at the metacarpophalangeal joints

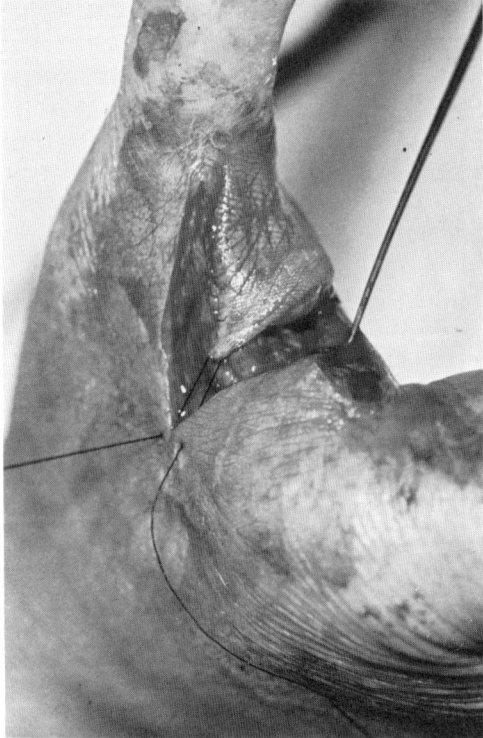

Fig. 11.14 The special stitch securing the apex of a flap in Z-plasty procedure

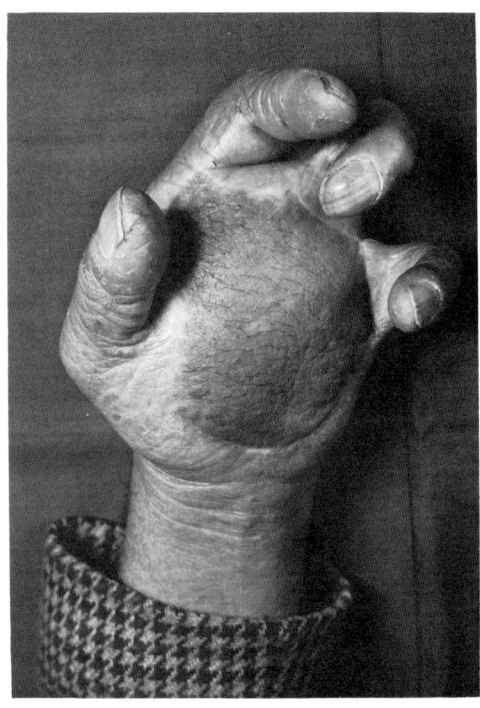

Fig. 11.15 Abdominal flap covering the palm. Note the excessive bulk and unsightly appearance

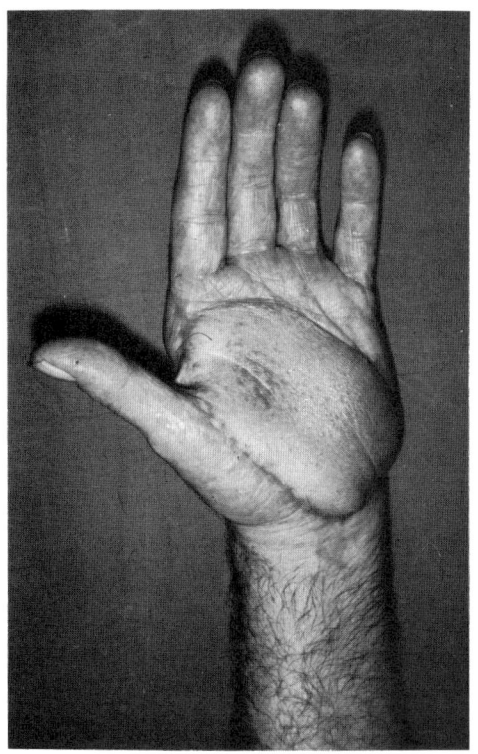 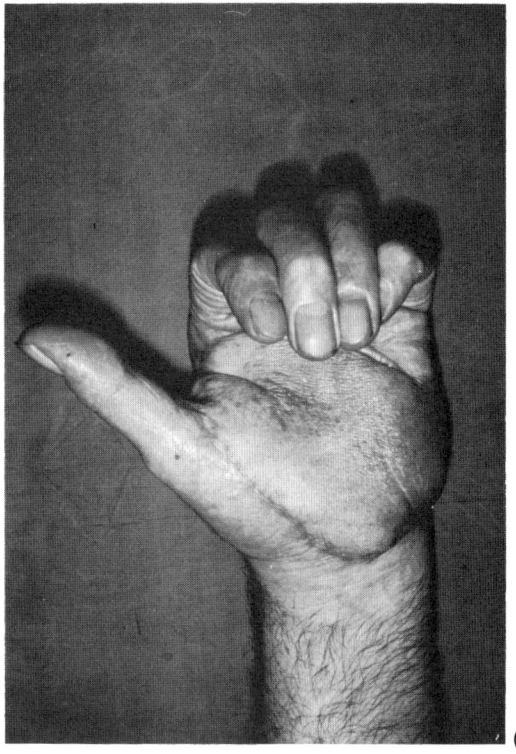

Fig. 11.16 (a) and (b) Primary replacement of skin defect in palm by a groin flap. The concavity of the palm has been largely preserved. No thinning of the flap has been undertaken

Bulky flaps

A useful technique when employing flaps in certain situations, for example, on the back of the hand or fingers, is the so-called crane principle (Millard 1968). A routine flap is raised and inset to the defect covering exposed tendons or open joints on the dorsum, as a primary measure. After 2 weeks, the flap is then carefully detached by dissecting it free but leaving a deep layer of viable tissue covering the defect. A split skin graft is then applied to this surface which is then managed in the usual way as for a free graft. The flap (crane) having performed its task is now returned to the donor site.

Excessively bulky flaps may be avoided to a certain extent by the use of those flaps with little subcutaneous tissue. Cross-finger flaps, cross-forearm or cross-arm flaps and groin flaps come into this category. Abdominal flaps give excessive bulk and the result of such a flap to cover the palm is extremely poor (Fig. 11.15). The groin flap in this situation is vastly superior (Fig. 11.16).

Treatment of unsatisfactory results

Flap necrosis

A limited area of necrosis may be treated by repeated saline dressings, and necrotic tissue progressively snipped away. A minimal raw area may be left to heal spontaneously but a larger one should be covered with a split skin graft as soon as the bed is healthy enough to accept it. It must be remembered that where a graft is applied, this will mean a further period of immobilisation of the hand. If there is the likelihood of severe stiffness developing, it may be better to continue with saline soaks and active mobilisation for a time. Extensive necrosis, for example, following a distally based avulsion flap inadvisedly sutured back in place,

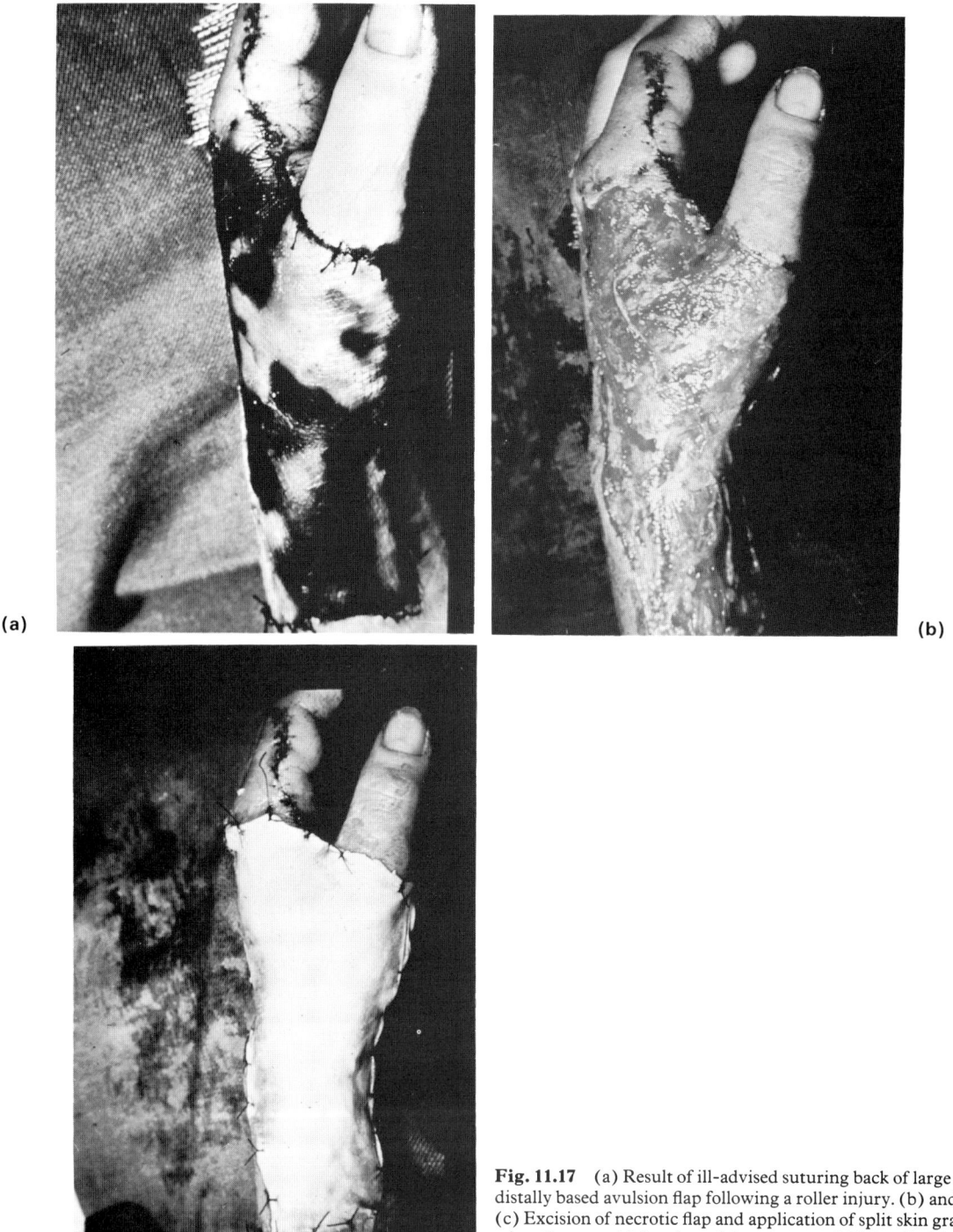

Fig. 11.17 (a) Result of ill-advised suturing back of large distally based avulsion flap following a roller injury. (b) and (c) Excision of necrotic flap and application of split skin graft when first seen 10 days later. Note the use of thick split skin as a single sheet. (d) and (e) Result 6 months later

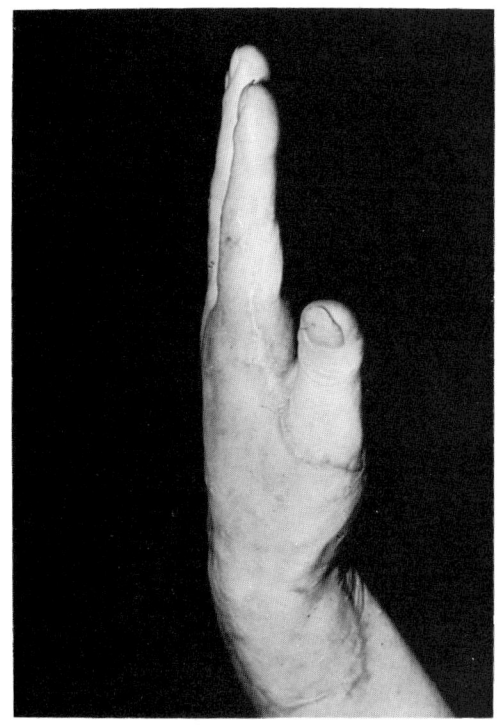
(d)

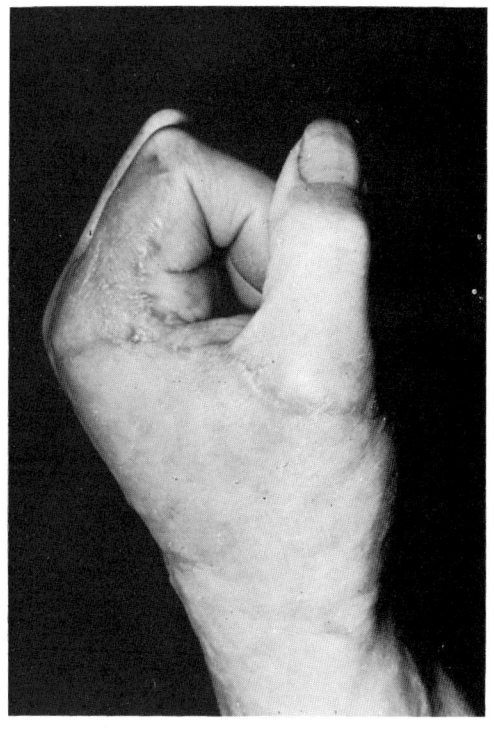
(e)

must be treated by excision of the slough and regrafting where feasible (Fig. 11.17). If the slough remains dry, infection is unlikely to become established for some time. If, on removal of this dry eschar, there is a satisfactory bed without exposure of tendons then a split skin graft should be applied at once. Where infection is established, the slough should be encouraged to separate by the use of repeated saline dressings or soaks. This process may be aided by cutting away dead tissue. Once the wound shows healthy granulations, split skin grafts should be applied.

If, following removal of slough, bare tendons are exposed, immediate flap cover is indicated but this is inadvisable in the presence of obvious sepsis. Should the latter be the case dressings should be continued and further desloughing undertaken as required until the bed is fit for grafting.

Excessive bulk

The majority of pedicle flaps are bulky on account of the subcutaneous tissue present though this varies according to the site from which the flap has been taken. Where excessive bulk is a problem, thinning may be undertaken. This must be done in stages raising one half of the flap at a time by incising either edge. In fact, it is better to excise the original scar at the inset of the flap in the process. The flap is elevated at the junction of the fatty tissue with the underlying bed, and excess fat removed from the deep surface of the flap using McIndoe's scissors. This should be performed under tourniquet control and subsequently careful haemostasis must be ensured prior to suturing. The other half of the flap may be similarly thinned after an interval. These thinning procedures are only successful up to a point.

An alternative procedure, and one well worth considering for bulky flaps on the backs of the digits and hand, is the crane method which has already been described as a means of providing skin cover at the time of injury. For an established flap, the whole of the flap is removed except its deepest layer and a split skin graft applied to the defect (Fig. 11.18). In fact, the surface of the

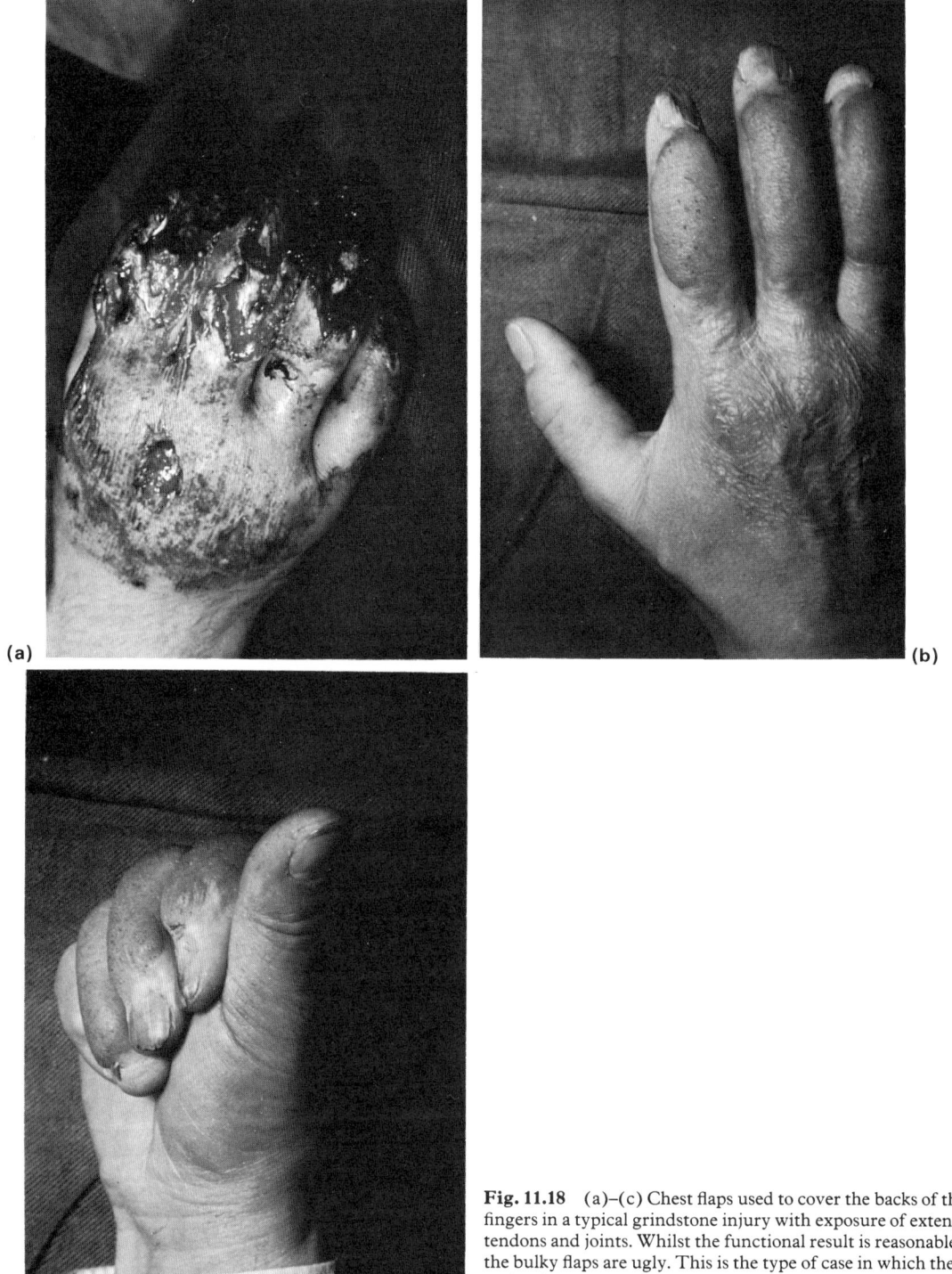

Fig. 11.18 (a)–(c) Chest flaps used to cover the backs of the fingers in a typical grindstone injury with exposure of extensor tendons and joints. Whilst the functional result is reasonable, the bulky flaps are ugly. This is the type of case in which the author has removed the flaps, except the deepest layers, which are then covered with split skin grafts producing a better cosmetic result than that achieved by routine thinning

original flap may be dissected off and reapplied as a Wolfe graft. The cosmetic result of such a procedure is superior to the simple thinning operation and the functional result is equally good. The colour match of a split skin graft used in such a way may also be superior to that of a flap used from a distant site. The cosmetic outcome of a flap repair is important to many patients.

Poor sensory innervation

Gnostic sensation is essential for the tactile surface of the thumb. Without this the thumb is virtually useless. A degloving injury of the thumb requires primary cover by means of a tubed flap. Whether a flap from the groin or the chest wall is used for this, the result is unsatisfactory because of the deficient sensation. Adequate sensation must be introduced by means of some form of neurovascular flap. An innervated cross-finger flap taken from the dorsum of the index finger has already been mentioned and provides an excellent method. Some aspects of the procedure merit further discussion (Fig. 11.19). The flap is marked out on the dorsal aspect of the proximal segment of the index finger and the adjoining part of the dorsum of the hand if necessary, with its base sited at the mid-lateral line. A longitudinal incision is extended proximally on the dorsal aspect of the thumb-index web from the base of the flap at its proximal extremity for a distance of 2 to 3 cm. This is in the line of the fibres of the terminal branch of the radial nerve. The flap is turned off the index finger at the level of the paratenon overlying the extensor expansion. The radial nerve fibres are now exposed over the thumb-index web, carefully mobilised and traced into the flap. The thumb defect is next created by removing the original pedicle skin from the volar tactile surface. A longitudinal incision is then made from the defect on the thumb along the dorso-ulnar aspect, to link up with the other longitudinal incision at the point of the V over the proximal part of the thumb-index web. The radial nerve fibres are then transferred to the thumb defect in continuity with the cross-finger flap which is now sutured to the tactile surface of the thumb. The longitudinal incisions are sutured and the secondary defect on the index finger covered with a split skin or full thickness graft. A full thickness graft may be fashioned from the part of the skin flap removed from the thumb. The cross-finger flap is divided and inset two weeks later. The functional results of these flaps are very good, and although the cortical representation of feeling in the transposed flap remains unaltered, the patient usually adjusts very well in time (Henderson & Reid 1980).

A modification of this technique (Sucur & Radivojedic 1985) involves severing the radial nerve on the dorsum of the hand and linking this by microsurgery to one of the digital nerves in the thumb. It is claimed that this gives excellent results and circumvents the problem of adjusting to a nerve supply coming from an adjoining part. Foucher & Braun (1979) have used a similar flap from the dorsum of the index finger which may be transferred to the thumb as an island, and has already been mentioned. It has the advantage of being a one-stage procedure. Transfer of a heterodigital neurovascular island flap may also give good results. This, too, has already been mentioned.

Acknowledgments

Figures 11.3, 11.9 and 11.11 appear by courtesy of the Editor of the *British Journal of Plastic Surgery*. Figure 11.6 is Mr. D. A. McGrouther's case and appears by courtesy of Butterworths. Figure 11.19 also appears by courtesy of Butterworths. Figure 11.17 appears by courtesy of the Editor of *The Hand*.

184 UNSATISFACTORY RESULTS IN HAND SURGERY

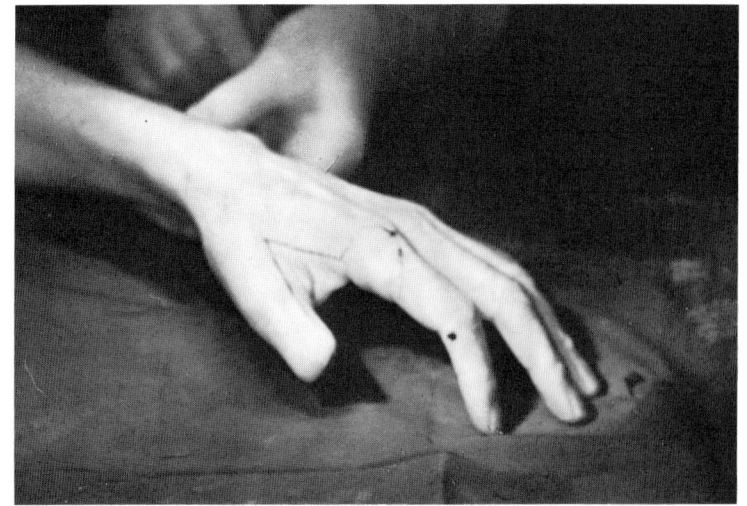
(a)

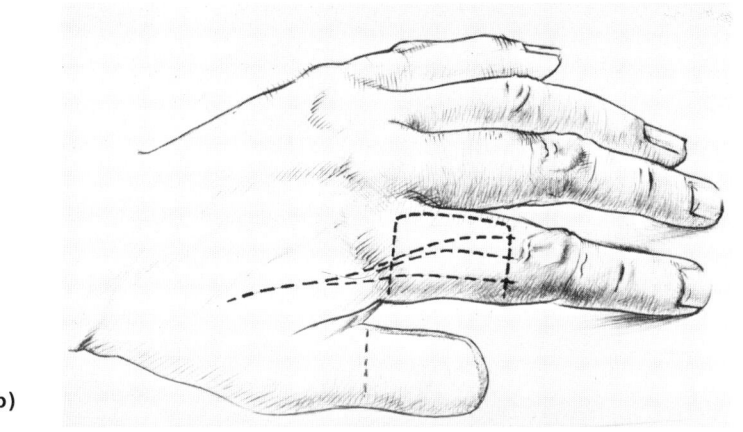
(b)

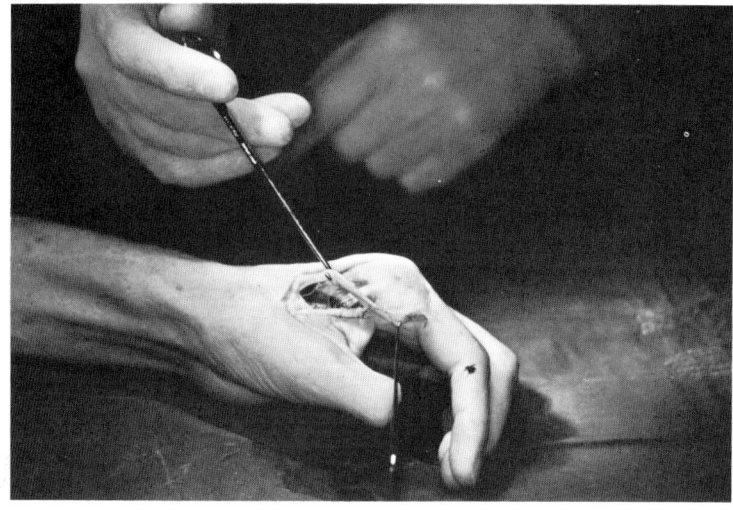
(c)

SKIN GRAFTS AND PEDICLE FLAPS 185

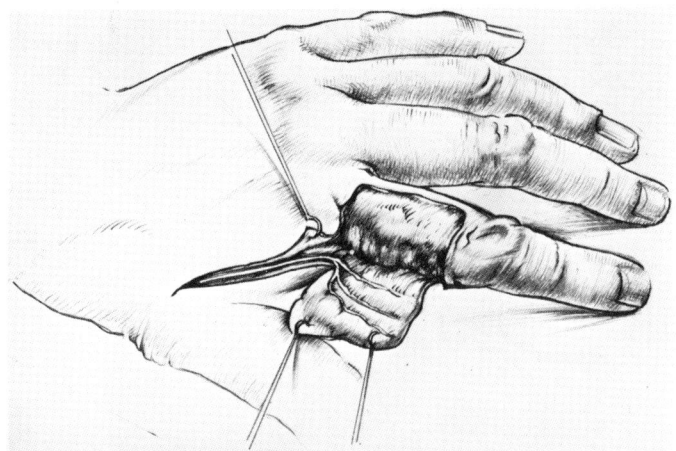

(d)

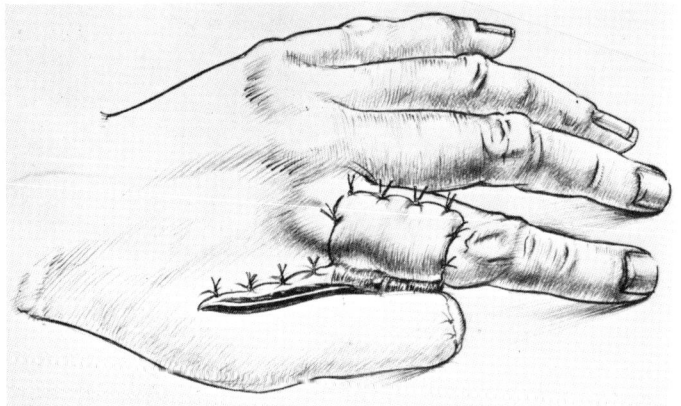

(e)

(f)

Fig. 11.19 (a) and (b) Innervated cross-finger flap marked out on the back of the index finger. (c) and (d) Radial nerve fibres being raised prior to being transferred with the flap to the thumb. (e) and (f) Suture of the flap to the thumb defect

REFERENCES

Atasoy R, Ioakimidis E, Kasoan M D, Kutz J E, Kleinert H E 1970 Reconstruction of the amputated fingertip with a triangular volar flap. A new surgical procedure. Journal of Bone and Joint Surgery 52A: 921

Climo S 1951 Dermal bleeding and the delay operation. Plastic and Reconstructive Surgery 8: 59–63

Dellon A Lee 1983 The extended palmar advancement flap. Journal of Hand Surgery 8: 190–194

Foucher G D, Braun J B 1979 A new island flap transfer from the dorsum of the index finger to the thumb. Plastic and Reconstructive Surgery 63: 344–349

Henderson H P, Reid D A C 1980 Long term follow up of neurovascular island flaps. The Hand 12: 113–122

Iselin F 1973 The flag flap. Plastic and Reconstructive Surgery 52: 374–377

Kutler W A 1947 A new method for fingertip amputations. Journal of the American Medical Association 133: 29

Littler J W 1961 Neurovascular skin island transfer in reconstructive surgery of the hand. In: Wallace A B (ed) Transactions of the International Society of Plastic Surgeons, Second Congress, London. E & S Livingstone Ltd, Edinburgh, p 175

McGregor I A, Jackson I T 1972 The groin flap. British Journal of Plastic Surgery 25: 3–16

Millard D R 1968 The crane principle for the transport of subcutaneous tissue. Plastic and Reconstructive Surgery 43: 451–462

Moberg E 1964 Aspects of sensation in reconstructive surgery of the upper extremity. Journal of Bone and Joint Surgery 46A: 817–825

Porter R W 1968 Functional aspects of transplanted skin in volar defects of the digits. Journal of Bone and Joint Surgery 50A: 955–963

Smith P J 1982 A sliding flap to cover the dorsal skin defects over the proximal interphalangeal joint. The Hand 14: 271–282

Sucur D, Radivojedic M 1985 Cross finger flap—A new technique. Journal of Hand Surgery 10B: 425–429

Vilain R 1952 Techniques élémentaires de réparation des pertes de substance cutanée des doigts. Semaine Hop. Paris 29: 1–7

Vilain R, Dupuis J F 1973 Use of the flag flap for coverage of a small area on a finger or the palm: 20 years experience. Plastic and Reconstructive Surgery 51: 397–401

D. M. Evans

12 Burns

The hand is particularly vulnerable to burn injury. This is because of its exposure, its use for manipulation, and the instinctive use of the hand to protect the face, or to remove burning clothes. The results of all but the most trivial burns are always to some extent unsatisfactory, and good management demands a constant effort to limit factors which may contribute to an unsatisfactory outcome.

It is not uncommon for a disappointing result to follow a hand burn in association with a generalised severe burn. One-third of burns of more than 50% surface area have hand involvement (Huang et al, 1975). Life-threatening problems elsewhere in the patient understandably distract attention from the hands, whereas a few minutes' attention in the early stages can establish a basis for early healing with optimal functional recovery. It is neglect of the posture, the effects of rising tissue pressure, and the proper treatment of the burned surface that leads to the appalling deformities and functional compromise that are sometimes still seen following hand burns in these circumstances.

The factors which can lead to an unsatisfactory result will be considered under the following headings: swelling, extension of skin destruction, damage to or reduced viability of deep structures, scar contracture, and tissue loss.

SWELLING

Increased formation of tissue fluid is an inevitable consequence of thermal injury. If the overlying skin retains its elasticity the hand swells and the loose skin over the dorsum of the hand and fingers can usually expand sufficiently to accommodate the rise in internal pressure. Following full thickness burns however the elasticity of the skin is lost and the rapid formation of oedema can lead to a serious rise in interstitial pressure.

Compression

As the interstitial pressure approaches diastolic blood pressure the circulation through the capillary bed becomes threatened and eventually ceases altogether, with extension of tissue death. Because of associated damage to the overlying skin it is extremely difficult to evaluate the extent to which the rise in interstitial pressure is contributing to distal ischaemia, and for this reason escharotomy should be carried out whenever raised pressure is suspected. Salisbury et al (1976) attempted to evaluate the benefit of digital escharotomy in burned hands. They used Doppler examination of the superficial palmar arch, and if there was no flow they included lateral digital escharotomy with the escharotomy of the limb, and this reduced the rate of digit loss from 21% to 7% in such cases. They found that the escharotomy had to be performed within 24 hours of the burn and they observed that the flow in the superficial arch on Doppler measurement did not always return immediately, even in cases where the escharotomy was effective. The need for escharotomy is usually associated with circumferential deep burns but Wexler et al (1974) suggested that it may even be necessary in some burns of the dorsal surface only, and in some cases more than one incision in each digit is required. It appears that the muscle microcirculation becomes compromised at an interstitial fluid pressure of 30–40 mmHg (Mubarak and Hargens, 1981).

The incisions for escharotomy in the hand should be placed with care, although in most cases in which it is necessary the skin that is being divided is dead, and exposure of underlying structures that would otherwise not become exposed is unlikely. Nevertheless it is reasonable to choose the sides of the fingers, and to place incisions on the dorsum of the hand parallel to but not overlying the extensor tendons. If the escharotomy incision passes from one section of the limb to another there must be continuity of decompression otherwise deceptively tight areas may be left to cause persistent constriction (see Fig. 12.4 below). The ultimate test of the need for an escharotomy is the extent to which the incision gapes.

Immobility

Immobility is the second important consequence of swelling which tends to hold the joints of the hand in an unfavourable position. The metacarpophalangeal joints become fixed in extension or hyperextension, the wrist and PIP joints tend to flex and the thumb adopts an adducted position. If this posture is not corrected by appropriate external splintage combined with elevation, the posture of the hand will become fixed in the worst possible configuration (see Fig. 12.8b below). The key to improving the posture of the hand at this stage is the maintenance of wrist extension which can be achieved with a simple external splint on the volar aspect of the hand and forearm. This must not extend beyond the distal palmar crease or it will limit metacarpophalangeal flexion. Nielsen & Sommer (1983) emphasise the need for these measures, and demonstrated in their series that the severe deformities that are seen at times can be avoided. They also used a K-wire across the metacarpal heads to allow skeletal traction for elevation. Maintenance of the thumb web can be more difficult but should be attempted from an early stage with a splint in the web space, or an intermetacarpal K-wire. Metacarpophalangeal flexion can often be maintained by a combination of physiotherapy at an early stage with wrist splintage, but in resistant cases there may be a place for percutaneous Kirschner wires passed from the dorsal aspect of each metacarpal head across the joint in flexion into the base of the proximal phalanx. If possible one should avoid passing the wire through the extensor tendon. Where it has been necessary to use this technique it is wise to keep the wires in place until skin grafts have been applied.

Persistent oedema

Persistent oedema may contribute to subsequent stiffness due to the gradual organisation and incorporation of the protein-rich exudate around joints and between gliding structures. Once this has become established it is extremely difficult to correct, another strong reason for limiting oedema as far as possible.

EXTENSION OF SKIN DESTRUCTION

Cell damage in the burned area continues until the heat is dissipated which may take many minutes, particularly if hot clothing is in contact with the skin. Clearly this aspect of management is beyond the reach of specialised burn care, but education of the public and of first aid workers in the need to remove hot clothing and to provide rapid cooling of the burnt skin is of value. There are other factors which can lead to an increase in the extent of cell destruction after the patient has come under specialised care and these include infection, vascular embarrassment of the skin, and persistent damage due to chemical burns.

Infection

The burnt surface is vulnerable to infection which may be introduced in the early stages or as a result of careless wound dressing technique. In most areas of the body the choice of treatment of the burn surface lies between closed dressings and exposure to the air. From the point of view of infection both of these methods have their advantages and disadvantages. Closed dressings carried out in an aseptic manner reduce the risk of contamination of the burned surface through cross-infection, but if infection does take place the warm moist atmosphere may provide the ideal environment for bacterial multiplication. Exposure has the advantage of maintaining a cool dry environment on the burned surface which inhibits bacterial colonisation. For the hand neither of these methods is ideal because they limit movement in the early stages. The use of polythene bags placed directly on the hand as an occlusive dressing was described by Slater & Hughes (1971) and has achieved wide acceptance. The bags should be sterile on the inside and bacterial growth is inhibited by the use of an antibacterial cream such as silver sulphadiazine. Sykes & Bailey (1976) compared the results of treatment with dry bags and bags containing sulfamylon or silver sulphadiazine, and found that hands in dry and silver sulphadiazine-containing bags healed in the same time, which was shorter than with the use of bags containing sulfamylon. The bacterial count was highest in the dry bags. The early resumption of movement is facilitated in a cool sterile environment and infection has not been a particular problem with this type of treatment.

Vascular embarrassment

This complicates hand burns where the effect of oedema on the circulation is not recognised and relieved by escharotomy (see above).

Chemical burns

Persistence of the chemical agent on the skin will continue to burn until it is removed, and therefore early copious washing is of great value. Hydrofluoric acid burns present a particular problem in this respect (Dibbell et al 1970) in that the effect of the acid on tissues is to liberate free fluorine radicals which in turn lead to further tissue destruction. If allowed to continue unchecked this process of burning is self-perpetuating and can lead to very extensive tissue loss. Such a burn should be irrigated copiously with iced water and the acid neutralized. The recommended method of treatment is by injection of a small volume of 10% calcium carbonate, but Hayashi (1981) has recommended soaking in 0.02% benzethonium chloride for 20–30 minutes, followed by daily 0.12% betamethazone-17-valerate ointment with gentamycin. This avoids painful injections.

DAMAGE TO DEEP STRUCTURES

Internal structures in the limb may be damaged by the thermal or electrical injury, or as a result of subsequent events. The extensor mechanism is far more vulnerable than the flexor apparatus because of the thin dorsal skin, the small amount of subcutaneous tissue, and the more frequent exposure of the extensor surface of the hand to thermal insult than the flexor surface. Over the dorsum of the hand a burn has to be very deep to involve the extensor tendons directly from the beginning, but in the fingers the extensor mechanism is very close to the surface, particularly when the fingers are flexed. The most vulnerable area is over the PIP joint, and boutonniere deformity due to loss of the central slip of the extensor mechanism is common in deep hand burns. It can be difficult to distinguish between direct burning as a cause and later exposure and drying of the extensor tendon. Whichever is the cause, any tendency for the hand to adopt the 'comfort' position with the MP joints extended will tend to increase the flexion deformity at the PIP joint and this makes it more difficult to correct later. Early recognition of this developing deformity should stimulate active steps to resist flexion at the PIP joint and this generally involves careful splintage and early physiotherapy. If the extensor tendon has actually been burned through, there is little that can be done to prevent a flexion deformity developing and secondary reconstructive surgery may be required. If the burn is a very localised one over the dorsum of the PIP joint, then a local skin flap might be appropriate to provide cover and preserve the underlying tendon.

Over the dorsum of the hand exposure is less of a problem but burns involving pressure in addition to heat often do lead to damage to the extensor mechanism. Wang et al (1985) have reviewed 60 cases and laid greater emphasis on early definitive surgery (within 3 days) than in either burns or crush injuries alone. This is because deep full-thickness loss is inevitable and stiffness can be limited only by early resumption of movement, which is not possible until reconstruction has been carried out.

Even if the tendons do not become exposed as a result of a dorsal full-thickness burn, in some patients the scar tissue that is laid down around the

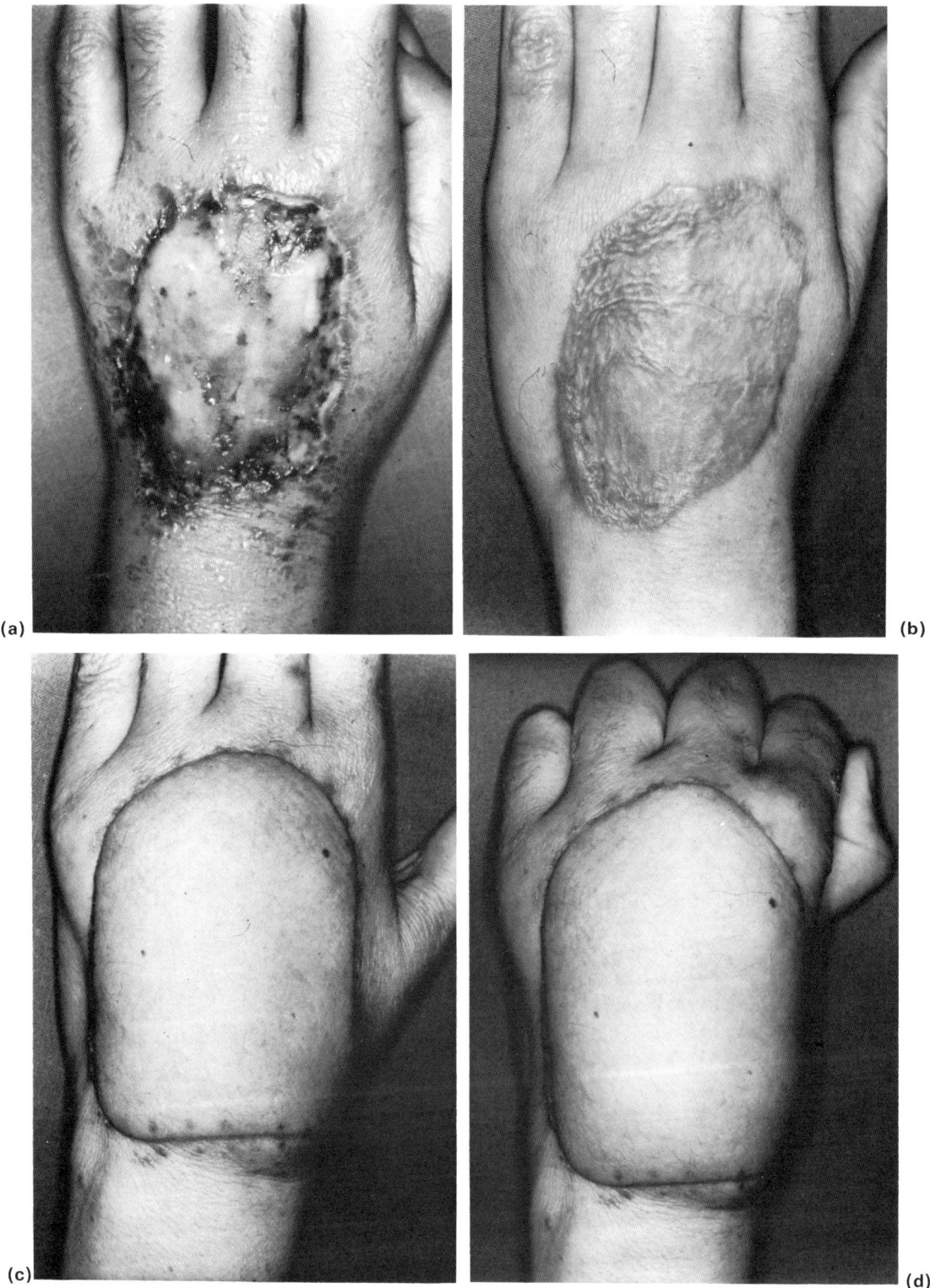

Fig. 12.1 (a) A full thickness dorsal hand burn due to combined heat and pressure. (b) The extensor tendons were not exposed, therefore a split skin graft was applied. The extensor tendons became adherent. (c) Free lateral arm flap cover after tenolysis and MP joint capsulotomy. (d) The degree of flexion possible in the early stages. This is improving with physiotherapy but further surgery will be needed to thin the flap. This case illustrates the disadvantage of skin flaps on the dorsum of the hand

tendons can lead to loss of gliding of undamaged tendons, and the stiffness resulting from this can be very difficult to overcome (Fig. 12.1). When it is clear from the outset that the extensor mechanism has been damaged the only hope of preserving function is through early full thickness cover. In some cases this will allow restoration of active extension without further surgery, even if the tendons themselves have been damaged, since the early contact with vascularised tissue can lead to tendon healing. Adhesions are likely to occur and may need tenolysis. If the burned tendons are allowed to remain exposed or to become infected they will have to be removed and management of the skin defect then depends on other factors, particularly whether or not there are exposed joints or cortical bone, in which case flap cover will very likely be necessary. This provides a suitable environment for later extensor tendon grafting. If the surface left behind after excision of the necrotic tendons is suitable for a free skin graft, healing can be more rapidly achieved. When the hand has been mobilised as far as it will go the decision can be made at leisure whether or not to undertake extensor tendon reconstruction, in which case a skin flap will usually be required to allow this. Occasionally when the defect involves a limited area of the dorsum of the hand the adhesion of the remains of the extensor mechanism to the skin graft allows sufficient active extension or tenodesis effect to make further tendon surgery unnecessary.

Muir (1970) emphasised the important difference between electrical and thermal burns. Electrical burns have a zone of diminished tissue viability which may survive if covered immediately with full thickness viable skin, but which would otherwise undergo necrosis. It follows from this that electrical burns should be excised early, to include the entire damaged zone. A typical electric burn has a red line around the central white area, and this should be excised completely. If loss of a free skin graft would expose important underlying

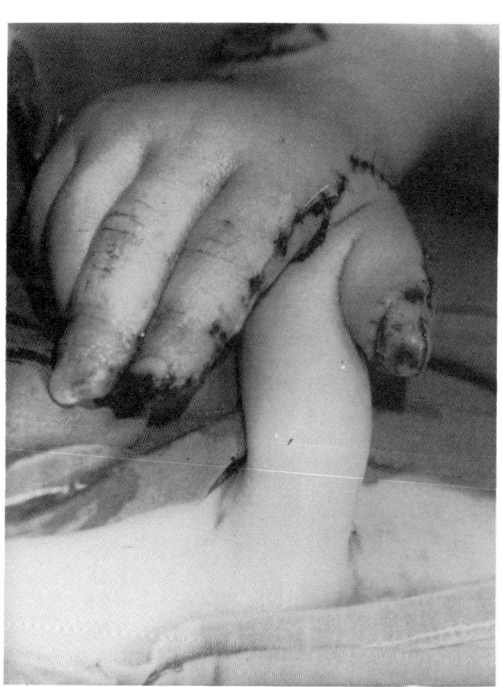
(a)

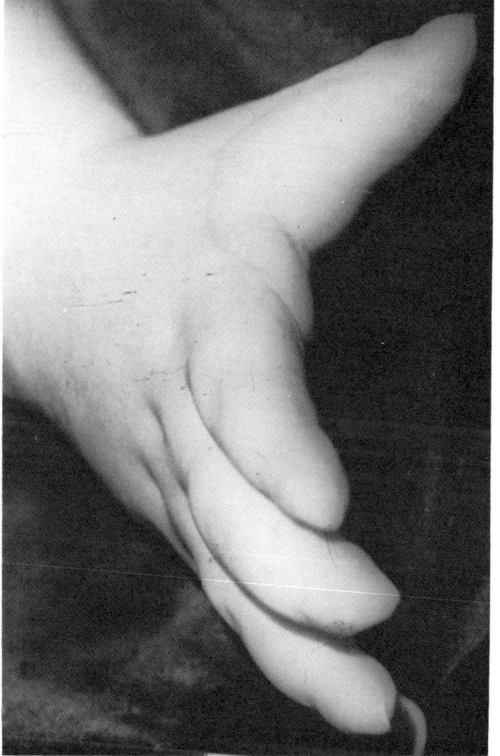
(b)

Fig. 12.2 (a) A full thickness electrical burn of the first web space, including the whole of the volar aspect of the thumb with damage to digital nerves and flexor pollicis longus. The patient is four years old. This has been resurfaced with a thin pedicled groin flap 24 hours after injury. There were ten other scattered full thickness burns on the hand and forearm. (b) The completed reconstruction

192 UNSATISFACTORY RESULTS IN HAND SURGERY

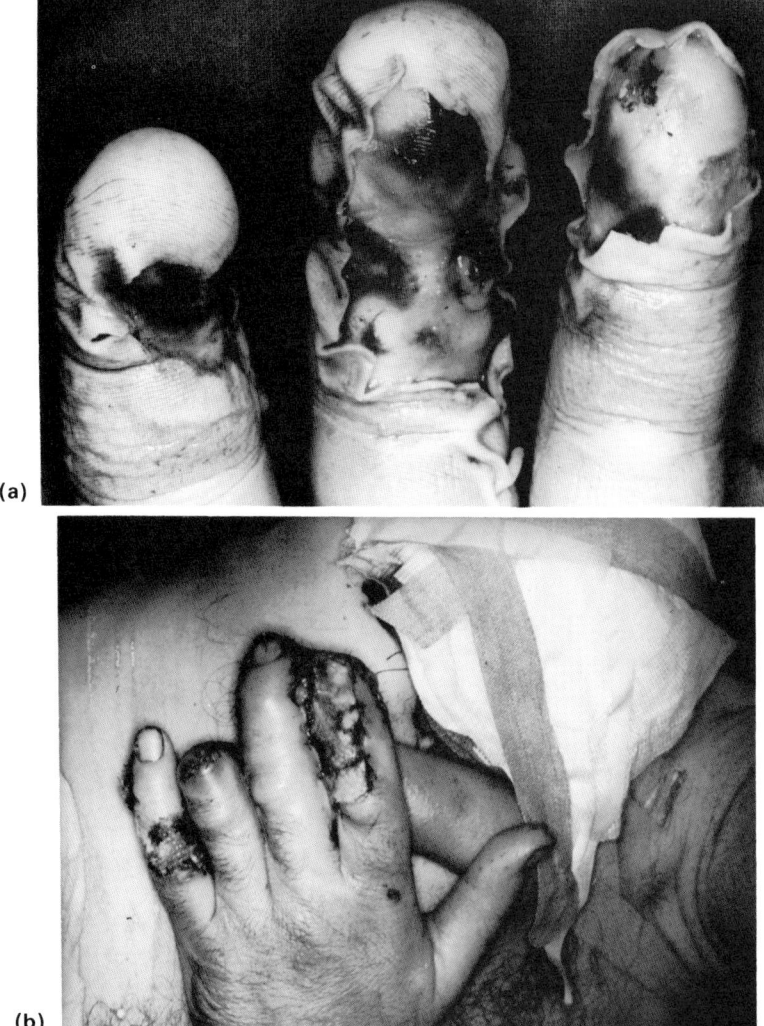

Fig. 12.3 (a) Electrical burn of the fingers with deep skin loss. (b) Local flaps were not available and a delto-pectoral flap was used for three skin defects. This flap cannot be raised thin as can a groin flap. (c) Early unsatisfactory fat flaps. (d) After one thinning procedure surprisingly good skin quality has been provided with some tactile sensation

structures such as tendons, it is wiser to use a flap for cover from the start. For small burns a local flap gives the best result, but for larger burns this may not be possible, and a distant flap is then required. Free flaps have many advantages in this situation (Fig. 12.1), but there is always too much subcutaneous tissue in free flaps transferred to the hand. A pedicled groin flap can be thinned in its distal portion so that there is almost no fat, particularly in children (Fig. 12.2), and this provides ideal skin cover in the first web space. Other pedicle flaps are difficult to thin primarily.

The deltopectoral flap has the advantage of better elevation of the hand during attachment, and when finally thinned can give an excellent result (Fig. 12.3).

Nerves

Peripheral nerves are particularly vulnerable to thermal and electrical injury, and evaluation of the significance of loss of nerve conduction is difficult. The commonest situation where this occurs is in localised electrical burns in the hand, particularly

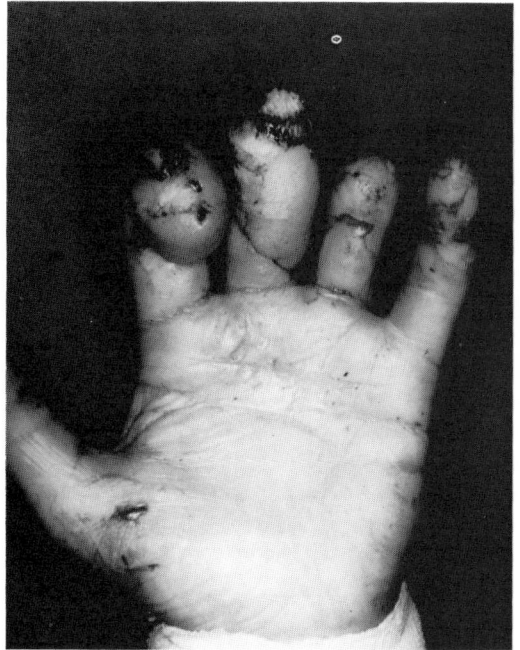
(c)

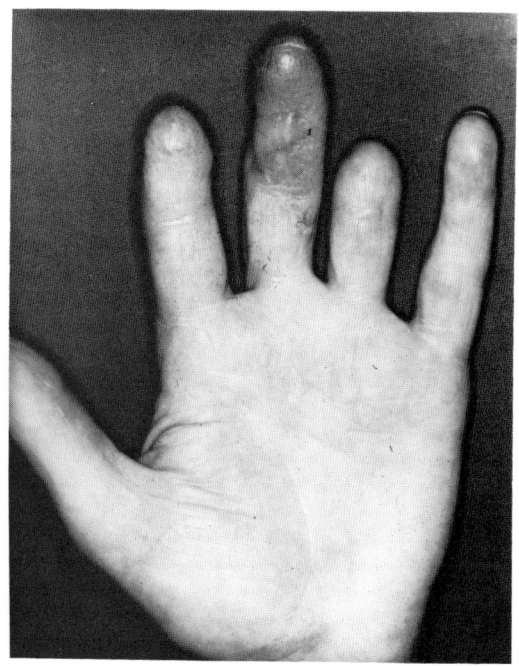
(d)

in the first web space or in the flexor aspects of the fingers. Occasionally a full thickness electric burn is excised and inspection of an underlying digital nerve reveals some discolouration. This may well mean that the nerve has been irrevocably damaged, but it is very reasonable to leave the nerve in place and graft over it, provided the surrounding tissue is healthy. If the nerve has been destroyed by the burn nothing is lost, if not, there may be some recovery. If a nerve graft is required subsequently it may be possible to re-route the graft beneath healthy surrounding skin, or a skin flap may be required. Major nerves can suffer a temporary conduction block following domestic tension electrical injury. If this happens it is reasonable to elevate the limb and wait provided there is no question of nerve compression at any site. This may be difficult to determine, and if there is any doubt it is better to decompress the nerve at vulnerable sites than allow compression to continue.

Muscle

Thermal burns with extensive muscle involvement always imply serious damage to the limb and may involve neurovascular structures with irrevocable consequences for the distal part of the limb. Since part of the muscle damage may be caused by compartment compression, fascial decompression should be carried out as a matter of course. Destruction of muscle due to heat is usually obvious and well demarcated from the start, and early debridement is advisable where circumstances permit, to avoid the danger of serious infection with systemic toxicity. Burns of this severity may involve other forms of trauma in addition, particularly due to crush.

High tension electric burns

These are the prime example of damage to deep structures of far greater extent than overlying skin damage, and this particularly affects muscle and neurovascular structures. Contact with the high tension source is usually made with one or both hands and the current passes up the limb, close to bone and often in the neurovascular plane. The distal part of the limb is usually mummified, but proximal to that there is apparently viable skin concealing massive deep destruction. There is enormous swelling in the muscle compartments which is revealed by fasciotomy which should be carried out immediately, and in contrast to escharotomy in thermal burns, requires a general anaesthetic, because skin sensation may be preserved initially. Fasciotomy should extend the whole length of the limb, well beyond the limit of superficial burning, because the swelling and its disastrous consequences extend proximally beneath viable skin (Fig. 12.4). Examination of deep muscle compartments during fasciotomy may reveal a cuff of necrotic muscle clothing the bone, extending up to the top of the limb and if this is present a high amputation is likely to be required, and should be carried out early to avoid the risk of infection and renal failure due to absorbed toxic products. Compression is not the only cause of extending necrosis. Wang & Zoh (1983) showed that the vascular occlusion that may occur is due to damage from within outwards, affecting the intima first, and is thus by inference due to the passage of current up the vessel. The same workers (Wang et al, 1982, 1984a) have demonstrated the value of early vein grafting of occluded arteries at the distal forearm level in such cases.

Another possible explanation for progressive tissue loss following electrical injury has been proposed by Robson et al (1984) who have identified a rise in tissue thromboxane after experimental electrical injury. They have demonstrated some useful effect of an anti-thromboxane agent experimentally.

If amputation is necessary after high tension burning, the stump should initially be left open and should only be closed when it is clear that all non-viable tissue has been removed (Fig. 12.4c).

Frequently there are other full thickness burns representing exit wounds and these need to be treated at the same time. They often require skin flap cover and the patient illustrated underwent three local flap procedures in addition to the amputation of the right upper limb, within the first week. Failure to treat high tension burns in this energetic way can result in loss of life of the patient or delayed healing and progressive functional damage due to infection.

Open joints

In the hand, joints are most vulnerable from their dorsal aspect. This usually involves damage to the extensor mechanism also over MP or PIP joints and occurs most commonly in severe burns involving the whole hand. Where an individual joint and extensor mechanism is involved it may be appropriate to cover the dorsal surface of the finger with a local or distant skin flap and this paves the way for later reconstructive surgery of the extensor mechanism. Where multiple fingers and joints are involved a conservative approach may result in healing, provided the circulation is intact and the burn does not extend into bone. Skin grafts can usually be successfully applied to the viable tissue surrounding the joint and will bridge across the joint if the capsular defect is small. This will leave a stiff joint and a decision can be made later as to whether skin flap cover and reconstruction of the extensor mechanism is justified in terms of the overall function of the hand.

SCAR CONTRACTURE

This is the principal source of unsatisfactory results following burns of the hand. All burns involving full thickness skin loss form scar tissue and all scars have a tendency to contract. One of the prime considerations in treating hand burns is to limit the extent to which scar tissue is required for healing and to control as far as possible the contracture. When the scar tissue has matured the range of movement and skin availability are assessed and remaining contractures released. These three processes, restriction of scar tissue, prevention of scar contraction, and release of contracture, will be considered in detail.

Restriction of scar tissue

Many people have emphasised the importance of early closure of burn wounds in the hand (Madden & Enna 1983). A full thickness burn that is allowed to remain unhealed beyond the first week is already on the road to contracture through the formation of granulation tissue which is eventually replaced by scar tissue, whether or not the surface is grafted. Therefore when circumstances permit, it should be a primary aim to achieve skin closure by whatever method is necessary before that time. The real problem in decision-making stems from

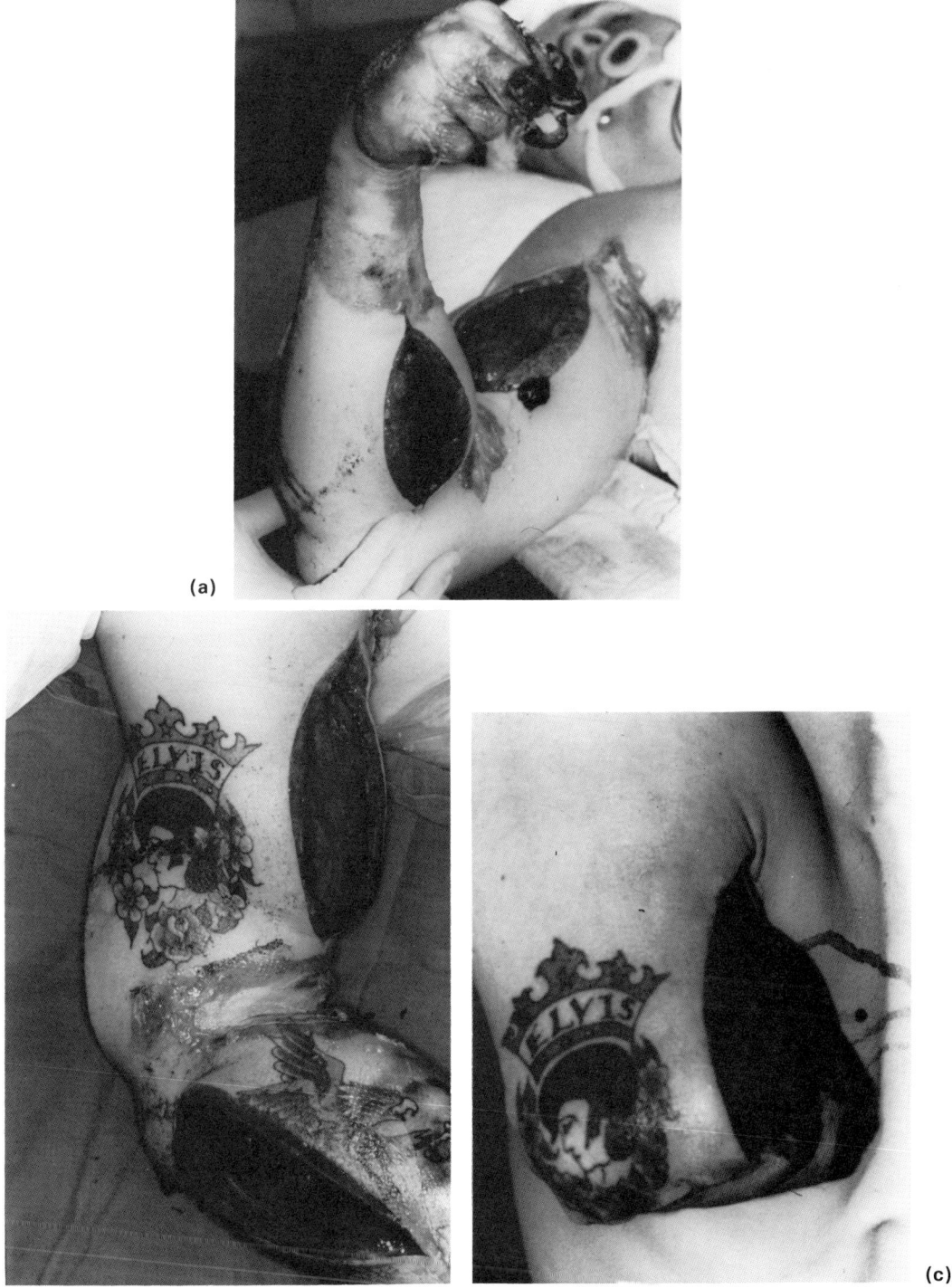

Fig. 12.4 (a) A severe high tension electrical burn of the right upper limb with total distal destruction. Inadequate fasciotomies have been performed. (b) The incision fails to cross the elbow region and should have been continuous across it. Nevertheless deep muscle destruction extended proximal to this area as far as the shoulder, so amputation would have been necessary even if a full fasciotomy had been performed. (c) Amputation was carried out four inches below the shoulder joint and was not closed primarily but grafted later. An additional full thickness burn in this axilla was repaired with a scapular island flap

the difficulty in diagnosing the depth of the burn, and in reliable prediction of early healing with or without grafting. Tangential excision (Janzekovic 1970) is one way of approaching this problem. The technique may be applied to any burn that is thought to extend into the deeper half of the dermis, and various criteria can be used to determine this, including the appearance of the burned surface, although this can be deceptive; Fig. 12.5 illustrates the difficulty of judging depth of a hand burn by appearance. Most surgeons regard the absence of pin prick sensation as a reliable sign that the burn is deep dermal or full thickness. If it is deep dermal spontaneous healing would be slow and it is Janzekovic's contention, supported by the research work of Lawrence & Carney (1973), that excision of the burned surface down to the level at which at least some viable tissue is present allows a skin graft to take and restore viability to those deep dermal elements that were threatened. Lawrence & Carney's studies of metabolic activity in the recipient areas for skin grafts showed that a skin graft can take on tissue with only 20–30% of normal metabolic activity.

Based on this concept tangential excision is performed by shaving the skin surface in successive layers with a skin graft knife until a layer is exposed in which the mesh of dermis is punctuated by healthy tissue. In other areas of the body this can be judged by the presence of bleeding, but in the hand it is ideal to carry out this technique under tourniquet, and the viability of the dermal surface has to be judged by its appearance without bleeding. Burned tissue is stained pink, in contrast to the healthy whiteness of dermis or yellow colour of fat. Another useful feature to observe is the presence of thrombosed small vessels, a sure sign that the tissue plane is within the burned zone. When a predominantly viable layer is reached a meshed skin graft is applied, and dressed before release of the tourniquet. Provided no major blood vessels are left open, good take of the skin graft will usually be obtained. If no tourniquet is used, or a tourniquet is released before application of the graft, blood loss can be considerable and may make the excision of remaining areas much more difficult. Furthermore it is unlikely that the graft can be applied without some haematoma being left beneath it.

Although tangential excision of hand burns of appropriate depth is widely practised, fully documented evidence of its advantage over good conservative management is not available. Labandter et al (1976) attempted to compare tangential excision and grafting with a regime of conservative treatment using dressings and intensive physiotherapy from the beginning. Their own conservatively treated cases were compared with the tangentially excised cases reported separately by Wexler et al (1974) and they were unable to detect a significant difference in the outcome. They emphasise the need for intensive physiotherapy from the beginning. Malfeyt (1976) loosely compared two series and felt that tangentially excised burns healed more quickly than conservatively treated burns of the dorsum of the hand, but he did not compare the final result and he makes no mention of the regime of physiotherapy in either group. Salisbury & Wright (1982) compared tangential excision and grafting with delayed treatment and grafting in dermal and full thickness burns of the dorsum of the hand and found no long term advantage in tangential excision. They suggested using this technique if the hand burn was the only injury, on the grounds that it was possible to discharge the patient from hospital more quickly. This advantage did not apply in more extensive burns. Wang et al (1984b) reported their experience of tangential excision of deep dermal burns in 156 patients and concluded that the procedure was worthwhile, and Pegg et al (1984) came to the same conclusion. There was no attempt at comparison with conservative treatment in these two series.

The grafted surface following tangential excision is usually free of contracture, provided some dermal components survive beneath the graft. Cysts frequently form in the grafted area (Stone & Lawrence 1973) and are thought to be the result of buried remnants of open ducts. If this is the case one could suggest that areas where cysts form in any numbers would have healed spontaneously without the need for skin grafting by epithelialisation from the edges of the open ducts. Another minor complication of tangential excision and grafting is the presence of overlapping frills of skin graft at the margin of excision, and these occasionally have to be shaved off in addition to the removal or dermabrasion of cysts.

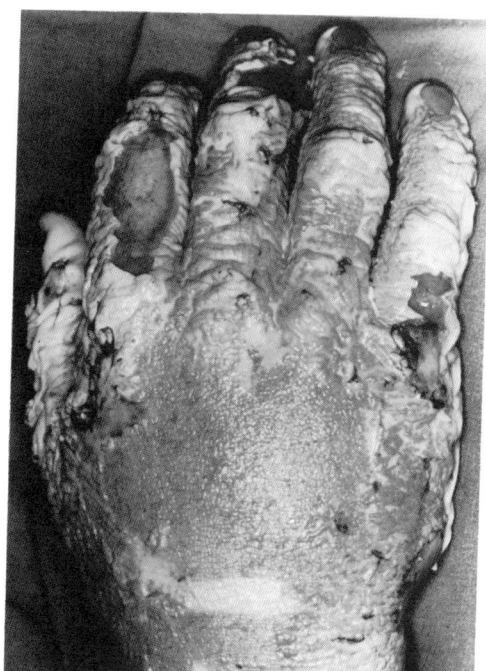

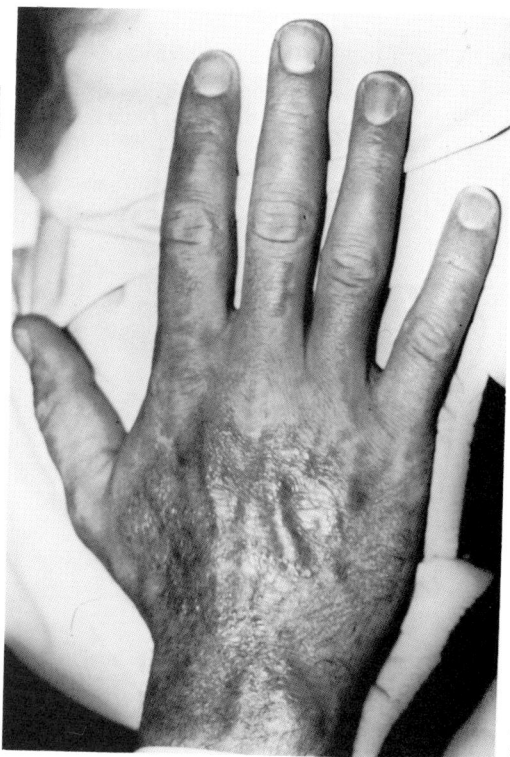

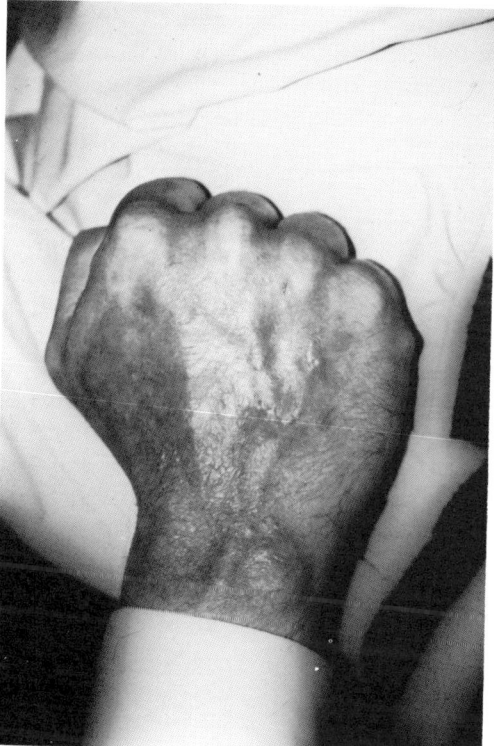

Fig. 12.5 (a) Mixed partial thickness and deep dermal burns of the hand. Early appearance suggested that dorsal aspects of the fingers might be deep-dermal and the dorsum of the hand partial-thickness. (b) and (c) The fingers healed spontaneously but the dorsal hand burn was shaved and grafted. The surface is scarred but allows full extension and flexion

An alternative approach to the deep dermal burn has been described by Holmes & Rayner (1984). They dress the burn for 2 weeks, and if the typical unhealed dermal web persists they use dermabrasion to remove the small granulations which protrude through the dermis, because they believe that these inhibit the growth of epithelial cells across the unhealed surface. Provided that the dermal honeycomb is still visible after dermabrasion they have found that no skin graft is necessary. In their series of 45 deep dermal burns treated in this way, only four failed to heal. Their incidence of hypertrophic and contracted scars is low.

On the palm of the hand a conservative policy is usually pursued when there is doubt about the depth of the burn, because the greater thickness of the skin increases the likelihood of survival of deep dermal and epidermal elements. When palmar burns are obviously full thickness, particularly in the case of electrical burns, the skin is excised with a scalpel rather than the skin graft knife and the principle of early replacement adhered to as discussed above. Thick skin grafts contract less than thin ones. A small full-thickness burn in a critical area can be replaced by the use of a local skin flap where the surrounding skin is completely undamaged. This can apply in the first web space where a skin flap is available from the dorsum of the index finger or the thumb, or at the palmar aspect of the bases of the fingers where a small skin flap can be taken from the side or dorsal aspect of the same or the neighbouring finger. This approach is usually only applicable in the treatment of small domestic-tension electrical burns. The use of large skin flaps for primary skin cover after burns is usually only indicated as a means of providing full thickness cover for important exposed structures.

Prevention of scar contracture

This requires constant attention from the beginning. Whenever the hand has to be immobilised the wrist should be maintained in extension. The first web space should be held abducted and the metacarpophalangeal joints of the fingers should be in a partially flexed position, and onto this basic posture has to be superimposed any special requirement dictated by the position of the burn or of the skin graft that has been used to replace it. Scars in any part of the hand may cause a contracture, particularly in children, where subsequent growth imposes an additional problem. As soon as the wounds and grafts are stable long term compression therapy is started, using individually made pressure gloves, and this limits scar hypertrophy. In doing so it helps with the prophylaxis of contractures, but must be combined with other specific preventive measures.

It is particularly on the flexor aspect of the hand and in the web spaces that contractures develop easily and have to be guarded against. For contractures to develop on the dorsal aspect of the hand there has to be a considerable amount of missing tissue and neglect. Where scars and grafts are situated in contractile areas such as the palm, palmar aspects of the hand and fingers, and the first web space, splintage may need to be maintained for many months, or even years, particularly in children. Electric bar fire burns of the hand are best treated by acrylic oyster splints (Olney 1983) which are made from plaster casts of the hand, and should be easily applied and maintained by the child's parents (Fig. 12.6). In addition to splintage, any tendency for burn scars to hypertrophy should be controlled as far as possible by a pressure glove made to fit the hand exactly. Web space contractures can be limited also by the use of interdigital compression. The first web space is best maintained by a moulded thermoplastic splint which may need to be altered as the web space opens out. This area requires attention from the earliest possible moment because the adductor pollicis muscle shortens as soon as a contracture becomes established, and this, combined with the mechanical advantage of the contracting skin, renders subsequent splintage valueless.

Flexion contractures of the PIP joints of the fingers are difficult to manage because there may be a simultaneous contribution from scar tissue on the palmar aspect of the finger and damage to the extensor mechanism on the dorsal aspect, giving a boutonniere type of deformity. When both of these contribute to the contracture it will only be successfully treated if both are corrected simultaneously. If the skin over the dorsal aspect of the PIP joint is also thin and scarred, correction may be impossible and the extent of functional impairment resulting from the deformity depends very much on the range of movement at the metacarpophalangeal joint. If that joint can hyperextend it is still possible to bring the tactile pulp of the finger into line with the other fingers; but if the MP joint is also flexed the finger sticks out in a palmar direction and gets in the way.

Surgical release of burn contractures

Particular areas where this is frequently required are the web spaces of the fingers, especially the first web space, the palmar aspects of the fingers, the dorsum of the hand, and the proximal part of the limb.

The first web space

An established contracture of the first web space significantly limits the functional capacity of the hand by preventing abduction of the thumb. In a localised full thickness burn resulting in this problem, such as may occur following an electrical burn, it is usually possible to release the thumb web and replace the skin of the web fold with a local flap from the hand. If the contracture results from a more extensive burn this may not be possible, in which case a distant pedicle flap may be required. Release of the contracted skin will allow some restoration of abduction but it is frequently necessary to release the deep fascia over adductor pollicis and between the adductor and the first dorsal interosseous, and frequently the adductor muscle itself needs release. This is done by extending into the thenar crease the incision by which the web space has been released, and exposing the palmar aspect of adductor pollicis down to its origin on the third metacarpal shaft. In doing this the motor branch of the ulnar nerve should be identified and protected as it emerges through the adductor, which is divided from its origin until the entire muscle can move with the thumb. This is preferable to the more simple procedure of release of the adductor tendon, because by releasing the origin the function of the muscle is retained. The ideal skin flap for web space reconstruction is a long dorsal flap from the index finger, extending almost as far as the PIP joint, with its ulnar margin extending proximally to the level of the base of the first metacarpal, and curving back towards the base of the thumb (Fig. 12.7). This flap is undermined to separate it from the index ray but dissection is not extended between the flap and the thumb since release of the web space will allow the flap to move into abduction together with the thumb, and the tip of the flap then flops over to restore the two layers of the first web fold. A split skin graft is applied to the donor defect on the dorsal aspect of the index finger and its metacarpal. This operation has to be followed up by splintage of the first web space until the scar softens.

Contractures may affect the thumb in other ways, described by Stern et al (1985). Extension and flexion contractures may require joint capsulotomies as well as skin release using grafts or local flaps.

Web spaces of the fingers

A web scar contracture may form on the dorsal or on the palmar aspect of the web space, or occasionally in both positions. Short dorsal webs can be corrected by a Z-plasty, or more effectively by a V-M plasty as described by Alexander et al (1982). Mild degrees of palmar syndactyly can be corrected by a procedure designed to allow the web skin to drop back without producing scarring on the free margin of the web (Scotland & Morris 1983). This is based on the concept that at least in some cases, the post-burn syndactyly is formed by traction on the web skin due to forced extension of fingers where there is some palmar tightness in a longitudinal direction. Tight web contractures may require a larger local skin flap than a Z-plasty will provide, and this can be taken from the adjacent side of an unburned finger (MacDougal et al 1976). A simple rhomboid design works well (Lister & Gibson 1972), but a small back-cut on the fourth side may be needed to allow the flap to transpose freely.

Flexion contractures of fingers

Once established these usually require additional skin for release, combined with joint capsulotomy at the PIP joint if skin release fails to free the joint. It is preferable to use a Wolfe graft or split skin graft if the underlying tissue bed allows (Alexander

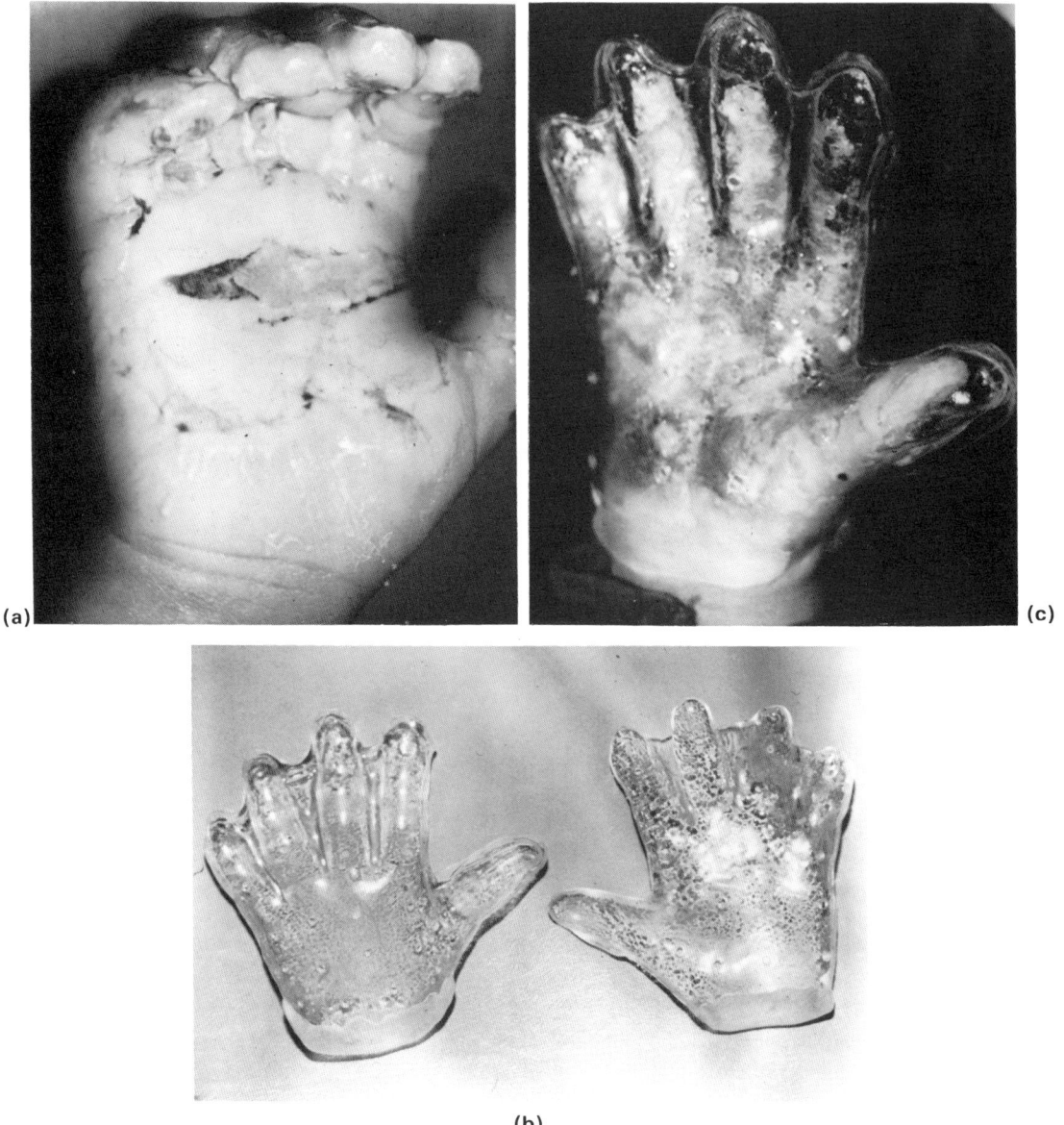

Fig. 12.6 (a) A typical electric bar-fire burn. This is a combined electrical and thermal burn, and is always full-thickness. The burn is excised primarily and must be splinted from the start. (b) Clear acrylic splints are made to fit accurately from a cast of the hand. (c) They should be fitted as soon as the skin is healed. (d) and (e) The splints should be worn for at least 6 months and if a splint for the first web space is needed this can be alternated with the acrylic splint. Full extension and flexion can be maintained by this technique

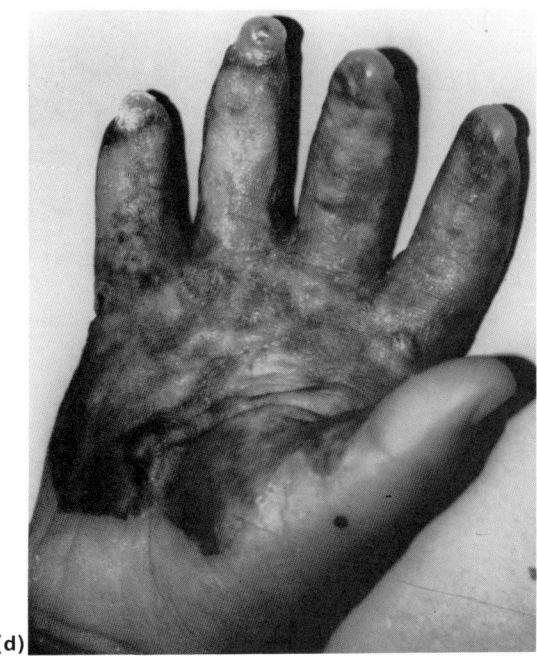
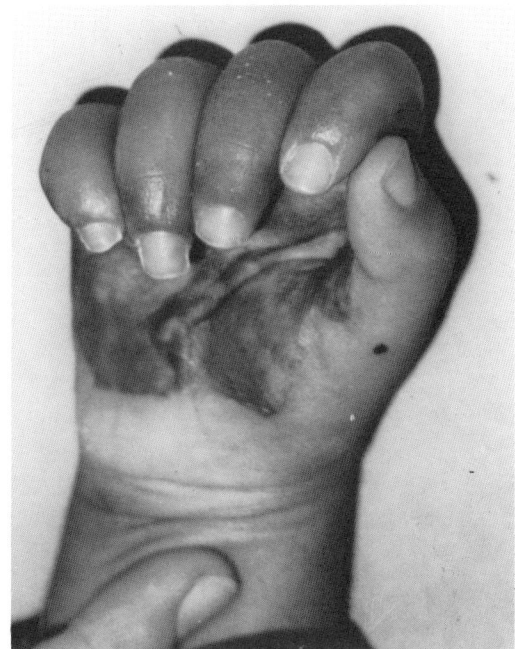
(d) (e)

et al 1981). They also showed that the insertion of temporary K-wires to maintain the correction tended to cause joint stiffness.

Dorsal contractures

It should be possible to prevent dorsal skin contractures by early skin replacement and correct splintage and physiotherapy during and after the healing period. When severe dorsal skin contractures occur, such as those shown in Fig. 12.8, it is very likely that there will be other joint contractures in the same limb or elsewhere in the body, because such contractures usually occur in extensive burns which have been inadequately cared for in the early stages. Tight hyperextension of the MP joints of the fingers limits prehensile hand function and also results in a flexion deformity at the PIP joint level even in the absence of palmar burns of the fingers. In addition the wrist is often held in a flexed position, and if there is a burn on the flexor aspect of the wrist this is likely to be tight also.

The ease with which this deformity can be corrected depends on the original depth of tissue damage, and it may not be possible to determine this until the burn scar is excised. In the case illustrated in Fig. 12.8 there was still soft tissue cover for the extensor mechanism after excision of the scar on both hands, and it was possible to divide the dorsal capsule of the metacarpophalangeal joints through a small incision in the lateral aspect of the extensor hood on each joint to allow MP flexion to be restored. The dorsal edge of the collateral ligaments had to be divided to allow full flexion, and a single sheet of Padgett dermatome graft was used to resurface each hand. When the right side was treated the graft was loosely meshed with the unfortunate result that each incision in the graft produced a small keloid scar; where possible meshing should be avoided in the use of thick skin grafts in pigmented people. The MP joints were held in 70° of flexion with a percutaneous K-wire brought out through undamaged skin beyond the area of grafting in each finger. An unusual problem was encountered in the left ring finger, which became painful and stiff after removal of the wire. An X-ray showed narrowing of the joint space and this suggested that the amount of compression that had been present when the finger was held in flexion for insertion of the K-wire had resulted in some cartilage necrosis. This was treated conservatively by gentle mobilisation and the joint

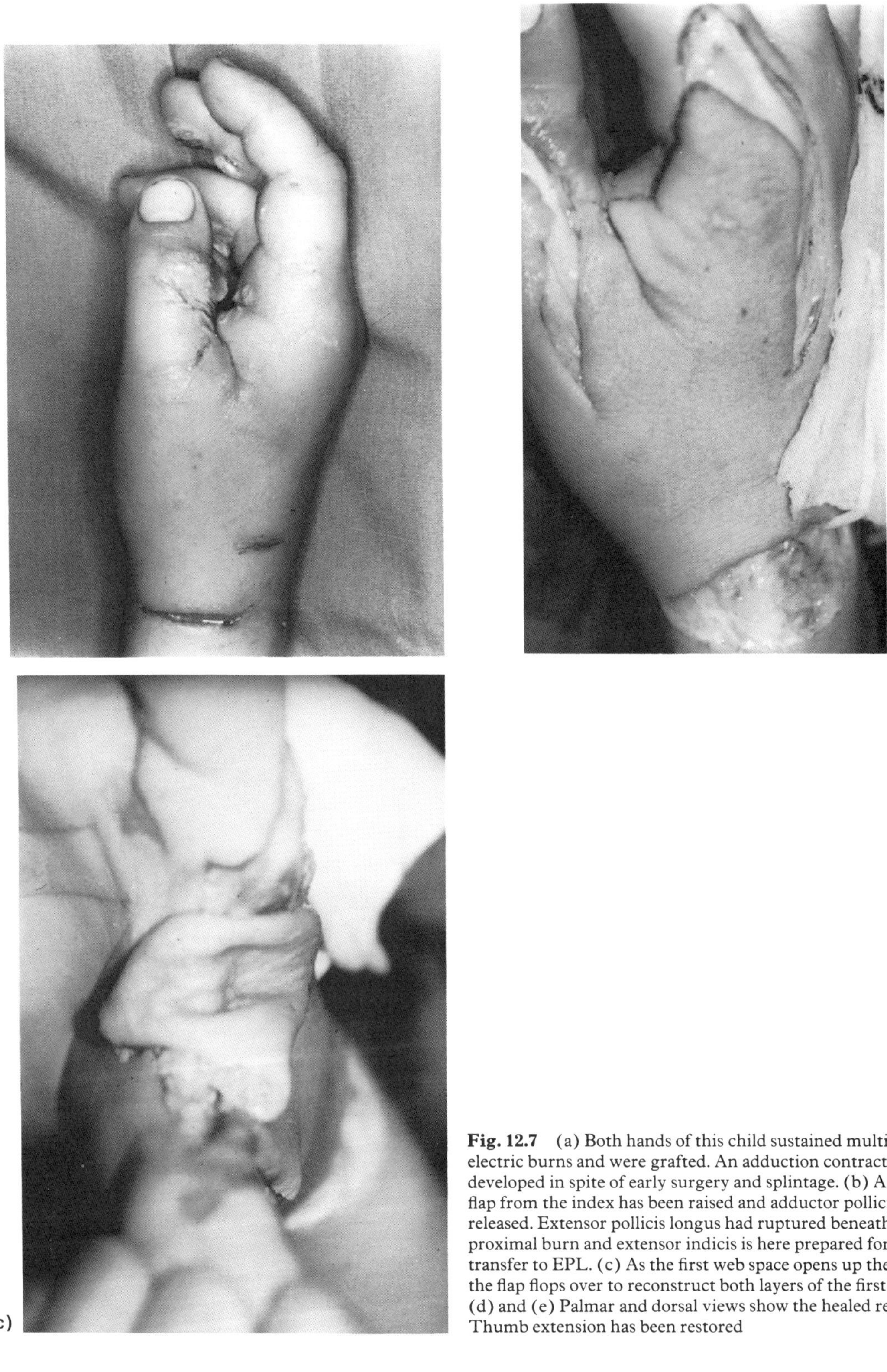

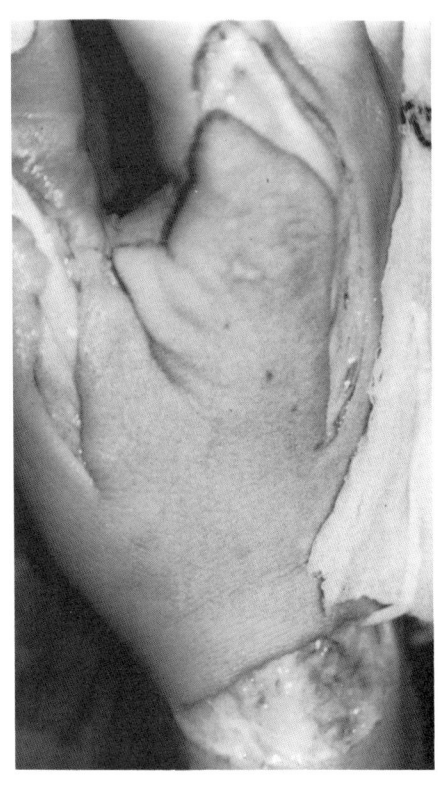

Fig. 12.7 (a) Both hands of this child sustained multiple electric burns and were grafted. An adduction contracture developed in spite of early surgery and splintage. (b) A dorsal flap from the index has been raised and adductor pollicis released. Extensor pollicis longus had ruptured beneath the proximal burn and extensor indicis is here prepared for transfer to EPL. (c) As the first web space opens up the tip of the flap flops over to reconstruct both layers of the first web. (d) and (e) Palmar and dorsal views show the healed repair. Thumb extension has been restored

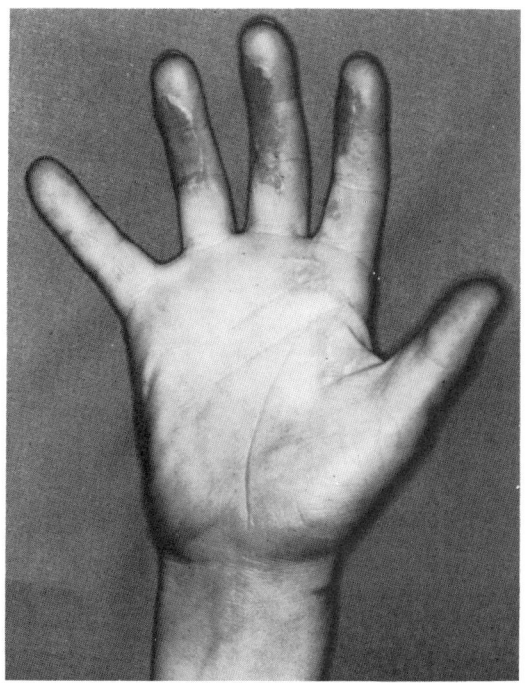
(d)

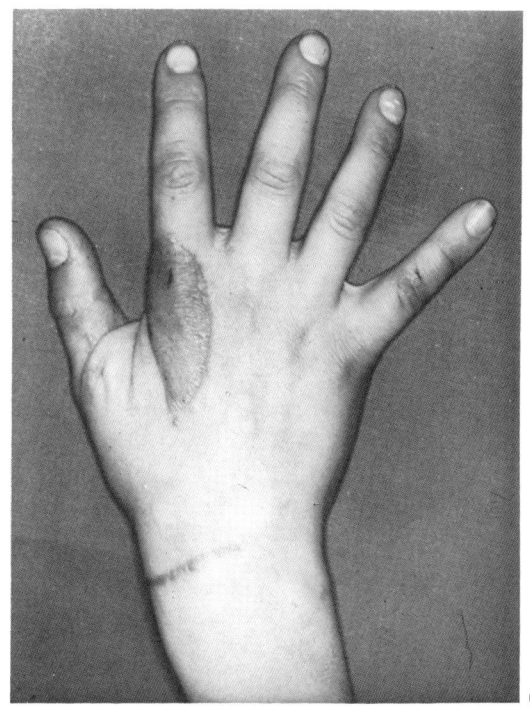
(e)

recovered, although it never regained as full a range of flexion as the other MP joints. If excision of the burn scar had resulted in exposure of extensor tendons, or if the tendons had been damaged, it is likely that a skin flap would have been required, using either a pedicle groin flap or a free flap.

Although flaps allow mobilisation of joints and tendons they frequently require subsequent thinning, and never give as good a result as a thick skin graft. An alternative exists in the form of the bipedicle dermal flap described by Colson et al (1967). This has been shown by Mercer (1985) to be applicable to defects of the whole of the dorsum of the hand. A bipedicle flap is raised on the lateral aspect of the opposite upper arm, with the central part of the flap raised to the depth of the deep surface of the dermis only so that no fat at all is taken with the flap. The hand is placed beneath this flap and the pedicles have to be sufficiently long to allow insertion of the hand without tension. The central part of the flap takes as a Wolfe graft but it will survive over an inhospitable surface because of the contribution to its survival from the pedicles. The extent to which this technique is applicable to large defects remains to be seen.

Proximal limb contractures

These will not be discussed in detail, but the risk of brachial plexus damage through traction or positioning during release should always be borne in mind (Law et al 1983). This problem can also be caused by a postoperative shoulder abduction splint. Abduction in front of the coronal plane avoids traction on the plexus.

An ingenious technique for contracture release at the elbow has been described (Dias 1983) where the tight band is incised transversely at two levels leaving a bridge of scarred skin crossing the flexion crease of the joint. This bridge of skin is not undermined, and a graft is placed in the elliptical defects above and below the bridge. The presence of the intact bridge lessens the likelihood of recurrent contracture.

Release of contractures can only be successful if followed by splintage and physiotherapy. Huang et al (1978) found a higher incidence of recurrent

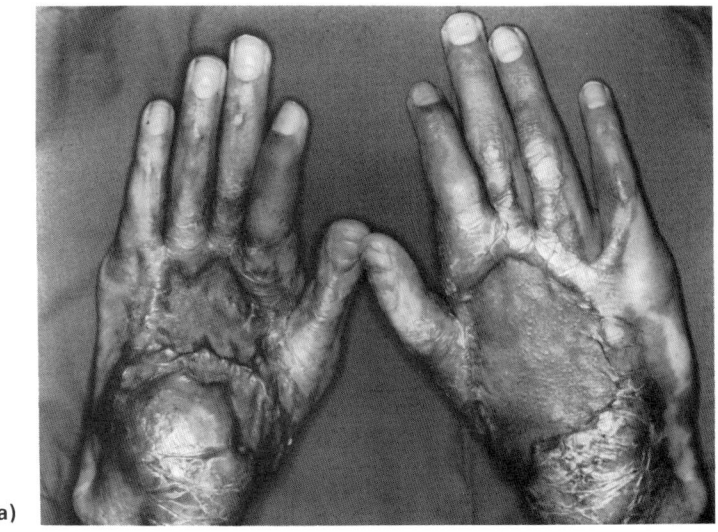

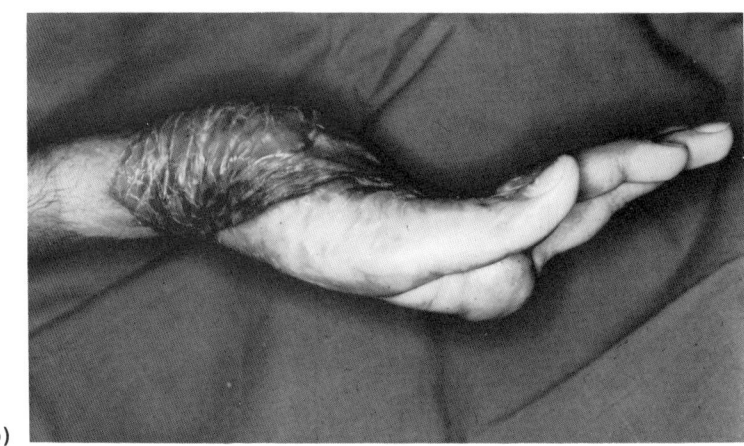

Fig. 12.8 (a) and (b) Bilateral dorsal hand contractures resulting from delayed healing and lack of splintage following full-thickness burns due to a gas explosion in a 12 year old girl. The wrists are flexed, MP joints hyperextended, PIP joints flexed and thumb adducted. (c) Excision of dorsal scarred skin and MP dorsal capsulotomy corrected the deformities while still preserving paratenon over the extensor mechanism, allowing the use of thick dermatome grafts. The MP joints were held flexed with K-wires. The result is shown in the right hand in extension and (d) in flexion. Note the additional scars of meshing incisions in the graft; these should be avoided if possible in pigmented skin

contracture if the splinting was discontinued before six months.

Underlying orthopaedic abnormalities

Joint ankylosis can take place in burned patients in the absence of skin flexion contracture (Fig. 12.9). Heterotopic calcification can cause elbow contracture in patients who are allowed to rest in bed with the elbows flexed for a long period of time (Cason 1981) and this can produce a joint ankylosis so severe that mobilisation of the joint can only be achieved by extensive capsulectomy and tendon release. The example shown is of a patient who was being treated for contractures of the neck and upper trunk, but the burns did not extend to the

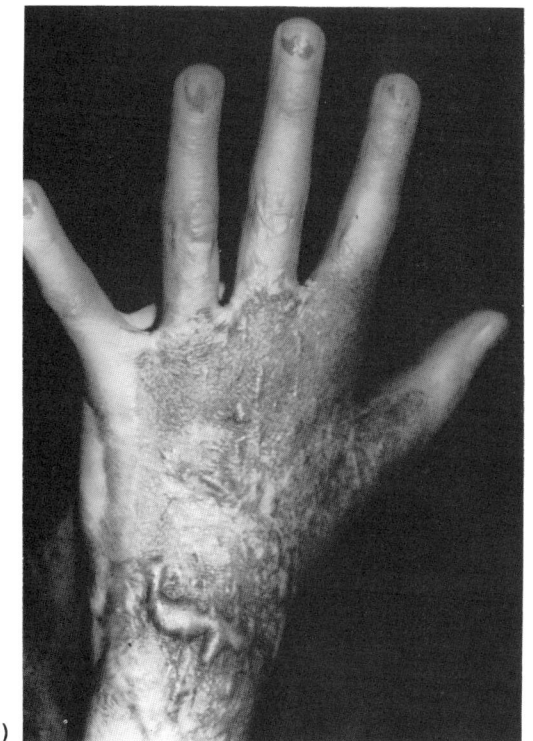 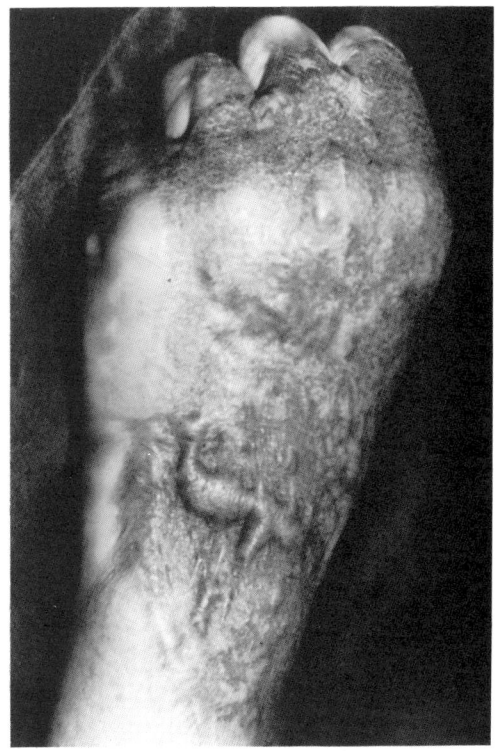

elbow. The cause of this type of contracture is not fully understood, but it is probably preventable by early physiotherapy to uninvolved areas.

Other orthopaedic abnormalities have been described resulting from burn contractures. Jackson (1978, 1981) described acquired vertical talus due to burn contractures in two babies, and this occurred because the sustentaculum tali is rudimentary at this age and the tight tendo achilles and burn scar were able to pull the talus to the medial side of the calcaneum. He also reported disordered growth due to epiphyseal injuries by burning, and a case of thumb dislocation caused by scar contracture. It is important to be aware of the possibility of these and other orthopaedic deformities when treating burn contractures in children.

TISSUE LOSS

Deep hand burns may result in loss of one or more digits or larger parts of the hand, and the principles of reconstructive surgery are no different from those applied to hand mutilation due to other causes. There is an additional problem however, in that the skin which clothes the amputation stump is usually thin and scarred and unsuitable for surgical manoeuvres involving local skin movement. For this reason it is often necessary to resurface the involved area with a skin flap to provide a suitable surgical environment for reconstructive surgery. The choice when faced with a hand such as that shown in Fig. 12.8 lies between a simple attempt to provide basic prehensile hand function by the formation of a cleft, with one mobile structure which can perform a simple gripping movement, and a more ambitious approach aimed at restoring two or more digits by digital transfer or free toe transfer. The decision cannot be made until the patient has fully recovered from the overall burn injury, which in most cases is extensive, and many factors have to be taken into account, including the patient's own wishes and motivation, the functional demands he will make on his hand, the age and general condition, the availability of undamaged toes, and the degree of damage to the limb proximal to the hand from the point of view of tendon and neurovascular recon-

206 UNSATISFACTORY RESULTS IN HAND SURGERY

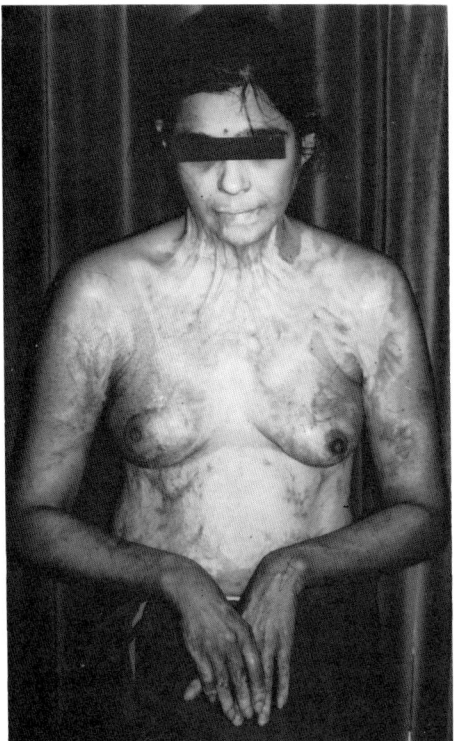

Fig. 12.9 This patient had contractures of the neck and axillae, due to burns, and 90° flexion contractures of the elbows not associated with burns of the overlying skin, but due to heterotopic calcification in the joint capsule and muscle insertions

struction, and the state of skin cover. The procedures that may be considered are as follows:

Deepening of the first web space

In the type of hand illustrated in Fig. 12.10 this will usually require skin flap replacement and frequently the second metacarpal has to be resected to open a wide enough first web space to provide a pinch grip. The skin flap used has to be as thin as possible because a bulky flap obliterates the space completely. It may be an advantage to place the flap only on one side of the cleft, and a skin graft on the other to avoid bulk, and the flap may need to be thinned later. From the functional point of view it is better to have a parallel-sided cleft than a v-shaped one, which tends to extrude the object being held. The disadvantage of this procedure is that there is little tactile sensibility, and where grafted areas have recovered sensation and there is

sufficient padding, it may be advisable to leave the original skin at tactile contact areas if possible. There is usually little scope for neurovascular island transfers in this type of post-burn hand but there may be occasions when an innervated toe pulp free flap would be of benefit.

Ray transfer

May et al (1984) have described their experience with advancement pollicisation of the second ray remnant which may be applicable in some cases. They emphasise the need for preliminary dorsal full thickness skin cover, and at operation the neurovascular structures are identified early and mobilised down to the level of the superficial palmar arch. The index metacarpal has to be mobilised completely. The difficulty with this operation is in releasing the mobilised index ray sufficiently to advance it distally over the end of the thumb. The first web space requires careful splinting postoperatively to prevent a contracture developing.

Distraction bone lengthening

In spite of the scarred overlying skin Stern & MacMillan (1983) have achieved a surprising amount of lengthening following osteotomy and the use of a bone distraction device.

Free toe transfer

Reconstruction of the thumb and or one or two digits is a possibility but the technical difficulties of this type of procedure in the severely burnt hand should not be underestimated. In particular the extensive deep scarring demands that the vascular pedicle has to be long, and if possible taken outside the zone of trauma. The reinnervation of the toe may present problems if the nerve branches in the palm are scarred, and the same difficulty may apply to the tendons. It is very likely that preliminary skin cover of the area for attachment to the toe will be required. There is little mention of the specific problems of the burned hand in the literature on toe transfer (Foucher et al 1984, Yoshimira 1980). Lister et al (1983) include one patient who had sustained electrical burns in their 54 patients on whom they had carried out toe transfers.

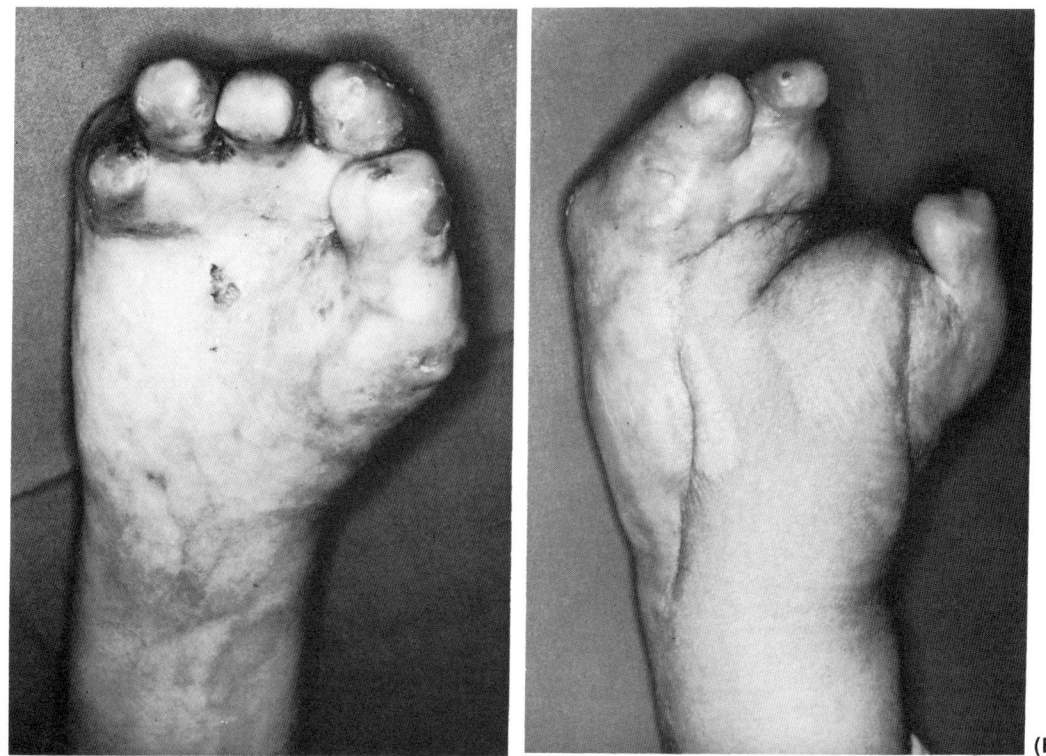

Fig. 12.10 (a) Severe mutilation with loss of all normal hand skin following very deep burns of the hand associated with extensive major burns. The loss of thumb mobility and first web space deprive this hand of any useful function. (b) Second metacarpal resection, web space release and flap skin cover have provided some prehensile function. The flap needs thinning

CONCLUSION

Unsatisfactory results are harder to correct than to prevent. This requires accurate assessment and primary treatment, good timing of surgical interference, and the ability to recognise failure of early treatment in time to remedy the situation before the patient becomes locked on the downhill path towards scarring, contracture and functional loss.

REFERENCES

Alexander J W, MacMillan B G, Martel L 1982 Correction of postburn syndactyly. Plastic and Reconstructive Surgery 70:345–352

Alexander J W, MacMillan B G, Martel L, Krummel R 1981 Surgical correction of postburn flexion contractures of the fingers in children. Plastic and Reconstructive Surgery 68:218–224

Cason J S 1981 Treatment of burns. Chapman & Hall, London, p 152

Colson P, Houot R, Gangolphe M, de Mourgues, Laurent J, Biron G et al 1976 Use of thin flaps (flap grafts) in reparative hand surgery. Annales Chirurgie Plastica 12:298

Dias A D 1983 A bipedicle flap in the correction of burn contracture. British Journal of Plastic Surgery 36:56–59

Dibbell D G, Iverson R E, Jones W, Laub D R, Madison M S 1970 Hydrofluoric burns of the hand. Journal of Bone and Joint Surgery 52A:931–936

Foucher G, Van Genechten F, Merle M, Denuit P, Braun F M, Debry R et al 1984 Toe to hand transfers in reconstructive surgery of the hand. Annales Chirurgie de la Main 3:124–138

Hayashi N 1981 Treatment of hydrofluoric acid burns. Burns 7:267–271

Holmes J D, Rayner C R W 1984 The technique of late dermabrasion deep dermal burns. Burns 10:349–354

Huang T T, Blackwell S J, Lewis S R 1978 Ten years of experience in managing patients with burn contractures of axilla, elbow, wrist, and knee joints. Plastic and Reconstructive Surgery 61:70–76

Huang T T, Larson D L, Lewis S R 1975 Burned hands. Plastic and Reconstructive Surgery 56:21–28

Jackson D 1978 Acquired vertical talus due to burn contractures. Journal of Bone and Joint Surgery 60B:215–218

Jackson D McG 1981 Destructive burns: some orthopaedic complications. Burns 7:105–122

Janzekovic 1970 A new concept in the excision and immediate grafting of burns. Journal of Trauma 10:1103–1106

Labandter H, Kaplan I, Shavitt C 1976 Burns of the dorsum of the hand: conservative treatment with intensive physiotherapy versus tangential excision and grafting. British Journal of Plastic Surgery 29:252–254

Law E J, Motz S M, Stern P J, MacMillan P G 1983 Intraoperative brachial plexus injuries during reconstruction of the burned axilla. Journal of Hand Surgery 8:585–589

Lawrence J C, Carney S A Tangential excision of burns: studies on the use of metabolic activities of the recipient areas of skin grafts. British Journal of Plastic Surgery 26:93–100

Lister G D, Gibson T 1972 Closure of rhomboid skin defects: the flaps of Limberg and Dufourmentel. British Journal of Plastic Surgery 25:3–16

Lister G D, Kalisman M, Tsai T-M 1983 Reconstruction of the hand with free microneurovascular toe-to-hand transfer: experience with 54 toe transfers. Plastic and Reconstructive Surgery 71:371–384

MacDougal B, Wray R C, Weeks P M 1976 Lateral-volar finger flap for the treatment of burn syndactyly. Plastic and Reconstructive Surgery 57:167–171

Madden J W, Enna C D 1983 The management of acute thermal injuries to the upper extremity. Journal of Hand Surgery 8:785–788

Malfeyt G A M 1976 Burns of the dorsum of the hand treated by tangential excision. British Journal of Plastic Surgery 29:78–81

May J W, Donelan M B, Toth P A, Wall J 1984 Thumb reconstruction in the burned hand by advancement pollicisation of the second ray remnant. Journal of Hand Surgery 9A:484–489

Mercer D 1985 The flap-graft. Paper read at the joint meeting of the British Society for Surgery of the Hand and the Eastern Mediterranean Hand Society, Cairo

Mubarak S G, Hargens A R 1981 Compartment syndromes and Volkmann's contracture. W B Saunders & Co, Philadelphia, p 77

Muir I F K 1970 Treatment of electrical burns. The Hand 2:137–139

Nielsen A B, Sommer J 1983 Surgical treatment of the deeply burned hand. Burns 9:214–217

Olney D B 1983 A review of the long term results of electric bar fire burns of the hand in children. The Hand 15:179–184

Pegg S P, Cavaye D, Fowler D, Jones M 1984 Results of early excision and grafting of hand burns. Burns 11:99–103

Robson M C, Murphy R C, Heggers J P 1984 A new explanation for the progressive tissue loss in electrical injuries. Plastic and Reconstructive Surgery 73:431–437

Salisbury R E, Taylor J W, Levine N S 1976 Evaluation of digital escharotomy in burned hands. Plastic and Reconstructive Surgery 58:440–443

Salisbury R E, Wright P 1982 Evaluation of early excision of dorsal burns of the hand. Plastic and Reconstructive Surgery 69:670–675

Scotland A D, Morris A M 1983 The trapezoid flap for the correction of burn scar contractures. British Journal of Plastic Surgery 36:291–294

Slater R M, Hughes N L 1971 A simplified method of treating burns of the hand. British Journal of Plastic Surgery 24:296–300

Stern P J, MacMillan B G 1983 Reconstruction of the burned thumb by metacarpal lengthening. Burns 10:127–130

Stern P J, Neale H W, Carter W, MacMillan B G 1985 Classification and management of burned thumb contractures in children. Burns 11:168–174

Stone P A, Lawrence S A 1973 Healing of tangentially excised and grafted burns in man. British Journal of Plastic Surgery 26:20–31

Sykes P J, Bailey B N 1976 Treatment of hand burns with occlusive bag: a comparison of three methods. Burns 2:162–168

Wang X-W, Liu H-C, Sung H-H, Gai S-L, Cheng X-X 1984a Early vascular grafting to prevent upper extremity necrosis after electrical burns. Burns 10:179–183

Wang X-W, Sun Y-H, Zhang G-Z, Zhang Z-M, Davies J W L 1984b Tangential excision of eschar for deep burns of the hand: analysis of 156 patients collected over 10 years. Burns 11:92–98

Wang X-W, Wei J-N, Sung Y-H, Li Y-N, Wang N-Z, Liu J-Q, Li S-M 1982 Early vascular grafting to prevent upper extremity necrosis after electrical burns. Burns 8:303–312

Wang X-W, Zhang X-Z, Song H-H, Zhang G-S, Davies J W L, Zapata-Sirvent R L, Robinson W A 1985 Thermal crush injuries of the hand and forearms: an analysis of 60 cases. Burns 11:264–268

Wang X-W, Zoh W-R 1983 Vascular injuries in electrical burns—the pathological basis for mechanism of injury. Burns 8:335–339

Wexler M R, Yeschua R, Neuman Z 1974 Early treatment of burns of the dorsum of the hand by tangential excision and skin grafting. Plastic and Reconstructive Surgery 54:268–273

Yoshimura M 1980 Toe to hand transfer. Plastic and Reconstructive Surgery 66:74–83

G. E. Omer

13 Nerves

Unsatisfactory results following nerve surgery may be expected to be within two categories: inadequate return of motor or sensory function, and a painful state as a complication of the surgical procedure. Both unsatisfactory results are avoided best by utilising an appropriate suture technique. The potential for optimal functional recovery is enhanced with re-education techniques. If pain dominates the clinical picture, the surgeon must differentiate treatment between reflex sympathetic dystrophy and a neuroma-in-continuity. If function is not recovered, appropriate motor and sensory transfers should be considered.

NERVE SUTURE TECHNIQUES

Microsurgery has improved our techniques for nerve suture, but the major lesson of the past decade has been that there are only two principles in nerve repair: (1) minimal tension at the suture line, both longitudinal and circumferential; and (2) careful matching of fascicular bundles within the nerve for appropriate longitudinal alignment of nerve cells (Millesi 1981).

Epineurial suture (Braun 1980, Omer & Spinner 1984)

This technique is well established (Fig. 13.1). The proximal and distal nerve stumps are mobilised and debrided to normal anatomy. The stumps are square-cut on the ends for a precise transverse surface match. The tourniquet is released to obtain hemostasis and to avoid intra surface hematoma. Large groups of fascicular bundles within the nerve are matched in longitudinal alignment and circumferential epineurium is approximated with a minimal number of fine (10–0) sutures. The epineurial technique is usually appropriate for immediate repair, especially proximal (high) nerve lesions where there are many fascicular groups which cannot be easily matched.

Complications result when the proximal and distal nerve stump transections do not obtain a flush joint for the anastomosis. There is hemorrhage and resulting fibrosis across the suture line. A running suture is not used, because it tends to constrict the circumference of the nerve trunk. The tourniquet should be released before the final sutures are placed, to evacuate any blood residue

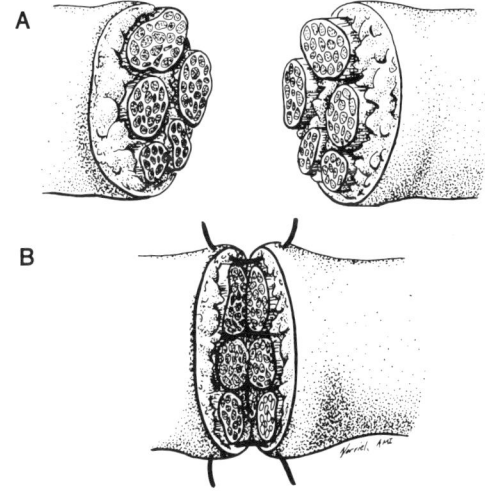

Fig. 13.1 Epineurial technique of suture placement for nerve repair (after Omer, G. E. Jr.: Complications of treatment of peripheral nerve injuries. In: Epps, C. H. Jr. (ed.) *Complications in Orthopaedic Surgery.* Philadelphia, J. B. Lippincott, 1985, with permission)

between the nerve stumps. If there is recognised tension at the suture line, Braun (1980) recommends holding sutures of 8-0 prolene placed through the epineurium to the surrounding tissue at a distance about 2 cm from the neurorrhaphy site.

Fascicular bundle suture (Omer & Spinner 1984, Urbaniak 1982)

The proximal and distal nerve stumps are mobilised and debrided to normal anatomy (Fig. 13.2). The circumferential epineurium is removed for 1 or 2 cm and the larger groups of fascicular bundles are isolated and cut at different levels. The tourniquet is released to obtain hemostasis. The isolated groups of fascicular bundles are matched by position in the nerve and by size and approximated by a minimal number of fine (10-0 or 11-0) sutures through the intra neural epineurium. The fascicular bundle suture is indicated when it is important to exclude one or more bundle groups from the others in the nerve, such as the thenar motor group in the median nerve, or the dorsal cutaneous branch of the ulnar nerve.

Complications arise when the suture needle penetrates the perineurium, which changes pressure within the funicular bundles and breaks the diffusion barrier. The operating microscope is indicated for fascicular bundle suture techniques. The suture line must be free of tension.

Electrophysiological techniques have been used to aid in fascicular bundle orientation in acute injuries. In the responsive patient, stimulation of the proximal stump elicits subjective sensations from the patient as long as the cells of origin in the dorsal root ganglia are intact. It is common to produce motor responses with electrical stimulation of the distal nerve stump for 4-7 days after injury. Anatomical dissection studies on the internal structure of nerve trunks are available to indicate the probable location of motor and sensory fascicular groups (Jabaley et al 1980, Sunderland 1978).

Autogenous nerve grafts (Moneim 1982, Omer & Spinner 1984)

Seddon popularised the cable graft, and his technique involved suturing multiple nerve segments to equal the diameter of the disrupted nerve, thus forming a multiple-segment cable (Seddon 1975). The cable graft is superior to grafting a single large-diameter nerve, because the multiple cables develop an adequate intergraft circulation, while a large-diameter nerve will undergo central necrosis. Millesi and associates have improved the multiple cable graft by developing a technique that emphasises no tension at suture lines, accurate group fascicular alignment and excision of the epineurium (Millesi 1981).

A practical indication for a nerve graft is when the tension at the suture line is too great for a single 8-0 suture to hold the nerve in approximation. Usually there is avulsion of nerve portions.

The proximal and distal stumps are mobilised and debrided to normal anatomy. The epineurium is removed for 1 to 2 cm and the larger groups of fascicular bundles are isolated and cut at different levels. It is important that the integrity of the perineurium be preserved during the dissection. A map is made of the cross-section of the nerve, both proximal and distal; and the number of grafts to match major fascicular bundles is calculated. The tourniquet is released and hemostasis is obtained.

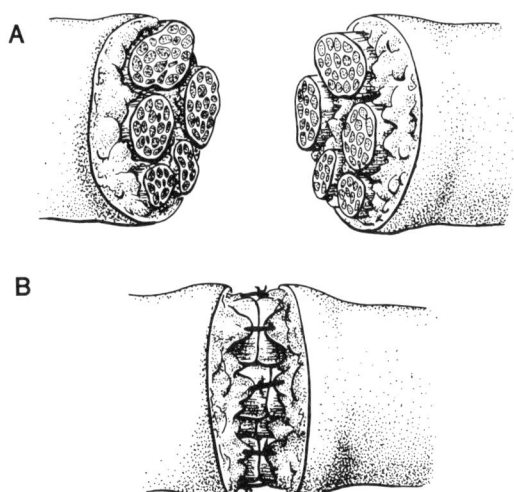

Fig. 13.2 Fascicular bundle (funiculus) technique of suture placement for nerve repair (after Omer, G. E. Jr.: Complications of treatment of peripheral nerve injuries. In: Epps, C. H. Jr. (ed.) *Complications in Orthopaedic Surgery*. Philadelphia, J. B. Lippincott, 1985, with permission)

The sural nerve is the donor of choice. Corresponding fascicular bundles from both the proximal and distal cut ends are joined by grafts. It is important that the size of the fascicular bundles joined correspond with the size of the graft. The 10–0 sutures are used for each graft at each end. The deep epineurium from the nerve stump is sutured to the epineurium of the donor graft with the adjacent joints in extension. The grafts should lie in the wound without tension.

Our experience indicates that a graft is needed if a sharp nerve laceration near a joint is left unsutured for more than 3 weeks. We prefer to remove the donor nerve through a Z-step longitudinal incision, although multiple transverse incisions are more often utilised.

After the nerve graft has been performed, the axons cross the proximal suture site and regenerate toward the distal suture site. In a long nerve graft the distal site may scar and block before the axons reach that level. Clinically, this becomes apparent as the Tinel's sign stops advancing. After a 60 day delay at this point, the distal suture site should be exposed in order to evaluate the neuroma-in-continuity by electrodiagnostic techniques (nerve action potentials). If there is no distal electrical conduction, the distal suture site should be resected and a second neurorrhaphy should be performed.

Following nerve suture, we immobilise the injured extremity for 3–4 weeks in a plaster circular cast or splint. Extreme flexion of any immobilised joint should be avoided. Antibiotics are indicated if there has been major dissection or a threat of infection. After the initial period of healing, joints are mobilised 10–15° per week.

RE-EDUCATION TECHNIQUES FOR IMPROVING RESULTS

Following nerve suture, static or dynamic splints can be utilised to place the hand in position to utilise the remaining active muscle-tendon units. External splints are sometimes awkward and often interfere with sensory input. Selected tendon transfers as internal splints enhance sensory re-education while awaiting the return of nerve control.

Muscle internal splints (Omer 1982a)

The muscle-tendon units used for internal splints should be synergistic with the muscle-tendon unit to be replaced, and must not cause subsequent imbalance with deformity when nerve function is recovered.

In radial palsy, the pronator teres transferred to the extensor carpi radialis brevis will produce active wrist extension, encourage metacarpophalangeal joint passive flexion, and allow ulnar-innervated intrinsic muscle finger extension (Fig. 13.3). The pronator teres, while producing active extension of the wrist, still performs as a pronator of the forearm.

The extensor indicis proprius transferred subcutaneously around the ulnar border of the wrist and into the dorsal apparatus of the thumb will provide adequate motion and power for opposition in low (distal) median palsy (Fig. 13.4). If the median nerve is lacerated by an oblique injury that spares the palmaris longus tendon, the tendon can be lengthened with a strip of palmar fascia and transferred to the insertion of the abductor pollicis brevis tendon.

An isolated tendon transfer cannot restore all the imbalance in a low (distal) ulnar palsy, but a single flexor digitorum superficialis tendon can improve the integration of metacarpophalangeal and interphalangeal joint flexion, key pinch for the thumb and improve the flattened metacarpal arch (Omer 1968, Omer 183a) (Fig. 13.5). The superficialis of the ring finger is preferred if the ulnar innervated portion of the flexor digitorum profundus is not paralysed. The superficialis first is split longitudinally well into the palm, and the ulnar half of the tendon is split again into two slips. If the finger interphalangeal joints cannot be actively extended when the metacarpophalangeal joint is stabilised in flexion, the two slips are directed volar to the deep transverse metacarpal ligament and then dorsal to be sutured in the central slip of the dorsal apparatus of the ring and little fingers. If a power grip is desirable, the two slips are passed distally through the flexor sheaths and sutured at the distal edge of the A-2 pulley. The radial half of the superficialis is directed transversely over the volar surface of the adductor pollicis muscle, but dorsal to the finger flexor tendons and neurovascular structures,

212 UNSATISFACTORY RESULTS IN HAND SURGERY

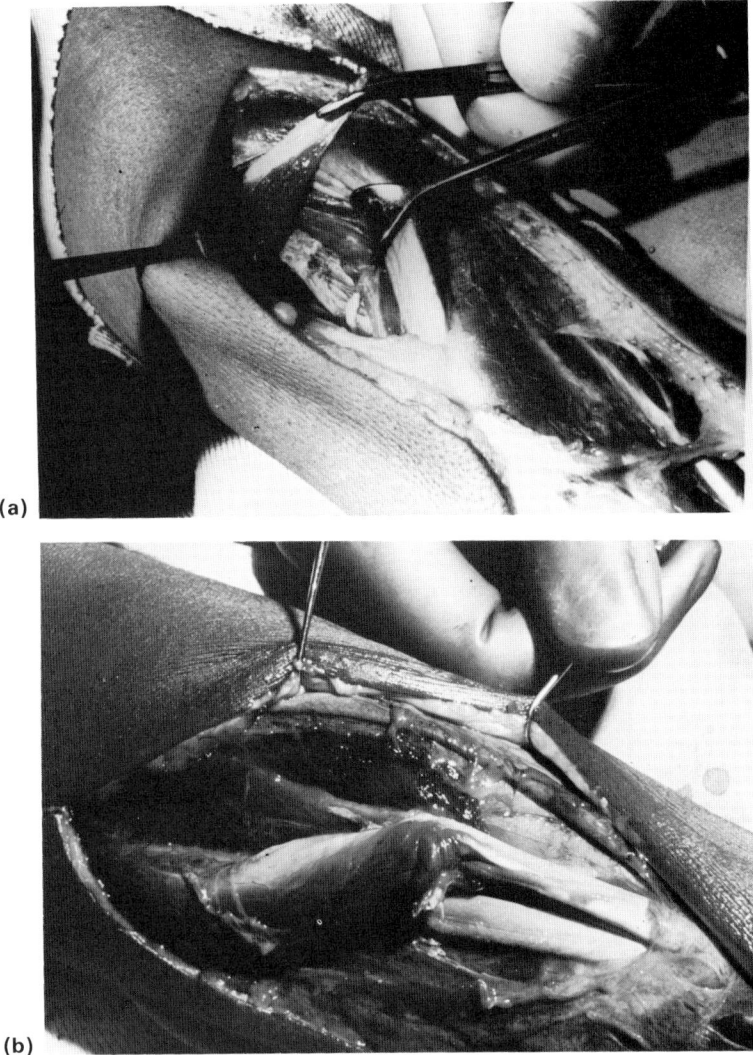

Fig. 13.3 (a) Release of the pronator teres muscle-tendon unit from the radius. (b) Transfer of the pronator teres superficial to the brachioradialis and the extensor carpi radialis longus into the tendon of the extensor carpi radialis brevis. The resting position at operation should be 20 to 25 degrees of wrist extension

and is sutured into the insertion of the abductor pollicis brevis. The pulley for this transfer is the distal edge of the palmar fascia inserted into the third metacarpal. Traction on the transferred tendon half should adduct and pronate the first metacarpal. Distal stability for pinch between the thumb and index finger is improved by arthrodesis of the matacarpophalangeal joint of the thumb, and is indicated when the patient develops a hyperextension deformity of the metacarpophalangeal joint following the superficialis tendon transfer.

Education for sensibility (Dellon 1981, Dellon & Jabaley 1982)

Recovery of perception of stimuli in the fingertip following nerve repair are in sequence: pain and

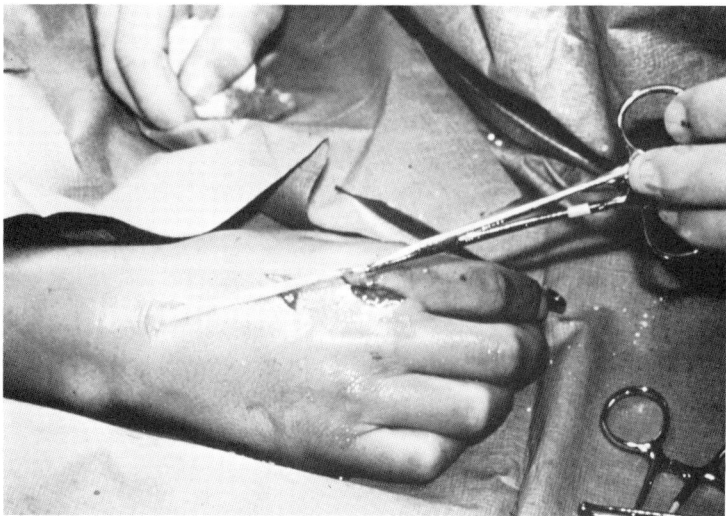

Fig. 13.4 Release of the extensor indicis proprius muscle for transfer around the ulnar side of the wrist and into the insertion of the abductor pollicis brevis tendon for abduction of the thumb. The resting position of the thumb at operation is 45 degrees of abduction with the forearm fully supinated and the wrist at zero degrees (after Omer, G. E. Jr.: Reconstruction of a balanced thumb through tendon transfers. Clin. Orthop. 195 (May): 104–116, 1985, with permission)

temperature, flutter-touch (30 cps) stimulus, moving-touch, constant touch, and vibratory (256 cps) stimulus (Dellon 1981). Dellon has related this pattern of sensory recovery as a time table on which to introduce sensory stimulating exercises. Instituting an exercise for sensory re-education before the appropriate fibre/receptor system has reunited can only lead to frustration and failure.

Sensory re-education should begin when perception of 30 cps vibratory stimuli and moving-touch stimuli are regained at the level of the proximal phalanx (Dellon & Jabaley 1982). Vibratory stimuli may be administered with the pronged end of a tuning fork held tangentially against the finger. A vibratory threshold has the same relation to the moving two-point discrimination test as the von Frey monofilament measurement has to the classic (static) two-point discrimination test (Dellon 1981). For moving-touch stimuli, the patient uses a soft instrument such as a pencil eraser, to stroke up and down the area being re-educated. This is done with eyes open and then closed.

As regeneration proceeds and the patient can perceive a constant-touch stimulus, an eraser is pressed as hard as necessary for the perception of constant-touch. Finally, 256 cps vibratory stimuli are added. The goal of sensory re-education is the achievement of the full potential for functional sensibility given by the nerve repair. The re-education programme should progress from the perception of moving touch and constant touch to identification of small objects. The patient can hold, move, and discriminate the difference between square and hexagonal nuts and small or large cap nuts. The exercise is performed with the eyes open and then closed to associate the new central sensation with the old activity. The exercise time should be 10–15 minutes per session, in a quiet room with the patient rested and prepared to concentrate. The exercise should be repeated 3–4 times each day. It is generally accepted that tactile gnosis cannot be present unless classic (static) two-point discrimination is less than 12–15 mm in the fingertip (Omer 1983b). If moving two-point discrimination is less than 6 mm a patient can identify objects by manipulating them.

PAIN PROBLEMS

Pain may develop after surgery for several reasons. The sutured portion of the nerve may develop

214 UNSATISFACTORY RESULTS IN HAND SURGERY

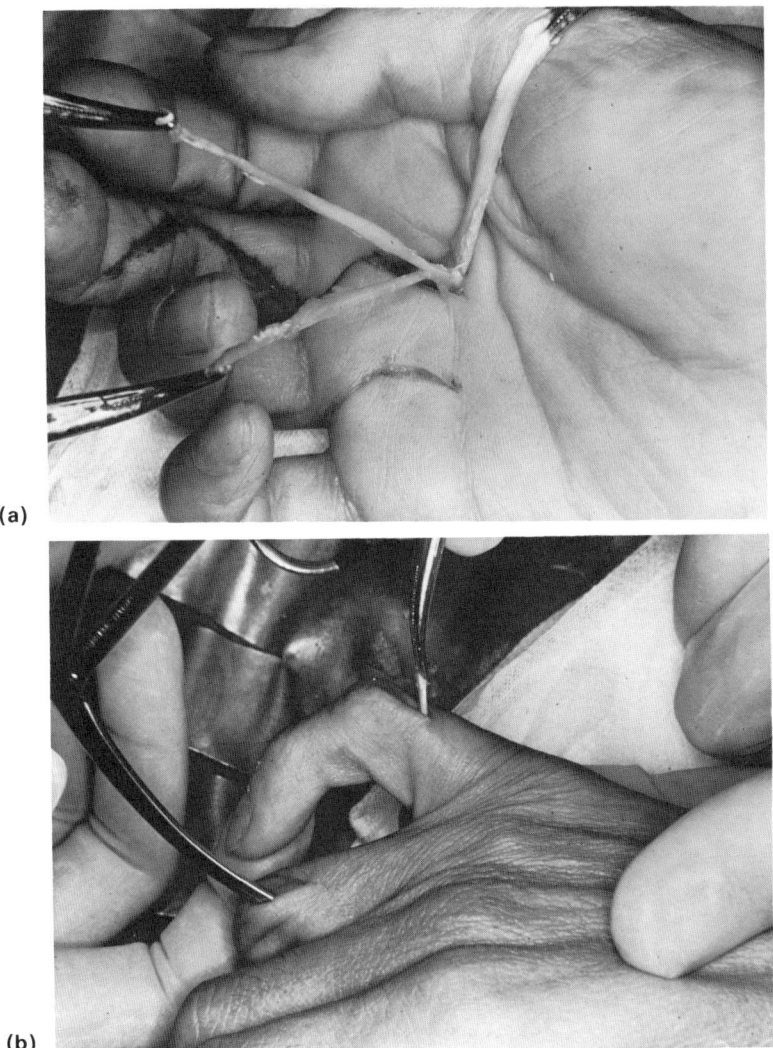

Fig. 13.5 (a) Release of the flexor digitorum profundus (of long finger) into palmar incision. The radial half of the tendon will motor thumb adduction, the ulnar slips of the tendon will prevent clawing of the ring and little fingers. (b) Insertion of the ulnar slips into the dorsal apparatus to stabilise extension of the ring and little fingers. (c) Insertion of the ulnar slips of the flexor digitorum profundus around the A-2 flexor pulley to stabilise extension of the ring and little fingers

intraneurial fibrosis, or external adhesions may transfix the nerve to its tissue bed. The compressed nerve will have venous stasis, capillary leakage, and perineurial edema (Rydevik et al 1981). This decreased blood flow can be associated with pain, as in any compression syndrome.

Several clinical syndromes have been described that include burning pain, abnormal vasomotor response, and dystrophy. Classic causalgia may have variants that are termed Leriche's post-traumatic pain syndrome (minor causalgia), Sudek's atrophy, or shoulder-arm-hand syndrome.

Reflex sympathetic dystrophy (Omer 1984)

Reflex sympathetic dystrophy may not develop immediately but may gradually increase to dominate the clinical picture. The syndrome is thought

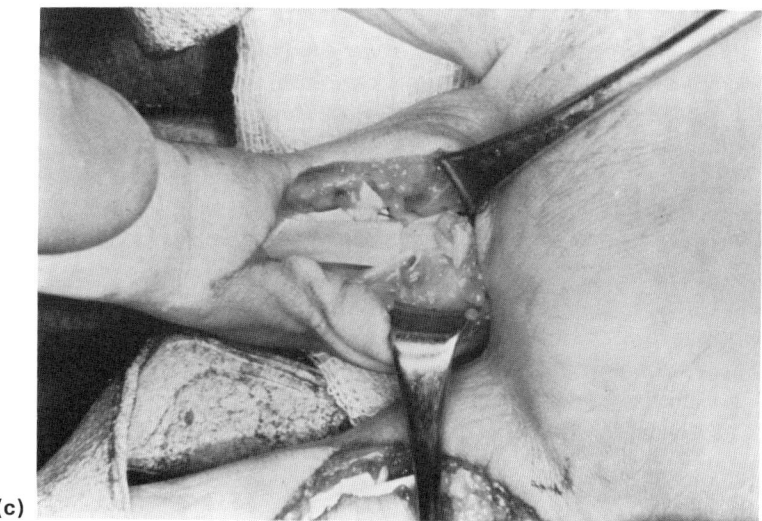
(c)

to be a prolongation of the normal sympathetic response to injury. There may be nerve trunk injury that results in abnormal cross-stimulation between sympathetic and sensory fibres, or there may be liberation of a vasodilator and chemical pain mediator at the periphery of the involved nerve. The loss of vascular, sudomotor, pilomotor, and muscle tone controls results in profound trophic changes with marked atrophy. In the early stages, the involved extremity is swollen and warm, with hyperesthesia to light touch and cold. After 2–3 months, there is fibrotic brawny edema. Antalgic contractures become fixed due to lack of active motion. Roentgenograms of the distal bones show patchy osteopenia. Six to nine months after the onset of pain, the extremity becomes pale and cool, with either hyperhidrosis or dryness. Pain may dominate, or the extremity may be completely rejected by the patient (Lankford 1980).

In those patients with vasospastic disorders, Hannington-Kiff (1974) introduced the regional intravenous sympathetic block technique with quanethidine. Under tourniquet control, 20 mg of quanethidine in 20 ml of normal saline is injected slowly into a dorsal wrist vein. The tourniquet is deflated in 20 minutes. Chuinard and associates (1980) have reported the use of reserpine for intravenous regional anaesthesia. One mg of reserpine in 50 ml of normal saline is injected and the tourniquet is released after 15 minutes.

Many patients do not have localised distal vascular involvement and early treatment for these cases includes chemical central interruption of the abnormal sympathetic reflex. A cervical sympathetic block should be performed as a diagnostic test as well as a therapeutic procedure. We use solutions of either 1% lidocaine hydrochloride or mepivacaine hydrochloride to produce peripheral warming, cessation of sweating, and relief of pain. A series of four or five blocks should be given on consecutive days, and the introduction of one placebo of normal saline solution during the series will confirm the effectiveness of the block.

Surgical sympathectomy should be performed when the burning pain completely responds to central chemical block, but requires repeated blocks for long-term relief. The effectiveness of surgical symathectomy is not related to interrupting a sensory pathway from the extremity, but to eliminating efferent discharge to the peripheral arteries. For a satisfactory result, postoperative precise sudomotor function tests should demonstrate complete sympathetic denervation of the involved extremity.

If the chemical blocks do not give relief longer than the duration expected from the anaesthetic agent, permanent improvement by surgical sympathectomy should not be expected. Transcutaneous electric nerve stimulation should be considered for these patients. Three sites may be utilised: proximal to the pain site over the involved nerve, at the periphery of a painful area, or directly over a pain site if proximal nerve trunks are not readily stimulated (Omer 1984). The intensity should be varied by the patient because stimuli that are too intense overcome the inhibition mechanisms and produce additional pain.

Neuroma-in-continuity

A neuroma becomes symptomatic, depending upon the quality and quantity of axon regeneration, and is influenced by the extent of fibrosis, vascularity, infection, foreign material, and other factors. Neuromas with inadequate numbers of large myelinated axons or outer fibrous layers develop hyperpathia, with over-reaction and after-sensation to stimuli. The extreme over-reaction is directly over the neuroma and the after-sensation is poorly localised but widely distributed over the area supplied by the nerve. Percutaneous injection about a painful neuroma should provide local anaesthesia. A peripheral chemical sympathetic block may be performed as an outpatient (Omer 1984, Omer & Thomas 1971). A 16-gauge needle is inserted just proximal to the 'trigger point', and a flexible 18-gauge polyethylene intravenous catheter inserted through the needle. The needle is removed, leaving the catheter in place. A solution of 0.5 ml of lidocaine hydrochloride, 0.5%, is injected. If the pain is relieved, the catheter is capped and taped to the skin, allowing exercise activity. Additional periodic injections of lidocaine solution are based on the length of time of pain-free activity. The periodic infusion has been continued for a few days up to 2 weeks under hospitalisation.

If local anaesthesia is unsuccessful, the neuroma-in-continuity should be explored and evaluated with an electrodiagnostic technique. Exposure well proximal and distal to the lesion is necessary. The nerve should be free to be lifted with Penrose drains. After exposure and hemostasis, the tourniquet should be deflated before recording is attempted. The exposed nerve is then suspended on bipolar platinum electrodes proximally and a recording electrode distally, as described by Kline (1982). The tip of one recording electrode is sharpened so that it may be placed in subcutaneous tissue to serve as a ground. The recording wires are directed through a standard amplifier and then to an oscilloscope. Stimuli are delivered to the proximal bipolar electrodes by a battery powered stimulator. The lowest threshold necessary to obtain a distal potential is determined, and the stimulus voltage is then increased until potentials of maximum amplitude and complexity are obtained. The recording electrode is then moved distally, and potentials at multiple points along the course of the regenerating nerve are obtained. If a distal nerve-action potential can be recorded within 2 to 6 months after suture, the lesion can be spared resection and resuture or graft repair. Absence of a nerve action potential indicates that the nerve is not regenerating, and will do better with resection and resuture than with neurolysis alone. It is appropriate to divide the nerve longitudinally, and assess fascicular groups before resecting the nerve trunk.

A painful partial nerve disruption may benefit from internal neurolysis and graft repair of some fascicular groups that are disrupted (Omer & Spinner 1984). If there is no useful distal sensory or motor function, an end-to-end anastomosis or nerve graft should be performed after removal of the neuroma-in-continuity.

PALSIED HAND

The objective of reconstructive surgery in the paralytic palsied hand is balanced performance, because these procedures redistribute existing assets rather than create new ones. Tendon transfers should eliminate a deforming force that will produce further imbalance or replace a single absent force to assist grasp, pinch, or release. Specific composite tissue transplantation is useful in sensory depleted glabrous skin areas required for precise pinch and grasp.

Homeostasis of the involved extremity must be established before elective reconstruction. There should be stable skeletal alignment with optimal joint motion. Tendon transfers performed across or distal to sites of bony non-union fail because the telescoping skeleton prevents the development of adequate amplitude for muscle power. Soft tissues should be free of scar contracture and have adequate circulation. Chronic wounds are a contraindication for elective surgery. The functional performance anticipated after tendon transfer should be possible to effect easily with passive movement before surgery.

Procedures to restore sensibility should be delayed until all indicated tendon transfers have been accomplished and the patient has supple tissues with an established range of motion. The foot is more variable in its blood supply than the hand, and arteriography or a Doppler probe is most helpful in previewing the anatomic variations. Preoperative planning is essential, but one must be prepared to insert segmental grafts into arteries, veins, or nerves as the situation dictates at the time of surgery.

The key to success in surgical technique is simplicity; complexity invites failure.

Tendon transfers are discussed in Ch. 17 and our transfer choices are simply outlined in Tables 13.1, 13.2 and 13.3 for the three isolated nerve injuries involving the hand (Omer 1983a).

Sensory reconstruction

Restoration of sensibility in the hand remains one of the greatest challenges in hand surgery. Neurovascular cutaneous island pedicle flaps have been utilised to restore median nerve sensation (Littler 1956). If the ulnar nerve is to be the donor, only the common digital nerve between the ring and little fingers is available, since sensibility along the ulnar aspect of the little finger is essential in total median nerve loss. The superficial vascular arch may have to be interrupted and the radial portion of the arch freed to swing with the cutaneous island. A double island along the ulnar border of the ring finger, across the distal edge of the palm, and along the radial border of the little finger has been transferred to the thumb-index web space (Omer et al 1970). A radial innervated cross finger flap from the dorsal index to the thumb pulp will provide a critical area of sensation (Gaul 1969). There is disorientation of sensitivity in all neurovascular island pedicle flaps. There is also a high incidence of cold intolerance and paresthesia is common at the margin of these flaps (Omer 1982b, 1983a). Littler (Omer 1983a) now believes that neurovascular island pedicle flaps that transfer sensation from one digit to another digit should be considered anachronistic procedures.

Microsurgical free flaps should provide donor skin that approximates the quality of the recipient skin with a sensory pattern predictable for precise sensibility (Hall & Buncke 1981) Morrison and associates (Morrison et al 1979) have described a modification of the toe-to-thumb transfer that is a free neurovascular wrap-around flap from the great toe. The trimmed nail and nail bed are included, as well as subcutaneous tissue, to prevent pulp swivel. The thumb skeleton is sculptured from the iliac crest, or the distal phalanx of the toe is utilised if there has been avulsion of the thumb. The dorsalis pedis artery and the long saphenous vein are retained in lengths to anastomose to the radial artery and the cephalic vein at the level of the snuff box of the wrist. The deep peroneal nerve is joined to the superficial radial nerve, and the plantar digital nerves must join the proximal median nerve. A long gap in the median nerve lessens the possibility for this type of transfer.

Taylor (1978) has demonstrated that a nerve can be isolated with an intact arteriovenous system by dissecting a neurovascular bundle with a sleeve of areolar tissue to preserve the direct and recurrent

Table 13.1 Radial nerve palsy

Needed action	Preferred motor	Alternate motor
Wrist extension	Pronator teres to extensor carpi radialis brevis	
Finger extension and thumb extension	Flexor digitorum superficialis (middle and ring) to extensor digitorum communis and extensor pollicis longus	Flexor carpi ulnaris to extensor digitorum communis and extensor pollicis longus
Proximal thumb stability	Split-insertion for flexor carpi radialis to abductor pollicis longus	Palmaris longus 'side-to-side stitched' to extensor pollicis brevis

Table 13.2 Ulnar nerve palsy

Needed action	Preferred motor	Alternate motor
Thumb adduction—key pinch (Add. Pol.)	Brachioradialis with free tendon graft between 3rd and 4th metacarpal to abductor tubercle 1st metacarpal	Flexor digitorum superficialis (middle)
Proximal phalanx power flexion (and) integration of M–P and I–P motion	Extensor carpi radialis longus to all four fingers with 4-tailed free tendon graft to either flexor sheath or central slip of dorsal apparatus	Flexor carpi radialis (if wrist flexion contracture); or flexor digitorum superficialis (ring)
Metacarpal (palmar) transverse arch (and) active adduction of little finger	Extensor digiti minimi to either flexor sheath or proximal phalanx of little finger (EDC to little finger must be active)	Flexor digitorum superficialis (middle) as split transfer—to little finger and as thumb adductor
Thumb-index-tip pinch (1st DI and 2nd PI)	Abductor pollicis longus slip with free tendon graft to insertion 1st dorsal interosseous (and) arthrodesis, M–P joint of thumb	Extensor pollicis brevis
Distal phalanx power flexion (ring and little fingers)	Flexor digitorum profundus (middle) 'side-to-side stitch' with ring and little profundi	Tenodesis, flexor digitorum profundus, D–I–P joint, ring and little fingers
Wrist flexion (FCU) (ulnar power)	Flexor carpi radialis to insertion of FCU	Palmaris longus to insertion of FCU
Volar sensation—ring and little rays	Free neurovascular cutaneous island flap—low lesion (plus) free vascularised nerve graft—high lesion	

Table 13.3 Median nerve palsy

Needed action	Preferred motor	Alternate motor
Thumb abduction for opposition	Extensor indicis proprius to tendon of abductor pollicis brevis and extensor pollicis longus tendon	Flexor digitorum superficialis (ring)—low lesion extensor carpi ulnaris—high lesion
Distal phalanx power for flexion (index and middle fingers)	Flexor digitorum profundus (ring and little) 'side-to-side stitch' with index and middle profundi	Tenodesis, flexor digitorum profundus, D–I–P joint, index and middle fingers
Distal phalanx power for flexion of thumb	Brachioradialis to flexor pollicis longus	Extensor carpi radialis longus
Volar sensation (thumb and index fingers)	Free neurovascular island flap—low lesion (plus) Free vascularised nerve graft—high lesion	Neurovascular cutaneous island pedicle from ring finger

vasa nervorum. Taylor has utilised a free superficial radial nerve vascularised graft to fill a gap in a median nerve.

However, there are few 'standard' or established procedures for transfer of sensibility to the hand, especially utilising free flaps. Experience should enlarge the available procedures for this difficult problem.

REFERENCES

Braun R M 1980 Epineurial nerve repair. In: Omer G E Jr, Spinner M (eds) Management of Peripheral Nerve Problems. W B Saunders, Philadelphia, Ch 21, p 366

Chuinard R G, Dabezies E J, Gould J S, Murphy G A, Mathews R E 1980 Intravenous reserpine for treatment of reflex sympathetic dystrophy. American Society for Surgery of the Hand Proceedings Journal of Hand Surgery 5: 289

Dellon A L 1981 Evaluation of Sensibility and Re-education of Sensation in the Hand. Williams and Wilkins, Baltimore, p 59

Dellon A L, Jabaley M E 1982 Re-education of sensation in the hand following nerve suture. Clinical Orthopaedics and Related Research 163: 75–79

Gaul J S 1969 Radial innervated cross finger flap from index to provide sensory pulp to injured thumb. Journal of Bone and Joint Surgery 51 A: 1257–1263

Hall E J, Buncke H J 1981 Microsurgical techniques to reconstruct irreparable nerve loss. Orthopaedic Clinics of North America 12:381–401

Hannington-Kiff J G 1974 Intravenous regional sympathetic block with guanethidine. Lancet 1:1019–1020

Jabaley M E, Wallace W H, Heckler F R 1980 Internal topography of major nerves of the forearm and hand: A current view. Journal of Hand Surgery 5:1–18

Kline D G 1982 Timing for exploration of nerve lesions and evaluation of the neuroma-in-continuity. Clinical Orthopaedics and Related Research 163:42–49

Lankford L L 1980 Reflex sympathetic dystrophy. In: Omer G E Jr, Spinner M (eds) Management of Peripheral Nerve Problems. W B Saunders, Philadelphia, ch 12, p 216

Littler J W 1956 Neurovascular pedicle transfer of tissue in reconstructive surgery of the hand. American Society for Surgery of the Hand Proceedings, Journal of Bone and Joint Surgery 38A:917

Millesi H 1981 Reappraisal of nerve repair. Surgical Clinics of North America 61:321–340

Moneim M S 1982 Interfascicular nerve grafting. Clinical Orthopaedics and Related Research 163:65–74

Morrison W A, O'Brien B McC, MacLeod A M 1979 The foot as a donor site in reconstructive microsurgery. World Journal of Surgery 3:43–52

Omer G E Jr 1968 Evaluation and reconstruction of the forearm and hand after acute traumatic peripheral nerve injuries. Journal of Bone and Joint Surgery 50A:1454–1478

Omer G E Jr 1982a Early tendon transfers in the rehabilitation of median, radial, and ulnar palsies. Annales De Chirurgie De La Main 1:187–190

Omer G E Jr 1982b Reconstructive procedures for extremeties with peripheral nerve defects. Clinical Orthopaedics and Related Research 163:80–91

Omer G E Jr 1983a The palsied hand. In: Evarts C M (ed) Surgery of the Musculoskeletal System, Vol 1. Churchill Livingstone, Edinburgh, ch 16:2, p 407, 2:, p 438

Omer G E Jr 1983b Report of the committee for evaluation of the clinical result in peripheral nerve injury. Journal of Hand Surgery 8:754–759

Omer G E Jr 1984 Management techniques for chronic pain of the upper extremity. Bulletin of the Hospital for Joint Disease Orthopaedic Institute 44:381–405

Omer G E Jr, Day D J, Ratliff H, Lambert P 1970 Neurovascular cutaneous island pedicles for deficient median-nerve sensibility. Journal of Bone and Joint Surgery 52A:1181–1192

Omer G E Jr, Thomas S R 1971 Treatment of causalgia: Review of cases at Brooke General Hospital. Texas Medical 67:93–96

Omer G E Jr, Spinner M 1984 Management of peripheral nerve problems. Instructional Course Lectures, American Academy of Orthopaedic Surgeons C V Mosby Co, Saint Louis. 33:461–530

Rydevik B, Lundborg G, Bagge U 1981 Effects of graded compression on intraneural blood flow. Journal of Hand Surgery 6:3–12

Seddon H 1975 Surgical Disorders of the Peripheral Nerves, 2nd edn. Churchill Livingstone, Edinburgh, p 1, 32–36

Sunderland S 1978 Nerves and Nerve Injuries, 2nd edn. Churchill Livingstone, Edinburgh, p 31, 83, 315

Taylor G I 1978 Nerve grafting with simultaneous microvascular reconstruction. Clinical Orthopaedics and Related Research 133:56–70

Urbaniak J R 1982 Fascicular nerve suture. Clinical Orthopaedics and Related Research 163:57–64

R. D. Leffert

14 Nerve compression

INTRODUCTION

The clinical manifestations of compressions lesions of nerves to the hand are often expressed in subtle signs and symptoms which may be difficult to detect or interpret. Nevertheless, the disorders that are clinically observed form an important area of interest to those who care for the hand. Although these lesions and their diagnosis may be considered as belonging within the realm of neurology, the hand surgeon should not be insecure in his ability to recognise them and offer definitive treatment. While he may receive either the patient or assistance in diagnosis from the neurologist, there should be no one better qualified by training and experience to deal effectively with compression lesions of nerves than one who literally handles them on a daily basis.

In order to define the scope of the problem, below are listed the loci of the compression lesions that are expressed as disorders of the hand:

1. Cervical spine
   a. Radiculopathy
2. Brachial plexus
   a. Subclavicular
   b. Thoracic outlet
3. Median nerve
   a. Carpal tunnel
   b. Pronator
   c. Anterior interosseous
4. Ulnar nerve
   a. Cubital tunnel
   b. Canal of Guyon
5. Radial nerve
   Radial tunnel syndrome

THE PATHOLOGY OF COMPRESSION LESIONS

Although there are an infinite number of circumstances that can surround a compression injury to a peripheral nerve, the distinctive and necessary one is of mechanical compression, which either by itself or by producing local ischemia within the nerve alters its ability to conduct impulses. The effects may vary depending on whether the deforming force is applied constantly or intermittently and to what magnitude over what area of the nerve. In normal nerves there are anatomical variations in intraneural topography or features of the regional anatomy that will either predispose or protect the nerve from compression. In patients who are systemically ill or debilitated, or those who have underlying and subclinical peripheral neuropathies, the effect of mechanical compression will be correspondingly greater than if these factors were not present. And, although compression can be brought about by many external forces or those that invade the body, this discussion will be applicable to those entities listed in the introduction since they are considered 'entrapments', lesions resulting from mechanical compression of adjacent and regional anatomical structures. Usually the affected nerve traverses a confined space that is either constricted due to a change in its external configuration or the presence of a space-occupying lesion that effectively reduces the available area. It should be noted, however, that not all entrapment lesions are caused by compression alone, since some of them may involve friction of the nerve against other structures or actual traction if the nerve should become adherent in the vicinity of a joint. There is a considerable literature devoted to the ongoing debate as to whether pure mechanical deformation of nerve is responsible for compression neuropathy or whether it is due to vascular insufficiency. In all probability (Sunderland 1978), both factors are operative since it would be hard to conceive of compressing a nerve without altering its blood supply.

DIAGNOSIS

Since many of the unsatisfactory results of treatment of compression lesions of nerves are directly attributable to errors in diagnosis, a brief review of diagnostic techniques is appropriate. And, although it hardly need be said, the simple lack of adequate history and physical examination accounts for the vast majority of such errors. Particularly when considering the circumscribed area of the hand, it is all too easy to omit examination of the remainder of the patient. Sterling Bunnell is often quoted as having said: 'The hand begins in the opposite cerebral cortex' and this truth should not be forgotten, since many signs and symptoms presenting in the hand will be manifestations of pathology actually located more centrally. In addition to a thorough motor and sensory examination, one should assess the circulatory status of the limb. The neck, shoulder and thoracic outlet should be examined before assuming that they are normal and that the lesion is indeed in the forearm or hand. When the history or physical findings point to the possibility of a generalised peripheral neuropathy, the lower extremities must be examined for motor and sensory function, something which can be accomplished quite adequately in about 90 seconds.

Electrodiagnosis

The techniques of electrodiagnosis are available to either aid the clinician in confirming a clinical diagnosis or to hopelessly becloud the issue and contribute to an unnecessary or inappropriate operative procedure. It therefore behoves the surgeon to have a working knowledge of the tests, their limitations, and particularly the interpretation of reports (Grundberg 1983, Bhala & Thoppil 1981, Iyer & Fenichel 1976, Buchthal et al 1974).

Electromyography is done with percutaneous needle electrodes in order to determine the integrity of the lower motor neuron. It can detect denervation and provide information about its chronicity, but it gives no information about etiology or where along the nerve the lesion is located unless multiple muscles are sampled in the context of the neurological examination. Nerve conduction velocity determination, by measuring conduction along the course of the nerve, can be used to demonstrate the level of the lesion. Both motor and sensory conduction velocities can be measured, and when combined with electromyography and clinical examination, can provide a high degree of diagnostic accuracy. The more proximal portions of the 'final common pathway' are inaccessible to the techniques of conduction velocity determination, but both F-responses and somatosensory evoked potentials can be used for this purpose. These applications are particularly important in the evaluation of lesions of the thoracic outlet, where conduction velocity, despite prior claims to the contrary, is often normal in cases of clinically manifest thoracic outlet syndrome. Hence, normal nerve conduction velocity through the thoracic outlet does not rule out a bona fide thoracic outlet compression (Lederman 1984) and the two more recent techniques of F-response and somatosensory evoked potential may help to pinpoint the lesion. Nevertheless, nerve conduction velocity determination is a valuable test which should be employed preoperatively, along with electromyography, in all cases of peripheral compression of nerves (Grundberg 1983, Harris & Tanner 1979). Since the normal values for nerve conduction may vary according to the laboratory wherein the test was performed, these standards should be consulted, despite the significant body of available normative data (Thompson 1981, Liberson 1963).

Radiological aids in diagnosis

All cases of compression of peripheral nerves should have adequate skeletal radiographs, and, when indicated, xerograms can be made. When there is evidence of a concomitant vascular lesion, arteriography may be indicated, although in thoracic outlet syndrome, unless there is a significant chance of a subclavian aneurysm or there has been previous surgery, non-invasive methods of evaluation will usually suffice. Myelography is, of course, useful in the evaluation of cervical radiculopathy, although by no means infallible. CT scanning, particularly when enhanced, is assuming greater importance as it becomes generally available. The practical value of magnetic resonance imaging remains to be determined.

CAUSES OF UNSATISFACTORY RESULTS

Misinterpretation of the nature of the pathological process

Generalised conditions, usually neurological but occasionally vascular, can become manifest in a single limb or expressed as a mononeuritis multiplex, and may be confused with multiple simultaneous compression lesions. Diabetes and neuropathies of other etiologies can be mistaken for mechanical lesions and can co-exist with them (Leffert 1969). Brachial neuritis is not uncommon and it, too, can sometimes be diagnosed as a compression lesion by the unwary, particularly if it is incomplete. Patients with congenital neuropathies are more sensitive to the effects of trauma that would not be noxious in other individuals. The various rheumatological entities can, in addition to nerve problems stemming from the intrinsic disease process, cause joint instability or swelling that can produce compression lesions of the nerves.

Local scarring, space-occupying lesions of both benign and malignant processes, including aneurysms, can be the underlying cause of compression lesions and ought well be identified prior to surgery, if at all possible. Tumours of peripheral nerves, when benign, are usually either neurofibromata which can occur in the absence of any of the stigmata of von Recklinghausen's disease, or neurolemmomas, which with the aid of magnification and microtechnique can be removed in many cases without damage to the fascicles surrounding them. The differential diagnosis is most important, since removal of a neurolemmoma is, in many cases, possible without sacrifice of the nerve, while a neurofibroma, being intrinsically part of the nerve fibres, cannot be removed without resection. When a tumour has assumed large proportions or is suspected of malignancy, then only an incisional biopsy should be done, with histological examination to determine subsequent treatment.

Mistaken level of pathology

The level of pathology can serve as a source of confusion and mis-diagnosis. As stated, a careful history and physical examination will usually eliminate most of these errors. A proximal lesion within the cervical spine, thoracic outlet, or about the shoulder or axilla can produce disturbances 'downstream' that are misinterpreted (Massey et al 1981). Commonly, patients with cervical radiculopathy in the C5–6 distribution will complain of nocturnal paresthesias in the thumb and index finger. These can be misinterpreted as representing carpal tunnel syndrome, particularly if no inquiry or examination regarding the neck is performed. Paresthesias of the little and ring finger with intrinsic weakness in the hand may immediately be ascribed to dysfunction of the ulnar nerve, whereas the unrecognised thoracic outlet compression may go unappreciated and the patient simply not respond to surgery done at the elbow. Sometimes the two lesions may co-exist, one proximally at the root of the limb or in the neck and one distally. This phenomenon, known as 'double crush syndrome' has been described by Upton & McComas (1973) and has been, in my experience, responsible for a number of failures to improve following surgery. Although Carroll & Hurst (1982) stated that the co-existence of thoracic outlet syndrome and carpal tunnel syndrome was extremely unlikely, that has not been my personal experience. Although the mechanism of double crush syndrome is not completely understood, it is helpful to think of it in terms of a proximal lesion sensitising the distal portions of the nerve to further compression.

The variations in innervation that are commonly encountered in post-mortem anatomical dissections of the forearm and hand should alert the clinician to the possibility that an atypical presentation of a nerve compression may be due to similar conditions in the living patient. By the use of careful physical examination, local anaesthetic block of adjacent nerves and electrodiagnostic techniques (Iyer & Fenichel 1976), most of these puzzles may be solved sufficiently to allow for appropriate surgical therapy.

Finally, one should not forget the possibility of intra-abdominal or intra-thoracic pathology with radiating pain producing symptoms that can be misinterpreted as coming from compression of peripheral nerves. Diaphragmatic irritation from diverse causes can produce this phenomenon with radiation into the shoulders and upper limbs. Apical lung tumours in particular, and especially in young women who smoke, must be included in the differential diagnosis of upper extremity neurological dysfunction, particulaly if it involves the outflow of the lower trunk of the brachial plexus.

Timing

The effect of continued compression on nerves varies according to several factors, including the extent and magnitude of the compression, as well as intraneural topography and the compliance of the surrounding tissues. Nevertheless, in most of these situations there is an initial period during which symptoms and signs may be detected but wherein complete reversal and restoration of full function are possible if adequate decompression is performed. The effects on the nerve, whether due to alterations in its circulation with stasis, or ultimately due to fibrosis, can reach a point beyond which recovery will be poor or at best, imperfect. This point in time varies with different situations and nerves. Moreover, the motor and sensory end organs are also subject to damage by denervation and if sufficiently impaired, will not recover. Significant motor weakness accompanied by profound muscular atrophy, particularly in an elderly individual, is likely to remain even after complete decompression although the prognosis is significantly better than it would be for a transected nerve with neurorrhaphy. It is, therefore, most important to advise the patient prior to any decompressive operation regarding the possibility of imperfect recovery. Tendon transfer may be performed at the time of decompression in selected cases (Braun 1978).

The operative procedure as a cause

Clearly, a mistake in diagnosis resulting in an operation done at the wrong level or location will almost invariably result in no alleviation of symptoms for which the procedure was done. In addition, inadequate operative procedures done at the proper level will similarly result in failure. The thoracic outlet decompression that is done by an inexperienced operator will often leave an excessively long posterior remnant of the first rib, which will then adhere to the lower trunk of the brachial plexus and not only fail to reduce symptoms, but actually increase them. Section of the transverse carpal ligament done blind or under a skin bridge can incompletely divide the most distal portion, which is considerably thinner, but which can still cause compression. Where the motor branch of the median nerve is separately compressed by a part of the transverse carpal ligament, failure to appreciate this variant will result in alleviation of sensory symptoms but no motor recovery (Bennett & Crouch 1982). For the ulnar nerve, an anterior transposition in the presence of a retained medial intermuscular septum or arcade of Struthers will produce not only failure of recovery, but significant local discomfort and an easily demonstrable Tinel's sign where the nerve is kinked over the fascia. And, if in a subcutaneous transposition of the ulnar nerve the nerve is not placed sufficiently anteriorly, it will be vulnerable to external trauma, or subjected to traction with movements of the elbow (Leffert 1982, Broudy et al 1978).

A decompressive procedure done at the correct level can still produce inadvertent damage to the nerve, caused either by surgical trauma, inadequate knowledge of the anatomy (Lanz 1977, Werschkul 1977, Kessler 1969), or unexpected variations in the path of the nerve and its branches. The peripheral nerves must be treated with the utmost delicacy in the operative field and great care taken not only to avoid direct damage to the fascicles, but to preserve as much of the segmental and longitudinal blood supply as is possible. Excessive mobilisation can be deleterious, even though normal nerves are relatively tolerant of such manoeuvres. Nerves that are already compromised and scarred are less so. Magnification with the operating microscope or loupe during surgery is necessary, as is the use of microtechnique. Although the ancients believed that dire consequences, seizures and death could result from touching nerves, the modern surgeon should know that lack of gentle retraction can result in paresthesias postoperatively or increased neurological deficit. The nerves must not be allowed to dry out and must be kept bathed in physiological solution, particularly if the procedure is lengthy. Finally, inadvertent damage to vascular structures in the vicinity of nerves can produce significant problems. Laceration of the palmar arch during the course of a carpal tunnel decompression can cause hemorrhage, which will not be apparent unless the tourniquet is deflated prior to closure. The proximity of the median nerve to the brachial artery at the elbow can predispose to arterial injury with subsequent aneurysm formation and gradual worsening of the neurological deficit with time. Scarring from the surgical procedure, fascial slings constructed to maintain the position of a transposed nerve, or intramuscular placement can produce significant damage.

Cutaneous nerves injured in the operative approach to compressed major nerves can become secondary sources of discomfort. The lateral cutaneous nerve of the forearm is encountered in the anterior approach to the radial nerve through the antecubital fossa and may sometimes be mistaken for it. The medial cutaneous nerve of the forearm is particularly vulnerable to injury during ulnar nerve transposition and should be sought and protected during this procedure. The intercostobrachial nerve, although considered of little importance in procedures done for cancer, is encountered during the performance of a transaxillary first rib resection (Roos 1971). If it is cut, the patient will complain, not only of a local neuroma, but of dysesthesia over the entire posterior aspect of the arm. Although with time the discomfort will subside somewhat, I have seen a number of patients who have had this as a permanent problem.

Many authors, including Denman (1981), Engber & Gmeiner (1980), Conolly (1978), MacDonald et al (1978), Das & Brown (1976), Carroll & Green (1972) and Eileen et al (1971) have commented on the avoidance of the palmar cutaneous branch of the median nerve during carpal tunnel decompression. Because this branch may be variable and may even travel within the transverse carpal ligament, great care is needed to avoid it. For this reason, a segment of the ligament should not be routinely excised during carpal tunnel release. Transverse incisions at the wrist, or those that cross the flexor carpi radialis tendon or go radial to it, are very likely to injure the nerve, resulting in a painful neuroma and dysesthesia in the palm. An interthenar approach such as has been suggested by Taleisnik (1973), with proximal extension as necessary, can be used to explore the area without producing a contracture across the volar wrist crease.

The occurrence of a reflex sympathetic dystrophy following decompression, particularly of the median nerve, can occur in several different ways. The first is to not recognise the presence of sympathetic dysfunction preoperatively and to cause an exacerbation of the condition by the operative procedure. Patients without sympathetic dystrophy can develop it postoperatively if the median nerve, which contains most of the sympathetic supply to the hand, is handled with less than optimal care, although I have observed this complication in a patient whose procedure was meticulously performed.

The aftercare of decompression of peripheral nerves should encourage wound healing with minimal scar, although this must be modified as necessary to prevent contractures of joints or adhesion of nerves to tendons. In subcutaneous ulnar nerve transposition, the nerve must not be allowed to return to its preoperative position. This requires 2 weeks of immobilisation with the elbow in flexion. Following carpal tunnel release, I immobilise the wrist in slight extension for 2 weeks to prevent prolapse of the nerve and tendons and adherence to the skin. The fingers must be gently exercised during this period to prevent adhesions to the nerve within the carpal canal, particularly if a synovectomy has been done.

Secondary gain factors

Because many of the effects of nerve compression are clinically expressed in terms of subjective complaint as pain, numbness or paresthesias, there is a small segment of the patient population that for secondary gain will continue to have symptoms or increased difficulty, even after an appropriately performed decompression of a peripheral nerve. The motivation may be subconscious, expressing a need for continued dependency or attention, or it may be more overt or deliberate in an attempt to achieve monetary compensation. Hopefully, the surgeon will have avoided operating on such patients by careful preoperative screening, but no surgeon is immune to this very human malady. Sometimes the postoperative neurological status may be unexplainable on the basis of known neurological patterns. At other times, the vehemence and vociferous embellishment of the symptoms in the absence of any appearance of discomfort may provide a necessary clue. Nevertheless, such patients continue to constitute a problem. In some cases, psychiatric evaluation and psychological testing can provide insights, but in many cases there is simply no way to achieve complete relief and resolution of the problem until the secondary gain factors have been satisfied. This may or may not be possible.

THE MANAGEMENT OF THE UNSATISFACTORY RESULT—PREOPERATIVE

Verification of diagnosis and documentation

The verification of the diagnosis both as to cause and the site of the pathology is central to investigation of the apparent failure of surgical therapy of a compression lesion. All of the prior medical records should be obtained if possible, including the detailed operative notes, as well as the electrodiagnostic studies, if they were done preoperatively. It is most important to attempt to ascertain the nature of the patient's socio-economic and family activities or hobbies prior to the surgery and to compare those with the present state of activity. The documentation of all of these facets of the problem is time-consuming at best, but necessary. As much insight as can be gained into the patient's emotional status and societal adjustment will be helpful. All of these data must be duly recorded in an orderly fashion to attempt to avoid falling into the same category of result if one chooses to re-explore the nerve.

Alternatives of therapy and informed consent

Once the surgeon has a clear picture of the patient and his problem, a frank discussion must be had so that the alternatives of therapy are clearly presented in as non-technical language as possible. In order for a patient to make a decision and render informed operative consent in many states, the language that is used and the explanations must be such that an attentive layman should be able to understand them. This is particularly important with patients who are already litigous or who do not need very much provocation to either sue their initial treating doctor or add you to the suit when the result is less than ideal. Most patients will ask for some type of numerical odds as to the possibility of their improvement if surgery is performed. I believe that to attempt to quote them exactly is to give the patient a false picture, and often leads to disappointment. I prefer to convey the general hoped-for results and indicate that each individual case, particularly for re-do surgery, must be taken on its individual merit. All the potential alternatives, both surgical and non-surgical, should be presented to the patient so that an informed decision may ultimately be made.

Non-surgical modalities of management

If there is an underlying disease process that is contributing to the symptomatology produced by the nerve compression, such as would be found with diabetic peripheral neuropathy, then appropriate medical management is instituted (Ellenberg 1968). However, it should be realised that there is not any assurance that treatment of diabetes will alleviate neuropathy, particularly if it is the mononeuritis multiplex that occurs in patients who are latent diabetics. Nevertheless, for those with symmetrical distal neuropathy, control of the diabetes may be of considerable benefit in terms of the neurological problem.

In some situations where there is a tender neuroma of a cutaneous nerve or where a major peripheral nerve has been left in a relatively subcutaneous position that is constantly traumatised, the use of supportive and protective orthoses can produce considerable symptomatic relief.

These orthotics may be worn at elbow and wrist with benefit, although they are obviously not curative.

In cases where activities of daily living or the patient's occupation constitute a noxious or aggravating factor in the perpetuation of symptoms, attempts ought to be made to change these circumstances. Consultations with vocational rehabilitation specialists and occupational therapists are often of great benefit in this sphere of treatment.

Pain management is a significant problem in patients who have had surgery for compression lesions and who continue to experience discomfort. One must be certain that the subjective sensations that the patients are reporting do not represent recovery of the nerve, since this is a common phenomenon, accompanied by cramping of muscles and paresthesias that may well not have been present prior to the decompression. Nevertheless, a patient whose compressed nerve has been decompressed should not have prolonged, significantly greater pain postoperatively, even though the sensations described above may come on even months after the surgery.

Assuming that all other causes for continued discomfort have been addressed, there remains the management of the symptom of pain. It is not rare to encounter patients who have been on narcotics prescribed by their doctors because of what appeared to be pain that could not be managed in any other way. Some of these patients have become frankly addicted and some of them may have had a history of drug abuse before the surgery. Nevertheless, it is very important to eliminate the use of narcotics for the continued treatment of pain following a decompression of a peripheral nerve. Very often the question is not raised until just before the end of my initial meeting with the patient, assuming that someone else has performed the initial surgery, and then a series of entirely predictable gambits takes place:

The patient states that the pain is unbearable and that the previous physician has provided narcotics to ease it. I have taken the position of prescribing nothing stronger than codeine, and even that very, very sparingly if the patient has already been on it. The various non-narcotic analgesics should be tried even though the patient maintains: 'Nothing works but Percodan'.

Dilantin is often suggested for pain relief in nerve injury, but in my experience, it is very rare that it has proved of benefit. Tegretol, an anticonvulsant that is used for painful states such as trigeminal neuralgia, is sometimes extremely effective in the treatment of discomfort from nerve injury, but it must be very carefully monitored. Before starting patients on Tegretol, a complete blood count, renal and hepatic function tests should be obtained because all of these may be adversely affected by the drug. These tests must be regularly repeated during the course of treatment.

Various combinations of antidepressants, tranquilizers and other psychopharmacological agents may be used according to the experience and preference of the physician. The combination of Elavil and Prolixin may sometimes be quite effective.

The transcutaneous nerve stimulator is a modality that, aside from local skin irritation, has virtually no downside risk. On the other hand, it must be used with significant support on the part of the prescribing and treating persons else the modality will fail. Although it may offer significant pain relief beyond that of a placebo and I have had a number of patients over the years who have been very grateful for the relief that it has afforded them, I am equally convinced that the manner in which the modality is prescribed is of importance.

Psychotherapy, when oriented toward helping the patient cope with the pain rather than attempting to 'talk him out of it' can be of benefit. However, in my experience, neither prolonged psychotherapy nor hypnosis have proved to be of significant benefit in relieving a patient of pain due to failed surgery for nerve compression, although they may well be able to cope better after such treatment. Along these lines, the techniques of behavioural modification do not address the primary pathology but seek to alter the patient's reaction to the pain. They are beyond the scope of this chapter.

OPERATIVE MANAGEMENT

Timing

The timing of the operative intervention following failed decompression of peripheral nerve lesions is crucial, yet often difficult to establish on the basis of rigorous criteria. There are some situations that demand immediate attention, such as a complete loss of neurological function following an operative procedure on a compressed nerve. Fortunately, these situations are rare, but they should be acted upon with dispatch lest the deficit be permanent rather than remediable. For most other patients, the need for immediate intervention will not be present, and one can have time to establish a rational algorithm for treatment. The preoperative status may be difficult to substantiate if the primary procedure was performed by another surgeon and the records cannot be obtained. Usually, with persistence, they can be, and at that time, the diagnostic work-up and what was done prior to surgery can be evaluated.

In some cases that I have personally observed, the problem was more apparent than real. Neither failure of the operative procedure nor actual worsening had occurred, and the problem was attributable to lack of communication between the surgeon and the patient as to what to expect in the postoperative period. In such situations, a tactful and reassuring explanation can put things right.

Those lesions that are neuropraxias may begin to improve almost immediately following decompressive surgery, and they will not be in the category of unsatisfactory results. The majority of the long-standing compressions will represent mixed lesions with a significant degree of axonotmesis. These, after an initial delay, should begin to recover in an orderly fashion that can roughly be calculated at the rate of an inch a month. The Tinel's sign can be useful in assessing recovery, but it must be realised that in order to be meaningful, the sign must be elicited distal to the point of compression and preferably on several occasions at different times. In some cases, the degree of compression can be so severe that regeneration will not occur following decompression, a true neurotmesis. Fortunately these situations are unusual in compression of nerves, although they may occur and they become manifest when the expected time for regeneration of an axonotmesis has passed. Preoperative electrodiagnostic techniques are of considerable benefit when integrated with solid neurological examination. However, the ability to define whether recovery has occurred over time is dependent upon the examiner's ability to document findings by means of careful clinical examination and the keeping of meticulous records.

Sequence of multiple operative procedures

Unfortunately, patients who have had unsatisfactory results from decompression of peripheral nerves often exhibit a series of operative scars up and down the limb with each site thought to be the culprit and ultimately found innocent. Such patients are generally very displeased at the inability of the surgeon to relieve their symptoms and go to another consultant who must now decide whether any of these sites was really pathological. Although both the 'double crush syndrome' and multiple areas of compression do exist, they are not nearly as common as these multiply operated limbs would have us believe. More often, rather than multiple compression lesions, these cases represent misdiagnoses. On the other hand, when one is presented with what would appear to be a case of multi-level compressions, it requires the utmost skill and diagnostic acumen to sort things out appropriately. From a purely practical point of view, for example, transposing an ulnar nerve is a considerably easier procedure than exploring the thoracic outlet, and common sense would have us accomplish that which has the least downside risk with the most potential benefit first. And, no matter what the order, if multiple compression lesions are suspected, it is wise to allow a hiatus of at least 2 months between procedures to assess the effect of the previous decompression. Prudence in the timing of procedures will, hopefully, protect the surgeon against the so-called Munchausen type of patient, who for some perverse and nefarious reason of psychiatric imbalance, actually enjoys being operated upon.

General operative therapy of the compressed nerve

From a simplistic point of view, nerves that are compressed and cause symptoms should be decompressed. As has been stated, a compression lesion that persists long enough can produce scarring beyond the epineurium to include the fascicles and result in a degenerative lesion. Grossly this process will cause a neuroma, which must be assessed in terms of the advisability of surgical manipulation. Where the epineurium is particularly scarred, it should be incised under magnification with care to protect the underlying fascicles, and if possible, removed in such a way as to preserve the superficial longitudinal blood vessels. If they are transgressed, then electrocoagulation by means of a bipolar device is judiciously employed. Usually it is desirable not to circumferentially denude a long segment of epineurium for fear of interfering with the blood supply. This is particularly applicable to the median nerve at the wrist, where, whenever possible, the dorsal surface should not be disturbed. The question of when epineurectomy is indicated remains somewhat controversial. In my experience with carpal tunnel release, longstanding symptoms, significant thenar atrophy, and profound sensory loss have become indications for epineurectomy as described. I believe that the routine use of intraneural lysis is potentially damaging to the fascicles and the intraneural blood supply. If this manoeuvre is employed for relief of intraneural scarring, it should be done only by an experienced operator using high magnification and micro-instruments. Curtis & Eversmann (1973) described their extensive experience with the procedure.

The transposition of decompressed nerves is a method of relocating a previously compromised nerve in a less scarred or better vascularised bed. It is particularly useful in ulnar nerve lesions of the cubital tunnel, although there is disagreement as to technique. My strong preference in most cases is for submuscular transposition, as described by Learmonth (Leffert 1982). Transposition may also be employed for the median nerve at the elbow, superficial to the pronator teres. The prevention of scarring by the use of various sheaths has had a long and unsavoury history. Suffice it to say that the presently preferred material is always the best one. None of the materials used have proved to have significant value in the prevention of scarring of a nerve that has undergone neurolysis. In addition, the mobilisation and isolation of such nerves may prove deleterious on the basis of

Table 14.1 Thoracic outlet syndrome

Unsatisfactory result	Symptoms and signs	Prevention	Treatment
Intercosto-brachial neuropathy	Hypaesthesia or dysaesthesia posterior brachium and axilla	Identification of nerve in axilla at third interspace—longitudinal fascial incision, gentle retraction, avoid laceration or avulsion	None other than time—in many cases, symptoms become less annoying
Lower trunk palsy or paresis	Long flexor and intrinsic weakness; hypaesthesia or anaesthesia over medial forearm and ulnar fingers and hand	Protection of nerve trunks at surgery from direct trauma or rib cutter or retractors. Gentle traction on arm during surgery—periodic relaxation of traction by scrubbed assistant	None for nerves. Reconstruction of hand by tendon transfers if palsy does not improve by one year.
Long thoracic nerve palsy	Winged scapula pain in shoulder	Avoidance of nerve at surgery in field—particularly if middle scalene is removed. Gentle traction on arm during procedure	None for nerve. Tendon transfer (pectoralis minor or major) for permanent palsy—greater than one year.
Failure of relief	Unchanged symptoms	Sufficient resection of rib Search for compressing bands, adventitious ribs, second rib compression	Re-exploration and neurolysis, resection of rib remnants, scalenectomy when scarring is severe
Delayed return of symptoms		Extraperiosteal resection of first rib, sufficient rib resection to prevent scarring of periosteal	(As above)
Persistent shoulder and neck pain	Lower trunk symptoms—usually sensory ptotic scapula trapezius, levator scapulae and rhomboid atrophy	Rapid resumption of progressive exercise programme for shoulder muscles and attention to postural abnormalities	Postural strengthening exercise programme for shoulder muscle

Table 14.2 Ulnar neuropathy at the elbow

Unsatisfactory result	Symptoms and signs	Prevention	Treatment
Nerve hypermobile or subluxating posteriorly over epicondyle or into olecranon groove	Local discomfort and tenderness. Painful clicking. Irritative neuropathy	Adequate anterior transposition, usually submuscular. Postoperative immobilisation 3 weeks	Neurolysis, usually external. Submuscular transposition
Local neuroma, medial cutaneous nerve of forearm	Local tenderness. Tinels referred to forearm. Forearm dysaesthesia	Identify and protect nerve in operative field	Repair if possible, otherwise excision of neuroma with placement in padded tissue
Failure of relief of symptoms	Local tenderness. Persistent ulnar neuropathy. Tinels sign above olecranon groove.	Excision of medial intermuscular septum and ligament of Struthers, if present	Neurolysis, usually external. Exploration for areas of impingement. Conversion of subcutaneous or intramuscular transposition to submuscular
Local clicking at elbow	Pain and click with flexion; no paraesthesias	Search for bands or aberrant muscles inspection of medial triceps at surgery	Lysis or fixation of aberrant muscle or bands as necessary
Stiff elbow	Flexion contracture	Mobilisation of elbow at 3 weeks	Gentle range of motion exercises. Avoidance of passive exercise or manipulation

Table 14.3 Median nerve at wrist

Unsatisfactory result	Symptoms and signs	Prevention	Treatment
Failure of relief	No change in median neuropathy	Complete division of transverse carpal ligament. Epineurectomy	Re-exploration, epineurectomy. ?? Intraneural lysis
Sensory relief only	Continued thenar muscle atrophy and weakness	Demonstration of clear decompression of motor branch and elimination of separate bands of transverse carpal ligament	Re-exploration if lesion was not longstanding—otherwise tendon transfer for opposition
Immediate worsening of sensory loss	Sensory loss, usually in common digital nerve distribution	Protection of nerves at surgery—avoidance of 'blind' incisions	Re-exploration, repair nerves
Immediate worsening of motor function	Paralysis of thenar muscles of opposition	Demonstration of thenar branch, search for aberrant takeoff from main nerve. Avoidance of radially placed incisions of transverse carpal ligament	Re-exploration with repair of nerve, if possible—otherwise tendon transfer for opposition
Tenderness in palm	Dysaesthesia and Tinel's sign—palmar cutaneous nerve	Proper placement of incision, interthenar. Avoid transverse, blind incisions or excision of segment of transverse carpal ligament	Exploration of palmar cutaneous neuroma—repair if possible, otherwise excision to point of origin in median nerve
Local pain at incision, paraesthesia with extension of wrist, shortening of flexor tendons	Recurrence of symptoms. Adherence of flexor tendons, local tenderness	Dorsiflexion splinting of wrist postoperatively for 2 weeks	Re-exploration, neurolysis and tenolysis. Splinting, partial reconstruction of ligament
Reflex sympathetic dystrophy	Pain. Vasomotor changes. Joint stiffness. Delayed return of function	Avoidance of trauma to nerve. Prompt mobilisation of all joints except wrist. Sympathetic blocks	Sympathetic blocks. IV Guanethidine. Physical therapy

Table 14.4 Radial nerve

Unsatisfactory result	Symptoms and signs	Prevention	Treatment
Failure of recovery of motor function	Persistent finger extensor weakness	Prompt decompression	Tendon transfer

interference with local segmental blood supply. Unless a new and well vascularised bed either between muscles (but not in) or in adipose tissue can be obtained, there is little reason to believe that scarring will not recur. When scarring has united the nerve to the skin, particularly in the region of a joint, a traction element will be introduced that can prove particularly vexing. Unless the nerve can be divorced from the skin by means of an interposed plane of other tissue such as muscle or fat, the condition will surely recur. Sometimes a pedicle of muscle can be of assistance, and in some cases, the cutaneous area must be resurfaced by means of a local or remote flap. Often these can be done as pedicle flaps, but sometimes free, microvascular techniques can be of advantage. Clearly there is no place for the use of split thickness skin in such situations, where an adequate thickness of soft tissue is essential to prevent constant trauma to the nerve.

The more common unsatisfactory results seen after surgery for treatment of nerve compression in the upper limb and hand are detailed along with their signs and symptoms, prevention and treatment in Tables 14.1–14.4. Clearly, prevention is most desirable.

REFERENCES

Bennett J B, Crouch C C 1982 Compression syndrome of the recurrent motor branch of the median nerve. Journal of Hand Surgery 7(4):407

Bhala R P, Thoppil E 1981 Early detection of carpal tunnel syndrome by sensory nerve conduction. Electromyography and Clinical Neurophysiology 21:155

Braun R M 1978 Palmaris longus tendon transfer for augmentation of the thenar musculature in low median palsy. Journal of Hand Surgery 3(5):488

Broudy A, Leffert R D, Smith R J 1978 Technical problems with ulnar nerve transposition at the elbow: Findings and results of reoperation. Journal of Hand Surgery 3:85

Buchthal F, Rosenfalck A, Trojaborg W 1974 Electrophysiological findings in entrapment of median nerve at wrist and elbow. Journal of Neurology, Neurosurgery, and Psychiatry 37:340

Carroll R E, Hurst L C 1982 The relationship of thoracic outlet syndrome and carpal tunnel syndrome. Clinical Orthopaedics and Related Research 164:149

Carroll R E, Green G P 1972 The significance of the palmar cutaneous nerve at the wrist. Clinical Orthopaedics and Related Research 83:24

Conolly W B 1978 Pitfalls in carpal tunnel decompression. Australian and New Zealand Journal of Surgery 48(4):421

Curtis R M, Eversmann W W Jr 1973 Internal neurolysis as an adjunct to the treatment of the carpal tunnel syndrome. Journal of Bone and Joint Surgery 55A:733

Das S K, Brown H G 1976 In search of complications in carpal tunnel decompression. Hand 8(3):243

Denman E E 1981 The anatomy of the incision for carpal tunnel decompression. Hand 13(1):17

Eileen O, Carston M, Eddeland A 1971 Anomalous distal branching of the median nerve. Case Reports. Scandinavian Journal of Plastic and Reconstructive Surgery 5:149

Ellenberg M 1968 Treatment of diabetic neuropathy with diphenylhydantoin. New York State Journal of Medicine 68:2653

Engber W D, Gmeiner J G 1980 Palmar cutaneous branch of the ulnar nerve. Journal of Hand Surgery 5(1):26

Grundberg A 1983 Carpal tunnel decompression in spite of normal electromyography. Journal of Hand Surgery 8(3):348

Harris C M, Tanner E et al 1979 The surgical treatment of the carpal tunnel syndrome correlated with pre-operative nerve conduction studies. Journal of Bone and Joint Surgery 61A(1):93

Iyer V, Fenichel G M 1976 Normal median nerve proximal latency in carpal tunnel syndrome: A clue to co-existing Martin-Gruber anastomosis. Journal of Neurology, Neurosurgery, and Psychiatry 39(5):449

Kessler I 1969 Unusual distribution of the median nerve at the wrist. A case report. Clinical Orthopaedics and Related Research 67:124

Lanz U 1977 Anatomical variation of the median nerve in the carpal tunnel. Journal of Hand Surgery 2:44

Lederman R 1984 Thoracic outlet syndrome: Letter to the editor. New England Journal of Medicine 310(16):1052

Leffert R D 1969 Diabetes mellitus initially presenting as peripheral neuropathy in the upper limb. Journal of Bone and Joint Surgery 51A:1005

Leffert R D 1982 Anterior submuscular transposition of the ulnar nerve by the Learmonth technique. Journal of Hand Surgery 7:147

Liberson W T 1963 Sensory conduction velocities in normal individuals and in patients with peripheral neuropathies. Archives of Physical Medicine and Rehabilitation 44:313

MacDonald R I, Lichtman D M et al 1978 Complication of surgical release for carpal tunnel syndrome. Journal of Hand Surgery 3(1):70

Massey E W, Riley T L, Pleet A 1981 Coexistent carpal tunnel syndrome and cervical radiculopathy (double crush syndrome). Southern Medicine Journal 74(8):957

Roos D B 1966 Transaxillary approach for first rib resection to relieve thoracic outlet syndrome. Annals of Surgery 163:354

Sunderland S 1978 Nerves and nerve injuries, 2nd edn. Churchill Livingstone, Edinburgh

Taleisnik J 1973 The palmar cutaneous branch of the median nerve and the approach to the carpal tunnel. Journal of Bone and Joint Surgery 55A(6):1212

Thompson L L 1981 The electromyographer's handbook. Little, Brown and Co, Boston

Upton A, McComas A J 1973 The double crush in nerve entrapment syndromes. Lancet 2:359

Urschel H C Jr 1972 Management of the thoracic outlet syndrome. New England Journal of Medicine 286:1140-3

Werschkul J D 1977 Anomalous course of the recurrent motor branch of the median nerve in a patient with carpal tunnel syndrome. Journal of Neurosurgery 47:113

F. D. Burke and R. G. Pulvertaft

15 Flexor tendons

GENERAL PRINCIPLES

The general principles of hand injury management have already been discussed in the opening chapter. Before considering those factors most relevant to tendon injury it is prudent to review the overall management policy of the surgeon. This will, of course, depend on available surgical skills, beds, emergency theatre time and facilities. Satisfactory results in flexor tendon surgery are not easily achieved. Delayed primary repair or tendon grafting later is indicated if immediately available surgical skills are poor, emergency operating facilities inadequate, or the wound conditions unsuitable.

The lacerated working hand is frequently covered with dirt or grease. Probing of the wound by inexperienced emergency room staff is unhelpful. Careful assessment for sensory loss precedes general or local anaesthesia. The hand can then be cleaned with soap or grease remover to avoid subsequent contamination of the wound. Exploration of the wound itself should be performed by an experienced person with the benefit of proper facilities; in particular, adequate illumination and sufficiently fine instruments. Loupe magnification is also of great benefit. A bloodless field is essential and a standard pneumatic tourniquet should be used. It is important to avoid desiccation of the wound during surgery. The wound edges should be kept moist with saline swabs throughout the procedure, their frequent use not only moistens the wound but helps to remove foreign debris from the laceration.

If the wound margins are permitted to become dry many cells lining the laceration die, increasing the risk of subsequent infection. It is usually necessary to extend the incision proximally or distally. This may be performed by using zigzag incisions or by a longitudinal incision at the midlateral line. It is important to achieve haemostasis before the wound is closed. This is best done by the use of a bipolar coagulator which produces a minimal amount of damage to the surrounding parts. Closure of the wound should be without undue tension. If the skin edges are drawn together too tightly their blood supply may be jeopardised and further tissue death may occur. Prophylactic antibiotics can never be a substitute for effective primary wound management. In the early postoperative period the arm is elevated to reduce the risk of oedema developing in the hand.

PRIMARY TENDON REPAIR

A prerequisite to the care of primary tendon injury is that the diagnosis is made at the first attendance. This requires an adequate knowledge of anatomy by the emergency physician, and sufficient experience to suspect when a tendon injury may have occurred. Alteration in the normal cascade of fingers is the most obvious clinical sign. The emergency physician must be capable of examining the hand; in particular, to assess the superficialis function to individual fingers. After careful clinical examination an experienced clinician can usually determine the extent of nerve and tendon injury. Exploration can then be performed with a clear impression of the structures requiring repair.

The cut crush ratio and evaluation of associated injuries is also required. Grossly contaminated lacerations or those presenting many hours after injury will merit debridement and skin closure with a secondary tendon graft. If damage involves both nerves and vessels with an associated fracture in a single finger, amputation may be the appropriate treatment.

The site of tendon injury is also an important prognostic indicator. Flexor tendon repairs in zone II (Fig. 15.1) remain the least satisfactory. In this zone the profundus tendon lies intimately related to the superficialis slips within the flexor tendon sheath (Fig. 15.2). Difficulties may also be experienced with zone I where the profundus alone traverses the distal flexor sheath. More satisfactory results are obtained in the palm and forearm, zones III and V respectively, but there is an increased tendency for adhesions to form between repaired tendons within the carpal tunnel (zone IV).

Tendon repairs in zones I and II

Satisfactory results in these zones remain the greatest challenge. After appropriate anaesthesia the limb is exsanguinated. The laceration is extended proximally and distally depending on the position of the finger at the time of tendon division. If the finger has been cut in flexion (for example—the hand slipping down a carving knife), distal exploration is required. However, lacerations in

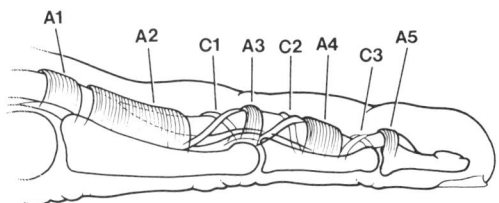

Fig. 15.2 The flexor pulley system

extension rarely require distal exploration as the profundus tendon is presented by flexing the distal interphalangeal joint. The proximal tendon stump has usually retracted but may be held by the long vincula. Extension of the sheath laceration should be minimal, and if further openings are required to retrieve tendon stumps they should be limited to cruciform portions of the pulleys. A small cuff or pulley should be left attached to the phalanx allowing resuturing of the sheath on completion of the repair. Although tendon retrievers on occasion succeed in delivering the proximal stump, the trauma they cause to the lining of the sheath may outweigh any advantages of a reduced exploration. A further incision may be required in the palm proximal to the A1 pulley. If the tendons have retracted to this level a fine silicone rubber catheter is passed down the sheath to the palm. The tendon ends alone are grasped with fine-tooth forceps and the repair suture inserted. A 4/0 braided non-absorbable polyester suture (Ethibond) is preferred by many surgeons. The Kessler locking suture (Fig. 15.3) maintains position well during the healing phase; the locking portions of the suture should be approximately 1 cm from the cut surface and the suture ends left long. The tendon ends are then aligned correctly and the sutures attached to the catheter. The tendons can then be reduced into the mouth of the A1 pulley and drawn down to the level of the repair with minimal damage to tendon and sheath. A similar stitch is applied to the distal tendon ends and the tendon sutured with knots buried in the cut surface. A running 6/0 nylon appositional suture may improve the contour of the repair. The tourniquet is released and haemostasis obtained. Where practical a careful sheath reconstruction with 6/0 nylon sutures reduces the risk of the tendon repair abutting against a pulley edge and helps to ensure retention of synovial fluid

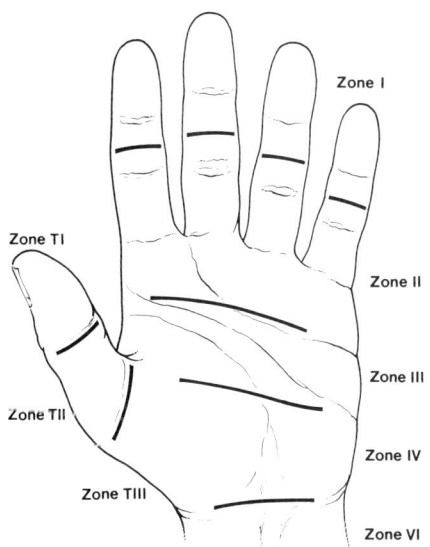

Fig. 15.1 The flexor tendon zones

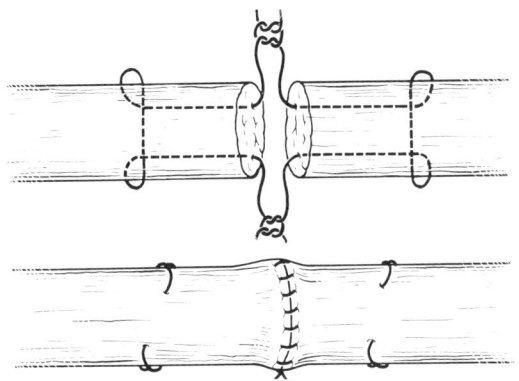

Fig. 15.3 The Kessler locking suture

within the sheath. Accurate skin apposition is particularly important if early mobilisation is planned. There is, at present, no agreement on the optimal rehabilitation programme. Immobilisation in a cast is preferred by some with progressive mobilisation at 3–4 weeks. Others prefer dynamic traction or passive/active mobilisation from the time of the repair. If early mobilisation techniques are used close supervision by the hand therapist is essential.

Delayed primary repair

A primary tendon repair may be delayed for 2 or even 3 weeks. If the repair is to be delayed more than a few hours the wound must be carefully cleaned and the skin sutured on the initial attendance. The suture line is dressed with paraffin gauze and dressing gauze. A plaster of Paris back slab in moderate wrist flexion reduces the chances of further proximal migration of the divided tendons.

Profundus avulsion

The ring finger is the most frequently involved. The injury usually occurs in rugby football or similar sports when attempting to grasp an opponent. The ring finger is forcibly hyperextended while the remaining fingers flex. The profundus may rupture at its insertion on the distal phalanx or detach a fragment of bone. If the fragment of bone is large proximal migration is minimal but there may be significant disruption of the articular surface of the base of the distal phalanx. Fixation of the fragment with Kirschner or pull-out wires will reconstruct the joint and permit early movement. The more common injury is for little or no bone to be attached to the avulsed tendon which is drawn forcibly into the palm. The patient is unable to flex the distal interphalangeal joint and careful palpation in the palm will often detect the retracted profundus tendon. The palm and distal phalangeal areas should be explored with minimal disturbance of the flexor tendon sheath. A fine silicone rubber catheter is passed from finger to palm and a modified Kessler wire suture inserted into the profundus stump. The suture is attached to the catheter and drawn through the pulley system. The tendon end is inserted into a drill hole in the distal phalanx and the wire suture passed through the nail and firmly tied over a button (Fig. 15.4). If the profundus stump is retracted into the palm the procedure can be performed through two small incisions, one over the distal phalanx and the other just proximal to the A1 pulley in the palm. If the profundus tendon has not fully retracted to the palm, exploration of the more proximal part of the finger is required and the tendon end retrieved through a window in a cruciate pulley. An alternative technique has the benefit of avoiding further disturbance of the pulley system. A fine catheter is passed from the palm to the distal sheath opening. The tendon and catheter are sutured together as they lie side by side just proximal to the A1 pulley. Traction on the catheter distally will usually return the proximal stump to the site of laceration. A modified Kessler suture can then be inserted and the tendon allowed to retract and the more proximal suture removed along with the catheter. Postoperative rehabilitation of an avulsed flexor tendon is similar to that of a primary flexor tendon repair although the firm distal tendon insertion obtained may encourage one to use early motion. Delay in diagnosis adversely affects the

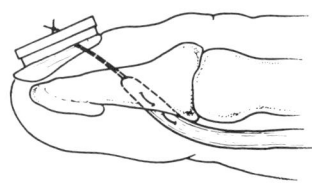

Fig. 15.4 Distal suture technique

results of surgery. Pulleys constrict if not occupied by tendon and it may prove impossible to re-insert the profundus tendon if exploration is delayed. At a later stage a tendon graft (which is slimmer) will be required.

Unsatisfactory results following primary tendon repair

Meticulous technique will reduce the density of adhesions. If the technique described above is employed the smooth surface of the tendon and sheath will be least traumatised. Ideally each stump should be picked up by the cut surface once only, to insert the repair stitch. The tendon should be kept moist at all times and not permitted to come into contact with skin or skin preparation solutions.

Rupture

Dehiscence may occur because of an inadequate repair or difficulties during rehabilitation. The Kessler locking suture technique is usually a satisfactory compromise in the conflict between strength of repair and tendon devascularisation. There are other suture techniques which produce a stronger initial repair (for example the Bunnell figure of 8 type). Unfortunately the greater exposure of the tendon required and the constricting effect of this suture are factors which increase the risk of devascularisation of the tendon ends. Polyester, nylon or stainless steel wire (4/0) are satisfactory suture materials. Wire is strong and inert and is preferred by some surgeons. It is more difficult to use being easily kinked and weakened.

Silk and absorbable sutures produce a greater inflammatory response with increased adhesions. At present there is no evidence that any absorbable suture material is as effective or inert as polyester, nylon or steel. Poor patient co-operation, inadequate splintage or excessive active motion in the early weeks following repair may be responsible for tendon rupture.

Wound infection

A wound infection following hand trauma is disastrous to the management of the injury. This is particularly true in the case of lacerations of the hand with associated tendon or nerve repair. Sepsis may damage repaired structures, delay mobilisation and lead to adhesions and contracture. Inadequate skin preparation or wound debridement may be responsible. Wound desiccation during surgery is a potent cause of cell death and possible wound infection. Inadequate haemostasis is followed by wound haematoma, which may become secondarily infected. The incidence of infection following hand lacerations should be very low and when cases do occur they merit investigation to establish the cause.

Flap necrosis

The adjacent skin may have been damaged at the time of injury. Great care must be taken when extending the original laceration; an adequate layer of fat should be raised with the skin flaps. This is most difficult at the level of the finger creases where the tendon sheath lies very close to the skin. If a zigzag (Brunner) incision is used (Fig. 15.5) it is unnecessary and unwise to extend the apex to the mid-lateral line. The flap should be short and broadly based. Flap ischaemia or necrosis will profoundly alter subsequent rehabilitation and is a sure cause of an unsatisfactory result (Fig. 15.6).

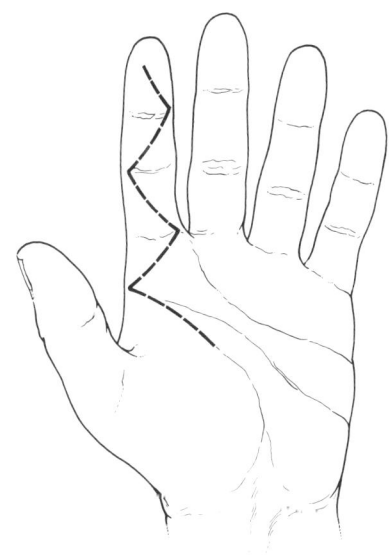

Fig. 15.5 The Brunner incision

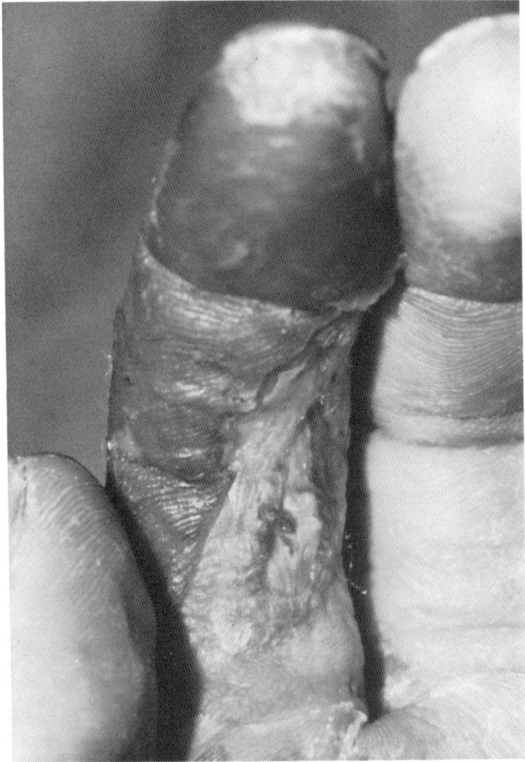

Fig. 15.6 An inappropriate incision with flap necrosis and exposed tendon

Joint contracture

The proximal interphalangeal joint is most at risk. The position in which the hand is placed during the immediate postoperative period following primary repair is of great importance. If the wrist and metacarpophalangeal joints are flexed to 40° the loading of the repaired tendons will be low enough to permit full interphalangeal joint extension.

Proximal interphalangeal joint contracture is a not uncommon complication of repairs in zones I and II. Constant vigilance is required to ensure that the joints remain in the appropriate position. Bulky dressings may permit the metacarpophalangeal joint to drift into extension with consequent proximal interphalangeal joint flexion. Particular care is required if dynamic traction is applied to the finger. The traction must permit full extension at proximal interphalangeal and distal interphalangeal joints. Early transfer to an appropriately moulded orthoplast splint with minimal dressings best maintains proximal joint flexion with the distal joints extended. Tenolysis is quite frequently required after primary tendon repairs in zones I and II; if the proximal interphalangeal joint must also be released the procedure is more complicated and less effective.

Primary flexor tendon repair in other zones

The management of zone III repairs is similar to the preceding section and the overall results are more favourable. Tendon adhesion is less frequent. Zone IV injuries are uncommon. These often require complete release of the flexor retinaculum to achieve adequate access. Associated median nerve injury is frequent. Intertendonous adhesions may be reduced by the repair of the synovial compartments (if feasible) and early passive finger motion. The wrist should be splinted in neutral position (if the wrist is flexed the tendons will bowstring close to the skin). Repairs in zone V require suturing muscle and tendon; there is a tendency for sutures to pull out of the muscle. A Bunnell double right angle suture (Fig. 15.7) achieves reasonable coaptation without serious tissue devascularisation. Early movement may jeopardise the repair. Closure of the synovial compartments and the deep fascia will reduce the likelihood of intermuscular or dermal adhesions.

TENDON GRAFTING

The development of tendon grafting stems from the teaching of Sterling Bunnell. In 1918, he reported the use of a toe extensor tendon to replace the flexor tendons of a little finger and a strip of triceps tendon for the flexors of the ring finger

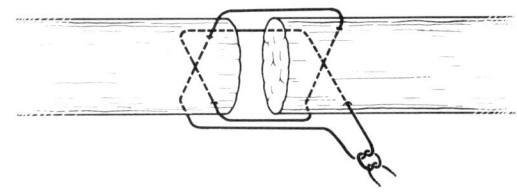

Fig. 15.7 The Bunnell double right angle suture

with a fair measure of success. He also described a case in which he had restored the extensor pollicis longus with a palmaris longus graft. In 1922, Bunnell reported several examples of thumb and finger flexor tendon injuries in which grafting had given good results. This classic paper, written over 60 years ago contains a wealth of advice which is still valid: 'Handling of the tissues should be reduced to a minimum... When handling a tendon or sheath, never should even a tiny scratch be made in the delicate membrane covering their surfaces, as here adhesions will form and prevent gliding... Free tendon grafts cause less reaction than foreign bodies. They subsist on surrounding lymph until they obtain their own blood supply... Often after a tendon repair it is necessary to do a second operation of freeing the tendon from adhesions. this is best deferred, however, for several months until the original postoperative induration has passed away, otherwise a summation of postoperative induration might defeat our purpose... The selection of the proper incision is very important ... Unless the joints are freely movable, it is useless to repair the tendon as it will not be able to move a stiff joint ... Co-operation by the patient is essential, and he must be willing to take some punishment in exchange for a good result.'

Bunnell's influence was worldwide and tendon grafting was widely practised for tendon divisions in the difficult region between the distal palmar crease and the middle finger crease (zone II). 'Poor results the world over follow suture of flexor tendons in what is called "no man's land", that is, between the distal crease in the palm and the middle crease in the finger' (Bunnell 1948). Secondary grafting became for many the method of choice for tendon divisions in zone II. However, there have been others, notably the Chicago School, Koch, Mason and Allen (Mason 1957) and Verdan (1972), who have consistently advocated suture when wound conditions are suitable. As surgical techniques improved with the use of magnification, finer instruments and suture materials, and as more surgeons were trained in hand surgery the emphasis has been placed upon tendon suture for the acute injury in this zone. It must be stressed that the high standards achieved by Verdan, Kleinert and his colleagues (Lister et al 1977) and others, are dependent upon suitable wound conditions and the availability of these facilities.

Indications for tendon grafting

The main indications for grafting in flexor tendon injuries are:

1. As an alternative treatment for an acute tendon division when wound conditions, operative facilities or surgical experience are unsuitable for primary, or delayed primary, suture. A wound toilet is performed with a view to grafting later.

2. As the treatment of election when a tendon injury has been overlooked or neglected. The patient may have been advised at the time of injury that there was no effective treatment for the condition.

A graft permits the distal junction to be sited beyond the distal interphalangeal joint, and the proximal junction in the palm or lower forearm where adhesions occur less readily and are more yielding than in the narrow confines of the finger. It also overcomes any gap which may have developed between the tendon ends because of local damage or muscle shortening. Single stage tendon grafting is an operation which yields good results when performed under favourable circumstances. Unfortunately, success cannot be guaranteed and some 25% have unacceptable results and require further treatment.

Factors influencing the result

1. Age
2. State of the hand
3. Surgical approach
4. Treatment of the tendon bed
5. The graft and the junctions
6. Choice of the mucle to act as motor
7. The hypermobile finger and the role of superficialis
8. Aftercare

(The general management and tissue craft will not be discussed in this section)

1. The very young and the elderly are rarely suitable subjects for tendon grafting. Children under the age of 3 or 4 years are unlikely to co-

operate in postoperative exercises. Skilled physical treatment, most valuable as it is, cannot substitute completely for lack of understanding and enthusiasm in the patient. It has been shown (Boyes & Stark 1971, Pulvertaft in press) that it is possible to obtain a satisfactory result from grafting after a lapse of several years since injury. The operation may safely be deferred for a year or longer without prejudicing the result.

2. Reconstructive surgery which has gliding as its goal should not be performed in a hand which has not recovered from the general effects of trauma. It is wise to wait for 4–6 months from injury before operating. The vascular and sensibility status of the finger must be adequate; if both digital nerves have been divided one at least should be repaired and be recovering. Full or nearly full passive motion is essential, but there is one interesting exception to this rule. The distal part of a profundus tendon divided in zone II acts as a piston within the cylinder formed by the digital theca; it may be prevented from gliding proximally by adhesions thus effectively blocking passive flexion. This piston effect vanishes when the distal profundus segment is removed allowing the return of passive motion.

3. An ill designed incision may ruin an otherwise potentially good result. There are three standard approaches to the digital sheath which have proved satisfactory and the choice is largely one of personal preference: the mid-axial incision deepened to pass posterior to the digital vessels and nerve (the method favoured by the authors), the same incision deepened to pass anterior to the neurovascular bundle, and the volar zigzag incision. Each of these incisions can be extended into the palm and affords an excellent exposure and leaves a trouble free scar.

4. The treatment of the tendon bed is influenced by the extent and nature of existing scar. The aim is to preserve the annular bands at the level of the metacarpophalangeal joint (A1), the proximal phalanx (A2), and the middle phalanx (A4). It has been our custom to excise the intervening parts of the fibrous sheath if they are involved in scar. Adaptations and formation of new pulleys may be needed according to prevailing circumstances. If possible, the distal part of superficialis is left in place giving a healed area over which the graft can glide. A severely scarred tendon bed or an ineffective pulley system is incompatible with a satisfactory result and should be treated by the staged operation.

5. The graft must be strong, slender and of sufficient length. It should be obtainable without risk of damage to its surface and should carry little or no paratenon. There are two tendons—plantaris and palmaris longus—which normally fulfil these requirements. Palmaris will not reach above the wrist except in the case of the thumb. If these tendons are not present or are of poor quality, an alternative is extensor digitorum longus in the foot which will provide three or possibly four grafts of ample length. Plantaris is removed through two small incisions, one on the medial side of the Achilles tendon and the other sited three finger breadths behind the medial border of the tibia in the upper calf. The border of the gastrocnemius muscle is lifted to expose plantaris lying upon the surface of soleus. Palmaris is removed in a similar manner. This technique is preferred to the use of a tendon stripper. In each case, the tendon is isolated and divided through the distal wound and drawn out through the proximal wound. The toe extensor is removed by open dissection. The graft is handled gently, is kept moist and placed in its new bed as soon as possible. The proximal junction is made by the weave fish-mouth technique (Fig. 15.8) which is secure and neat. The distal attachment is made to the profundus tag or direct to bone (Fig. 15.4).

We prefer to suture the proximal end of the graft first, using a convenient method of distal attach-

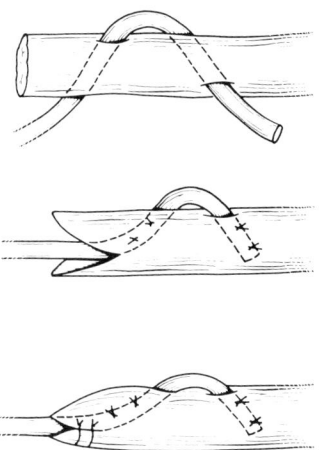

Fig. 15.8 Proximal suture by weave fish-mouth technique

ment by which the graft tension can be adjusted. The graft, which needs to be slender, is drawn through the stub of the profundus tendon and on through the finger pulp by a Reverdin needle. The graft is held by an arterial clamp (Fig. 15.9) to permit the tension to be judged before stitching it to the profundus remnant. The finger is then flexed and the graft drawn through a little further and cut short. The finger should lie, on completion of the operation, in the functional position, or slightly more flexed, in relation to the other fingers (Fig. 15.10). Damage to the graft surface, insecure attachments and incorrect length of the graft may each contribute to failure.

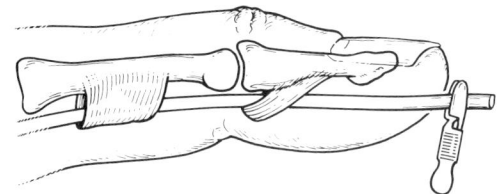

Fig. 15.9 Distal suture technique

6. The choice between superficialis and profundus to serve as motor to the graft is of significance. Superficialis is likely to have retracted further and shortened more than profundus because of the check rein effect of the lumbrical muscle on the latter, but this is not always the case. Clearly, it is logical to choose the mucle with the greater amplitude, but if there is little or no detectable difference it should be appreciated that superficialis, being an independent muscle, has the advantage of being able to adjust itself more readily to the prevailing circumstances. If the profundus is chosen, the junction being made in the proximal palm, the lumbrical muscle should be examined to ensure that it is not fibrotic, the significance of which is mentioned later.

7. The naturally hypermobile finger is in danger of locking in hyperextension if superficialis action is lacking causing a swan-neck deformity. This is more likely to happen if the distal part of superficialis is excised and is another good reason for leaving it in place. If there appears to be a likelihood that this may develop, either for the reasons given or because of damage to the volar plate (Fig. 15.11), it is wise to forestall it by tenodesing the joint in slight flexion. It is not unusual for fingers after flexor tendon grafting to develop a slight flexion contracture at this joint which serves to prevent this complication.

8. For many years there have been differing opinions regarding the relative merits of rest and early mobilisation after tendon grafting and the argument is not yet resolved. In a recent questionnaire (Strickland 1984) submitted to the members

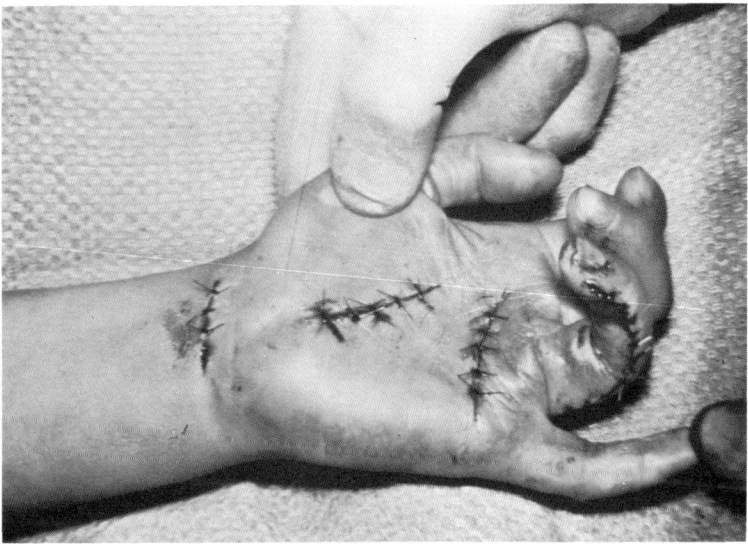

Fig. 15.10 The recommended tension of a tendon graft

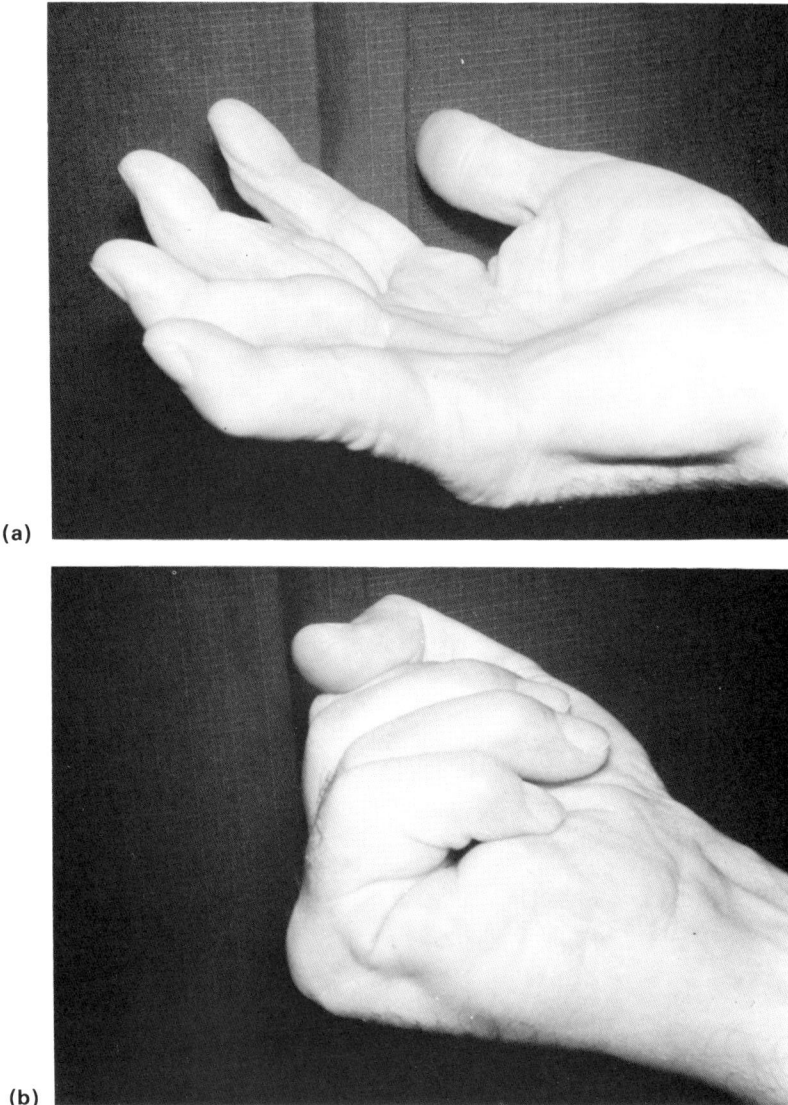

Fig. 15.11 (a) and (b) Divided both flexor tendons in zone 2 of middle, ring and little fingers. Result after tendon grafts and tenolysis. Demonstrates swan-neck deformities due to division of volar plates of proximal interphalangeal joints. Capsulorrhaphy or tenodesis was recommended but refused

of the American Society for Surgery of the Hand 37% favoured splintage for 3 weeks, 30% encouraged controlled motion within the first postoperative week, 15% within the second week and 18% during the third week. Our personal practice has been splintage for 3 weeks; RGP has held all three joints of the fingers in moderate flexion after grafting, while FDB prefers flexion of the metacarpophalangeal joint with the interphalangeal joints extended as after tendon suture. Movements are then commenced under the control of an elastic check rein strap. The skills and enthusiasm of a hand therapist are of outstanding help in the aftercare; it is beneficial to readmit to hospital some adults and most children for assisted exercises at this stage.

Special circumstances

1. Flexor profundus loss with a normal superficialis
2. Flexor pollicis longus loss
3. The Bunnell bridge graft

1. Inability to flex the distal phalanx is not a significant disability for the average labouring man, but it can cause a serious problem for one who needs perfection. A musician is a prime example. Suture is effective for an isolated profundus division if the patient is seen within a week or two after injury, or later if the division has occurred at a distal level and retraction has been prevented by intact vincula. At a late stage the choice lies between acceptance of the condition, arthrodesis or tenodesis of the distal joint, or a graft to replace profundus. The operation of tendon grafting if unsuccessful can place the existing function at risk and is justifiable only if the patient's requirements are sound and he is determined to seek perfection, the general state of the finger is good and the surgeon is experienced in this work. The operation has a special application to the little finger in those persons in whom superficialis action is poor and flexion is largely dependent upon flexor profundus.

Several techniques have been practised; passing the graft through superficialis along its anatomical course (Pulvertaft 1960, 1984), by-passing the superficialis decussation (McClinton et al 1982), and using the staged method of grafting (Honner & Meares 1977).

2. It has been our experience that grafting for flexor pollicis longus loss has a good prognosis. There is only one tendon involved and, although the normal flexion range of the interphalangeal joint is 80 to 90 degrees, a controlled range of 30 to 40 degrees restores a strong pinch and is adequate for most function. Three incisions are used; midaxial in the thumb, in the thenar crease to give access to the difficult palmar region, and proximal to the wrist. The graft extends from the distal phalanx to above the wrist and any one of the three grafts mentioned are suitable. It is convenient to use palmaris longus. Alternative techniques are elongation of flexor pollicis longus in the forearm, or transfer of a superficialis unit to act as a thumb flexor (Posner 1983). We do not regard the former to be as reliable as a free graft; the latter is an effective procedure and is clearly the method of choice when flexor pollicis longus has a poor excursion.

3. The Bunnell bridge graft (Bunnell 1944a) is a useful treatment for the late repair of tendons divided in the palm and wrist in which muscle shortening prevents end-to-end contact. A Bunnell figure of eight stitch is inserted in the proximal part of the profundus tendon and passed through a short length of graft taken usually from the injured superficialis tendon to enter the distal part of profundus in the manner shown (Fig. 15.12). Continuity is restored without the necessity of replacing the whole distal part of profundus.

Unsatisfactory results following tendon grafting

The more common complications are tendon adhesions or joint contractures, rupture of the graft or its attachments, bow-stringing of the graft, lumbical plus syndrome and swan-neck deformity.

Treatment of the unsatisfactory result

1. Adhesions. We known that intrinsic healing of tendon does occur, but the major healing process

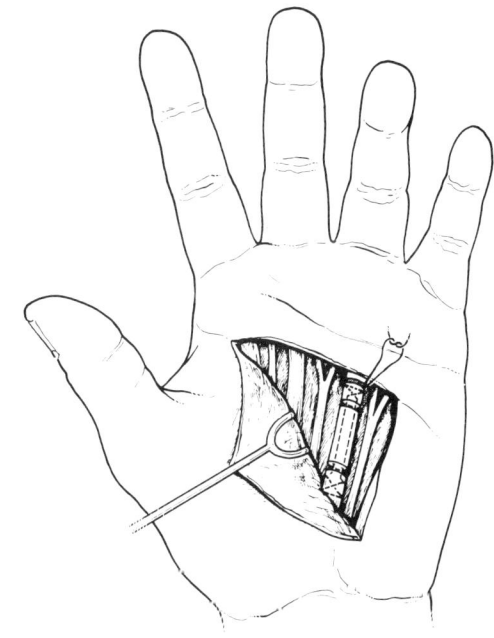

Fig. 15.12 The Bunnell bridge graft

arises from extrinsic sources. Fibroblasts grow out from the surrounding synovium or paratenon to injured tendon which in practice means the junctions and any damaged surface of a graft. There is a good reason to keep these adhesions to a minimum by careful surgery. If these bands do not resolve or stretch, the tendon will remain closely anchored to its surroundings. Peacock (1981) tells of an occasion when he had the rare opportunity to examine a finger after death in which there had been a good functioning flexor tendon graft. 'The tendon graft was surrounded by fibrous adhesions, but the graft moved over a relatively large amplitude of motion in spite of the adhesions. Careful examination revealed that the fibrous tissue connecting the tendon and surrounding bed was long enough to permit motion of the tendon'. Exercises and corrective dynamic splintage under the care of a therapist are useful until the maximum increase in active range is obtained. Progress may be slow and regular measurements are recorded. If, after 6–9 months, the active range remains obstinately less than the passive range, a tenolysis should be considered.

Tenolysis is an exacting operation and likely to be more difficult than the original procedure. Should other corrective measures such as skin or joint release, or pulley reconstruction be necessary it is better to plan for a staged tendon graft. Tenolysis requires that the graft, or tendon, is fully freed from all adhesions, interfering as little as possible with the blood supply and preserving the pulley system. The operation is not complete until it is clearly established that the finger will extend well and will flex to its full passive range when traction is applied. The use of a sedative and local anaesthesia gives the advantage of observing the gain in active range while the operation is in progress. Should the operation be prolonged, it is more acceptable to both patient and surgeon to use general anaesthesia. At one time it was considered advisable to cover the liberated graft with paratenon, but this is a misconception as it probably turns to scar and does not remain as gliding material. It is no longer used. The injection of triamcinolone (Whitaker et al 1977) at the time or of local anaesthesia during the first postoperative week (Schneider & Mackin 1984) are not within the authors' experience.

The result depends upon the extent of the operative measures required, the gentleness and the efficiency with which they are performed, the quality of the aftercare and, not least, the character of the patient. When the adhesions are localised, there is likely to be a dramatic improvement, but when a graft is bound down throughout its length the prognosis is less favourable. In some cases (Fig. 15.13) it may be wise to concentrate on the restoration of proximal interphalangeal joint control and accept a less satisfactory distal joint action. The conclusions of Fetrow (1967) are worth recalling: 'Tenolysis is a useful procedure to improve function of tendons bound down in scar tissue when the indications and technique are carefully followed. Tenolysis is unsuccessful when done in the face of poor indications, when the tendon is not freed completely, or when the tenolysis is performed in association with complex orthopaedic procedures which do not permit early postoperative active motion'.

2. Rupture of a tendon suture or of a graft is a major disaster. It is a rare occurrence and is the result of an accident or of excessive zeal on the part of the patient or the treatment staff. There is no doubt of the diagnosis because of the change in stance of the finger and the abrupt loss of active flexion, but there is some doubt as to the right action to take. In our experience of this complication it appears that the rupture usually occurs at the proximal or distal attachments and very rarely in the substance of the graft. It is tempting to advise exploration and repair of the rupture but as the danger of causing more tissue reaction exists— the summation of induration as Bunnell puts it— we advise that the tissues are rested for 6 months before a new grafting operation, possibly a staged operation, is performed.

3. Bowstringing (Fig. 15.14) is due to the lack of the essential pulleys A1 (or A2) and A4 as the result of the original injury or due to stretching of a newly constructed pulley. Occasionally, the wearing of a ring will give sufficient relief but reconstruction is usually required and is described later.

4. The 'lumbrical plus' syndrome has been described by Littler (1960) and by Parkes (1970) who pointed out that if the lumbrical muscle is scarred or its limit of stretchability is reached, any

FLEXOR TENDONS 243

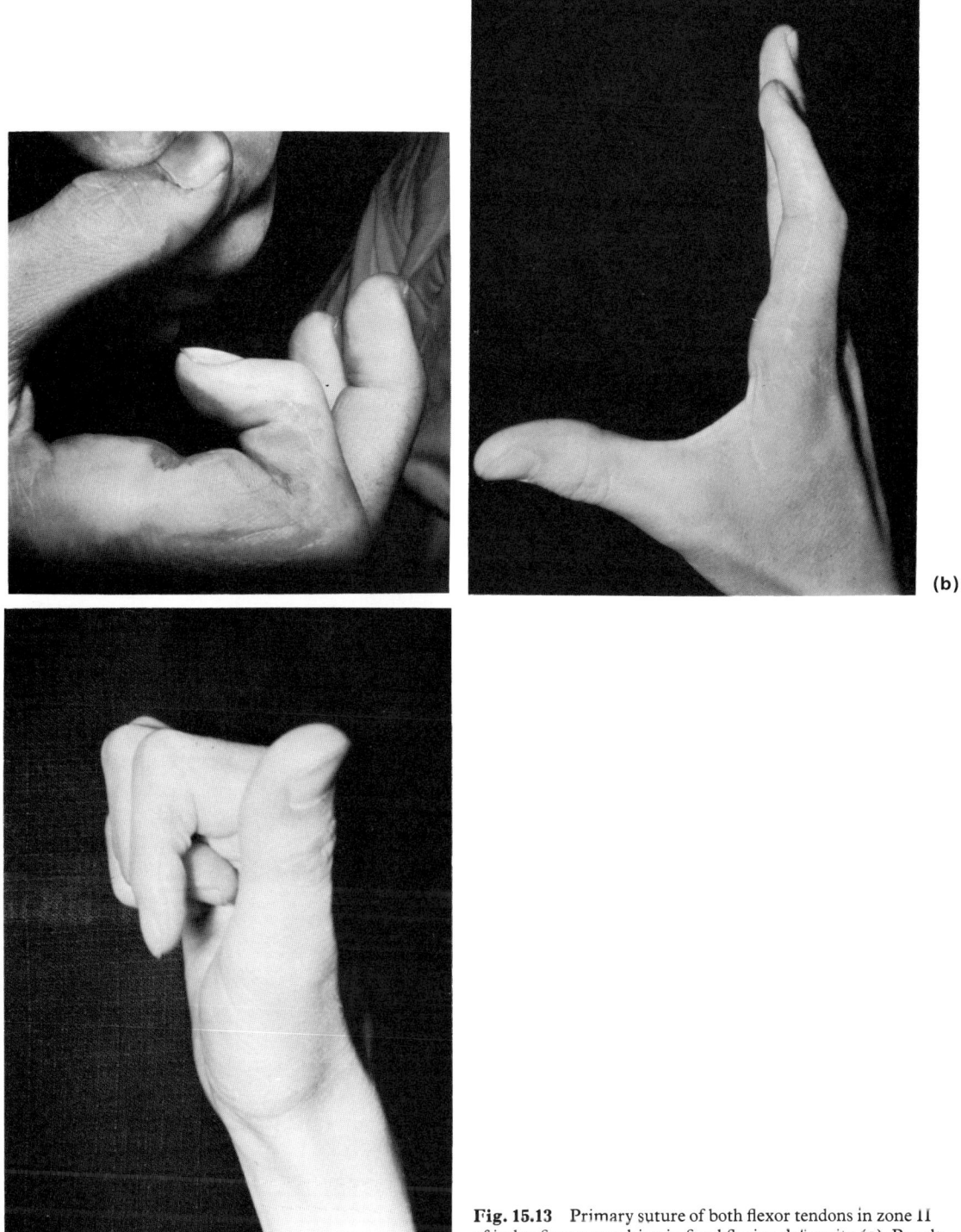

Fig. 15.13 Primary suture of both flexor tendons in zone II of index finger, resulting in fixed flexion deformity (a). Result of tenolysis (b) and (c)

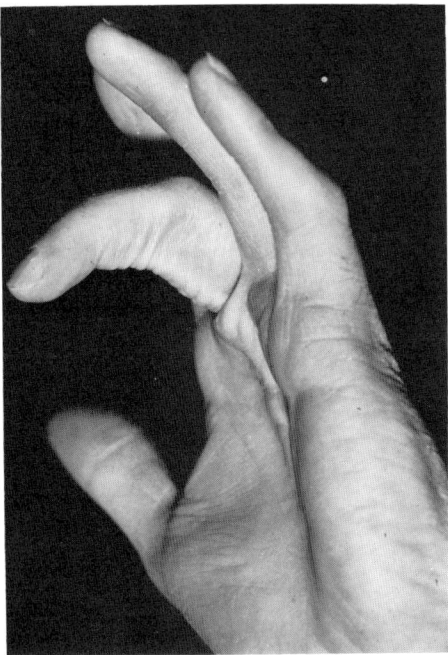

Fig. 15.14 Bowstringing of tendon graft due to defective pulleys

further proximal shift of the profundus tendon will exert traction on the lumbrical insertion and extend the interphalangeal joints. This effect may also be seen if the profundus tendon beyond the lumbrical origin has been replaced by an overlong graft. The patient finds that when attempting final flexion of the finger the interphalangeal joints extend instead of flexing. The middle finger is the one more commonly affected. It may be corrected by division of the lumbrical muscle.

5. Swan-neck deformity is a complication which may reveal itself as the finger regains motion. It may not be sufficient to require treatment, but if it is ugly or disabling it should be treated as already mentioned.

Staged tendon grafts

Single stage grafts are contraindicated when the tissue bed is inadequate or when the pulley system is extensively damaged. Although it is possible to reconstruct a pulley system around a tendon graft the postoperative management of the graft may prematurely overload the pulley. This may lead to attenuation or rupture of the pulley. It is more sensible to reconstruct the pulley system around a silicone rubber rod. The pulleys can mature without loading and a satisfactory passive joint range can be regained. The tendon graft then replaces the rod at approximately 4 months in a supple, mobile digit.

The insertion of the implant is the more extensive procedure. The finger is explored through either a mid-lateral or zigzag incision. The flexor tendons are excised preserving as much of the annular pulley system as possible. A stump of profundus is left attached to the distal phalanx. The more proximal one-third of the tendon insertion is raised from the bone to accept the distal end of the implant. Three, four or five mm rods are used, depending on the digital pulley size. Four mm is ideal for many hands. The rod is passed down the sheath and should be of such a size that it slides easily with finger motion. The distal end is bevelled and sutured firmly to the under surface of the profundus stump (Fig. 15.15). It is essential that the junction lies well distal to the volar plate of the distal interphalangeal joint. Several separate non-absorbable sutures are used. If pulley reconstruction or release of a joint contracture is required it is performed at this stage. The tendon of the chosen muscle is attached to the rod in the palm, identified proximal to the wrist, and both are then drawn through the carpal tunnel to wrist level. The implant is released from the tendon end and laid alongside the superficial flexors. The tendon of the

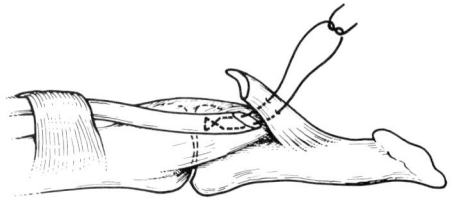

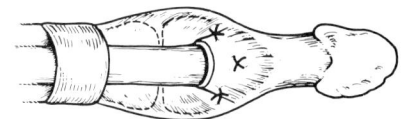

Fig. 15.15 Distal rod attachment

chosen muscle is shortened and 'parked' in an accessible position (usually sutured to flexor carpi radialis or flexor carpi ulnaris and appropriately documented in the operation note). The tourniquet is released, haemostasis obtained and the wounds closed with interrupted fine nylon sutures. The hand is rested on a splint to allow the skin to heal and passive mobilisation commenced approximately one week later.

The first stage is performed in this way to ensure that the subsequent stage involves minimal exploration. The second stage should be performed when full passive motion has been regained and the finger is supple. This is usually about 4 months later. A preoperative radiograph will indicate the position of the rod and confirm that the distal end is beyond the distal interphalangeal joint. Small incisions are made over distal phalanx and wrist and the ends of the implant identified. Exposure distally should be minimal and not extend proximal to the distal interphalangeal joint. This reduces the chances of adhesions proximal to the distal interphalangeal joint. The tendon graft is harvested, sutured to the implant at wrist level and drawn into the digit. The distal end is firmly attached to the profundus stump or to the distal phalanx ensuring that all sutures lie distal to the volar plate. Traction on the graft at the wrist will indicate whether the distal attachment is satisfactory (Fig. 15.16). The distal interphalangeal joint should flex easily through its passive range. The motor is freed from any adhesions at the wrist. The proximal end of the graft is firmly sutured to the motor using a fish-mouth weave. Tension is adjusted so that there is mild over-correction of the normal cascade posture of the affected finger. The wrist should be flexed and extended to ensure that the range of motion of the involved digit is satisfactory before the operation is completed. If the hand is rested on a splint for 4 weeks and then mobilised, a position of mid-flexion at wrist and metacarpophalangeal joints with more distal joint extension is chosen. Early passive/active motion in a similar splint may be considered if there is close supervision by a hand therapist. We have no experience of permanent artificial tendons and their role remain, as yet, unclear.

Unsatisfactory results following staged tendon grafting

The possible complications following the first of the two stages are wound infection, flap necrosis, rod detachment and synovitis in the flexor tendon sheath. Flexion contracture is uncommon although

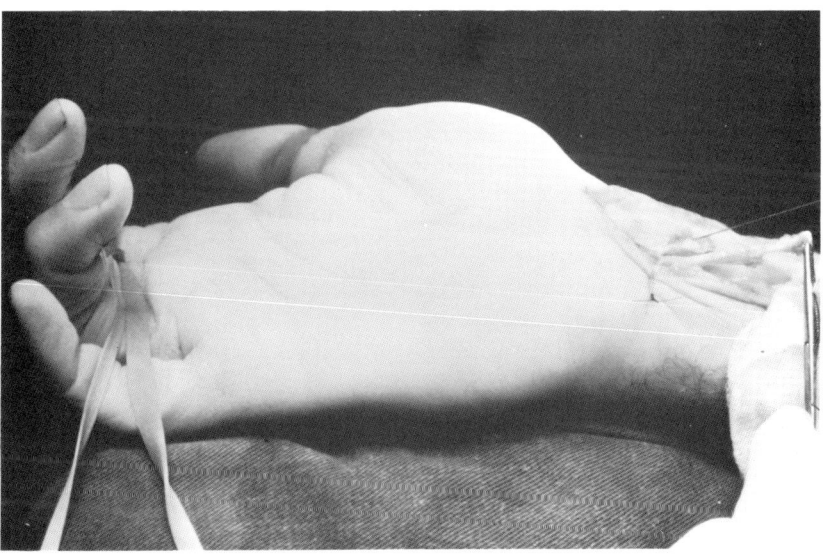

Fig. 15.16 Second stage tendon grafts to middle and ring fingers. Proximal traction on the grafts demonstrates flexion at the distal interphalangeal joints

a therapy programme is frequently required to regain full passive flexion.

Infection

Infection may arise from inadequate haemostasis with secondary infection of retained haematoma. An over-large rod will not slide proximally in flexion and may buckle at areas in the finger unsupported by pulleys, and if skin flaps in this area are thin an infection may be introduced into the finger.

Rod detachment

If the rod is inadequately attached to the distal phalanx it will migrate proximally in the sheath. Careful distal suturing with a satisfactory grasp of both rod and profundus stump should obviate the problem. An over-large rod that will not glide during passive motion is at increased risk of distal detachment. A lateral radiograph prior to the graft insertion will identify the problem. If distal detachment has occurred the involved portion of the pulley system narrows and a more extensive distal exploration is required. This increases the likelihood of adhesions and reduced mobility.

Synovitis

A minority of patients develop swelling and inflammation in the sheath during the early postoperative period (Hunter 1984). The incidence of this complication is reduced by inserting the rod using the no-touch technique which reduces the accumulation of electrostatically charged particles. The rod should move readily through the pulley system. If a sterile synovitis does develop in the early postoperative period swift progression to the second stage is advised. Continuing synovitis may result in progressive joint contracture if the normal 4-month period is allowed to pass before the tendon graft is inserted.

Complications of the second stage are tendon adhesion or rupture, infection or joint contracture. Flap necrosis should not be a problem as the incisions are small and have been previously used. Infection and contracture have been dealt with previously under complications of primary tendon repair, and graft adhesions and rupture under tendon grafts.

PULLEY RECONSTRUCTION

What constitutes an adequate pulley system? Experiments involving segmental division of pulleys indicate that the A2 and A4 are essential for full digital flexion (Doyle & Blythe 1975). If all other pulleys are excised the fingertip will still come to the distal palmar crease. However, when considering sheath reconstruction it is wise to spread the load as broadly as possible. If all the force of the flexor tendons are applied to two narrow pulleys at A2 and A4 they will tend to stretch. In practical terms every effort should be made to preserve as much of the existing system as possible and, where necessary, to supplement it with broad additional pulleys.

Techniques of reconstruction

Weilby's technique as described by Kleinert & Bennett (1978) makes use of the pulley remnants which are attached to the proximal phalanges. reconstruction is performed with the use of a thin tendon weave. A narrow curved needle with a large eye is required. A palmaris longus tendon split longitudinally is of appropriate size. If the tissues permit, the weave should extend the length of the phalanx ensuring broad support to the tendons. Bunnell (1944b) passed tendon around the phalanges to recreate a pulley. Lister (1979) described the use of extensor retinaculum passed around the phalanx and firmly sutured to itself. If tendon graft and sheath reconstruction are both required it is desirable to perform a staged tendon graft and reconstruct the pulley at the first stage.

AMPUTATION

In a severe compound injury, the tendon division is only part of the total damage and the expectation of a functioning digit may be remote. When a single finger alone is affected, amputation may be the best solution and thus avoid the embarrassment of an indifferent finger in an otherwise normal hand.

In general, our observations have been based on the asumption that we are discussing single finger injuries. Multiple digit injuries and specially those involving the thumb raise other considerations. When the flexor tendons of all fingers are divided in zone II with severe accompanying injuries, amputation is not an acceptable alternative treatment. It is better to possess four fingers without motion of the interphalangeal joints than a hand without fingers. Assuming the wound conditions are satisfactory, is it wiser for the surgeon to perform tendon suture, primary or delayed primary, in all fingers or do no more than a wound toilet with a view to grafting later? The answer must depend upon the facilities and the personal experience and ability of the surgeon.

It is important at all times to keep a sense of proportion and allow wisdom to guide our decisions. The mention of two unsatisfactory results within our knowledge may not be out of place. The first was that of a young man who attended hospital having already received primary care for multiple zone II 'tidy' tendon divisions. This had consisted of excision of all flexor tendons and their replacement by silicone rods. All fingers were healed but they were swollen, very stiff and offered little hope of improvement. It would, we believe, have been wiser to have performed primary tendon suture or, if in doubt, do no more than a wound toilet and prepare the hand for tendon grafting after a suitable delay as was done in this case (Fig. 15.17). The other, also a young man, had suffered division of the profundus tendons and digital nerves in zone 1 of the index, middle and ring fingers. He had been treated at a late stage by amputation of the distal phalanges because of lack of active flexion and diminished sensibility (Fig. 15.18). Fusion of the distal joints and the passage of time would have led to a less unsatisfactory result.

We have expressed our views upon the care of flexor tendon injuries with emphasis upon the causes of unsatisfactory results, how they can be avoided and sometimes cured. Our remarks are offered in humility for we have, in the main, drawn from our personal experience. The restoration of useful function after tendon injuries in the hand continues to present its problems. Increased knowledge of the factors influencing tendon healing and the high level of technical ability now attainable

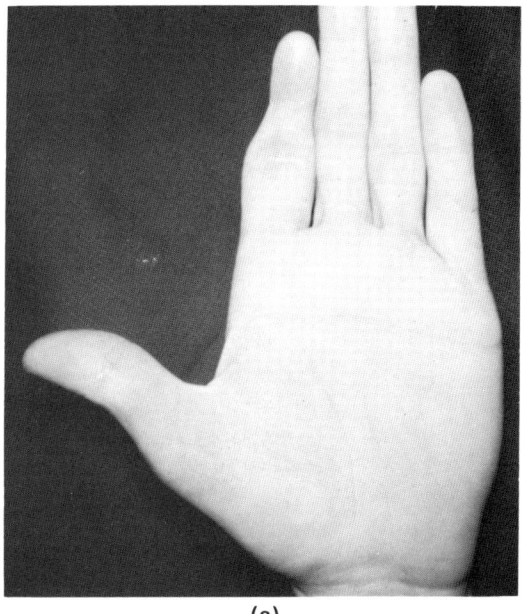

(a)

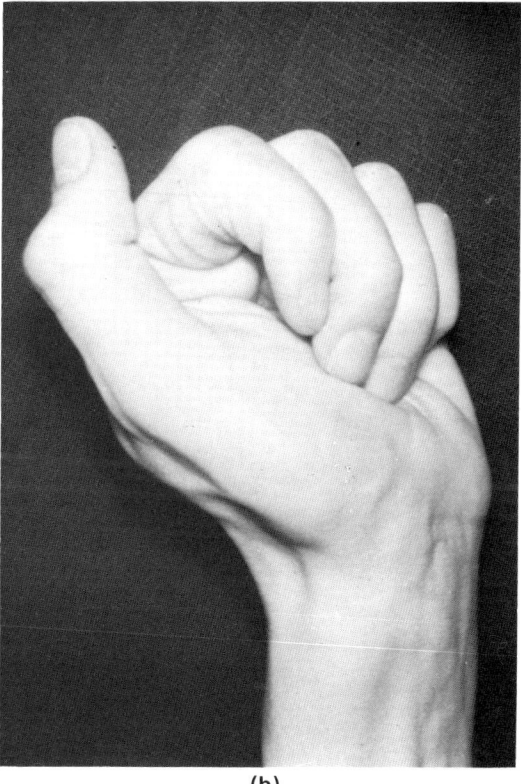

(b)

Fig. 15.17 (a) and (b) Divided both flexor tendons in zone II of all fingers. Also fracture neck of proximal phalanx of index finger. Result after tendon grafts to middle, ring and little fingers 4 months after injury and to index finger 4 months later

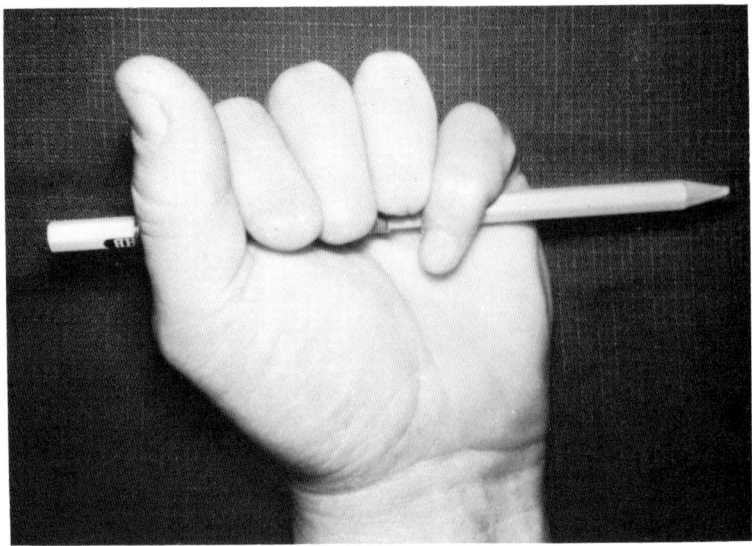

Fig. 15.18 An unusual form of treatment for profundus division (see text)

have improved the standard of results, but we do well to remember the words of Mayer (1938) 'Reconstruction of a severed tendon constitutes one of the most delicate problems in surgery—a challenge to the ingenuity and dexterity of the surgeon'.

Acknowledgements

The authors are grateful to Mr Patrick Elliott, medical artist and to Mr Barry Wilks and his staff of the Medical Illustration Department of the Derbyshire Royal Infirmary for their assistance.

The following illustrations are reproduced by courtesy of the publishers: Figs 15.7, 15.8, 15.9 and 15.12 from *Operative Surgery*, 3rd edn. The Hand, Butterworth & Co., Ltd. London; Fig. 15.10 from the *American Journal of Surgery*, 109: 350 and Fig. 15.17 from the *Journal of Bone and Joint Surgery*, 55-B: 45.

REFERENCES

Boyes J H, Stark H H 1971 Flexor-tendon grafts in the fingers and thumb. Journal of Bone and Joint Surgery 53-A: 1332–1342

Bunnell S 1918 Repair of tendons in the fingers and description of two new instruments. Surgery, Gynecology and Obstetrics 26: 103–110

Bunnell S 1922 Repair of tendons in the fingers. Surgery, Gynecology and Obstetrics 35: 88–97

Bunnell S 1944a Surgery of the hand. Lippincott, Philadelphia, ch 12, p 301

Bunnell S 1944b Surgery of the hand. Lippincott, Philadelphia, ch 12, p 315

Bunnell S 1948 Surgery of the hand, 2nd edn. Lippincott, Philadelphia, ch 12, p 626

Doyle J R, Blythe W 1975 The finger flexor sheath and pulleys: anatomy and reconstruction. A.A.O.S. Symposium on tendon surgery in the hand. Mosby, St Louis, p 81

Fetrow K O 1967 Tenolysis in the hand and wrist. Journal of Bone and Joint Surgery 49-A: 667–685

Honner R, Meares A 1977 A review of 100 flexor tendon reconstructions with prosthesis. The Hand 9: 226–231

Hunter J M 1984 Staged flexor tendon reconstruction. In: Hunter J M, Schneider L H, Mackin E J, Callahan A D (eds) Rehabilitation of the Hand, 2nd edn. Mosby, St Louis, p 288–313

Kleinert H E, Bennett J B 1978 Distal pulley reconstruction employing the always present rim of the previous pulley. Journal of Hand Surgery 3: 297–298

Lister G D, Kleinert H E, Kutz J E, Atasoy E 1977 Primary flexor tendon repair followed by immediate controlled mobilisation. Journal of Hand Surgery 2: 441–451

Lister G D 1979 Reconstruction of pulleys employing extensor retinaculum. Journal of Hand Surgery 4: 461–464

Littler J W 1960 Discussion on Extensor Habitus, White W L. Journal of Bone and Joint Surgery 42-A: 913

McClinton M A, Curtis R M, Wilgis E F S 1982 One hundred tendon grafts for isolated flexor digitorum profundus injuries. Journal of Hand Surgery 7: 224–229

Mason M L 1957 The treatment of open injuries to the hand with particular reference to tendon repair. Postgraduate Medicine 22:157–164

Mayer L 1938 Repair of severed tendons. American Journal of Surgery 42:714–722

Parkes A 1970 The 'lumbrical plus' finger. The Hand 2:164–165

Peacock E E 1981 Research in tendon healing. In: Tubiana R (ed) The Hand. Saunders, Philadelphia, vol 1, ch 52, p 516

Posner M A 1983 Flexor superficialis tendon transfers to the thumb—an alternative to the free tendon graft for treatment of chronic injuries within the digital sheath. Journal of Hand Surgery 8:876–881

Pulvertaft R G 1960 The treatment of profundus division by free tendon graft. Journal of Bone and Joint Surgery 42-A:1363–1371

Pulvertaft R G 1984 Tendon grafting for the isolated injury of flexor digitorum profundus. Bulletin of the Hospital for Joint Diseases Orthopaedic Institute 44:424–434

Pulvertaft R G (1987) Flexor tendon grafting after long delay. In: Tubiana R (ed) The Hand. Saunders, Philadelphia, vol 3

Schneider L H, Mackin E J 1984 Tenolysis: dynamic approach to surgery and therapy. In: Hunter J M, Schneider L H, Mackin E J, Callahan A D (eds) Rehabilitation of the hand, 2nd edn. Mosby, St Louis, ch 26, p 280–287

Strickland J W 1984 Flexor Tendon Surgery Panel. American Society for Surgery of the Hand. Private publication.

Verdan C 1972 Half a century of flexor-tendon surgery. Current status and changing philosophies. Journal of Bone and Joint Surgery 54-A:472–491

Whitaker J H, Strickland J W, Ellis R K 1977 The role of flexor tenolysis in the palm and digits. Journal of Hand Surgery 2:462–470

S. L. Biddulph

16 Extensor tendons

INTRODUCTION

Considering the absence of a complicated pulley system, the anatomical simplicity and the limited excursion required from the extensor mechanism, the results of extensor tendon repair should be excellent. Unfortunately this is not so. Surgical repair is only successful if performed skillfully, carefully and atraumatically. Postoperative care is as important as the procedure itself.

ANATOMY AND PATHOMECHANICS

The fact that the extensor mechanism lies on the convex aspect of the hand is responsible for its special characteristics (Fig. 16.1). These affect both structure and function. There is no tendency for the tendons to bowstring thus no complicated pulley mechanism exists in the digits. The absence of a fibrous sheath like that of the flexor tendon simplifies the anatomical structure, but this very simplicity has led surgeons to believe that no great care or skill is required in repair.

The extensor tendons tend to spread over the underlying bones, forming aponeuroses. Thus they develop adhesions to the joint capsule and the periosteum with relative ease. However, these flattened tendons heal faster because their nutrition is better.

Wrist joint level

Because of the existence of a pulley system and an associated synovial sheath, gliding is of great importance at the wrist level. The extensor retinaculum tends to hold the extensor tendons close to the radius where they may be damaged by spicules of bone, nutritional interruption or trauma. Although retinacular release results in bowstringing, it can prevent rupture in some cases.

Metacarpophalangeal joint level

Over the metacarpophalangeal joint the extensor tendon retains its individual structures but extends laterally to form the extensor hood. This helps maintain the tendon's central alignment over the dorsum of the joint.

Proximal interphalangeal joint level

At the proximal interphalangeal joint the flattened extensor tendon trifurcates after it has been joined by the tendons of the lumbricals and interossei. None of these divisions has any individual contractibility (Fig. 16.1). The central slip cannot retract after dehiscence from its insertion into the middle phalanx unless permitted by the lateral slips. Inserting as it does so close to a joint the central

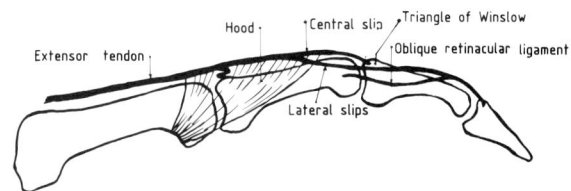

Fig. 16.1 The relevant anatomy. Salient features are the interdependancy of the central and lateral slips as far as length is concerned. Insertion of the tendon so close to the joint exposes it to great stress hence the tendency to rupture at this level

slip is subjected to great stress when forcefully flexed. The resulting tension may cause the tendon to rupture or avulse with a fragment of bone. An avulsion fragment is a useful radiological guide to the degree of elastic recoil. If the triangle of Winslow is not disrupted it maintains the dorsal alignment of the lateral slips over the proximal interphalangeal joint and contributes to healing if early effective splinting is applied.

Distal interphalangeal joint level

At the distal interphalangeal joint the lateral slips join to form a single conjoint tendon through which is transmitted the major extensor force at the joint. Here again the tendon is similarly exposed to great stress on forced flexion. It is joined on either side by the oblique retinacular ligaments which produce a certain degree of passive extension of the distal interphalangeal joint when the proximal interphalangeal joint is extended. These flimsy structures make no significant contribution to extension of the distal interphalangeal joint (Harris & Rutlege 1977).

Over the shafts of metacarpals and phalanges

The tendon lies close to the skin and the bone. It is covered by a layer of synovium which provides nutrition via blood vessels and a loose areolar tissue in which the tendon can glide. Injuries may involve both synovium and periosteum and result in adherence of skin to tendon, and tendon to bone.

COMMON REASONS FOR FAILURE OF TENDON REPAIR

1. Delay in treatment

Delay in the institution of treatment may be the fault of the patient or the doctor. Patients are often ignorant of the serious nature of the injury: it may be perceived to be a simple sprain that will heal with time. Incomplete recovery or the development of a secondary deformity such as a flexion contracture may persuade the patient to consult a doctor. Unfortunately flexion or extensor contractures are usually fixed by this stage.

The diagnosis may be missed by the doctor at the time of injury. A boutonniere deformity may take anything from a few days to some weeks to become established. As stated above the surrounding soft tissues may temporarily maintain some continuity of the tendon and alignment of the lateral slips. With time the soft tissues stretch and the typical deformity develops. At this stage simple splintage may be ineffective.

Having made the diagnosis the surgeon may not appreciate the urgency of the condition: delayed treatment may allow secondary contractures to become established.

2. Faulty immobilisation

Most closed ruptures of tendons, especially over the digit proper, will heal with simple, early and adequate splintage.

Faulty splintage promotes the development of a deformity rather than preventing it! A splint may be incorrectly applied or fail to immobilise the correct joints in the appropriate position. In an early boutonniere deformity, the metacarpophalangeal joint should be left free and the proximal interphalangeal joint splinted in a fully extended position or even in some hyperextension if it is possible. The distal interphalangeal joint may be left free or immobilised in flexion. In mallet deformity the distal interphalangeal joint should be immobilised in extension but the proximal interphalangeal joint need not be immobilised.

Excessive splinting may result in unnecessary stiffness of normal joints. A short splint which fails to keep the injured tendon in a fully relaxed position is quite ineffective as it allows the immature reparative tissues to be stretched or torn.

The most common reason for failure of splintage is removal of the splint too soon. On average a tendon heals in 3 weeks. In the hand there is an inverse relationship between the healing time and the size of the tendon. The smaller the tendon the longer it takes to heal. The small slips of the extensor tendon need approximately 6 weeks to heal and splintage should be continued for this period. Any compromise raises the failure rate.

3. Delayed wound healing

Delayed wound healing may be due to skin loss at the time of injury or it may be secondary to wound infection or sloughing. Injudicious incisions such as z-shaped incisions with acute angles may cause skin to slough with exposure of the underlying tendon.

4. Infections

Because of the excellent blood supply, sepsis is rare in hand surgery and usually follows delayed and inadequate primary wound care. Prevention is achieved by adequate debridement and prophylactic antibiotics.

5. Failure to correct established fixed contractures

Tendon repair should never be attempted unless all the joints over which the tendon acts are fully mobile. Failure to obey this rule gives poor results. Before tendon repair, joint contractures should be corrected by physiotherapy, splinting, and even surgery (Rothwell 1976, Tubiana 1968).

PROBLEMS AT THE LEVEL OF THE WRIST JOINT

The extensor retinaculum is the only pulley system along the extensor tendons. It is responsible for a set of postoperative complications similar to those seen following flexor tendon surgery.

At the wrist extensor tendon excursion is at its maximum, that is about 3 cm. When the gliding mechanism is interfered with, extension is significantly affected.

Unlike the flexor muscles, extensor muscle bellies shorten rapidly and cause excessive retraction of cut tendons. Two to three weeks after injury, it may not be possible to get the muscle out to full length for an end to end anastomosis, therefore it is important to repair these tendons early.

Closed extensor tendon rupture at this level may be due to a variety of reasons:

(i) Fractures around the wrist.
(ii) Rheumatoid arthritis.
(iii) Cortisone infiltrations.

A common lesion is rupture of extensor pollicis longus following fracture of the distal radius. Rupture may be due to vascular insufficiency because of swelling within the third compartment or to fraying of the tendon over a sharp spicule of bone projecting into the third compartment (Engkvist & Lundborg 1979). Fraying and compression will be accentuated if the third compartment is intact and this situation is more likely to be seen with fractures with minimal displacement (Helal et al 1982).

In five of my own patients with Colles' fractures, the onset of tenderness along extensor pollicis longus a few weeks after the injury raised the suspicion of tendon damage. All were explored prophylactically. In each case the tendon of extensor pollicis longus was found to be severely frayed within the compartment. A small spicule of bone was found projecting into the compartment and was apparently responsible for the damage. The fragment was removed and the tendon released from its compartment. In two cases it was necessary to reinforce the weakened tendon with a suture. Untreated these tendons would certainly have ruptured completely.

Where multiple tendons are severed each one should be repaired individually using a technique similar to that appropriate for flexor tendons. Obviously care must be taken to anastomose corresponding tendons. Should the retinaculum interfere with excursion, it should be resected until free gliding is achieved, but part of it should be preserved to prevent bowstringing (Fig. 16.2). The limb should be splinted for 3 weeks postoperatively.

In dealing with a shortened extensor pollicis longus, extra length may be obtained by rerouting the tendon directly (Fig. 16.2). If this fails, a tendon transfer using extensor indicis proprius is indicated. The transfer should be performed under a fair degree of tension so as to restore full extension of the thumb. It may take some months postoperatively before full opposition and flexion is regained.

Depriving the index finger of its extensor indicis proprius may cause the digit to lose full extension.

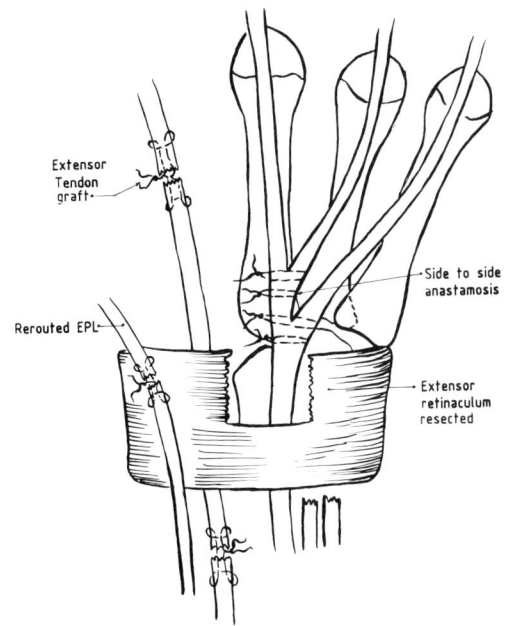

Fig. 16.2 Repair at wrist level. The extensor retinaculum should be resected in part should it impinge on the site of tendon repair. A tendon graft may be used to make up length but the results are generally disappointing. Extra length can be gained by rerouting a ruptured and shortened extensor pollicis longus

This complication can be minimised by shortening the tendon of extensor digitorum communis to take up the extensor lag.

Functional loss due to chronic lesions of single tendons of extensor digitorum communis is best restored by side to side anastomosis of the distal end of the severed tendons to an intact neighbouring tendon (Fig. 16.2). Again sufficient tension is important: the affected digit should be in 30 degrees hyperextension after the anastomosis. If all the digital extensors have been severed, extension may be restored by transferring a wrist flexor in as much tension as possible.

In a long standing lesion one might be tempted to consider a tendon graft to make up tendon deficit in single or multiple tendon lesions (Fig. 16.2). Unfortunately the procedure often fails because of the development of adhesions and because the shortened muscle belly will have lost some of its excursion. Where the muscle belly has been damaged retraction is even more of a problem and tendon transfers may have to be considered

because of the difficulty in achieving satisfactory repair of muscle tissue.

PROBLEMS AT THE METACARPOPHALANGEAL JOINT

Lesions of the extensor mechanism over the metacarpophalangeal joint are generally transverse or longitudinal. Transverse lesions usually involve the extensor tendon proper whereas longitudinal lesions are commonly seen in the dorsal hood on either side of extensor tendon.

Transverse lesions are usually the result of open injuries and may be partial or complete. As the extensor expansion is very wide, transverse lacerations are usually incomplete. Indeed the extensor tendon proper may be completely severed while full extension of the proximal phalanx is preserved by an intact extensor hood which also prevents significant tendon retraction. Under these circumstances spontaneous healing may occur. However, any subsequent sudden stress may tear the fragile fibres of the hood and result in a complete lesion with loss of extension of the proximal phalanx. The diagnosis may be missed when the hood is intact: a diagnosis may be obscured by the fact that the intrinsic muscles extend the interphalangeal joints of the digit.

Transverse lesions commonly result from fist fights: a man punches another on the mouth striking a tooth which penetrates the skin and tendon. A serious additional complication of this kind of injury is septic arthritis of the underlying metacarpophalangeal joint, a condition which must be diagnosed early and treated immediately.

Transverse lesions due to closed rupture are rare and are usually seen in patients in whom the extensor tendon has been weakened by disease.

Longitudinal lesions are generally closed and follow a forceful manoeuvre. These lesions present with pain, swelling and even bruising over the dorsum of the joint. The tear of the hood is more common on the radial side of the tendon: the normal digit lies in slight ulnar deviation, imposing greater stress on the radial side of the hood. Initially there may be no functional loss but as the remaining intact fibres stretch, the tendon tends to dislocate ulnarward with flexion of the metacarpophalangeal joint. This movement may be accompanied by a disturbing snap. Later the tendon may become permanently fixed in the ulnar valley producing ulnar deviation of the digit and even a flexion contracture should the tendon have slipped far enough towards the volar side of the joint.

Open transverse lesions are best managed by thorough debridement of the wound and repair of the cut tendon. Several interrupted sutures will suffice (Fig. 16.3).

Postoperatively the tendon must be protected by splinting the joint in full extension for not longer than 3 weeks. Longer immobilisation may result in stiffness. The proximal interphalangeal joint need not be immobilised.

Closed longitudinal lesions are best treated by splinting the metacarpophalangeal joint in extension for three weeks. Open lesions are managed like transverse lesions (Fig. 16.3).

Poor results are usually caused by inadequate immobilisation and disruption of the suture line. A second repair using the principles outlined above is usually successful.

Where the extensor tendon is dislocated, open repair of the hood is indicated. If the ulnar aspect of the hood has become contracted it must be released to allow relocation of the tendon over the mid-dorsal line of the joint and repair of the thinned radial hood.

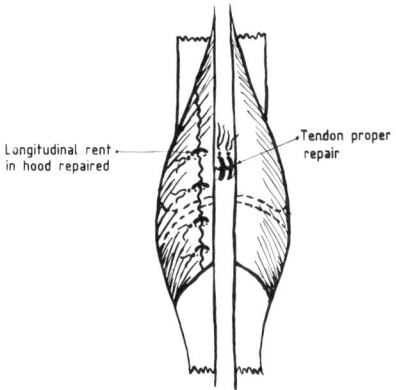

Fig. 16.3 Repair at MP joint level. Several interrupted sutures are used to repair a transverse lesion of the extensor tendon extending onto the dorsal hood if need be. Longitudinal rents are similarly repaired using interrupted sutures. In longstanding cases the contracted hood on the opposite side must be released sufficiently to allow the tendon to be realigned dorsally prior to repair

Complicated procedures such as those described by Harrison (1971) are rarely indicated and may interfere with motion of the joint.

PROBLEMS AT THE PROXIMAL INTERPHALANGEAL JOINT

The boutonniere deformity is common and is significantly disabling when fixed. The extensor tendon trifurcates over the proximal interphalangeal joint: one or more of the three slips may be severed.

As stated above unless all three divisions are severed, the proximal end of the tendon is unable to retract to any significant extent. Closed rupture generally involves only the central slip and may accompany volar dislocation of the proximal interphalangeal joint. However other soft tissue elements such as Winslow's triangle are frequently intact and strong enough to aid the elastic recoil of the lateral slips to their normal position dorsal to the joint, temporarily maintaining a near normal range of extension.

On the other hand, with open laceration particularly if the tendon lesion is complete, the loss of extension and development of the deformity is immediate.

Both closed ruptures of the central slip and undisplaced avulsion fractures respond well to adequate external or internal splintage. External splintage, although simple, has the disadvantage of being interrupted by the patient. The splint is exposed to use, moisture and sweating. Patients tend to remove the splint for toilet activities. If the patient fails to understand the importance of avoiding any flexion when the splint is removed, he may tear freshly formed reparative tissue and interfere with healing. Because of the disadvantages of external splintage, it is preferable to use internal fixation, using a Kirschner wire introduced percutaneously. This permits the patient full use of the digit while ensuring adequate immobilisation. As the central slip is slender, the period of immobilisation should be 6 weeks. There is no need for the metacarpophalangeal or distal interphalangeal joints to be splinted as well. Simple splinting can be tried at any stage up to 6 weeks following the injury but the patient should be warned that the success rate is lessened by delay.

In cases with minimal deformity a tenotomy of the lateral slips at the distal interphalangeal joint, proximal to the junction with the oblique retinacular ligaments may give sufficient retraction of the extensor mechanism to correct the deformity (Fowler 1949).

Significant proximal retraction of the central slip occurs only when associated with gross volar migration of the lateral slips and hyperextension of the distal interphalangeal joint. In these cases and with displacement of an avulsion fragment of more than 2 mm, open reduction and re-insertion of the tendon is indicated.

In longstanding cases any flexion deformity at the proximal interphalangeal joint and/or hyperextension at the distal interphalangeal joint should be corrected prior to re-insertion of the central slip. This can be achieved by physiotherapy, splinting or surgery. Care should be taken not to excise too much scarred tendon as this, together with further umbrication caused by the suture material, may produce so much shortening that the tendon can no longer reach the middle phalanx.

Surgery consists of re-insertion of the central slip (Fig. 16.4) relocation of the volarly displaced lateral slips and narrowing of the triangle of Winslow. Postoperatively the joint should be splinted with a Kirschner wire for a minimum of 6 weeks (Fig. 16.4).

Treatment of those cases in which initial surgery has failed is similar to that of the established case. If the joints are mobile and postoperative care is adequate, tendon grafting or one of the more complicated tendon repairs is rarely necessary.

The presence of a very short central slip together with fibrosis of the lateral slips may prevent subsequent full extension. In such cases a tendon substitution procedure is indicated (Matev 1964).

PROBLEMS AT THE DISTAL INTERPHALANGEAL JOINT

Both traction and incisional injuries cause loss of active extension with a resulting mallet finger. In traction injuries the lesion is generally distal to the confluence of the oblique retinacular ligament and the lateral slips, and either involves the tendon

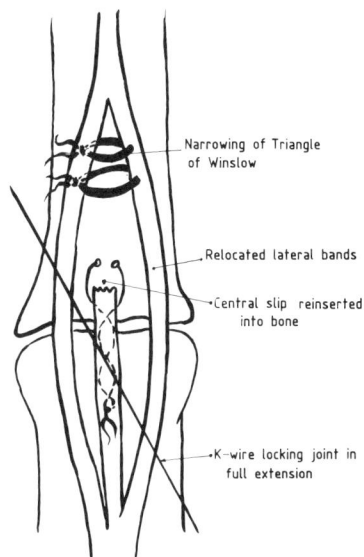

Fig. 16.4 Repair at PIP joint level. Repair of the established boutonniere deformity consists of (a) Release of any established joint contracture. (b) Re-insertion of the central slip into bone. (c) Relocation of the lateral slips dorsally and narrowing of the triangle of Winslow. (d) Splinting of the joint in full extension using a Kirschner wire for 6 weeks

proper, or is associated with an avulsion fracture. The fracture may be small involving only the dorsal edge of the base of the distal phalanx or it may be quite large extending through half of the base of the distal phalanx. It may or may not be displaced. Whatever the type of tendinous interruption, the degree of immediate loss of extension depends on the completeness of the lesion and the extent of soft tissue injury.

The conjoint tendon is reinforced by lateral reflections which, if intact, may maintain extension to some degree. In avulsion fractures these soft tissues and the periosteum may prevent displacement of the fragment. (Should they be torn, extension will be lost and an imbalance in favour of flexion will result.) With disruption of the tendon maximum extensor force is centred on the proximal interphalangeal joint and if the joint is lax, swan-necking may occur. Under these circumstances greater shortening of the disrupted tendon is possible.

The correct management of the mallet finger deformity is immediate and adequate splintage for 6 weeks. Splinting may be either external or internal using a Kirschner wire for reasons outlined above. Although immediate splinting is ideal it can be instituted at any stage up to 6 weeks after injury with a reasonable chance of success.

Small undisplaced avulsion fractures may be treated in the same way. If the fragment is displaced or involves a significant portion of the articular surface, open reduction and internal fixation is indicated (Tubiana 1968).

Larger fragments may result in both loss of extension and volar subluxation of the distal phalanx. After reduction the distal interphalangeal joint should be immobilised in full extension for 6 weeks. Following closed rupture immobilisation of the joint in hyperextension should be avoided because of the risk of ischaemia of the skin over the immediate dorsal aspect of the joint and consequent sloughing of skin and exposure of the underlying tendon.

Arthrodesis of an established mallet finger is no longer widely used. Loss of movement in the joint may constitute a severe disability in many patients and an attempt should be made to restore active extension. As explained above, the lateral slips do not retract individually to any extent. Thus, except for the rare cases in which actual traumatic loss of tendon tissue has occurred, there is generally no need for tendon graft.

My preferred method of treatment is as follows:

Through a dorsal Y-shaped incision, the tendon is exposed and re-inserted into the base of the distal phalanx. As with repair of the boutonniere, excessive shortening of the tendon should be avoided (Fig. 16.5).

The tendon is best anchored by means of a pull out suture and the joint locked in full extension for 6 weeks (Fig. 16.6). To produce a dermodesis, in addition a transverse elipse of skin is excised over the dorsum of the joint.

Small fragments may be excised and the tendon re-inserted as described above, footing being into the defect left by the fragment (Fig. 16.6). In cases where the joint has been severely damaged, arthrodesis is best.

PROBLEMS OVER BONY SHAFTS

Where tendons lie in close proximity to bone, both tissues may be injured simultaneously. Further-

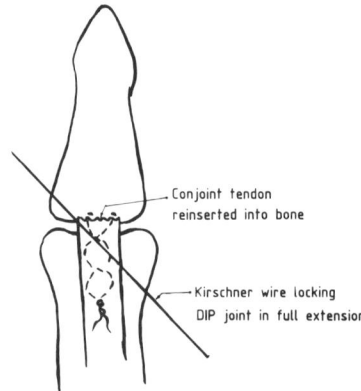

Fig. 16.5 Repair at DIP joint level. Repair of the established mallet finger deformity consists of: (a) Release of established joint contracture prior to repair. (b) Shortening of the lengthened conjoint tendon. If no proper grip can be achieved distally, a pull-out suture should be used. (c) The joint should be splinted for 6 weeks using a Kirschner wire introduced either longitudinally or crosswise. (d) An elliptical piece of skin is resected dorsally to produce an element of dermodesis. This will further help to prevent a recurrence

more tendon damage may be aggravated or even caused by the bony injury. A serious complication of this kind of injury is tendon adherence. Once the protective qualities of the synovial covering of the tendon and the periosteum have been interrupted, dense cross adhesions may develop. They are not easily broken down by physiotherapy or use. Tendon adherence results in loss of tendon excursion and presents as a loss of extension or flexion. The patient may be unable to make a fist, or a deformity resembling a mallet or boutonniere deformity may be seen.

Management

To minimise the adhesions resulting from this type of injury, one should aim for early repair and early

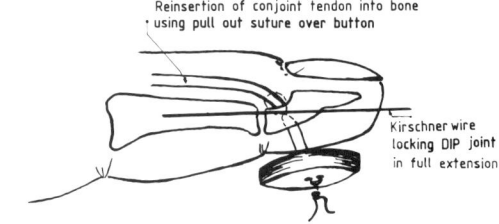

Fig. 16.6 With avulsion fragments it is better to resect the fragment and re-insert the tendon into bone. Footing should be into the defect left by the fragment and held in position by a pull-out suture over a button

gentle mobilisation. When there is an associated boutonniere or mallet deformity or some other contraindication to early mobilisation, it is prudent to await tendon healing and to accept incomplete mobility and the need for later tenolysis.

All unstable fractures should be stabilised by internal fixation so as to facilitate early mobilisation of the tendon. I prefer Kirschner wires which are easy to introduce, need little or no periosteal or soft tissue stripping, and are simple to remove. Clearly one should aim to achieve early adequate skin cover: this permits better mobilisation and enhances the quality of tendon healing.

Improvement in mobility will continue for many months as long as the scar tissues have not matured. Thus surgical mobilisation such as tenolysis should be delayed for at least 6 months. A tenolysis may be followed by a recurrence of adhesions or tendon rupture: adhesions may be prevented by the interposition of a sheet of silicone rubber between tendon and bone. The tendon must be mobilised early. Prophylactic antibiotics are advisable.

LESIONS ASSOCIATED WITH SKIN LOSS

Because of the paucity of subcutaneous soft tissue a blow or crushing injury to the dorsum of the hand damages the skin and tendons against the underlying bone. Skin may be lost and the tendons may be exposed, stripped of synovium, abraded, severed and even lost. Exposure of tendon results in rapid dessication which may lead to dense fibrosis and even tendon necrosis.

In the management of these injuries it is important to achieve immediate skin cover because airtight or vaseline gauze dressings may not prevent tendon necrosis. The tendon should be repaired immediately by simple end to end anastomosis, primary tendon transfer or grafting. Tendons with an intact synovial lining will support a split skin graft and function adequately afterwards. If synovium has been lost vascularity is poor and the tendon will no longer support a split skin graft: full thickness skin cover is therefore essential to prevent dessication and to assist revascularisation and healing. This may be achieved by local rotation flaps or an inguinal flap (MacGregor 1972). Inguinal flaps should not be taken too far laterally as they are bulky and unsightly and require later defatting. Flaps taken from the region of the anterior superior iliac spine or the inguinal area are generally satisfactory and cosmetically acceptable, particularly if the defect to be covered is of moderate size. The skin is thin and pliable and permits a fair degree of mobilisation.

Tenolysis of extensor tendons may necessarily be extensive. The procedure is extremely difficult if skin cover is poor. Areas with split skin cover may slough exposing the freshly mobilised tendon, thus compromising the result.

Where the dorsum of the hand has been covered by a good split skin graft without restoration of tendon continuity, it may be possible to perform a tendon graft using a two-stage technique such as described by Hunter (1977). This avoids the need to replace the split skin graft by a full thickness flap.

The use of silicone sheeting to prevent adherence to phalanges and metacarpals should only be used if the skin cover is adequate. Skin breakdown leads to secondary infection and even tendon loss.

Healing by secondary intention and gradual epithelialisation should be avoided as it results in dense adhesions. The ideal management of the composite lesion is as follows:

A thorough wound toilet and debridement of devascularised tissue is performed, followed by internal fixation of associated bone and joint injuries. Tendons are repaired by direct suture, transfers or grafting. Skin cover is achieved by primary suture, skin graft or composite flap. Prophylactic antibiotics are advised.

REFERENCES

Engkvist O, Lundborg G 1979 Rupture of the extensor pollicis longus tendon after fracture of the lower end of the radius—a clinical and microangiographic study. The Hand II: 76–86

Fowler S B 1949 Extensor apparatus of the digits. Journal of Bone and Joint Surgery 31B: 477

Harris C, Rutledge G L 1972 The functional anatomy of the

extensor mechanism of the finger. The Journal of Bone and Joint Surgery 54A: 713–726

Harrison Stewart H 1971 Reconstructive arthroplasty of the metacarpo-phalangeal joint using the extensor loop operation. British Journal of Plastic Surgery 24: 307–309

Helal B, Chen J C, Igweby G 1982 Rupture of the extensor pollicis longus tendon in the undisplaced Colles' type of fracture. The Hand 14: 41–47

Hunter J M, Jaeger S H 1977 Tendon implants primary and secondary usage. Orthopaedic Clinics of North America 8: 473–489

MacGregor I A 1972 The groin flap. British Journal of Plastic Surgery 25: 3–16

Matev I 1964 Transposition of the lateral slips of the aponeurosis in the treatment of long standing Boutonniere deformity of the fingers. British Journal of Plastic Surgery 17: 281–286

Rothwell A G 1976 The repair of established boutonniere and mallet finger deformities. Journal of Bone and Joint Surgery 58B: 384

Stack H G 1969 Mallet finger. The Hand I: 83–89

Tubiana R 1968 Surgical repair of the extensor apparatus of the fingers. Surgical Clinics of North America 48: 1015–1031

Zancolli E A 1979 Structural and Dynamic Bases of Hand Surgery, 2nd edn. J B Lippincott Company, Philadelphia, p 3–104

D. C. Riordan

17 Tendon transfers

There are many different types of complications in the surgery of tendon transfers, and one commonly thinks of postoperative infections. This is a serious complication but will not be discussed here. This discussion will center on the various factors that must be considered in performing tendon transfer. A great many different factors influence the result of such tendon surgery.

The hand surgeon planning tendon transfers should know what factors influence the results of such surgery before carrying out the surgery. There must first be an evaluation of the individual, his personality, the type of soft tissues, the amount of development of the normal muscles of the extremities, the presence or absence of scar, and the sensibility of the part or parts involved. An evaluation of the muscles paralysed or the muscle function missing from trauma must be determined in order to know what types of function must be restored.

PATIENT EVALUATION

An evaluation of the individual can be determined in a limited way by the interview, history taking and examination of the patient during the first examination. If there are some doubts, a second examination of the patient could be arranged for, or further information could be obtained from those who may have previously treated the patient. The cooperation of the patient during the examination is frequently an excellent clue. If the patient should try to feign weakness, stiffness or contractures, one can usually determine this during the examination.

TISSUE STATUS

It is extremely important to determine the pliability of the soft tissues in the involved extremity prior to performing any type of tendon transfers (Fig. 17.1(a) and (b)). This can be done by palpating

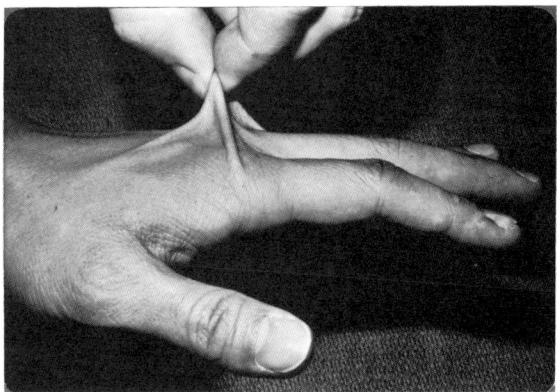

(a)

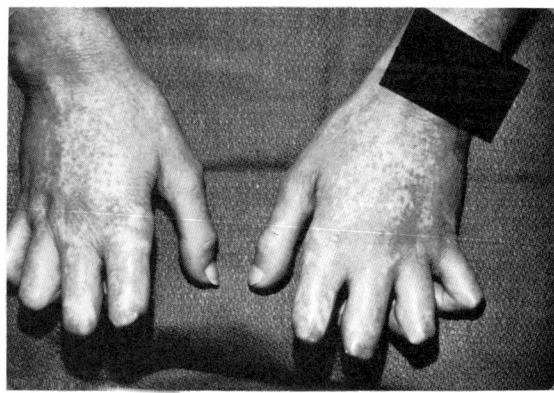

(b)
Fig. 17.1 (a) Normal pliability of skin and subcutaneous tissues is best illustrated on the dorsum of the hand and fingers. (b) Taut skin and hard subcutaneous tissues as seen in scleroderma. Skin is so tight it may be shiny.

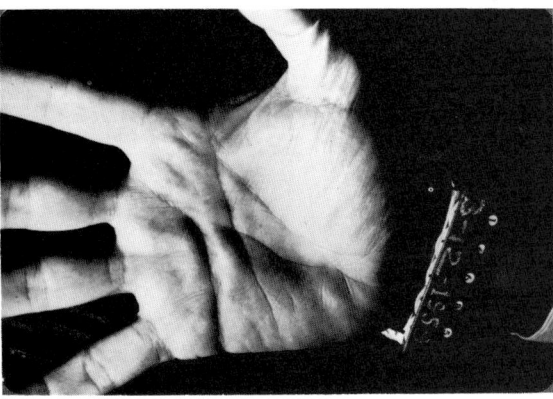 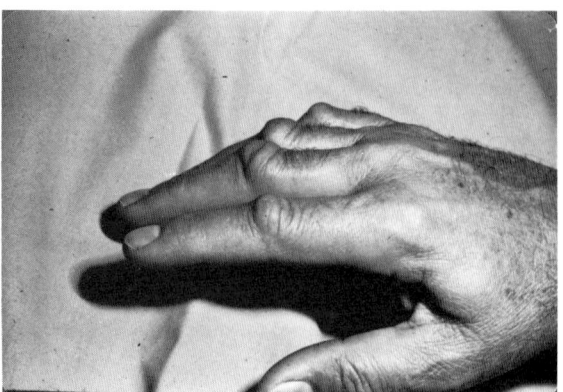

Fig. 17.2 (a) Slight thickening of the palmar fascia and early nodule formation as seen in Dupuytren's disease. (b) Hard nodules seen and felt on the dorsal aspect of the middle joints of the fingers usually indicate an increased possibility for stiffness after surgery and immobilisation.

the soft tissues of the upper extremity (Fig. 17.2(a) and (b)) for any signs of scleroderma, by palapating the palmar aspect of the hands and the skin over the dorsum of the middle joints of the fingers looking for nodules or thickened bands of palmar fascia from Dupuytren's disease. If there is a thickening on the involved and the uninvolved hand, one should know that the patient may be more likely to have postoperative stiffness following surgery than someone without the Dupuytren's tendency. It may also help to look at other scars the patient may have had from previous surgery or systemic disease. If there are scars on the involved extremity, these should be carefully inspected (Fig. 17.3 (a)–(c)). The examiner should also inspect the nails for any abnormalities or scars around the nails that may suggest circulatory problems such as Raynaud's disease, or grooves in the nails which may indicate some serious illness (Fig. 17.4). The examiner should have a general idea of whether or not tendon transfers are going to be necessary and what route they would take, and if that route would be likely to go through any of the scar present on the involved extremity (Fig. 17.5(a)–(d)).

SKELETAL INTEGRITY

The integrity of the skeleton must be considered first. Are there any fractures in the area being considered for the transfers, and if so, are they healed? Are the joints stable and in good alignment are the joints mobile enough to consider doing tendon transfers and if the transfer has to go through the interosseous membrane is it clear and free of scar or bone? Is the hand mobile enough to go through the postoperative immobilisation without resulting in considerable stiffness?

MUSCLE EVALUATION

After these factors have been determined, a muscle evaluation must be done. The normal or uninvolved extremity should be examined first for comparison. A list of the functioning muscles from proximal to distal should be made, and their relative strength recorded (Fig. 17.6). The same evaluation, in the same order, is then done on the involved extremity. Of those muscles that are functioning, some can be borrowed for the transfer and others cannot. Some must be left in the original position to perform necessary functions that are needed to stabilise or move the parts of the extremity. The ones that can be borrowed are noted in Figure 17.6. It is not usually possible to restore each individual muscle function that is missing. For example, in the loss of the finger extensors, a single muscle may be called upon to power all four of the finger extensors. It must be determined which muscle functions have to be restored and which can be overlooked or substituted for.

On the list mentioned above, one can decide which muscles can be moved to perform a new

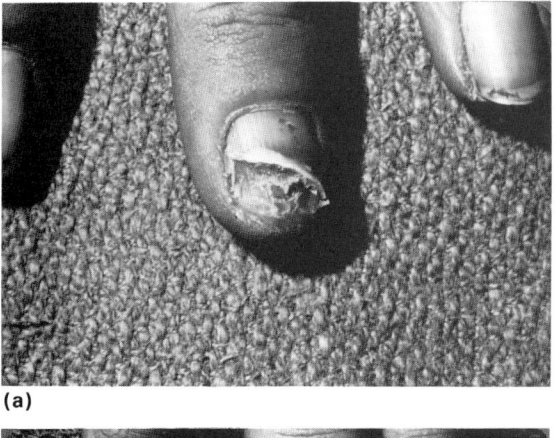
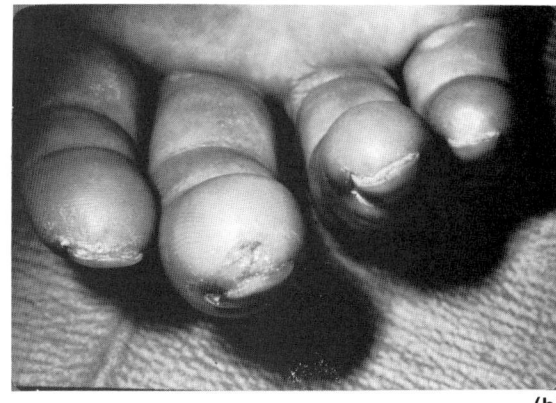
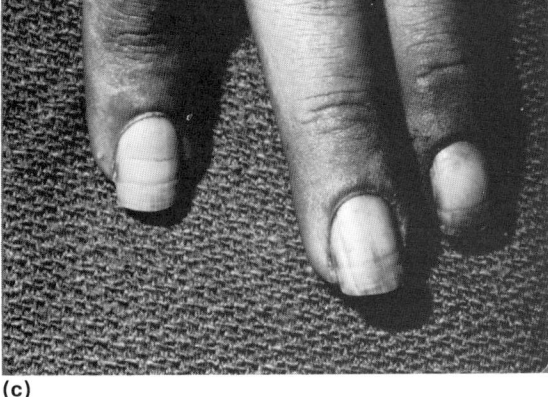

Fig. 17.3 (a) Nail deformity resulting from small necrotic avascular areas as seen in Raynaud's disease. (b) Healed scar at the tip of the finger typical of healed ulcer of Raynaud's disease and an indication for caution in performing any type of surgery. (c) Transverse grooves seen in all nails at same level is an indication of some serious illness (in this case, severe hepatitis).

function and a line is drawn from the donor to the recipient muscle or muscles (if multiple). Thus one has a 'picture' of the transfer or transfers that can be performed in order to restore some of the missing function. During this examination of the muscles on the involved extremity, the examiner should determine if the damage has been to the muscle bellies or to their tendons or to the nerve supply. In some cases a proximal muscle belly may be present and functioning. If so, the muscle belly will have a limited range of excursion and should not be used in the transfer as its excursion will be inadequate or it will check rein and limit another tendon if added on to another transferred muscle to 'reinforce it'.

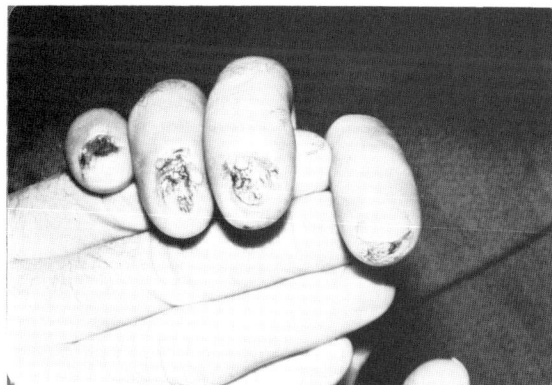

Fig. 17.4 Nail bed infections in an anaesthetic hand of a median and ulnar nerve laceration and excessive nail biting in an unstable personality. This resulted in osteomyelitis of the distal phalanges which had to be treated before the nerves could be repaired.

SENSIBILITY

The sensibility of the normal and the involved extremity must be carefully evaluated. It is important to realise that nerves should have been repaired before any type of tendon transfer is performed. The only exception to this are those cases needing tendon transfers who have Hansen's

262 UNSATISFACTORY RESULTS IN HAND SURGERY

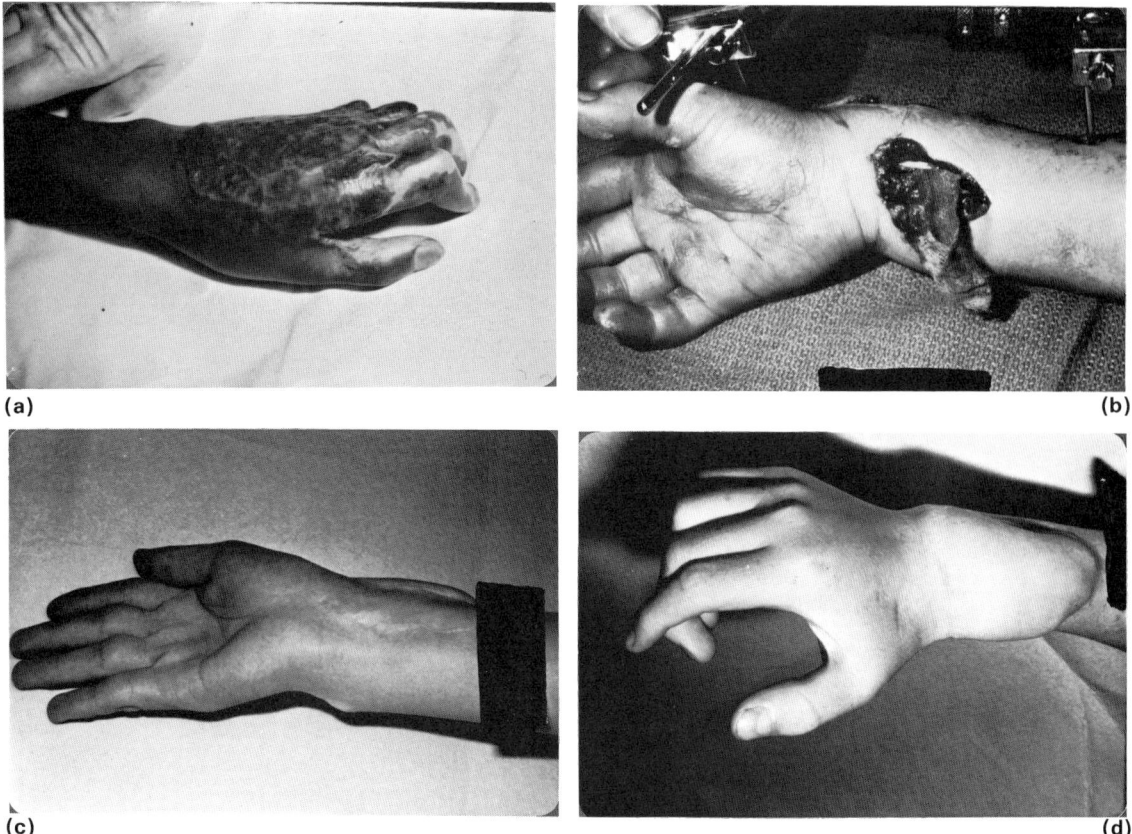

Fig. 17.5 (a) Burn scars over stiff joints must be covered with better skin and subcutaneous tissues before joint releases and tendon transfers can be done. (b) Shot gun injury through skin, tendons, bone and nerve (Same case as (a)). (c) Same case, local sliding flap used to cover volar skin defect. (d) Same case, abdominal flap used to cover large defect on dorsal side of hand and wrist prior to bone, tendon or nerve repair.

disease, syringomyelia, or rarely some cases of Charcot–Marie–Tooth disease. If there is deficient sensation one should determine the cause. If trauma to the nerves has occurred, one should determine if an adequate nerve repair was carried out and how long ago. If the nerves have been adequately repaired and the reaction from that repair has quieted down, one may proceed with the tendon transfers while waiting for the sensation to improve. The patient can be taught to substitute eye sight for the absent sensation and make muscles work even though the distal parts may not have complete sensibility.

The techniques of nerve repair will not be discussed here. If a nerve to a muscle or group of muscles can or has been repaired, there is a good chance that some motor function may recover. If it does recover function, it will not be as strong as it was before the injury nor will it be under independent voluntary control as it was before the injury. It will usually function as a mass action muscle since the same nerve fibres do not go to the same muscle bundle and the independent control is missing or unlearned in adults. In addition, the range of excursion will be less than a normal muscle, probably due to the prolonged time from repair to recovery which allows for shortening of the nonfunctioning muscle fibres.

MUSCLE REQUIREMENTS

The surgeon examining the extremities for the functioning muscles should have a knowledge of

TENDON TRANSFERS 263

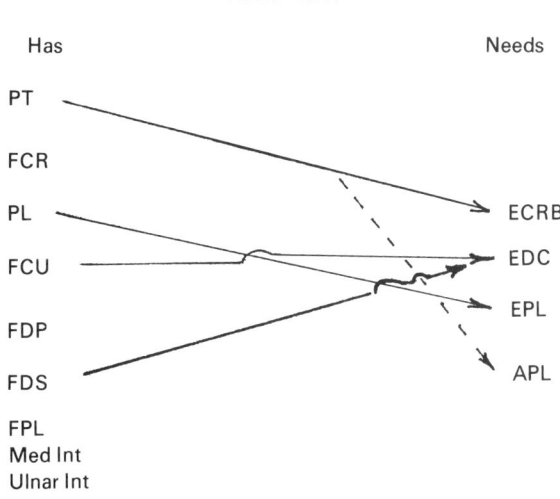

Fig. 17.6 Muscle evaluation chart

the relative power of the paralysed muscles (when they were normal), and of the relative power needed in their new position when they are transferred. The ranges of excursion in the normal position, as well as the range of excursion expected of them in their new position must be known and evaluated. (Fig. 17.7(a) and (b)). A muscle with an excursion of 1.5 cm will not produce the desired range of motion for a muscle tendon unit that normally moves 2.5 cm. If the involvement is unilateral, the normal can be used to compare the involved extremity with, but if there is bilateral involvement, then each must be judged on its own merits.

JOINT MOBILITY

When evaluating the joint mobility, the amount of contracture as well as the type of contracture must be determined. If a contracture is present but it

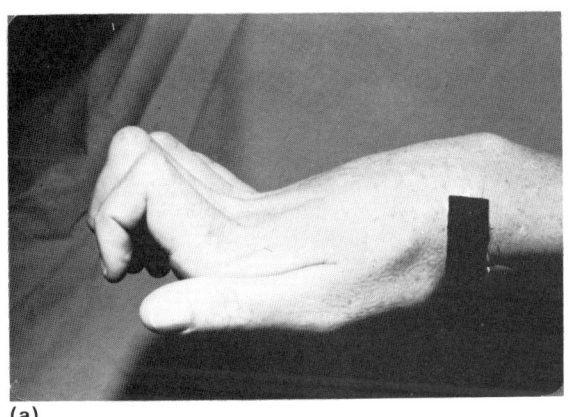

(a)

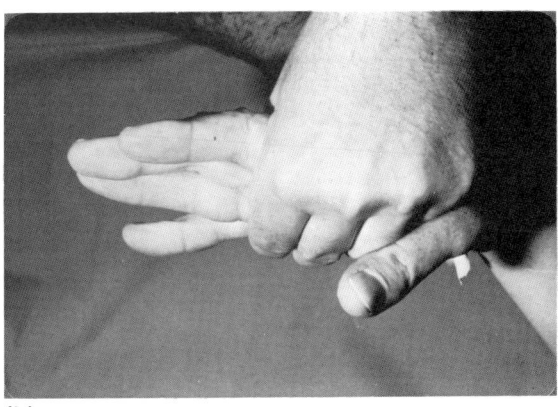

(b)

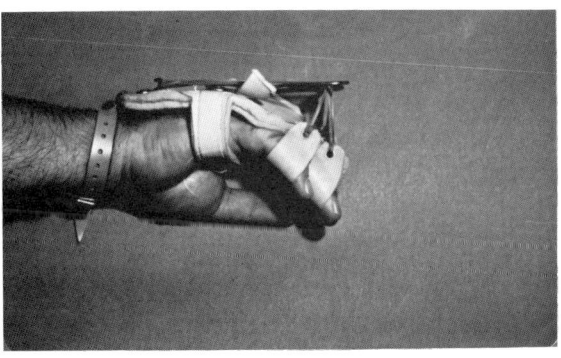

(c)

Fig. 17.7 (a) Median and ulnar nerve paralysis attempting to extend fingers, showing inability to extend middle and distal phalanges without intrinsic muscle function on fingers and thumb. (b) Test for extensor tendon mobility by blocking hyperextension of proximal phalanges shows that the extensor mechanism is still sliding and capable of extending the middle and distal phalanges. This function must be present before attempting a tendon transfer to restore intrinsic function. (c) When the test shown in (b) shows that the extensor mechanism cannot extend the fingers because of joint contractures, then traction splints must be used to overcome the joint contractures before the surgery is performed.

264 UNSATISFACTORY RESULTS IN HAND SURGERY

can be slowly stretched out, it can be overcome by splinting or traction or a combination of both. (Fig. 17.7(c)) Some contractures, however, are so rigid that they defy correction except by surgical release of the joint. These contractures must be corrected before the tendon transfers are attempted. In some cases a differentiation between joint contracture and contracture caused by shortened or fibrotic muscles, or those caused by adhesion of the tendons must be differentiated and corrected before tendon transfers can be considered. A period of time for recovery of the tissues after joint release must be given and this can be aided by appropriate physical therapy until tissue recovery has occurred.

ROUTE OF THE TRANSFER

The route of the tendon transfer must then be considered. A straight line is the preferred route for a transfer (Fig. 17.8(a)). This results in the least amount of loss of power of a transferred muscle tendon unit. A muscle tendon unit in its normal unscarred bed probably has a slight loss of power from the 'friction' of the gliding tendon surrounded by its paratenon and lubricated by the synovial fluid, but this is probably not measurable. When a tendon is transferred to a new bed, it becomes surrounded by scar and is attached to scar throughout its length. This will result in loss of excursion and power as well. It is necessary for the surgeon to be as 'atraumatic' as possible in using tendon tunnelers for passing the tendon through the tissues and to avoid scar or non-yielding septa or interosseous membranes if possible. Physical therapy and patient education after the immobilisation is discontinued will usually result in a satisfactory range of motion for the transfer.

A straight line for the route of the transfer is not always possible. In some cases, a pulley is needed to change the angle of the approach of a tendon, as in an opponens transfer from the volar side. In some transfers, the route of the tendon will have to be around the radial or ulnar border of the forearm. (Fig. 17.8(b) and (c)) This means that a septum or septa may have to be penetrated by the transfer. Sometimes the scarring on the border of the forearm may be so severe that this route cannot be used and the interosseous membrane route may be necessary (Fig. 17.8(d) and (e)). In all three of these examples, a pulley, the border of the forearm and the interosseous membrane, there will be a lesser loss of motion or power if the paratenon can be preserved and transferred with the tendon so it will line the pulley, the border of the forearm or the interosseous membrane area. Thus the adhesions will stick to the paratenon and allow the tendon to glide more freely inside the sheath and allow a greater range of motion and less loss of power. Great care must be taken to preserve this paratenon around the tendon and to transfer it intact on the tendon being transferred. In going around the border of the forearm, care must be taken to not disturb or elevate the periosteum or this will add to the amount of adhesions to an immovable structure. Care must also be taken in transferring through the interosseous membrane to cut a wide opening in the structure to allow the muscle belly or bellies to pass through the structure (Fig. 17.9(a) and (b)) so that the adhesions will be to the muscle belly and not to the tendon itself. Although there will be some restriction by adhesions to the muscle belly, they will not be nearly so restrictive as if they were adherent to the tendon itself. In making the wide opening in the interosseous membrane in the forearm, care must be taken not to damage the interosseous vessels and the anterior interosseous branch of the median nerve. When the transfer has to go around the borders of the forearm it is sometimes possible to use the dorsal or volar fascia of the muscles to turn down as a flap and cover the bone with a smooth slippery lining as demonstrated by the work of Bielsalski & Mayer (Bielsalski & Mayer 1916, Mayer 1916) on tendon sheaths and their blood supply. Care must be taken to observe all these factors mentioned.

Figure 17.10(a) shows a method of constructing a fixed pulley when restoring opposition of the thumb using a sublimis tendon when the normal adductor pollicis is present (Riordan 1953). The tendon transfer must also be maintained at the axis of motion on the radial side of the abductor pollicis brevis. Its insertion should be into the extensor pollicis longus tendon to assist in simultaneous extension of the distal phalanx of the thumb as the normal abductor pollicis brevis does. Examples of

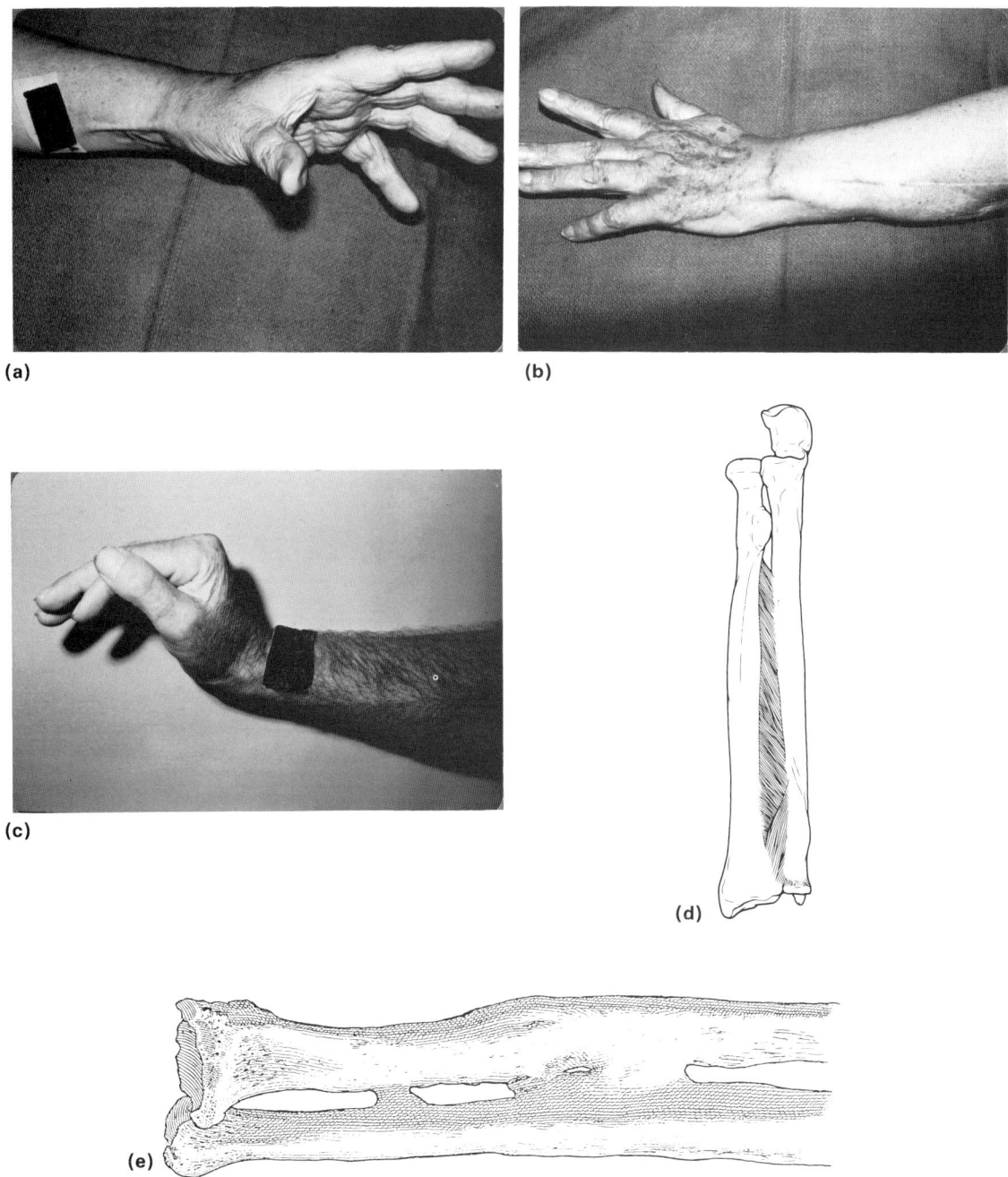

Fig. 17.8 (a) Radial nerve palsy showing a transfer of the palmaris longus into a rerouted extensor pollicis longus as a straight line transfer. (b) Radial nerve palsy showing a transfer of the flexor carpi ulnaris around the ulnar border of the forearm, a little more distal than usual to avoid the scar from previous bone repair. It shows the unsightly bulge that this transfer around the ulnar border of the forearm produces because of the size of the muscle mass that must be transferred. Function was adequate, however. (c) Radial nerve palsy with adequate wrist extension from transfer of pronator into extensor carpi radialis brevis. Adhesions to the interosseous membrane of the transfers of flexor digitorum sublimis of the long and ring fingers into the extensor digitorum communis through the interosseous membrane resulted in incomplete extension of the fingers when the wrist was in extension. (d) Sketch of the fibrous structure of the interosseous membrane in the forearm. (e) Sketch of X-ray showing cross union between radius and ulna preventing interosseous route of transfer.

266 UNSATISFACTORY RESULTS IN HAND SURGERY

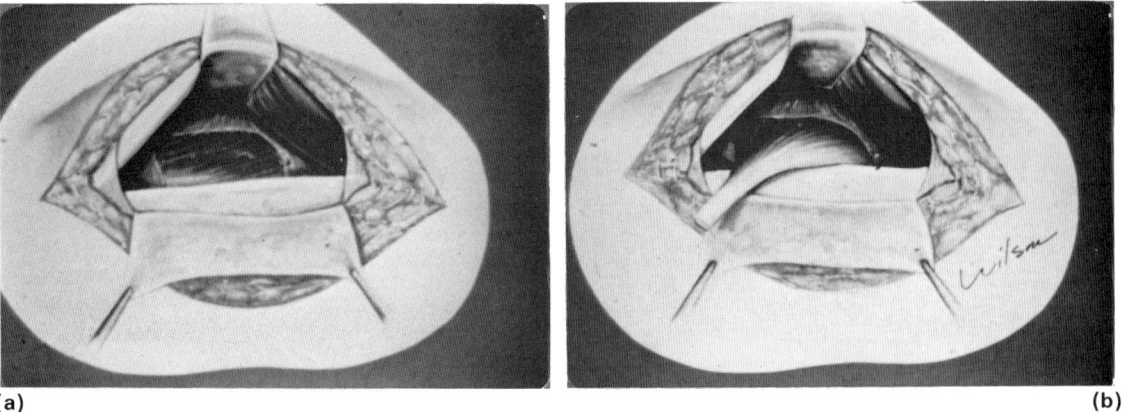

Fig. 17.9 (a) Sketch of large hole cut in interosseous membrane with muscle to be transferred through the hole showing after the excision of the membrane. (b) Sketch showing the muscle and tendon coming through the hole in the interosseous membrane giving adequate room for the transfer.

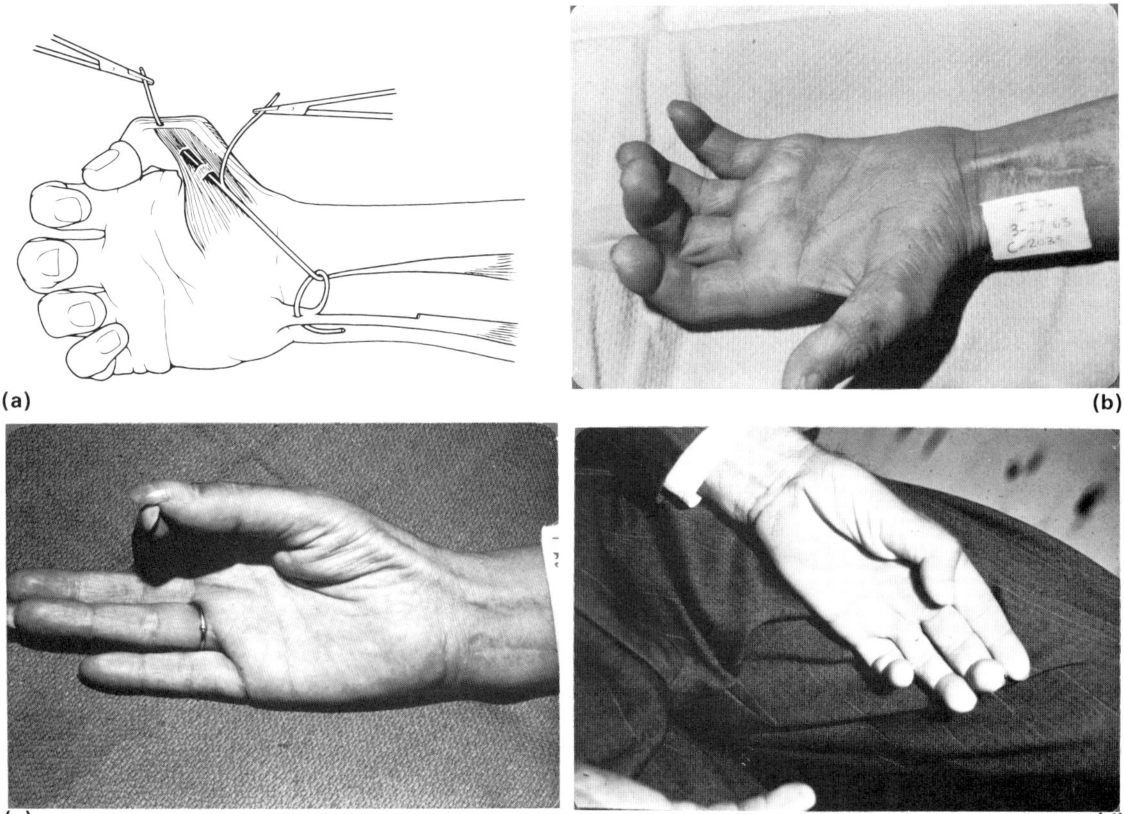

Fig. 17.10 (a) Sketch showing fixed pulley made from one-half of the flexor carpi ulnaris, making the change of direction occur approximately at the centre of the wrist and the tunnel made through the tendon of the abductor pollicis brevis to keep the transfer at the centre of the axis of motion of the metacarpophalangeal joint of the thumb. (b) Case showing adhesion of the transfer at the pulley preventing full opposition of the thumb. (c) Case of polio showing radial shift of the pulley and inadequate opposition because of improper alignment to produce abduction and opposition. (d) Case of an original Steindler (1923) opponens with the transfer passed through the shath of the flexor pollicis longus and having no angle of approach on the metacarpal to do anything except flex the metacarpal. There is no rotation or abduction of the metacarpal.

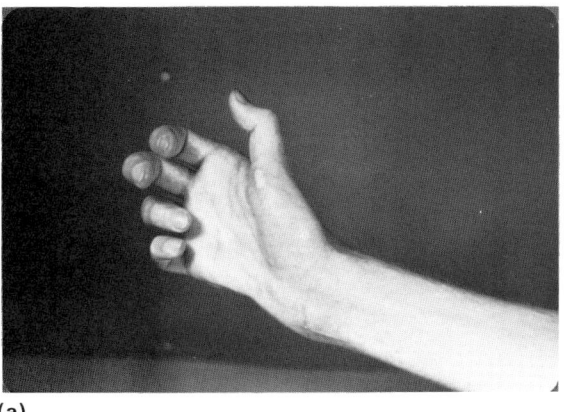
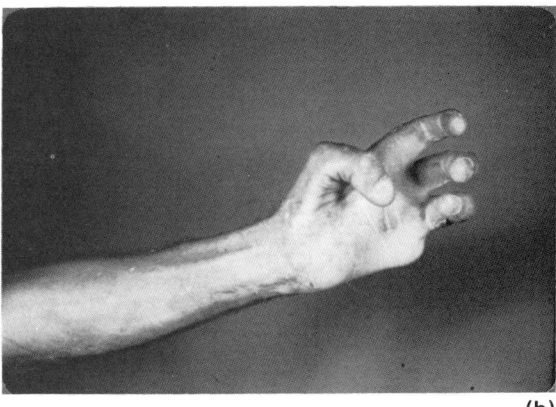

Fig. 17.11 (a) Case with hyperextension of the metacarpophalangeal joint of the thumb because of the shift of the tendon transfer behind the axis of motion at the joint. This resulted from not determining before surgery that the joint was hyperextensible and that no tunnel was made through the tendon of the abductor pollicis brevis to hold the transfer at this point and therefore prevent hyperextension. (b) Case with flexion deformity at the metacarpophalangeal joint produced by migration of the tendon transfer anterior to the axis of motion of the joint.

failure to observe these mechanical points are shown in Figs 17.10(b)–(d) and Figs 17.11(a) and (b). Failure to diagnose or appreciate the importance of a normal hand showing hyperextensibility (Riordan 1984) of the joints as shown in Fig. 17.12(a) can result in deformities as shown in Fig. 17.12(b).

The amount of tension a tendon transfer is placed under when being joined to a distal tendon or tendons of insertion is important. Brand (1985) has discussed using a radian as a means of determining range of motion needed in grafts and transfers and uses this method in judging tension in doing tendon transfers. My method has been to determine the range of tendon excursion of the tendon being transferred in its transferred position. This means stretching it to its maximum excursion and then releasing it to see its maximum range of retraction. This range of motion is then fitted into the middle two-thirds of the range of excursion of the tendons into which the transfer is to be inserted. This means determining the maximum range of excusion demonstrated by making the tendons fully extend and flex the parts they move, and then putting the tendon transfer into the tendons so that the range of the transferred tendon is in the

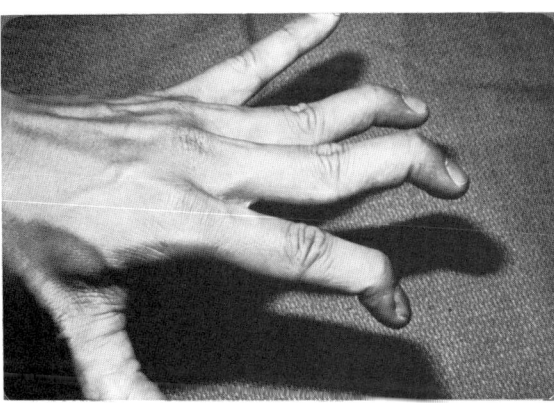
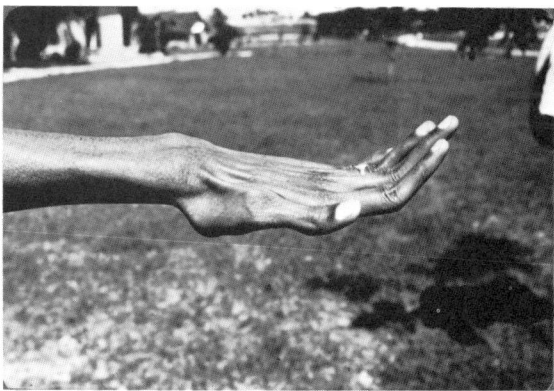

Fig. 17.12 (a) Normal hand showing marked tendency to hyperextend joints which means that intrinsic tendon transfers cannot be inserted into the lateral bands of the fingers or this swan neck type of deformity will result. (b) Case showing the swan neck deformity of all fingers resulting from insertion of the intrinsic transfer into the lateral bands in normally loose, hyperextensible joints.

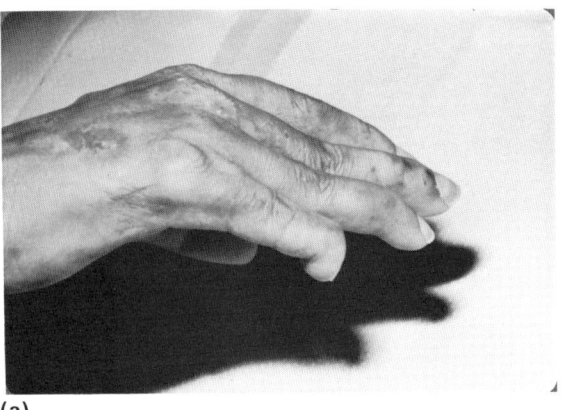 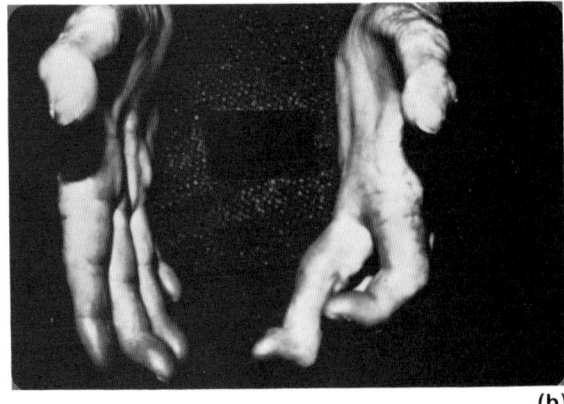

Fig. 17.13 (a) Case showing an intrinsic plus deformity (swan neck plus flexion contracture of the metacarpophalangeal joints) resulting from too much tension on a Fowler type of intrinsic transfer and from having to advance the tendons distal to their normal insertion thus resulting in the limited range of motion. (b) Case of bilateral ulnar-median palsy with Bunnell sublimis intrinsic transfer done on both hands 10 years previously. The right hand shows good correction of the deformity but the left hand shows swan neck of the long and ring fingers and flexion deformities of the index and little fingers. This is probably from improper tension of the four slips of the single sublimis tendon to the individual fingers.

middle two-thirds of the range of motion desired to achieve the distal function of the part or parts.

Figures 17.13(a) and (b) and Figs 17.14(a) and (b) show examples of errors made in determining this tension on multiple tendons. An error in making the proper incisions is demonstrated in Fig. 17.15.

The importance of the pulley systems in the hand is best shown when these systems are violated or ignored and not reconstructed when necessary. Figures 17.16(a)–(e) show a combination of factors which combined to produce the deformities shown 25 years after surgery. Doing the Bunnell pulley advancement (Bunnell 1948) (which lengthens or removes the A-1 pulley) plus the added increase in the flexor moment arm of the long flexors, plus the off centre pull of a Bunnell (1944) sublimis intrinsic transfer gives the intrisic plus and ulnar drift of the fingers. Then, 2 years after the surgery, a return of interosseous muscle function following ulnar nerve repair results in all of these factors combining to produce the deformities shown in this case.

Proper evaluation of causes of contractures

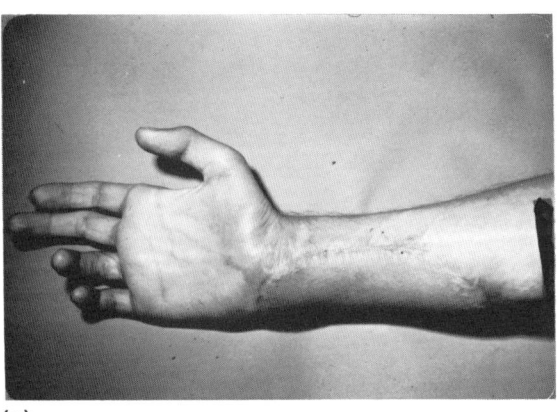 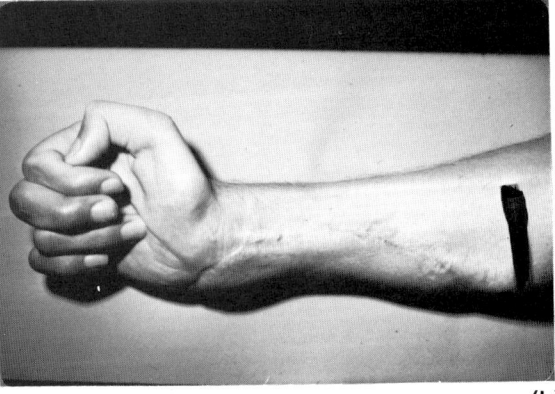

Fig. 17.14 (a) Case showing loss of skin and tendons covered by abdominal flap. The tendon transfer of extensor carpi radialis longus to restore finger flexion shows too much tension on the profundus of ring and little fingers resulting in inadequate extension of these two fingers but adequate extension of the index and long fingers. (b) Same case showing adequate finger flexion of all four fingers. This shows error in judging the proper tension placed on all four tendons to a single transfer when the four fingers have a different length and therefore a different range of excursion.

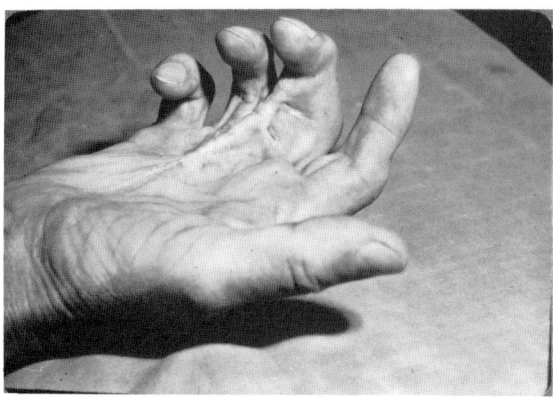

Fig. 17.15 Case showing severe contracture resulting from longitudinal incisions without doing Z-plasties for excision of fascia in a case of Dupuytren's contracture

produced by fibrosis of the muscles from vascular causes shown in Figs 17.17(a) and (b) is the same as would result from a tendon transfer being placed under too much tension (Enna & Riordan 1973) so that a full range of excursion could not be obtained because of the inability of the muscle to lengthen to that degree.

In hyperextensible fingers, when removing a sublimis for transfer, one slip of the sublimis must be left long to produce a tenodesis across the middle joint to prevent hyperextension of the middle joint (Fowler 1946) (Fig. 17.17(c)).

Another cause for failure in tendon transfers is that some surgeons fail to realise that muscles that are reinnervated after motor nerve repair are no longer able to be brought under individual control so that they are not good muscles for transfer to restore missing muscle function. In the majority of cases only mass action of such recovered muscles such as interossei is possible and they function only as a unit in doing mass action functions such as extending all fingers or flexing all fingers at the same time. One is unable to independently use a single interosseous as in pointing the index finger or wagging it from side to side. Occasionally in the very young this independent function can apparently be relearned but I have not seen it in adults. An example of this is shown in Fig. 17.18(a)–(e). The same is true when doing tendon transfers in cases of spastic paralysis. The purpose of doing the tendon transfers is not to get an independent muscle function but mainly to try and balance the stronger flexors by transferring an expendable wrist or finger flexor and using it to reinforce the weaker extensors of the wrist or fingers. Since all muscles function mostly at the same time in spastics, the main function of transfer is to balance the forces acting on the extremity.

METHOD OF TENDON INSERTION

After the route of the transfer has been decided upon, one must consider the type of insertion that should be used. There are many ways described for tendon insertions, not only tendon to tendon, but tendon into bone. The majority of time, a tendon to tendon suture can be done which gives more strength. Occasionally a bony insertion is necessary and this can be as a single hole, burying the tendon into the bone, or by passing a tendon into one hole and bringing it out through another hole in the bone and suturing the tendon to itself thus making it unnecessary to use pull out wire technique. In the lower extremity, one should be very careful in inserting a tendon into a hole in the bone since this creates a permanent weak spot in the bone. In cases with diminished sensation, as in Hansen's disease or diabetes, this may result in a fracture and result in a Charcot foot (iatrogenically produced). When suturing tendon to tendon, an end to end type may be used or a multiple weaving type of suture may be used. Most prefer the weaving type because there is probably less likelihood of the suture coming apart or stretching a little to change the length relationships. If this occurs, a less than satisfactory range of excursion will result because of the relative lengthening this produces.

IMMOBILISATION

The next problem to be considered is how long should the extremity be immobilised to allow for healing of the tendon transfer. Equally as important is what position the extremity should be immobilised in so there is not undue stress on the tendon suture lines during the healing period. The position of the immobilisation should be one that uses wrist flexion or extension to take the tension off the transferred tendons and to allow the fingers to be

270 UNSATISFACTORY RESULTS IN HAND SURGERY

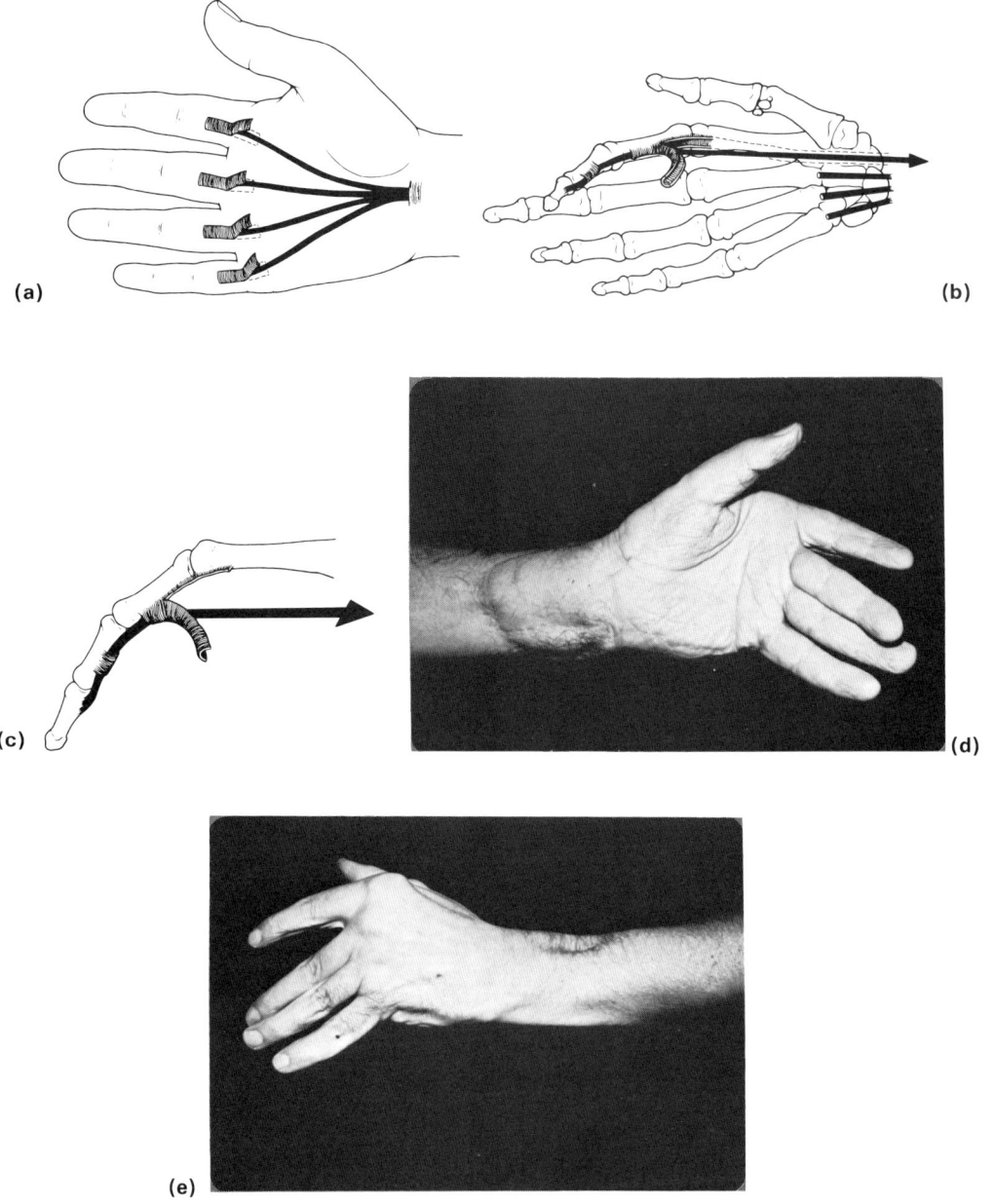

Fig. 17.16 (a) Sketch showing Bunnell pulley advancement which he advised doing when doing intrinsic replacement operation in the 1940–42 era to 'get mechanical advantage' and have the long flexors also flex the proximal phalanges. (b) Sketch showing how this allows flexors to ulnar drift after removal of the A-1 pulley. (c) Sketch in the lateral plane showing how this allows volar displacement of the flexor tendons and a marked increase in the flexion moment of the flexor tendons. (d) Palmar view of a case in which the Bunnell pulley advancement was done in addition to a Bunnell sublimis intrinsic transfer, as seen 25 years after the surgery. The result of the transfer plus the pully release and a partial recovery of the interossei after the ulnar nerve suture all made for the development of severe intrinsic plus-ulnar drift type of deformity. (e) Same case, dorsal view, showing marked ulnar drift.

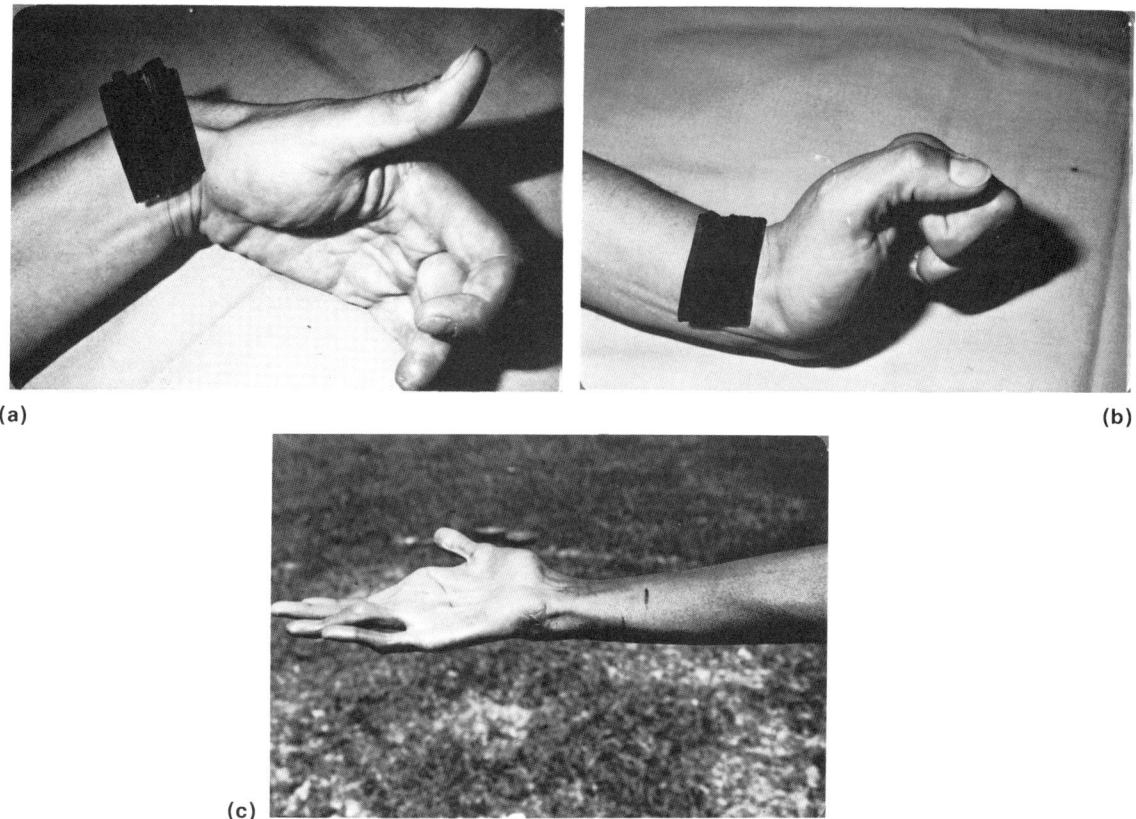

Fig. 17.17 (a) Case showing incomplete finger extension due to muscle fibrosis and shortening due to intra-arterial drug injection. (b) Same case showing that wrist extension produces tight flexion of the fingers in spite of the non-contractility of the muscles (tenodesis of profundi). (c) Case showing swan neck deformity of ring finger resulting from removal of both insertion slips of sublimis tendon used for opposition of the thumb. One slip should be left long enough to tenodese across the interphalangeal joint to prevent hyperextension.

mildly flexed at all joints. Fingers should never be immobilised in complete extension at all joints at the same time. The middle and distal joints can be kept in extension if the proximal joints are flexed 70 or more degrees. It is preferred to have some 20 or 30 degrees of flexion of the middle and distal joints as well as the proximal joints if at all possible. Three weeks of immobilisation is used followed by changing the splints and bringing the wrist partially out of its flexed or extended position and reimmobilising the wrist. If the elbow has been included in the immobilisation it may be left out at this time. Also at this time, limited flexion or extension of the fingers can be allowed depending upon whether the transfers were for flexion or extension. About 50% of the possible range of motion is allowed but the fingers must always rest on a splint preventing full flexion if the tranfers were for restoration of extension or prevention of full extension if the transfers were for restoring finger flexion. At 5 weeks the same splint can be removed and saved as a half cast for resting splinting and the patient can be allowed to gradually achieve full flexion or full extension (Fig. 17.19(a) and (b)) At no time during this time frame should motion against resistance be allowed. This moving against resistance (such as squeezing a ball) (Fig. 17.20) cannot be safely allowed unless a full 8 weeks has been allowed for mature healing of the sutured tendons. If resistance is allowed too early, grandual stretching of the tendon suture or sutures may occur and the result will be a limited range of

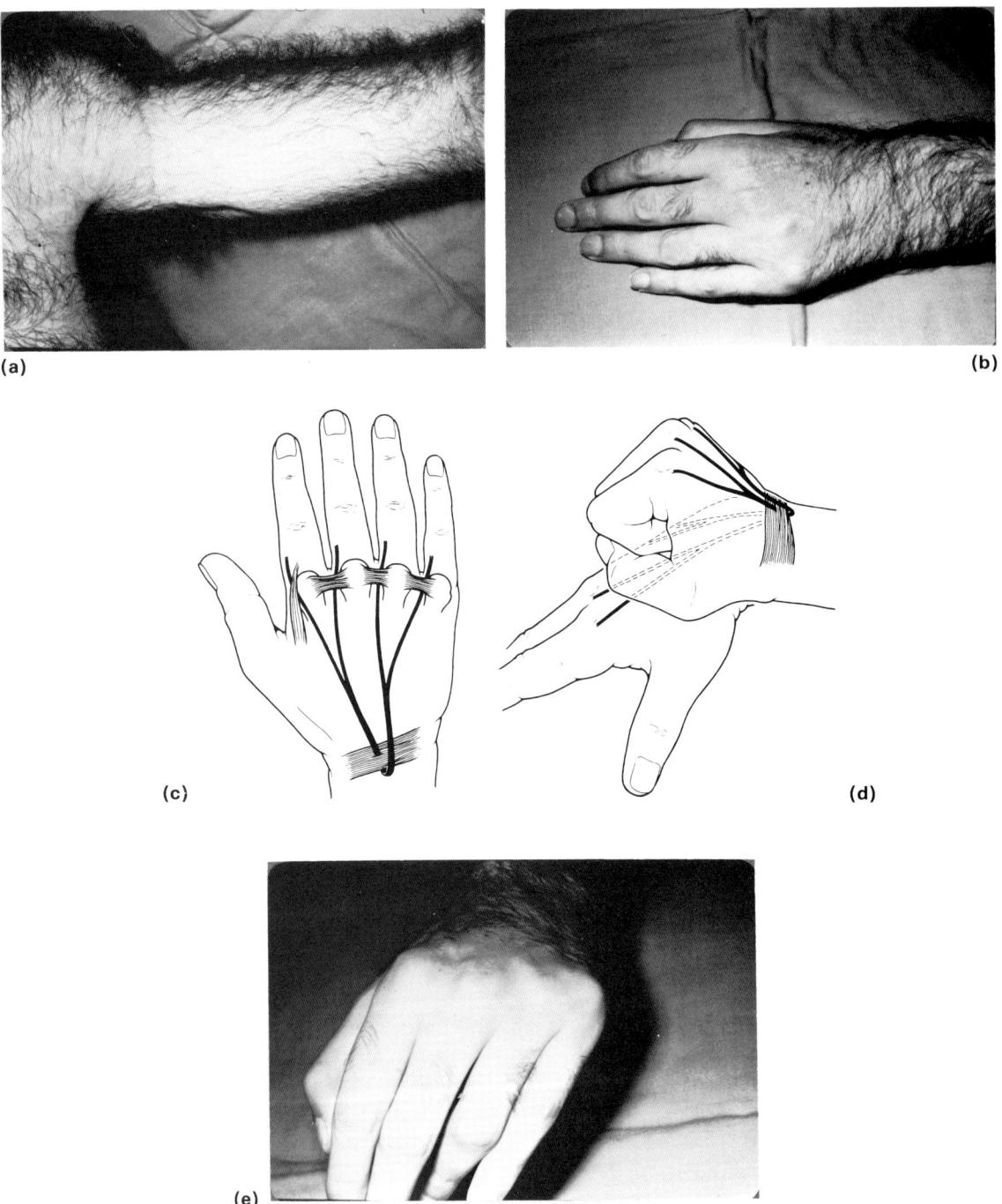

Fig. 17.18 (a) Circular scar at upper arm where water ski tow rope encircled arm and cut through all vessels and nerves. Vessels repaired primarily, nerves repaired at 6 weeks. (b) Muscle recovery followed in 2 years with fair sensation and fair voluntary control over muscles. (c) Sketch of Fowler intrinsic tenodesis used for paralysis of the interossei and lack of active controllable muscle to transfer to the interossei. (d) Lateral sketch of how a Fowler intrinsic tenodesis works with flexion and extension of the wrist. (e) Same case showing how the fourth and fifth metacarpals rise dorsally when the intrinsic tenodesis is made to work by wrist motion. This same reversal of the metacarpal arch has been noted on active intrinsic transfers from the dorsal side on modified Fowler or Riordan type of transfers.

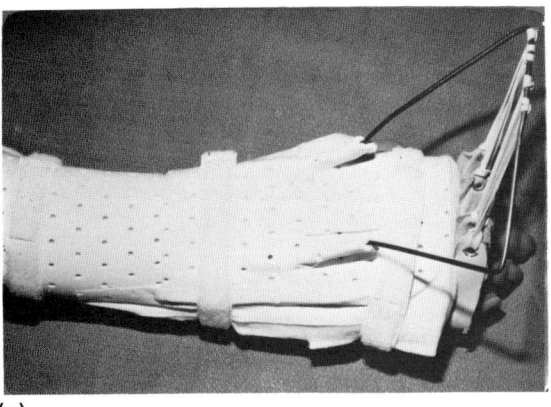 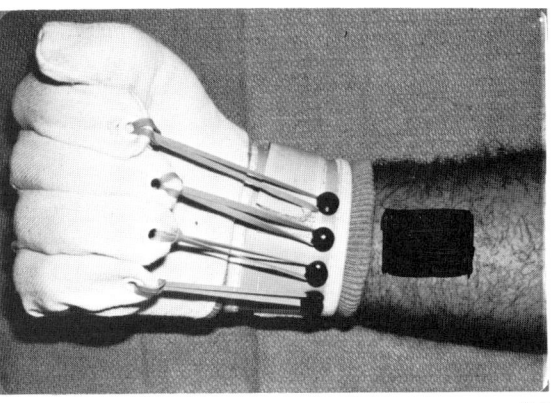

Fig. 17.19 (a) Traction splint used in post operative period to prevent hyperextension of proximal joints and give extension assist to middle and distal joints. (b) Traction glove used to assist in gaining flexion after 6 weeks following transfers for extension of fingers if flexion is not progressing satisfactorily.

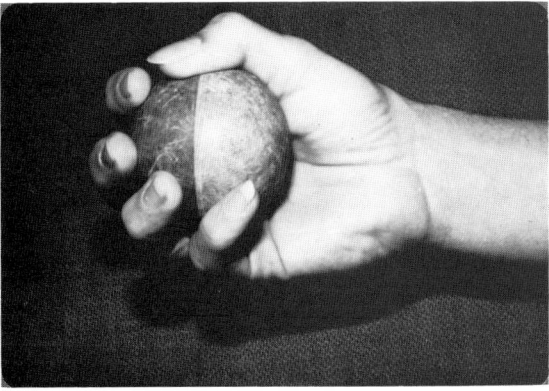

Fig. 17.20 Squeezing a ball offers complete resistance to movement and puts too much stress on tendon healing if done before 8 weeks postoperative

excursion or the tendon suture may come apart and the total result will be lost necessitating a revision or repair of the transfer.

PHYSICAL THERAPY

Physical therapy after the initial mobilisation can be carried out and some limited therapy can be instituted during the period of partial activity and splinting. After the 8 week period, physical therapy and occupational therapy can both be used to help rehabilitate the patient and return him to his former occupation or train him for a new occupation if he is unable to perform his former occupation.

REFERENCES

Bielsalski K, Mayer L 1916 Die Physiologische Sehnen Verpflanzung, Springer, Berlin, p 218–250

Brand W 1985 Clinical Mechanics of the Hand. Mosby, St Louis, p 41–55

Bunnell S 1944 Surgery of the Hand. Lippincott, Philadelphia, p 367–369

Bunnell S 1948 Surgery of the Hand, 2nd edn. Lippincott, Philadelphia, p 489–490

Enna C, Riordan D C 1973 The Fowler procedure for correction of the paralytic claw hand. Plastic and Reconstructive Surgery 52:352–360

Fowler S B 1946 Personal communication.

Mayer L 1916 The physiological method of tendon transplantation. Surgery, Gynecology & Obstetrics. 298–304

Riordan D C 1953 Tendon transplantation in median and ulnar nerve paralysis. Journal of Bone & Joint Surgery 35A:312–320

Riordan D C 1984 Intrinsic paralysis of the hand. Bulletin of Hospital for Joint Diseases, Orthopaedic Institute, 44:435–441

Steindler A 1923 Reconstructive Surgery of the Upper Extremity. Appleton, New York. p 85–88

E. A. Zancolli

18 Tetraplegia

The function of the upper limb of the tetraplegic patient can be improved by reconstructive surgery. Such improvement depends fundamentally on the level of the spinal cord lesion and, consequently, the number of functioning muscles available for transfer. Improving the function of the upper limbs in tetraplegic patients not only offers them greater independence in daily activities but also manifestly improves their psychological condition.

The factors that favour good surgical results are:

1. Lesions with functioning muscles available for tendon transfer.
2. The absence of spasticity in the upper limbs.
3. The presence of two-point tactile discrimination.
4. Flexible joints.
5. Adequate operative planning.
6. Technical precision.
7. Adequate postoperative control.

If any one of these factors is interpreted incorrectly or executed inadequately reconstructive surgery can have unsatisfactory results, which will not only aggravate the functional condition of the limb that has undergone surgery but will also, to an even greater extent, affect the patient's psychological condition.

The most important surgical improvements have been achieved by restoring:

1. Active extension at the elbow when the triceps muscle has been paralysed in high and some middle level spinal cord lesions.
2. Prehensile function of the hand particularly with middle and low level lesions. Reconstruction of the prehensile function of the hand is always very weak with high level spinal cord lesions.

I will discuss, in particular, the commonest causes of unsatisfactory results and suggest ways of preventing them. However, firstly I shall present the clinical data that has been collected from patients examined and treated at the Institute of Rehabilitation, Buenos Aires.

CLINICAL MATERIAL

We have seen 172 patients with traumatic tetraplegia, 114 of whom have been evaluated over a period of 24 years. The statistics referred to below relate to a group of 97 who underwent surgery on their upper limbs (Zancolli 1975). These patients had sustained their initial spinal cord injury through: motor accidents (51%); diving into water of insufficient depth (40%), bullet wounds (3%), and other causes (5%). The ages ranged between 15 and 43 years.

Sixty-two per cent underwent upper limb surgery between 7 and 18 months after the initial accident. Fifteen per cent had spasticity in their upper limbs. Taken altogether, 90% had two-point discrimination in at least one of their digits. Taking different levels of spinal cord lesion separately, two-point discrimination was found in 32% with high level lesions, 76% with middle level lesions, and 97% with low level lesions. Six patients could stand up with orthoses. All patients had in common adequate motivation, few psychological problems, and good function in their triceps muscles (middle and low level lesions).

CAUSES OF UNSATISFACTORY RESULTS

We have analysed, according to our own experience, the causes of unsatisfactory results in reconstructive surgery performed in patients with traumatic tetraplegia. These can be placed into three groups:

1. Defects in the preoperative evaluation and selection of patients.
2. Defects in operative planning.
3. Defects in operative technique.

Defects in preoperative evaluation and selection of patients (Table 18.1)

These generally represent a defective preoperative study of the patient. Such study requires a detailed analysis of each factor that the surgeon must take into account before deciding on surgery to restore the function of the upper limbs. These factors are:

1. The patient's general condition

This includes pressure sores, problems with urinating and defecating, psychological condition, motivation, and neurovegetative syndromes (temperature regulation, autonomic dysfunction, orthostatic vasodilatation). The result of surgery will be complicated if the patient suffers from severe psychological problems or shows inadequate postoperative cooperation. Patients who still cannot accept that there can be no further recovery from their spinal cord injury will find it difficult to accept an indication for reconstructive surgery. This attitude may change if they see good surgical results in similar cases. It is therefore necessary to expose them to good surgical results, especially in a rehabilitation centre, where patients can talk and observe each other.

2. The condition of the muscles

Before beginning reconstructive surgical procedures on the upper limbs the spared muscles must have recovered their maximum possible function. From the start it is possible to define with sufficient accuracy the level of the spinal cord lesion in patients with traumatic tetraplegia.

The muscles that have kept their function must undergo intense retraining to acquire their maximum possible power before they are used for transfer. They can be evaluated according to Highet's scale of 0 to 5 (Zancolli 1975). Those with a strength of 4 or more can be used for transfer. The strength of the spared muscles depends upon the level of the spinal cord lesion as their innervation originates from more than one spinal segment. Thus the triceps, which will be able to contract if the seventh spinal segment has been preserved (stong active extension of the wrist with preserved function of the pronator teres and palmaris longus) acquires greater strength if, in addition, motor function exists in the fingers on the radial side of the hand, which in turn indicates that the eighth spinal segment has in part been preserved (see Table 18.1 below).

Table 18.1 Preoperative evaluation and selection

1. The patient's general condition
2. Condition of the muscles
3. Ability to sit
4. Sensation in the hand
5. Condition of the joints (elbow, wrist, digits)
6. Daily activities (in bed and in the wheelchair)
7. Functional tests of progressive ability
8. Classification (clinical group)

As severe spasticity constitutes a contraindication to surgery, it is important to know whether there is spasticity in the upper limbs. Minor spasticity does not constitute a contraindication. The muscular spasticity of traumatic tetraplegia generally has characteristics that distinguish it from cerebral paralysis:

1. Its presentation tends to be sporadic and this is influenced above all, like cerebral paralysis, by emotional stimulants.
2. It may be shaky in character.
3. It occurs irregularly in the muscles of the upper limb, sometimes in the finger flexor muscles, sometimes in the extensor muscles, or sometimes in both.

Muscular spasticity tends to occur most often in patients who have partly recovered or who have partial spinal cord lesions. Severe spasticity was found in the intrinsic muscles of the hand in one of our patients.

3. Ability to sit

It is important that the patient can sit before the hands are operated on. Thus, patients who can actively extend, but not flex, their wrists can improve the opening of their hands by using gravity. To do this the patient rests the pronated forearm on the arm-rest of the wheelchair and allows gravity to flex the wrist. This manoeuvre is particularly useful for tendon transfers carried out on the extensor tendons of the fingers. The forearm can be pronated, to achieve this effect, passively in high level spinal lesions or actively by the pronator teres in middle and low level lesions. Wheelchair handling and propulsion will be helped by the ability to pronate the forearm actively. With tendon transfers for extension of the elbow correct postoperative retraining of the muscles can be achieved without the patient previously being able to sit.

4. Sensation in the hand

We have previously referred to our statistics on the preservation of motor function (conscious control of position, movement and strength) and sensory function (two-point discrimination and Seddon's coin test). It is interesting to emphasise that in tetraplegics the area of skin where sensation is preserved usually does not coincide with the metameric muscular level. Thus with high level spinal cord lesions cutaneous sensation may be preserved more distally than in motor function. In our experience the area of cutaneous sensitivity varies in relation to a given level of the spinal cord lesion much more than does motor function; only rarely does the level of muscular paresis or paralysis not coincide with the level of the spinal cord lesions.

Variations in sensory and motor function between one hand and the other are common, making it necessary to examine each hand separately. Moberg (1978) states that there are differences between one side and the other in one half of all patients.

5. Condition of the joints

The state of the joints is important when considering surgery. All tetraplegics should undergo constant articular mobilisation to avoid rigidity. In our experience we have observed flexion contracture of the elbow (seven cases), supination contracture of the forearm in high level lesions (two cases), intrinsic contracture of the fingers (one case) and flexion contracture of the fingers (one case). In two of our patients there was supination of the forearm but passive pronation was possible because there was no contraction of the interosseous membrane. These patients were unable to move the hand to the wheel of the wheelchair. This complication occurs with high level lesions because there is no resistance to the supinating action of the biceps. In these patients the biceps can be transferred to a new insertion, giving it a pronating action. In fixed supination contracture the interosseous membrane must be completely freed in the forearm before transfer of the biceps muscle to gain pronation.

6. Daily activities

The tetraplegic patient's ability to carry out basic daily activities, and consequently his capacity to function independently, must always be evaluated. This allows a correlation with the results achieved by surgery. Daily activities performed in bed and in the wheelchair must be considered.

1. In bed: moving; rolling; lifting the body; grabbing objects from the night table; hygiene; dressing; feeding; and reading.
2. In the wheelchair: passage from wheelchair to bed, chair or car; control and management of wheelchair; balancing the body; accommodation of the legs; hygiene; dressing; eating; and writing.

It must be recorded for each of these activities whether the patient can perform it independently; only with the help of a special aid; or not at all.

7. Functional tests of progressive ability

These tests evaluate function and strength particularly of extension of the elbow and the prehensile action of the hand (opening the hand, power grip, and lateral pinch) before and after surgery. These tests are used to evaluate the results obtained (Tables 18.2 and 18.3).

Table 18.2 Five point progressive ability test: extension of the elbow

Function	Points
Reaching raised objects	1
Ability to drive	1
Ability to propel wheelchair	1
Ability to raise self in seat	1
Body transfer	1
Total*	5

*5 = excellent; 4 = good; 2 = fair; 1 = poor.

Table 18.3 Nine point progressive ability test: hand function

Function	Points
Power grip	
Drink from glass/cup	1
Turn taps	1
Manage wheel chair	1
Lateral pinch	
Comb hair or eat with spoon or fork	1
Use key	1
Handle matches or coins	1
Open hand	
Typewriting	1
Wash and dry face and extremities	1
Shake hands	1
Total*	9

*9 = excellent; 7-8 = good; 4-6 = fair; 1-3 = poor.

8. Classification

Classically, patients have been grouped in relation to the level of spinal cord lesion (metameric level) according to which muscles are paralysed and which cutaneous areas have retained their sensitivity. Lipscomb et al (1958) classified their patients according to the level of the cervical skeletal injury. This does not give a true picture, however, as the skeletal lesion often does not coincide with the level of the spinal cord lesion. Lamb & Landry (1972), and later Freehafr et al (1974), classified their patients according to which muscles retained their function.

Moberg (1975, 1978) developed a classification based on eight clinical groups according to which muscles retained their active function, and two clinical groups based on afferent stimuli available to control the pincer action of the hand: 1. with ocular afferent stimuli alone; 2. with ocular afferent stimuli and two-point cutaneous discrimination.

According to Moberg, the grasping function of the hand could be used without the help of sight only if the digits could distinguish two points of touch at 10 mm or less apart.

Participants at the last conference on tetraplegia, which took place in Giens, France in 1984, attempted to arrive at a standard classification for all patients. To help reach a general agreement all data on sensibility and function were taken into account.

We (Zancolli 1968, 1975, 1978) classify our patients according to the most distal spared motor function. Since the meeting in Giens we have decided to add to this classification the hand's sensation and whether or not muscular spasticity is present (Tables 18.4 and Fig. 18.1). We classify sensation (two-point discrimination) in the hand as positive (Cu+) or negative (Cu−). Two-point discrimination is considered to be positive when the two points are 10 mm or less apart. Spasticity is said to be positive (Sp+) or negative (Sp−). Each upper limb is evaluated separately (right and left). James House (Tetraplegic Group Meeting 1984) has accepted a similar classification.

According to this classification a patient with active wrist extension (group 3: wrist extension II) and two-point discrimination of 10 mm or less, and without muscular spasticity, in both upper limbs would be recorded as: Group 3, Cu+, Sp−, (right and left). The classification comprises nine functional groups of which one is irregular. This final group is irregular because motor function does not correspond to the level of the spinal cord lesion. This is very rare.

Motor function is taken as the principal factor in the classification presented here for the following reasons:

a. It is an easy way of determining the level of the spinal cord lesion. The motor function of the upper limb is determined by asking the patient to try to perform the following basic actions: raising the shoulder girdle; neutral, external and internal abduction of the shoulder; flexion and extension of the elbow; pronation and supination of the forearm; flexion and extension of the wrist; flexion and extension of the digits; intrinsic movements of the digits. Each of these movements should be attempted with and without passive resistance. After the performance of these movements it is easy, through the surgeon's observation alone, to

Table 18.4 Classification of tetraplegia

Group (most distal function preserved)	Most distal muscles preserved	Sensibility	Spasticity
1. Elbow flexion	Without brachioradialis With brachioradialis		
2. Wrist extension I (complete ROM. Power 4−)	Ext. carpi. rad. longus. supinator	↓	↓
3. Wrist extension II (complete ROM. Power 4+)	Extensor carpi radialis brevis		
4. Forearm pronation	Pronator teres	Cu (tactile gnosis):	Sp (spasticity):
5. Wrist flexion, elbow extension	Flexor carpi radialis Triceps	+positive (<10 mm) negative (>10 mm)	+positive −negative
6. Finger extrinsic extension	Finger extensors Extens. carpi ulnaris	↓	↓
7. Thumb extrinsic extension	Thumb extrins. extensors		
8. Digits extrinsic flexion (partial or complete)	Flexor extrinsics 　Without flex. superficialis 　With flex. superficialis		
9. Irregular			

*High level lesion = group 1, Middle level lesion = groups 2, 3, 4 and 5, Low level lesion = 6, 7 and 8.

know the level of the spinal cord lesion. With all these movements, above all when they are met with passive resistance, it is convenient to keep the patient's trunk stable.

b. Spared muscular function varies very little with any given level of spinal cord lesion. We have already mentioned that cutaneous sensation varies much more often with a given level of lesion.

c. The main problem for a tetraplegic patient is the motor defect, even for those without two-point discrimination.

d. We operate on both sides even in patients without cutaneous sensation in both hands, trying to achieve prehensile function. In these cases sight can compensate for the action of the hands when these are used independently of each other.

e. Finally, surgery is planned in relation to motor, and not to sensory, deficit.

Defects in surgical procedure

Unsatisfactory results due to defects in surgical procedure depend basically on: 1. inadequate staging of the procedure; 2. wrong selection of the type of operation in relation to the clinical group. In patients without active extension of the elbow, this movement must be restored before considering functional reconstruction of the hand. All patients with high level spinal cord lesions (group 1), and some with middle level lesions (groups 2, 3 and 4) are unable to extend their elbows. Upper limb function is markedly improved in tetraplegic patients by reconstruction of active elbow extension. This can be seen in the case of the following activities: a. reaching raised objects with the hand; b. controlling flexion of the elbow, particularly when the patient is in bed and wants to raise his hand to his mouth; c. raising and moving the body when in a sitting position; d. ability and strength to manage the wheelchair; e. better use of the brachioradialis when this muscle has been transferred to achieve extension of the wrist.

The stabilising function of the triceps is important for the functions of the brachioradialis. We choose the type of tendon transfer for elbow extension according to the clinical group. Moberg's technique is used in patients in group 1 (elbow flexion, with or without brachioradialis): the posterior deltoid, extended by tendon graft, is transferred to the olecranon process. In groups 2, 3 and 4 (wrist extension I and II, and forearm pronation) we prefer biceps-to-triceps transfer. This is a method which has given us very satisfactory results and which makes postoperative recovery very easy.

Biceps-to-triceps transfer requires good functioning of the supinator muscle. Otherwise, supination of the forearm would be lost. The function of the supinator muscle will be normal if active extension of the wrist is present, even if it is weak (group no. 2). Obviously the supinator muscle will always be active with more distal spinal cord

TETRAPLEGIA 279

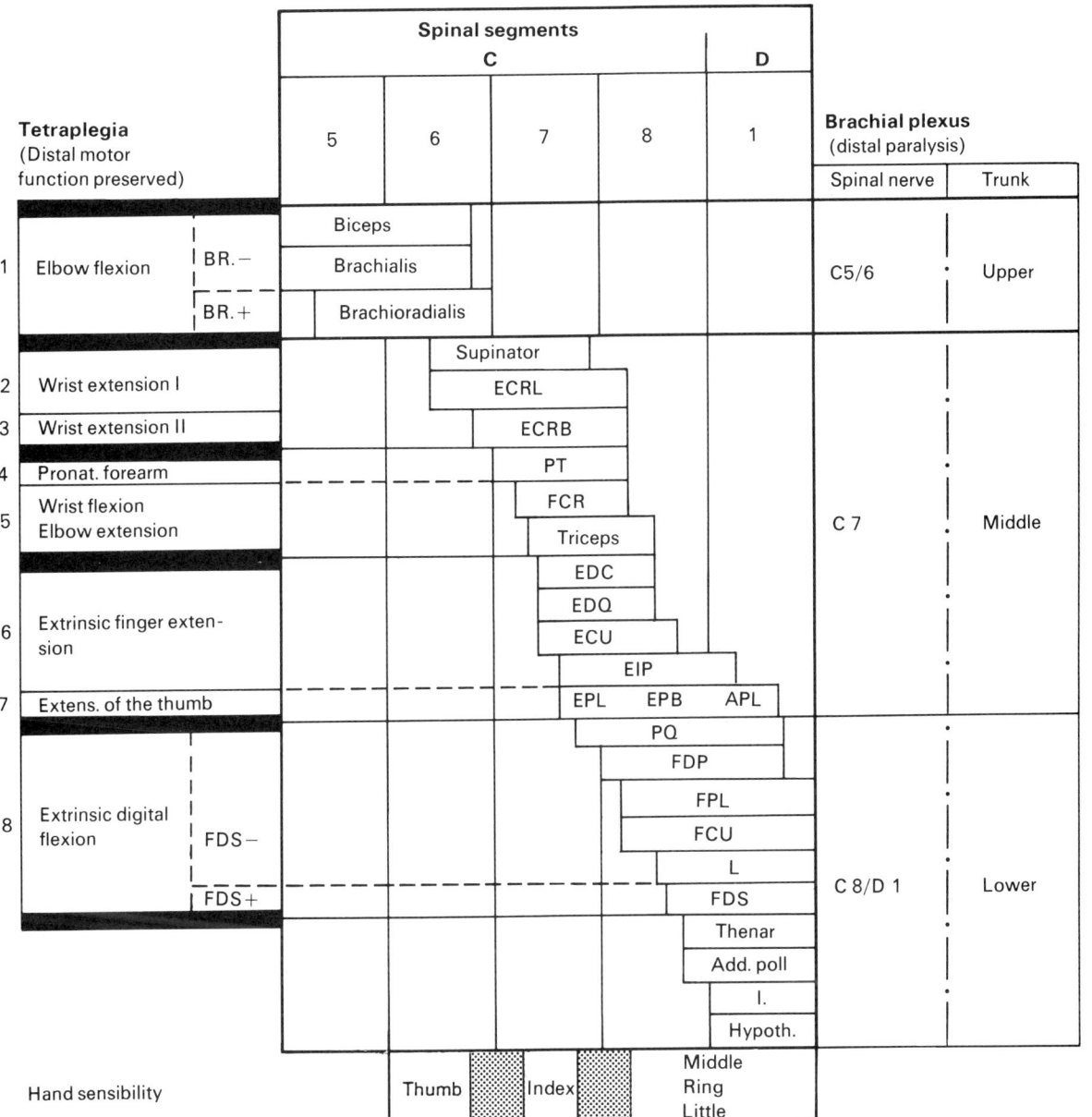

Fig. 18.1 Grouping of tetraplegic and brachial plexus lesions to spinal segments

lesions. Electromyography can also be used to evaluate the activity of this muscle.

Thirteen of our patients underwent biceps-to-triceps transfer and were followed for an average of 37 months. We obtained the following results:

a. Elbow extension (5 point test): excellent 28%; good 52%; fair 30%; poor 0. The mean power of extension was 2400 kg.

b. Elbow flexion: in all cases this function was completely preserved. Its strength was reduced in comparison with preoperative level in 24% but none of the patients complained about this or found it inconvenient.

c. Forearm supination: active supination was preserved in all patients. One patient sustained postoperative paralysis of the radial nerve; this had completely recovered by 4 months and was the result of surgical trauma to the radial nerve.

Reconstruction of hand function must take place after reconstruction of elbow extension as stated above. It is indicated when there are muscles with a strength of 4 or more available for transfer. Only in patients who have elbow flexion without the brachioradialis muscle is reconstructive hand surgery not indicated.

The lower the spinal cord lesion the better will be the results. The surgical procedure must correspond with the clinical group of spinal cord lesions. With high level lesions only weak lateral pinch of the thumb can be achieved, based on the automatic action of the wrist.

With middle level lesions lateral pinch, power grip and opening of the hand can be achieved. These actions are improved when the function of the flexor carpi radialis muscle is present. It is wrong in such cases to attempt to achieve only lateral pinch and flexion of the fingers (Lamb & Chan 1983). Extension of the fingers must, and can (Zancolli 1978), also be achieved. This not only produces better function but avoids flexion contracture of the fingers. With low level lesions even better function can be achieved: pinch with the pulps of the digits, power grip, and good finger extension.

With any level of lesion, the better the sensory condition of the hand the better will be the motor function achieved.

CONCLUSIONS

When indicated and well executed, upper limb reconstructive surgery in tetraplegic patients is so effective that no one can dispute its place in treatment. No splint can be a substitute for successful surgery. However, surgery must be avoided if there are general or local contraindications.

Unsatisfactory results are caused by defects in preoperative evaluation and selection of patients, defects in operative planning, and technical defects in surgery.

With high and middle level lesions only lateral pinch, not pulp pinch, should be attempted. Pulp pinch requires many tendons for transfers, and these are not available in such patients. The restoration of pulp pinch should be attempted only in patients with low level spinal cord lesions.

REFERENCES

Freehafer A A, Vonhaam E, Allen V 1974 Tendon transfers to improve grasp after injuries of the cervical spinal cord. Journal of Bone and Joint Surgery 56A:951–959

Tetraplegic Group Meeting, Giens 1984 (Second small group international conference) Hyeres, France, 1984

Lamb D W, Landry R M 1972 The hand in quadriplegia. Paraplegia 9:204–212

Lamb W D, Chan K M 1983 Surgical reconstruction of the upper limb in traumatic tetraplegia. Journal of Bone and Joint Surgery 65B:291–298

Lipscomb P R, Elkins E C, Henderson E D 1958 Tendon transfers to restore function of hands in tetraplegia, especially after fracture-dislocation of the sixth cervical vertebra on the seventh. Journal of Bone and Joint Surgery 40A:1071

Moberg E 1975 Surgical treatment for absent single-hand grip and elbow extension in quadriplegia. Journal of Bone and Joint Surgery 57A:196–206

Moberg E 1978 The upper limb in tetraplegia: a new approach to surgical rehabilitation. George Thieme, Stuttgart

Zancolli E A 1968 Structural and dynamic bases of hand surgery, 1st edn. J B Lippincott, Philadelphia

Zancolli E A 1975 Surgery of the quadriplegic hand with active strong wrist extension preserved. A study of 97 cases. Clinical Orthopaedics 12:101–113

Zancolli E A 1978 Structural and dynamic bases of hand surgery, 2nd edn. J B Lippincott, Philadelphia

… R. G. Eaton and S. Z. Glickel

19 Fractures and dislocations

The dynamic anatomy of the osseous and soft tissue structures of the hand provides an exquisitely balanced mechanism which allows rapid, synchronous movement of its component parts while maintaining stability. What is perhaps most impressive about the relationship between the soft tissue and skeleton is the direct proximity of one to the other yet the necessity that they move with sufficient independence of each other to allow full excursion in flexion and extension. Prosecting a fresh cadaver digit clearly demonstrates that the extensor mechanism not only lies adjacent to the proximal phalanx but that there are soft tissue connections between it and the periosteum of the phalanx itself. Injury to bone is only one element and often not even the most important element of the injury created by a fracture. Fractures must be thought of as physiologic insults both to the bones and the soft tissues which envelope them throughout the forearm, wrist and particularly within the digits. Similarly, injuries to the soft tissues around the joints must be thought of within the context of the adjacent articulating surfaces.

No fracture or dislocation within the hand should be thought of as so simple that it cannot become complicated. Even tuft fractures of the distal phalanx have on occasion failed to unite becoming painful to the patient when pressure is applied. This can be particularly disabling to the manual labourer. The most basic question which we must address, then, is why 'unsatisfactory' results may occur in the treatment of fractures and dislocations. In light of the discussion of the dynamic anatomy of the hand above, it should be apparent that a certain percentage of less than optimal results are inevitable whenever the bony and soft tissue architecture is disrupted, regardless of how meticulously and expertly the anatomy is restored. Proliferation of scar tissue about injured structures cannot be prevented and may result in the adherence of moving parts, diminishing active motion. This may certainly be the case in injuries of the proximal phalanx in which the extensor mechanism becomes fixed to the underlying bone either by fibrous tissue or callous. Intra-articular fractures may result in a diminished arc of motion of the involved joint and an increased propensity to develop future degenerative changes despite what would appear to be anatomic reduction. Open injuries have an increased likelihood of going on to develop suboptimal digit or hand function due to fibrosis resulting from the severity of the injury or the initial contamination. If infection supervenes, the chance of losing function is even greater. Crush injuries, with the additional diffuse type of soft tissue trauma and interstitial edema which they create, are not infrequently complicated by prolonged swelling and periarticular or peritendinous adhesions. Fractures and joint injuries accompanied by tendon lacerations and/or nerve injuries are more likely to become complicated by tendons which do not glide well within an injured fibrosseous sheath or joints with restricted range of motion. The chance of an unfavourable result occurring in clinical settings such as these can certainly be diminished by meticulous wound and fracture care and diligent efforts at post-injury rehabilitation but an excellent or good result cannot always be achieved even in the best of hands.

Other reasons for unfavourable results can be divided into several broad categories. Some appear so obvious that their mention may seem an affront to the intelligence of the conscientious practitioner. However, as often as not, it is as the result of a fairly simple oversight, seemingly minor error in judgment, or slight inattention to detail that an injury becomes complicated. A fracture or dislocation cannot be appropriately treated primarily if it is not recognised. The need for adequate radiographs cannot be stressed too strongly or too frequently (Fig. 19.1). In the course of a day in every emergency room, a primary care physician may see a patient with a swollen finger or hand and almost reflexively order radiographs of the hand. This mundane chore is often relegated to the triage nurse prior to the physician ever seeing the patient. A busy emergency practitioner might look at a patient without carefully examining the injured extremity and order radiographs based upon gross physical appearance. Needless to say, every injured hand or finger should be examined prior to deciding upon which radiographs need to be ordered. If the injury appears to involve the hand, as in the case of a metacarpal fracture, radiographs of the hand should be obtained in three planes, namely, anterior–posterior, lateral and oblique. If the predominant swelling and tenderness is within a digit or the thumb, AP, lateral and oblique radiographs of the injured digit should be obtained. It should be very clearly stated on the X-ray requisition that a radiograph of the injured digit and not the hand is being requested. Lateral radiographs of the hand are often taken with the fingers held in full extension and superimposed upon each other. It can very easily be seen how an injury to a phalanx could be obscured by the overlying shadows of adjacent digits. More than one malpractice attorney has funded his sailboat from the settlement of a case in which a fracture dislocation of a proximal interphalangeal joint was missed because a radiograph of the hand and not the involved digit was obtained and interpreted as normal. There are those who would argue that obtaining AP, lateral and oblique radiographs is excessive and that an AP and lateral are sufficient. The authors have certainly seen instances in which a fracture was either not demonstrated on the two basic views or the degree of displacement of a fracture fragment was underestimated on a lateral view and more clearly demonstrated on an oblique view or vice-versa.

There is a wide spectrum of opinion concerning the criteria for adequacy of reduction of many fractures. Failure to reduce a fracture which would optimally have been treated with anatomic or near anatomic reduction may result in a persistent deformity and diminished function. Hopefully, it is more commonly the generalist and less commonly the hand specialist who opts to accept a degree of fracture angulation or rotation which is

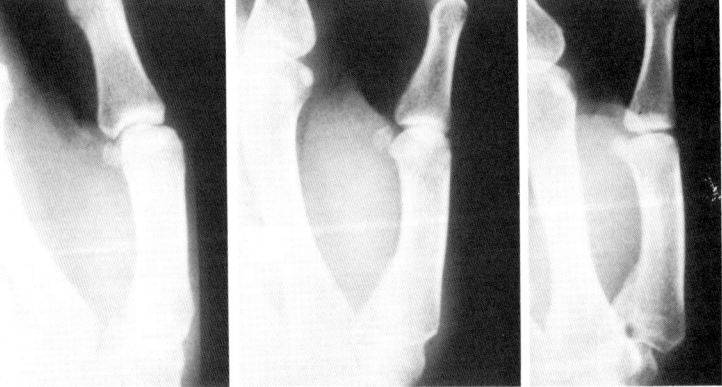

Fig. 19.1 Left: An oblique view of the carpometacarpal joint of the thumb shows no definite evidence of a fracture. Centre: An 'obliqued' lateral view is suggestive of an old fracture of the volar aspect of the base of the thumb metacarpal but does not demonstrate any incongruity in the articular surface. Right: A true lateral of the thumb metacarpal demonstrates a malunited Bennett's fracture with a significant step off in the articular surface. Note that on the true lateral radiograph the metacarpophalangeal volar plate sesamoids are superimposed on each other

likely to create problems when union is achieved. Fractures of the proximal phalanx and metacarpal fit squarely into this category. Essentially no rotational deformity of a proximal phalangeal or metacarpal fracture should be accepted because of the potential for crossing over of adjacent digits when taken through an arc of motion (Fig. 19.2). More specific examples will be discussed later.

One of the leading causes of complications related to fracture care is the failure to recognise fractures which are inherently unstable. Many fractures in the hand and digits can be treated well with fairly simple devices like aluminum splints, customised plaster of paris splints and even buddy taping. However, the same modalities applied to unstable fractures will result in loss of reduction which, if unrecognised, may go on to malunion. In this same vein it is incumbent upon the treating physician to closely follow fractures which are likely to be unstable particularly if they are treated without internal fixation and to obtain follow-up radiographs at appropriate intervals to be certain

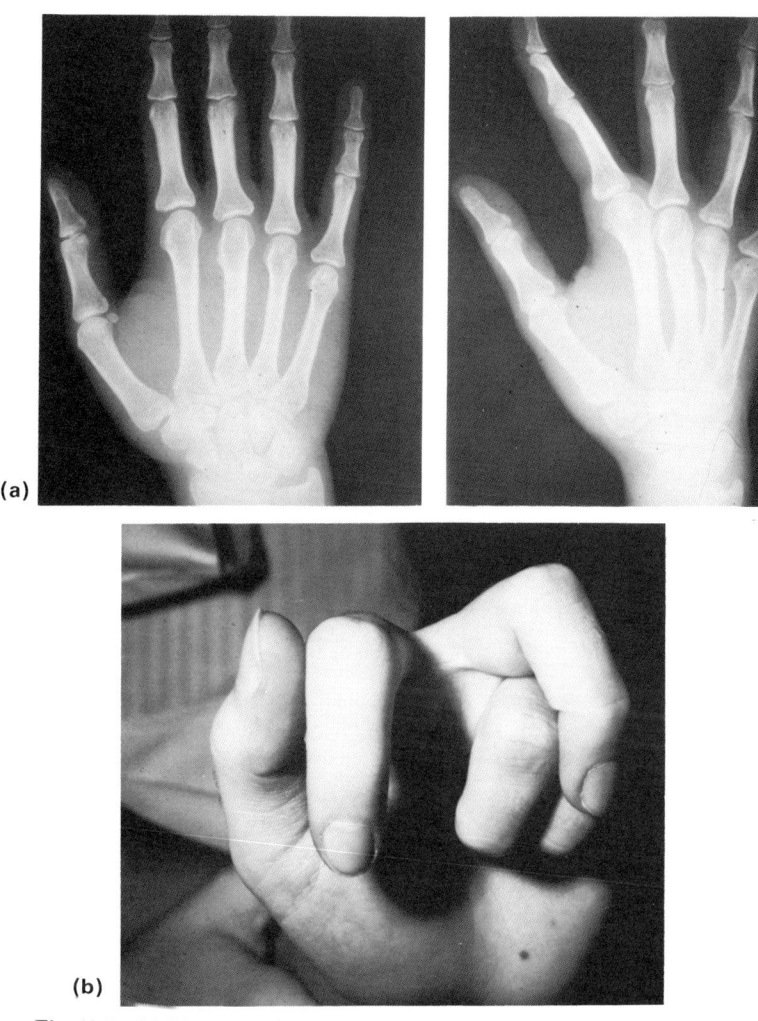

Fig. 19.2 (a) Malunion of a mid-shaft third metacarpal fracture with rotatory deformity. Left: Note shortening of the third metacarpal and thickening of the diaphysis. Right: On the AP radiograph the condyles of the metacarpal and proximal phalanx are rotated in comparison with the adjacent rays. (b) There is gross rotation of the middle finger with flexion. (Reproduced with permission of Lea and Febiger, Philadelphia: Kilgore E S, Graham W P 1977 *The Hand. Surgical and non-surgical management.* Lea and Febiger, Philadelphia)

that reduction is being maintained. Unstable fractures in the hand should be re-X-rayed within 3–5 days of reduction so that if reduction is lost, re-reduction can be performed relatively easily. Many fractures, particularly those in children, become 'sticky' within a week to 10 days making re-reduction difficult and traumatic to the tissues. A similar logic applies to the treatment of joint dislocations and subluxations which all need to be reduced (Fig. 19.3). Most dislocations, including simple dislocations of the PIP and DIP joints, are stable once reduced. That, however, is not always the case and occasionally an unstable interphalangeal joint dislocation will redislocate if inadequately immobilised. This is especially true with fracture dislocations of the proximal interphalangeal joint treated with dorsal splinting.

It is quite widely accepted that mobilising the joints of the hand as early as possible after injury is desirable. A significant contributing factor to unsatisfactory results is holding fractures for excessive periods of time. The negative effect of prolonged immobilisation is seen at the adjacent joints and even adjacent fingers which become stiff. As a rule, hand long bone fractures which are treated with cast or Kirschner wire immobilisation rarely need to be immobilised for more than 3–4 weeks. Specifically, metacarpal fractures can be held for 3–3½ weeks after which gentle active range of motion exercises may be begun. A similar interval applies for immobilisation of proximal and distal phalangeal fractures. Middle phalangeal fractures take slightly longer to heal and should be held for 4–4½ weeks. Radiographic evidence of fracture healing often becomes apparent after clinical stability occurs. One of the best criteria for when immobilisation can be discontinued and motion begun is whether the fracture site is tender. Fractures which are not tender to palpation are usually healed enough to begin mobilisation. A corollary of the problems created by holding joints immobilised for too long are those created by holding a joint in an incorrect position for any period of time (Fig. 19.4). Metacarpophalangeal joints should be immobilised in flexion between 60 and 90 degrees. In the flexed position the MP collateral ligaments are on maximal stretch and therefore will not shorten. The interphalangeal joints should be immobilised in extension or flexion

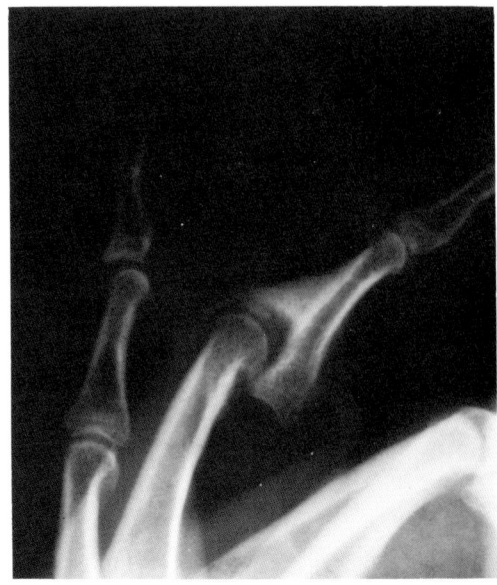

Fig. 19.3 An unrecognised volar dislocation of the proximal interphalangeal joint resulted in proximal migration of the middle phalanx and formation of a 'false' joint dorsally with the proximal phalanx articulating with periosteal new bone of the middle phalanx

of no more than 20 degrees except in the case of certain very specific injuries to or about the joint (James 1966). Immobilisation of the MP joints in extension or the PIP joints in marked flexion can result in stiffness which may be irreversible. The 'pancake' splint in which the wrist, metacarpophalangeal and interphalangeal joints are all held in full extension is never indicated.

There has been a recent trend toward very early mobilisation of fractures following rigid internal fixation. The basic tenet of this approach is that rigid fixation can be achieved in most hand fractures using scaled down plates and precision tapped screws (the AO small fragment equipment). The application of this hardware requires accurate open reduction and additional dissection of the soft tissue. The theoretical advantage of the technique is that the fracture is rendered rigidly stable permitting motion to be instituted almost immediately postoperatively. The theoretical concept of immediate mobilisation of joints after fracture fixation is appealing. However, it is gained at the expense of additional periosseous trauma and requires above average skill to achieve this theoretical advantage. Unsatisfactory results will be

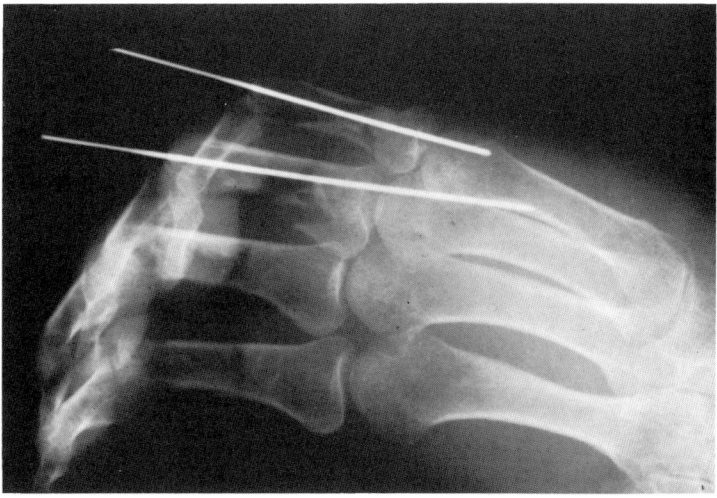

Fig. 19.4 Grossly unstable comminuted fractures of the fourth and fifth proximal phalangeal bases were partially reduced and internally fixed with Kirschner wires passed from distal to proximal. The PIP joints were immobilised in approximately 60 degrees of flexion and the metacarpophalangeal joints held in full extension by the Kirschner wires. If the position of the joints is not corrected by changing the internal fixation, extension contractures of the MP joints and flexion contractures of the PIP joints are likely sequelae

minimised if this technique is reserved for unstable fractures according to the specific indications of the AO group who have developed the technique. Otherwise the simplest treatment available to stabilise the fracture should be used.

Just as overzealousness in treating fractures can be problematic, so too, underzealousness can cause unfavourable results. Attempting to hold an oblique fracture of either a proximal phalanx or metacarpal with a single transverse Kirschner wire has a high likelihood of failure. A single pin provides inadequate fixation and the distal fracture fragment is likely to migrate proximally pivoting along the pin. Similarly, closely spaced crossed Kirschner wires used to transfix long oblique fractures are likely to fail (Fig. 19.5). While early motion is desirable, Kirschner wire fixation cannot be discontinued before the fracture is reasonably solid. Guide lines for immobilising fractures of the specific bones in the hand were mentioned previously and these same rules of immobilisation apply to fractures treated with pin fixation. There are clearly situations in which the fixation afforded by a stable construct using K-wires can allow motion of an adjacent joint before complete immobilisation is discontinued. For example, condylar fractures of the proximal phalanx transfixed with two or three transverse K-wires can often be moved within a week or so of fixation providing that the patient is reliable. It is preferably done under the guidance of either the surgeon or hand therapist. Having outlined some of the etiologies of unsatisfactory results we will now discuss specific problems in the treatment of fractures and dislocations which can cause untoward sequelae.

DISTAL PHALANX

In general, fractures of the distal phalanx heal readily and without complications. The most common fracture is of the tuft of the distal phalanx resulting from a crush injury. These rarely need fixation other than a splint protecting the distal phalanx and immobilising the distal interphalangeal joint. Transverse fractures of the distal phalanx can however, be unstable and may angulate most often with the apex volar. This can result in an occasionally painful or cosmetically unappealing deformity of the fingertip and a possible nailplate abnormality as well. The problem may be obviated by fixing the fracture with a longitudinal Kirschner

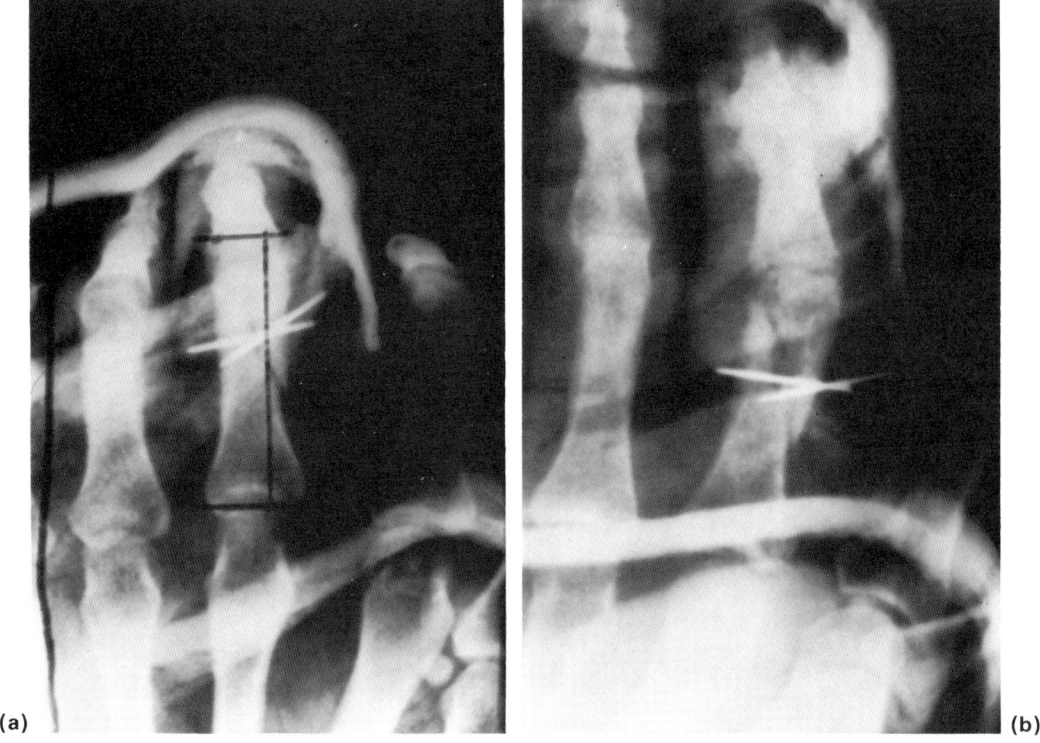

Fig. 19.5 (a) Demonstrates an oblique fracture of the proximal phalanx fairly well reduced and internally fixed with two closely spaced, crossed Kirschner wires. (b) Fixation is inadequate for an oblique fracture which displaces with the distal fragments sliding proximally along the obliquity of the fracture line

wire passed down the intramedullary canal of the distal phalanx and, if deemed necessary for proximal fixation, across the distal interphalangeal joint. Although most fractures of the distal phalanx heal readily it is incorrect to assume that non-unions never occur. Comminuted fractures including longitudinal components through the shaft of the phalanx caused by severe crush injuries are often accompanied by significant soft tissue trauma. In order to prevent non-union in widely displaced fragments one may reduce the fragments by gentle transverse pressure with a fracture clamp and transfix them with small (0.028 inch) Kirschner wires.

If a non-union does result, the patient may be symptomatic, experiencing pain with pressure on the finger tip. On the rare occasion where the patient is persistently symptomatic, union may be achieved with bone grafting. One of the authors (S.G.) has successfully treated a non-union of a fracture of the distal phalanx with electrical stimulation. The EBI (Electro Biology) company makes a small coil within which the finger can be placed to stimulate fracture healing. The patient developed a non-union of a distal phalangeal fracture which prevented him from doing his customary work as a mechanic. After treatment for 4 months with electrical stimulation the fracture healed and the finger became asymptomatic (Fig. 19.6).

Transverse fractures of the distal phalanx resulting from crush injuries can be complicated by interposition of the nail matrix between the fracture fragments preventing reduction and union. Any significant nail bed laceration should be meticulously debrided and repaired and, specifically in the presence of a transverse fracture of the distal phalanx, it should be very clearly demonstrated that the lacerated end of the nail matrix is not interposed between the fracture fragments. If it is, it may be gently withdrawn using either a dental probe or fine forceps and carefully repaired.

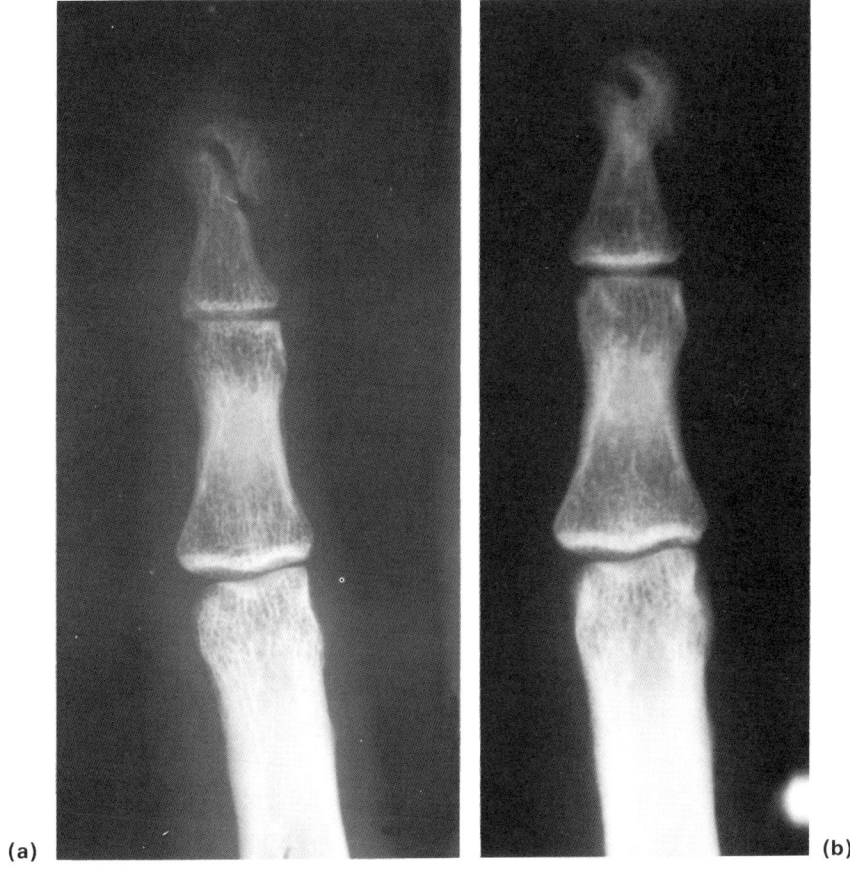

Fig. 19.6 (a) A 28 year old labourer with a non-union of an oblique fracture of the tuft of the distal phalanx of his dominant index finger 8 months after crush injury. (b) The non-union has healed after treatment for 4 months with noninvasive electrical stimulation

The fracture should then be reduced and, if necessary, transfixed with a small Kirschner wire (Fig. 19.7).

Dislocations of the distal interphalangeal joint are usually easily reducible but irreducible dislocations have been reported (Palmer & Linscheid 1977). Adequacy of reduction of a DIP dislocation must be confirmed radiographically and failure to achieve satisfactory reduction and stability should alert the surgeon to the possibility of volar plate or flexor digitorum profundus tendon interposition between the middle and distal phalanges. Irreducible dislocations must be opened, anatomically reduced and the volar plate repaired.

Suboptimal results in the treatment of mallet deformities occur with greater frequency than most hand surgeons would like to admit. The leading cause of failed treatment of soft tissue mallet fingers is patient non-compliance with the prescribed splinting regimen. The distal interphalangeal joint must be held in full extension for between 4 and 6 weeks with a splinting device of the practitioners choice. The patient is then gradually weaned from the splint. If the patient removes the splint during the course of treatment and allows the distal interphalangeal joint to flex the healing of the extensor tendon may be disrupted and a residual lag in the DIP joint result. Minor extension lags are tolerable as long as a swan-neck deformity does not result. A significant lag with or without an accompanying swan-neck deformity may require correction. Our preferred treatment

288 UNSATISFACTORY RESULTS IN HAND SURGERY

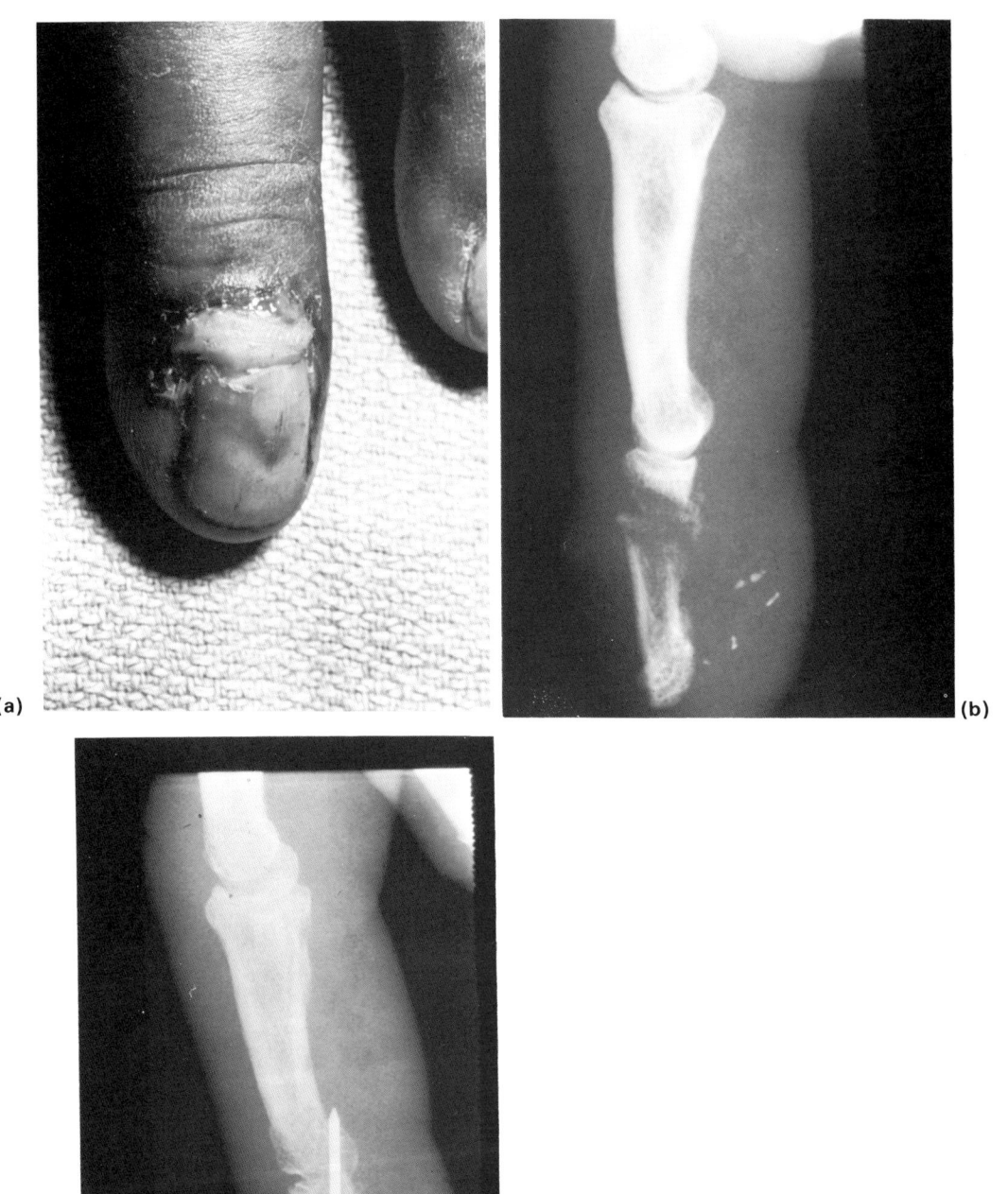

Fig. 19.7 (a) Previously untreated crush injury of the fingertip with nail matrix interposition between the fragments of a distal phalangeal fracture. (b) The fracture fragments are held apart by the interposed nail matrix preventing reduction and fracture healing. (c) The nail matrix has been removed from the fracture which has been reduced and internally fixed with a longitudinal Kirschner wire. (Reproduced with permission of Lea and Febiger, Philadelphia: Kilgore E S, Graham W P 1977 *The Hand. Surgical and non-surgical management*. Lea and Febiger, Philadelphia)

would be a spiral oblique retinacular ligament reconstruction as described by Littler (Thompson et al 1978). A significant lag with distal interphalangeal joint pain but without a swan-neck deformity may be definitively treated with distal interphalangeal joint fusion. Most bony mallet deformities with dorsal fragments representing less than 30% of the articular surface heal uneventfully with the same treatment program as a soft tissue mallet. If, however, the fracture fragment is larger, there is a step off in the articular surface and especially if there is volar subluxation of the distal phalanx a suboptimal result may follow. Most agree that subluxation of the distal phalanx should be corrected (Stark et al 1962). Persistent volar subluxation and incongruity in the articular surface is likely to result in painful degenerative changes in the DIP joint and may require an arthrodesis.

MIDDLE PHALANX

Most fractures of the middle phalanx result from crush injuries. This fact, combined with the thickness of the cortical bone and relative paucity of cancellous bone cause fractures of the middle phalanx to take longer to heal than those of the other phalanges. Fractures that can be adequately reduced should be immobilised for at least 4 weeks and if they appear unstable at the time of reduction may be internally stabilised with Kirschner wires. The simplest technique for fixing a transverse fracture of the middle phalanx is to pass a single longitudinal Kirschner wire down the intramedullary canal of the distal phalanx, across the distal interphalangeal joint and down the intramedullary canal of the middle phalanx. The DIP joint should be transfixed in slight flexion. In difficult circumstances, the PIP joint may be flexed and the wire introduced across the PIP joint, down the canal of the middle phalanx and across the DIP joint into the distal phalanx. The wire is then withdrawn distally so that its proximal end lies within the subchondral bone of the base of the middle phalanx and the PIP joint is left free. Another option would be crossed Kirschner wires with careful attention paid to assuring that the wires do not distract the fracture. Either inadequate fixation or too short a period of immobilisation may result in delayed or non-union. If the digit is mobilised too rapidly and the fracture is unstable, an angulatory malunion may ensue. If this is treated within 2–3 months of the original injury the fracture site may still be identified and gently teased apart with a scalpel or a slender osteotome. The angulatory deformity should be corrected and the osteotomy bone grafted and fixed with Kirschner wires. The likelihood of developing some stiffness of the DIP joint after such a procedure is significant.

PROXIMAL PHALANX

Fractures of the proximal phalanx are common. Their treatment may be fraught with problems. As previously discussed, both the flexor and extensor mechanisms are intimately applied to the periosteum of the proximal phalanx. Significant fibrosis resulting from a fracture or a bony spike projecting dorsally or volarly may result in adherence of the extensor or flexor mechanisms, respectively (Fig. 19.8). Whenever possible, fractures of the proximal phalanx should be treated closed in order to avoid the additional insult to the soft tissue created by the dissection necessary to achieve open reduction. Contrary to the opinion held by many authors (Huffaker et al 1979, James 1966), most fractures of the proximal phalanx can be treated by closed reduction and percutaneous internal fixation with Kirschner wires (Belsky et al 1984). In our experience, it is rare that a fracture of the proximal phalanx need be opened to be reduced. Reduction can almost always be accomplished by longitudinal traction with flexion, utilising intact soft tissue structures including the dorsal periosteum, flexor sheath, and the extensor mechanism to guide reduction. Transverse fractures most commonly occur in the junction of the proximal and middle third of the phalanx and tend to angulate volarly. Failure to reduce these fractures or failure to maintain their reduction will result in persistent angulatory deformity. If treated by plaster immobilisation, careful follow-up with serial radiographs must be obtained to document maintenance of the reduction. Our preferred method of treatment of these fractures is to reduce and transfix the fracture with a longitudinal Kirschner wire passed across

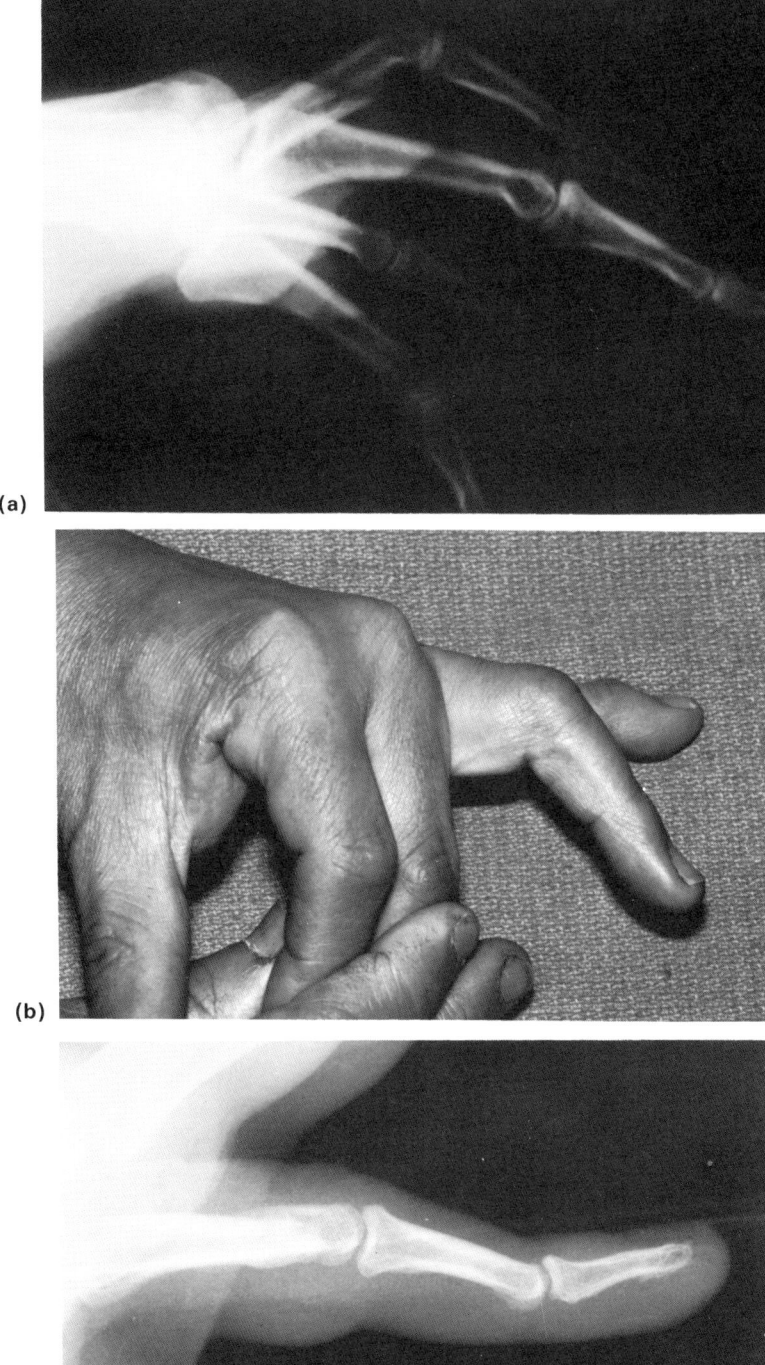

Fig. 19.8 (a) Lateral radiograph shows a fracture of the proximal phalanx with a large volar spike. Failure of reduction with persistence of the volar spike can result in adherence of the flexor digitorum superficialis tendon. (b) The result may be a flexion contracture of the PIP joint. (c) Another consequence of malunion of proximal phalangeal fractures with shortening of the phalanx is functional lengthening of the extensor mechanism and a boutonniere deformity

the metacarpophalangeal joint and down the intramedullary canal. Rotational control is provided by the dressing and cast.

Oblique fractures of the proximal phalanx are also common and can lead to poor results. These fractures are frequently unstable and have a potential for rotational deformities of the digit. Rotation often cannot be assessed radiographically and must be determined by clinical examination. With the digit anaesthetised, the patient should pass the affected finger through an arc of motion and the alignment be assessed. If there is any rotational deformity, as manifested by crossing over of two adjacent digits, this must be corrected. During flexion of the digits, the fingernails, particularly the middle fingernail, tend to point toward the distal pole of the scaphoid when they are anatomically aligned. The goal of reduction is anatomic alignment. It is very difficult to hold reduction with plaster alone. Our preferred treatment is to reduce the fracture with flexion of the MP and PIP joints and longitudinal traction. Reduction can be held with a fracture clamp applied transversely transfixing the two fracture fragments. Two or more transversely oriented Kirschner wires usually adequately fix the fracture. The pins should remain in place for approximately $3\frac{1}{2}$ weeks. Failure to achieve or maintain reduction may result in a persistent rotational deformity which would have to be corrected by osteotomy. If necessary, the osteotomy should be performed through the proximal flare of the proximal phalanx. Osteotomy through the metacarpal may result in malalignment of the metacarpophalangeal joint.

Intercondylar fractures of the proximal phalanx are unstable (James 1966, Steel 1978, Strickland et al 1982). The distal fracture fragment may slide proximally along the obliquity of the fracture line. This results in incongruity of the joint and, if allowed to heal unreduced, a transverse tilting of the articular surface which is manifested by an angulatory and sometimes rotatory deformity of the digit through the PIP joint (Fig. 19.9). If undisplaced, it is frequently wise to pass a percutaneous wire across the condyles to prevent displacement. If displaced, intercondylar fractures of the proximal phalanx should be reduced either closed or, if necessary, opened and transfixed with either Kirschner wires or an AO mini fragment screw. Early mobilisation of the PIP joint can be instituted if the fixation is stable.

Fractures of the neck of the proximal phalanx which angulate volarly result in dorsal displacement of the distal fragment. If allowed to heal, one consequence of the malunion can be a bony block to flexion caused by the prominent volar spike projecting into the retrocondylar space, blocking PIP flexion. If a malunion is recognised early on, it can be carefully taken down by gently osteotomising the phalanx along the line of the previous fracture. If union and remodelling has occurred and the problem is treated months after the injury, the volar spike preventing full flexion can be removed through a midaxial approach. One or both collateral ligaments may need to be resected if full flexion is not gained. Any intra-articular fracture of the proximal or middle phalangeal components of the proximal interphalangeal joint which results in a significant step off in the articular surface must be reduced and fixed anatomically. Otherwise, there is a strong potential for developing degenerative changes in the joint.

Most dislocations of the PIP joint are dorsal and can be easily reduced (Eaton 1971). Dorsal dislocations result in disruption of the volar plate which must be allowed to heal. This is most easily accomplished by splinting the joint with a dorsal block splint in 20 to 30 degrees of flexion for approximately 3 weeks. If dorsal dislocations are not maintained in flexion, incompetence of the volar plate resulting from this situation or simple hyperextension injury of the PIP joint rupturing the plate can be successfully treated with a superficialis tenodesis (Adams 1959, Swanson 1960). Volar dislocations of the PIP joint are less common and must be recognised as distinct from dorsal or lateral dislocations. In volar dislocation, there may be avulsion of the insertion of the central tendon from the base of the middle phalanx or a longitudinal rent in the extensor mechanism. Such volar or rotatory dislocations are often described as irreducible. The majority, however, can be reduced closed using traction with flexion and rotation to disengage the 'buttonholed' condyle from between the lateral band and central slip of the extensor mechanism. Once reduced, the finger is tested for active extension which is usually possible through the contralateral lateral band. The finger is then either splinted in full extension or a dynamic extension splint (e.g. spring splint) is applied maintaining the PIP in full extension but permitting some active flexion to prevent stiffness.

If closed reduction or full active extension and flexion cannot be achieved, open reduction to remove interposed soft tissue must be done and the extensor mechanism repaired. The collateral ligament does not need to be repaired.

Fracture dislocations of the proximal interphalangeal joint may be fraught with difficulty and frequently there is some loss of motion in the joint. These injuries may be difficult to treat primarily and, when missed, are even more difficult to treat secondarily. If the volar fracture fragment of the middle phalangeal articular surface is less than 40% of the articular surface, dislocation may be able to be reduced and will be stable as long as the PIP joint is held in flexion during the initial period of immobilisation. PIP fracture dislocations which are stable after reduction in flexion can be treated by dorsal extension block splinting as described by McElfresh et al (1972). Beware of inadequate radiographs which may not demonstrate the dorsal subluxation of the middle phalanx. Healing in this position results in a serious incongruity of the PIP articular surface. Patients, athletic trainers and many physicians have a tendency to dismiss injuries to the PIP joint as 'jammed fingers'. As a result, PIP fracture dislocations not uncommonly present

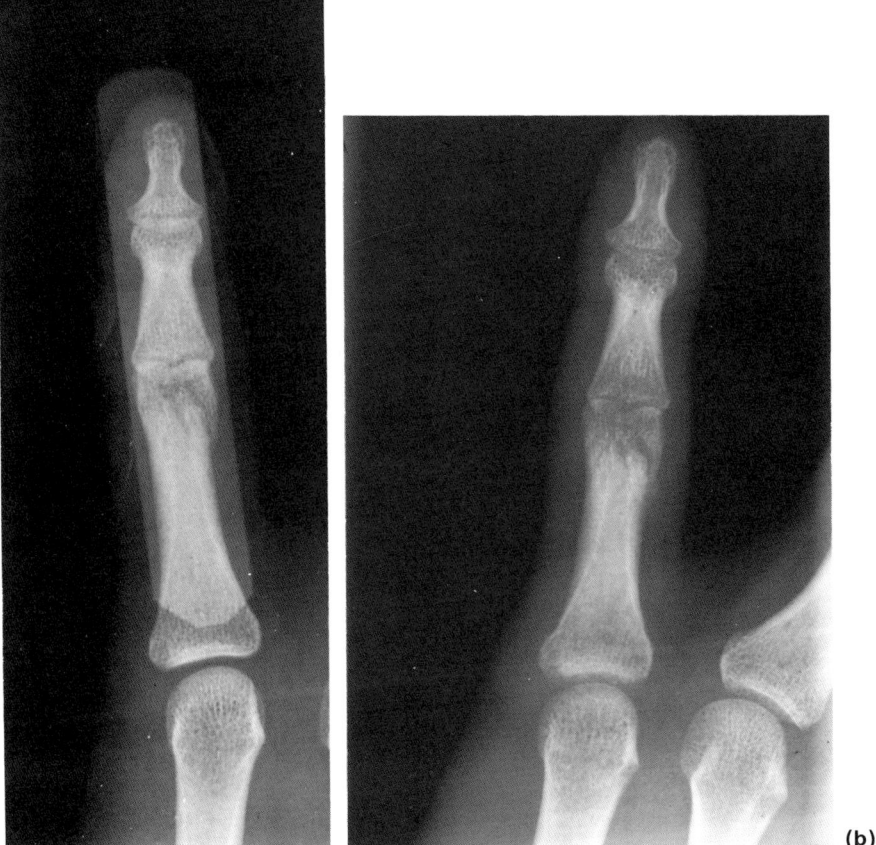

Fig. 19.9 (a) Intercondylar fractures of the proximal phalanx are unstable. This fracture in a professional athlete was treated with a dorsal aluminum splint. (b) After 3 weeks of splinting the fracture of the condyle had subsided proximally slightly but was felt to be healed. (c) The patient returned to athletics and the condyle grossly displaced. (d) At 5 weeks post-injury an open reduction and internal fixation with transverse Kirschner wires was performed. Because of the inherent instability of these fractures, they should be percutaneously pinned with transverse wires at the time of injury

long after the injury. In this instance, or in the case of an acute injury in which the subluxation cannot be reduced, correction must be achieved or limited motion in the joint and eventual osteoarthritis is likely to result. The authors' recommended treatment of this problem is the volar plate arthroplasty described by Eaton (1980). The fracture fragments of the volar base of the middle phalanx are removed and the volar plate is advanced into the defect. This effectively resurfaces the joint and provides stability to prevent recurrent dorsal subluxation.

METACARPAL

Fractures of the shaft and neck of the metacarpals generally angulate dorsally with the distal fragment displaced volarly. There is considerable debate about what degree of angulation of metacarpal fractures, particularly of the metacarpal neck, is acceptable. This discussion is centred principally around the ring and little metacarpals in which some dorsal angulation can be tolerated. The same is not true of the index and middle metacarpals which are part of the fixed unit of the hand having minimal potential for compensatory realignment. Fractures of the ring and little metacarpals often occur during altercations and patients may be reticent about seeking treatment. Most shaft and neck fractures of the ring and little finger metacarpals are treated by closed reduction and immobilisation in either an ulnar gutter splint or a short arm cast incorporating the ring and little fingers. The deforming forces which created the initial angulation, i.e. the flexor tendons and intrinsic muscles, may cause reangulation of the fracture in plaster. This is particularly true in the hand which is swollen at the time of cast application and becomes less edematous with immobilisation and elevation. If these fractures are not followed radiographically

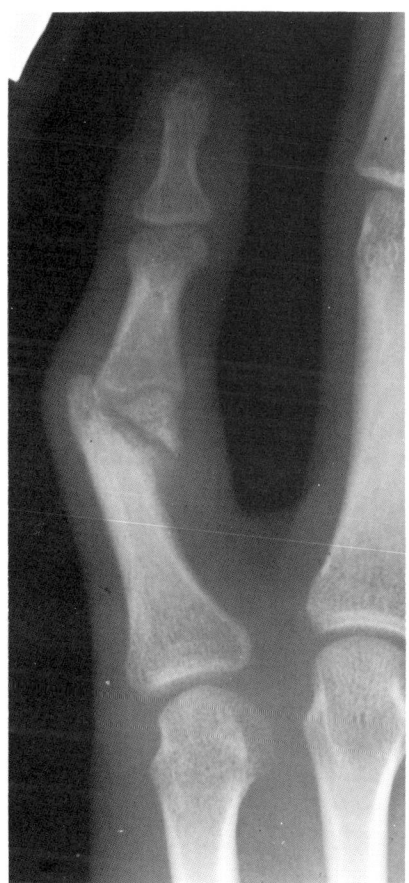

(c)

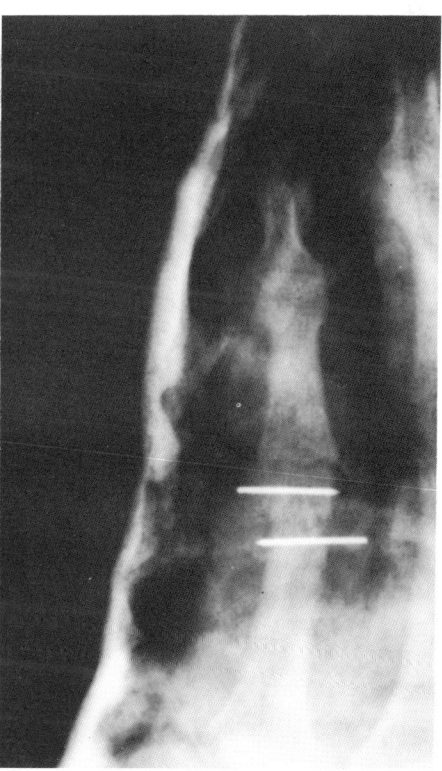

(d)

at short intervals after reduction, an angulatory malunion can occur. The degree of deformity obviously depends upon the degree of angulation and upon the level in the metacarpal at which the angulation occurs. Dorsal angulation in the midshaft results from flexion of the distal fragment creating a considerable depression of the metacarpal head with prominence of the fracture on the dorsum and of the head in the palm. This may represent a significant cosmetic deformity with loss of normal contour of the metacarpophalangeal joint and a dorsal prominence at the fracture site. Dorsal angulation of fractures of the metacarpal neck may present less of a problem. Many authors accept up to 40 degrees of angulation and others even accept as much as 70 degrees (Hunter & Cowen 1970). Nevertheless, dorsal angulation of the metacarpal neck of the ring or little fingers may not be as trivial a deformity as assumed. Here too, there is a loss of the normal contour of the metacarpophalangeal joint with the head depressed into the palm. This prominence in the palm can be uncomfortable in manual labourers who must perform power gripping particularly using tools like hammers and pliers. Athletes such as baseball players and golfers also find prominence of the metacarpal head in the palm uncomfortable. Dorsally angulated metacarpal neck and shaft fractures may result in a zigzag deformity at the adjacent PIP joint with hyperextension of the MP joint and compensatory flexion at the PIP joint. These fractures should be primarily reduced as anatomically as possible. The reduction should be maintained either by cast immobilisation in a well moulded plaster or, as is our preference, by a Kirschner passed down the intramedullary canal of the metacarpal. This form of K-wire fixation is simple, easy to perform and rarely accompanied by complications. The result can be an anatomic reduction with none of the attendant problems mentioned above.

Oblique fractures of the metacarpals have a tendency to shorten and may rotate as well. Any rotational deformity must be corrected. Whereas shortening of the metacarpal theoretically can reduce power grip if the shortening is of significant proportions, this shortening is also apparent as a cosmetic deformity with a 'sunken' metacarpal. It may be difficult to hold reduction of oblique metacarpal fractures. A fracture clamp may be applied transversely across the fracture and transverse Kirschner wires placed percutaneously. Sometimes sufficient contact between the proximal and distal fragments is achieved by the reduction so that a longitudinal pin placed down the intramedullary canal of the metacarpal will maintain longitudinal alignment and the interlocking of the bony spicules of the fracture will prevent rotation. The AO group recommends open fixation of oblique fractures of the metacarpals using interfragmentary screws. Immediate motion may be begun postoperatively.

Metacarpal head and neck fractures may be accompanied by human bite injuries when the fracture results from metacarpal tooth contact. These wounds are contaminated with mouth bacterial flora which may have inoculated the joint at the time of impact. Patients who suffer this kind of injury are sometimes hesitant to admit the circumstances of the injury or do so only after significant infection has developed. If the tooth injury is only subcutaneous a localised cellulitis may result. If, however, the joint has been inoculated, septic arthritis often caused by virulent organisms may ensue. If untreated, the result can be catastrophic for the joint. The articular cartilage may be destroyed within as brief a period as 48 hours. If the patient does present primarily after the injury, the wound must be carefully inspected and debrided. If there is any doubt about the joint having been inoculated it should be explored, debrided and irrigated and the wound left open. The patient should be admitted to the hospital for intravenous antibiotics, splinting and elevation.

Fractures of the base of the metacarpals may occur in the metaphysis or may be intra-articular. There is a tendency for fractures of the metaphysis to dorsally angulate. It is important in any fracture or dislocation of the base of the metacarpal to obtain good radiographs. A lateral of the hand may obscure angulation at the fracture site or subluxation of the metacarpal base. A 20 degree pronated lateral may help demonstrate the deformity. Unreduced intra-articular fractures or, less commonly, dislocations of the CMC joint can produce progressive degenerative changes in the joint with significant pain and disability. Attempts should be made to reduce dislocations of the CMC joint even if they are several weeks old. The reduction should be performed open and fibrous tissue which has accumulated within the joint space removed. Fixation should be maintained with Kirschner wires for at least 4 weeks. Late arthritic changes may be treated either with fusion (Clendenin & Smith 1984) or interposition arthroplasty.

THE THUMB

Sir Charles Bell in 1833 noted that 'on the length, strength, free lateral motion and perfect mobility of the thumb depends the power of the human hand'. Compensation boards customarily attribute 40% of hand function to the thumb alone. The ability to position the thumb in space with dexterity and force is crucial for both power grasp, pinch and fine manipulation with the opposing digits. Unsatisfactory results in the treatment of fractures and dislocations of the thumb can detract from that delicate balance of form and function which is so critical to the integrity of the hand. Particular attention must therefore be paid to the prompt recognition and appropriate primary treatment of injuries to the thumb axis.

Fractures of the distal phalanx of the thumb are less common than in digits. Tuft fractures occurring as the result of crush injuries usually respond to conservative treatment with splinting and go on to heal uneventfully. However, a laissez faire approach to fractures of the base and shaft of the distal phalanx may lead to an unsatisfactory result of treatment. Transverse fractures of the shaft are often dismissed as being stable injuries with the fracture fragments constrained by the vertical fibrous septae of the thumb tip. Such fractures may be inadvisably splinted by the primary care physician and the patient told to return in 3–4 weeks for follow-up. In the interim, the fracture becomes less and less tender and the patient is inclined to use the tip of the thumb more liberally for activities requiring forceful key and tip pinch and gripping. Direct pressure on the tip of the thumb tends to displace the distal fragment dorsally and efforts to flex the interphalangeal joint of the thumb cause the proximal fragment to be displaced volarly because of the pull of the insertion of the flexor pollicus longus on the base of the distal phalanx. The consequence is to create volar angulation at the fracture. Repetitive overuse can cause delayed union of these fractures and failure to obtain follow-up X-rays in a splint can allow volar angulation to go unrecognised and malunion to result. If these fractures are treated with a simple dorsal aluminium splint or a Stack splint it is imperative that radiographs be obtained at frequent intervals in the first 2 weeks after injury in order to assure that the fracture is not displacing. In the less compliant patient more satisfactory immobilisation of the distal phalanx and distal interphalangeal joint may be achieved at the expense of immobilising the entire thumb and wrist for a 3–4 week period in a thumb spica cast brought out to the tip of the thumb. The most definitive way to immobilise these transverse distal phalangeal fractures is to pass a Kirschner wire down the intramedullary canal of the distal phalanx and across the distal interphalangeal joint. This should be augmented by external support either with a splint over the proximal and distal phalanges or a cast as described above. If a tendency toward volar angulation of a conservatively treated transverse fracture is recognised during the first 2 weeks of treatment, it may well be able to be corrected by a closed reduction manoeuver. If a volarly angulated malunion has occurred it can either be accepted if the angulation is minimal and asymptomatic or corrected with a volar closing wedge osteotomy if the volar prominence is tender with the use of the thumb or if an unacceptable cosmetic deformity results.

Intra-articular fractures of the interphalangeal joint of the thumb may result from crush injuries. Failure to achieve anatomic reduction may presage the development of osteoarthritis in the joint. If the fracture is a non-comminuted disruption of either the head of the proximal phalanx or base of the distal phalanx reduction can often be achieved closed utilising the lateral compression which may be achieved with a fracture clamp. When the fracture gap has been closed it can be transfixed with transverse Kirschner wires. These fractures should be opened only if closed reduction cannot be achieved. In that event, internal fixation can be achieved either with Kirschner wires or mini fragment screws applied perpendicular to the long axis of the phalanx. Collateral ligament and volar plate injuries of the interphalangeal joint of the thumb can cause instability and degenerative changes in the joint if they are unrecognised initially. Primary healing of a disrupted collateral ligament or volar plate can almost invariably be achieved by splinting the interphalangeal joint in 20 degrees of flexion. The only instance in which open treatment need be considered is if the ruptured soft tissue structure has become interposed within the joint which cannot be reduced closed.

Unlike ligament injuries of the interphalangeal joint, collateral ligament injuries of the metacarpophalangeal joint frequently need to be opened. Failure to recognise or appropriately treat ulnar collateral ligament injuries of the metacarpophalangeal joint of the thumb can result in permanent disability due to degenerative changes in the joint if instability results. This can be avoided by recognition of complete tears. This assessment can almost always be made clinically. If the metacarpophalangeal joint of the injured thumb opens 30 degrees more than the uninjured thumb MP joint with radially directed stress and if this opening of the ulnar joint line has no firm end point, the ligament should be considered ruptured until proven otherwise. In the setting of an acute injury, an occasional patient is too anxious and guarding too much to allow a satisfactory exam. This problem may be obviated by placing radial and median nerve blocks and repeating the exam. Stress radiographs may be used to add confirmatory evidence of opening of the ulnar joint line but are only helpful if the exam is performed by the clinician. In our experience which coincides with Stener's observation, a large majority of complete tears of the ulnar collateral ligament of the MP joint are accompanied by Stener lesions (Stener 1962). In this instance the distal stump of the ruptured ligament lies deep and the proximal stump lies superficial to the adductor aponeurosis. The torn collateral ligament cannot heal if a Stener lesion is present. Therefore, clinical evidence of a complete tear is an indication for operative repair. The Stener lesion does not occur on the radial side of the thumb metacarpophalangeal joint.

If the radial joint line opens 30 degrees more on the injured than the uninjured side with ulnar directed stress, that is strongly suggestive of a complete tear of the radial collateral ligament. If there is no evidence of volar subluxation of the proximal phalanx on the lateral radiograph, these can be treated by immobilisation in a thumb spica cast. If, however, there is volar subluxation of the proximal phalanx on the lateral radiograph, this is indicative of a more extensive tear which involves the dorsal capsule as well as the ligament. These should be opened and repaired surgically. If a ruptured MP collateral ligament is unrecognised or inadequately treated initially late instability results. If the instability has not progressed to degenerative disease of the metacarpophalangeal joint, our preferred treatment is ligament reconstruction using a palmaris longus tendon graft passed through two vertically oriented drill holes on the base of the proximal phalanx and a single drill hole in the neck of the metacarpal. The same form of reconstruction can be used on the radial or ulnar side. If degenerative changes have supervened, MP arthrodesis is a very satisfactory solution.

Fractures of the thumb metacarpal occur most commonly in the proximal third of the bone. Attempts to treat transversely oriented fractures of the base of the thumb metacarpal with plaster or splint immobilisation alone is a potential cause of an unfavourable result. These fractures tend to angulate dorsally because the abductor pollicus longus tends to extend the proximal fragment and the intrinsic muscles tend to flex the distal fragment. In order to prevent angulation, these fractures should be internally stabilized. This can usually be done with closed reduction and percutaneous pin fixation passing a 0.045 inch Kirschner wire down the intermedullary canal of the metacarpal from distal to proximal through the dorsal aspect of the metacarpal head (Fig. 19.10).

Fractures of the base of the thumb metacarpal involving the articular surface can easily become complicated if treatment is not optimal. The first step in optimal treatment is recognition of the fracture. It is crucial that a true lateral radiograph of the thumb metacarpal be obtained. To be certain that a radiograph is a true lateral one should see superimposition of the MP volar plate sesamoids.

Closed reduction and plaster immobilisation of Bennett's or Rolando's fractures may be complicated by loss of reduction in plaster and resultant

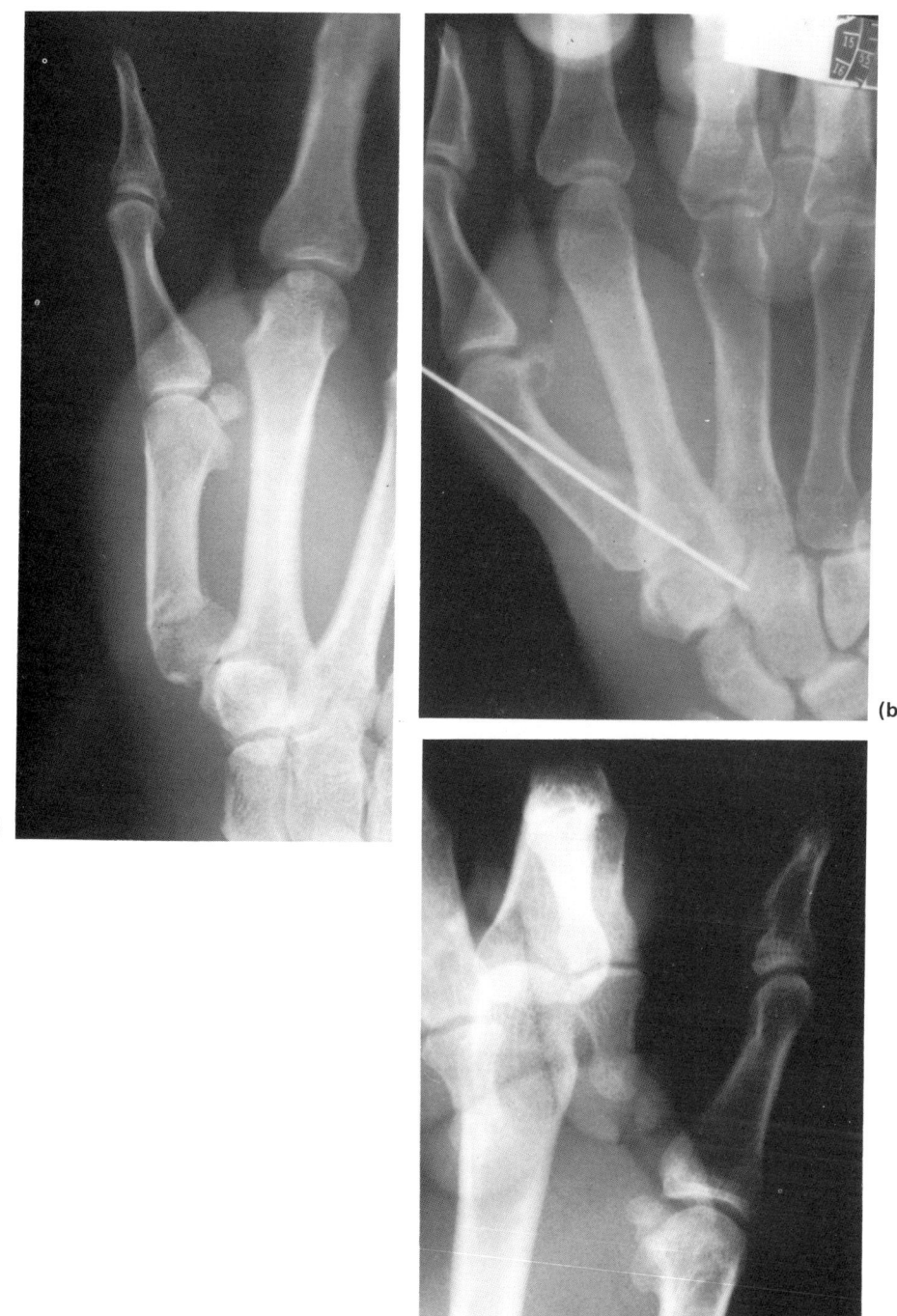

Fig. 19.10 (a) Nonarticular fractures of the base of the thumb metacarpal tend to angulate dorsally. The proximal fragment is extended by the abductor pollicus longus and the distal fragment is flexed by the flexor pollicus brevis. Plaster immobilisation is often inadequate to control these muscle forces and progressive angulation ensues. (b) These fractures should be internally stabilised to prevent angulation. (c) Failure to reduce and fix fractures of the thumb metacarpal base can result in malunion which may be first noticed when cast immobilisation is discontinued if serial radiographs have not been obtained

incongruity of the articular surface. The end result of significant incongruity or a step off in the joint surface is osteoarthritis. Internal fixation is indicated in most of these fractures. Whether or not this is done closed or opened depends on the adequacy of the closed reduction. The reduction manoeuvre entails longitudinal traction, extension and pronation of the thumb metacarpal along with direct pressure on the base of the metacarpal. Anatomic reduction should be strived for. Any step off of the fracture fragments causing incongruity in the articular surface is considered unacceptable. A small gap between the two fracture fragments in a Bennett's fracture or a non-comminuted Rolando's fracture is not ideal but can be accepted as long as the gap is no greater than 2 mm. Our preferred fixation of Bennett's fractures which can be adequately reduced is done in one of two ways. In the first and more difficult technique, the dominant metacarpal fragment is reduced to the volar fracture fragment and the two are transfixed with a transverse Kirschner wire. The metacarpal is held reduced on the trapezium with a longitudinal or oblique Kirschner wire transfixing the metacarpal and trapezium. The second technique which is simpler and quite satisfactory is to achieve a closed reduction and secure fixation by passing a longitudinal Kirschner wire down the intramedullary canal of the thumb metacarpal transfixing it in a reduced position to the trapezium. Since the volar fragment is usually small and stable and the longitudinal pin holds the dominant, dorsal frag-

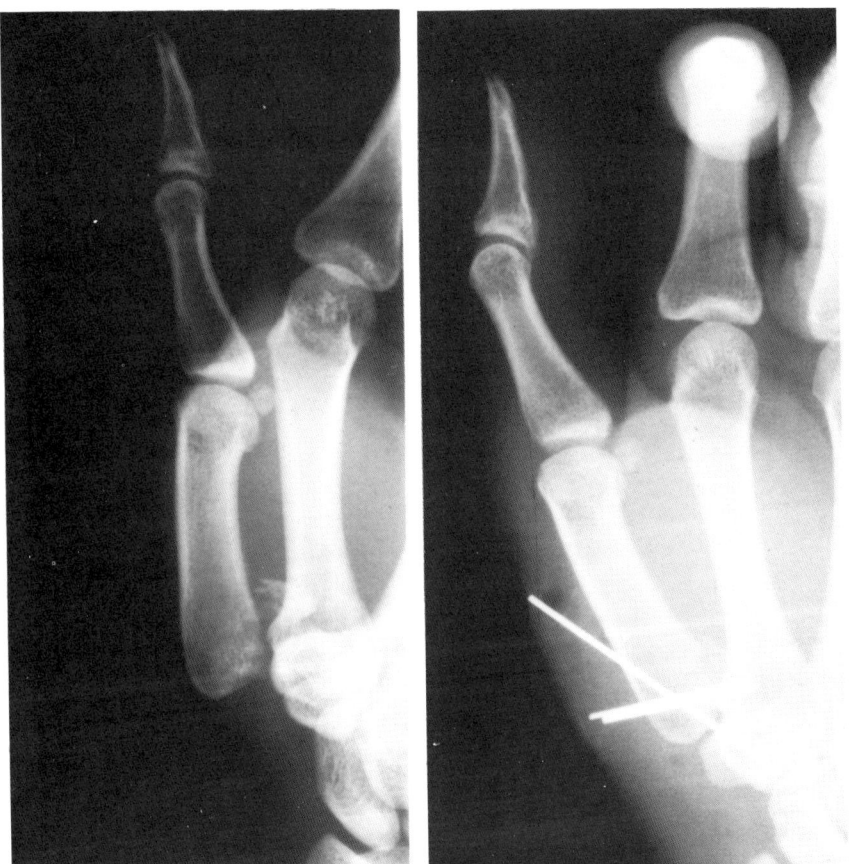

(a) (b)

Fig. 19.11 (a) A 28 year old bicyclist suffered a Bennett's fracture of his dominant thumb which was untreated for 7 weeks. The thumb metacarpal is grossly subluxed. (b) Open reduction allowed the thumb metacarpal to be reduced and transfixed to the intact volar fracture fragment. (c) and (d) The fracture healed and the trapeziometacarpal joint remains stable. The patient has full painless range of motion

ment, this fixation is adequate. Unsuccessful efforts at closed reduction necessitate open reduction and internal fixation of a Bennett's or Rolando's fracture. We prefer to expose the carpometacarpal joint of the thumb using a modified Wagner approach (Wagner 1950). The degree of comminution of the fracture is invariably worse on direct examination than it is radiographically. Reduction may not be easy even under direct vision. After reduction, internal fixation can be achieved using Kirschner wires in a manner similar to that described above. The only modification is that the transverse wire fixing the volar fragments can be passed from within the intramedullary canal of the bone out through the dorsal cortex of the metacarpal and skin and then retrogradely passed across the volar fracture fragment after reduction is achieved. The thumb metacarpal should be transfixed to the trapezium to prevent loss of reduction. Another method of fixation is the use of an interfragmentary AO mini-screw fixing the base of the dominant metacarpal fragment to the volar fragment. The use of AO mini-plates has been described but has the disadvantage of involving more significant stripping of the soft tissues to apply the hardware than the other techniques mentioned.

Failure of recognition or inadequacy of treatment of a Bennett's fracture can have disastrous consequences. Incongruity of the carpometacarpal joint of the thumb may lead to degenerative changes with ensuing pain, weakness and loss of motion. If an unreduced Bennett's fracture is recognised reasonably early, attempt can be made to do a 'delayed primary' or 'secondary' reduction and internal fixation. The limits of 'reasonably early' recognition are by no means well defined. Previously untreated Bennett's fractures can be open reduced as late as 7 weeks after the injury with achievement of a satisfactory reduction and

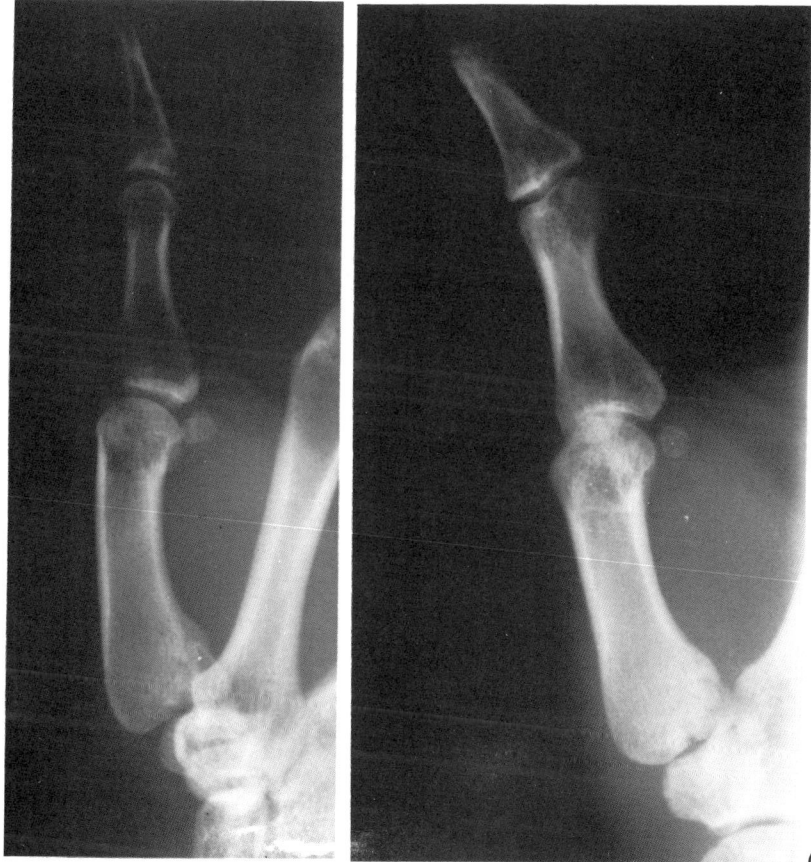

(c)   (d)

excellent clinical result (Fig. 19.11). If a secondary reduction is impossible, an alternative is to excise the volar fragment and reconstruct the volar ligament of the CMC joint. If the articular cartilage of the joint is in good condition at the time of exploration the volar ligament can be reconstructed using the technique described by Eaton & Littler (1973). If there is significant erosion of the articular cartilage of the CMC joint, it is necessary to resurface the joint using a fascial interposition arthroplasty and reconstruct the volar ligament (Eaton et al 1985). In this technique, the same approach is used as in the ligament reconstruction but the proximal portion of the flexor carpi radialis tendon strip used for the reconstruction is interposed in the joint space as an arthroplasty. The distally based portion of the strip of the FCR is used for the ligament reconstruction. Other techniques of resurfacing of the trapeziometacarpal joint of the thumb have been described with good results reported (Ashworth et al 1977). However, if the metacarpal is subluxed to any degree, reconstruction of the volar ligament should be considered.

Dislocations of the trapeziometacarpal joint are uncommon. If such a dislocation is reduced primarily but there is persistent laxity in the joint due to incompetence of the ligaments, there may be late subluxation and eventual degeneration. After reduction of a dislocation of the trapeziometacarpal joint, the patient should be allowed to take the joint through a range of motion and the joint should be gently stressed by the examiner to assure clinical stability. If the joint is stable, it should be immobilised in a short arm thumb spica cast for 4–5 weeks. If, however, the joint remains unstable after reduction, a primary volar ligament reconstruction is an effective way to restore stability.

REFERENCES

Adams J P 1959 Correction of chronic dorsal subluxation of the proximal interphalangeal joint by means of a criss-cross volar graft. Journal of Bone and Joint Surgery 41A:111

Ashworth C R, Blatt G, Chuinard R G, Stark H H 1977 Silicone rubber interposition arthroplasty for the carpometacarpal joint of the thumb. The Journal of Hand Surgery 2:345–351

Belsky M R, Eaton R G, Lane L B 1984 Closed reduction and internal fixation of proximal phalangeal fractures. The Journal of Hand Surgery 9A:725–729

Clendenin M B, Smith R J 1984 Fifth metacarpal/hamate arthrodesis for post-traumatic osteoarthritis. The Journal of Hand Surgery 9A:374–378

Eaton R G 1971 Joint Injuries of the Hand. Charles C Thomas, Springfield, Illinois

Eaton R G, Glickel S Z, Littler J W 1985 Tendon interposition arthroplasty for degenerative arthritis of the trapeziometacarpal joint of the thumb. The Journal of Hand Surgery 10A:645–654

Eaton R G, Malerich M M 1980 Volar plate arthroplasty of the proximal interphalangeal joint: A review of ten years' experience. The Journal of Hand Surgery 5:260–268

Eaton R G, Littler J W 1973 Ligament reconstruction for the painful thumb carpometacarpal joint. Journal of Bone and Joint Surgery 55A:1655–1666

Huffaker W H, Wray R C, Weeks P M 1979 Factors influencing final range of motion in the fingers after fractures of the hand. Plastic and Reconstructive Surgery 63:82–87

Hunter J M, Cowen N J 1970 Fifth metacarpal fractures in a compensation clinic population. Journal of Bone and Joint Surgery 52A:1159–1165

James J I P 1966 Fractures of the phalanges and metacarpals. Proceedings of the British Club for Surgery of the Hand, London

McElfresh E C, Dobyns J H, O'Brien E T 1972 Management of fracture-dislocation of the proximal interphalangeal joints by extension block splinting. Journal of Bone and Joint Surgery 54A:1705–1711

Palmer A K, Linscheid R L 1977 Irreducible dorsal dislocation of a distal interphalangeal joint of the finger. The Journal of Hand Surgery 2:406–408

Stark H H, Boyes J H, Wilson J N 1962 Mallet finger. Journal of Bone and Joint Surgery 44A:1061–1068

Steel W M 1978 The A.O. small fragment set in hand fractures. The Hand 10:246–253

Stener B 1962 Displacement of the ruptured ulnar collateral ligament of the metacarpophalangeal joint of the thumb—a clinical and anatomical study. Journal of Bone and Joint Surgery 44B:869–879

Strickland J W, Steichen J B, Kleinman W B, Hastings H, Flynn N 1982 Phalangeal fractures. Factors influencing digital performance. Orthopaedic Review 11:39–50

Swanson A B 1960 Surgery of the hand in cerebral palsy and the swan-neck deformity. Journal of Bone and Joint Surgery 42A:951

Thompson J S, Littler J W, Upton J 1978 The spiral oblique retinacular ligament (SORL). The Journal of Hand Surgery 3:482–487

Wagner C J 1950 Method of treatment of Bennett's fracture dislocation. American Journal of Surgery 80:230.

20 Wrist injuries

F. M. Howard

Watson and associates (1984) demonstrated that the mechanics of wrist motion require a stable, functioning radio-lunate joint. Fortunately, this joint often is the last to undergo degenerative change in the series of destructive changes associated with osteoarthritis and traumatic arthritis (Fig. 20.1). Why is it that a wrist with severe traumatic changes can function surprisingly well over many years (Fig. 20.2), yet a wrist which has seemingly minor changes becomes painful and disabling?

WRIST KINEMATICS

For the wrist to function properly Kauer (1974) has stressed the importance of each carpal bone maintaining its own space. Once this territorial imperative is lost, the mechanics of the associated carpals are altered and the wrist falls into a pathological state with ensuing degenerative changes. The anatomical relationship between the scaphoid and lunate, triquetrum, hamate, and capitate should be accurately maintained to provide

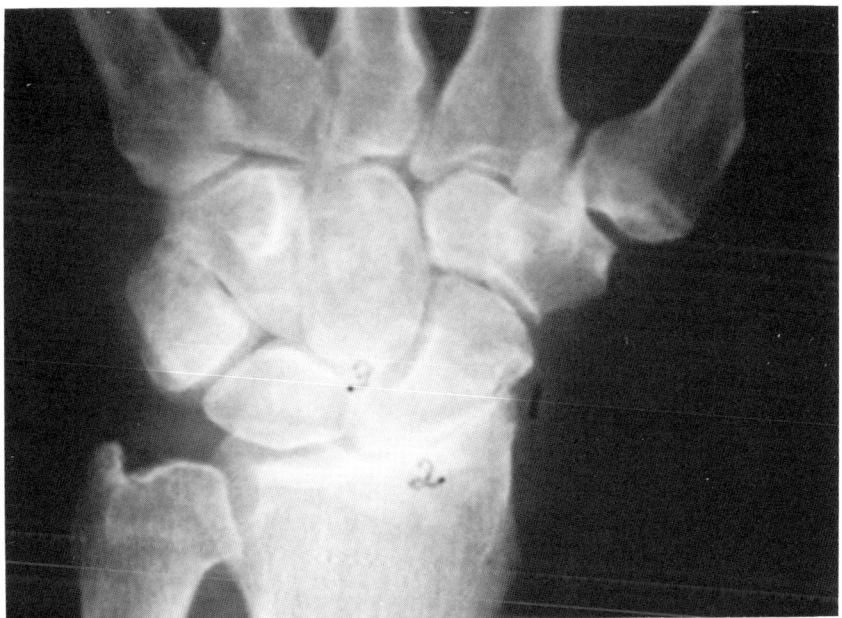

Fig. 20.1 Progression of degenerative arthritis of the wrist. The disease starts at the tip of the radial styloid (1) and adjacent waist level of the scaphoid (2) and skips to the lunate-capitate articulation (3). The radial-lunate joint is frequently spared

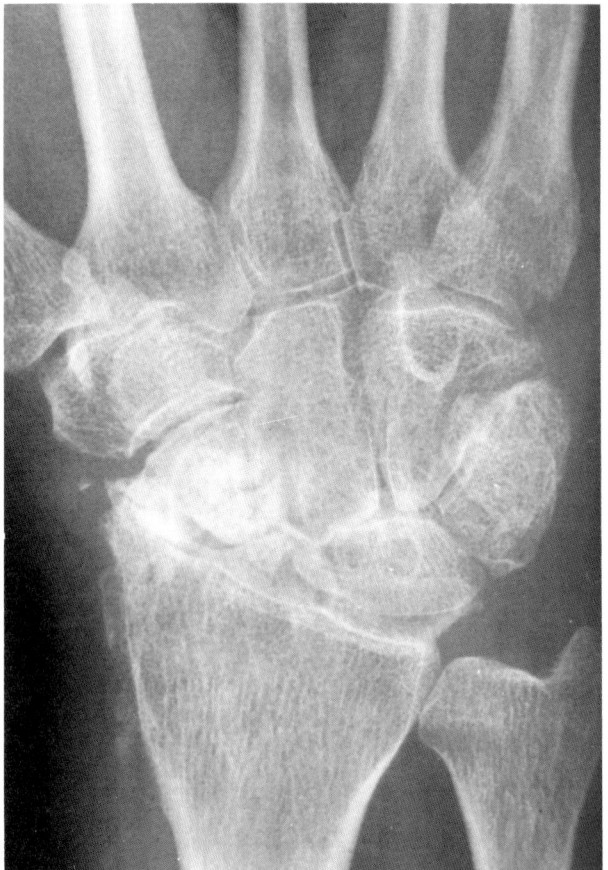

Fig. 20.2 55 year old ex-army pilot who incurred a fracture of the scaphoid 40 years before. He was unaware of this fracture until a second injury 40 years later caused pain and X-ray evaluation; grip strength and range of motion was about 40% normal. Note degenerative areas cited in Fig. 20.1 with functioning radial-lunate joint

on gross measurements of carpal motion and function. For the most part, our understanding came from the pathological and injured wrist while our understanding of the normal wrist is still elementary and pedestrian. Often, our measurements of the X-ray films can be off by 10 to 15 degrees of error. Hopefully, more accurate, precise measurements of carpal motion will be forthcoming as Weeks (1985), Belsole (1985), and others pursue the mathematical manipulation of three dimensional images offered by the computered tomogram scanner (Fig. 20.5). The shape, motion, contact, and position changes in the carpals must be thoroughly understood before we can grasp the abnormal, distorted kinematics of wrist motion (Fig. 20.6).

Faced with our primitive knowledge of the

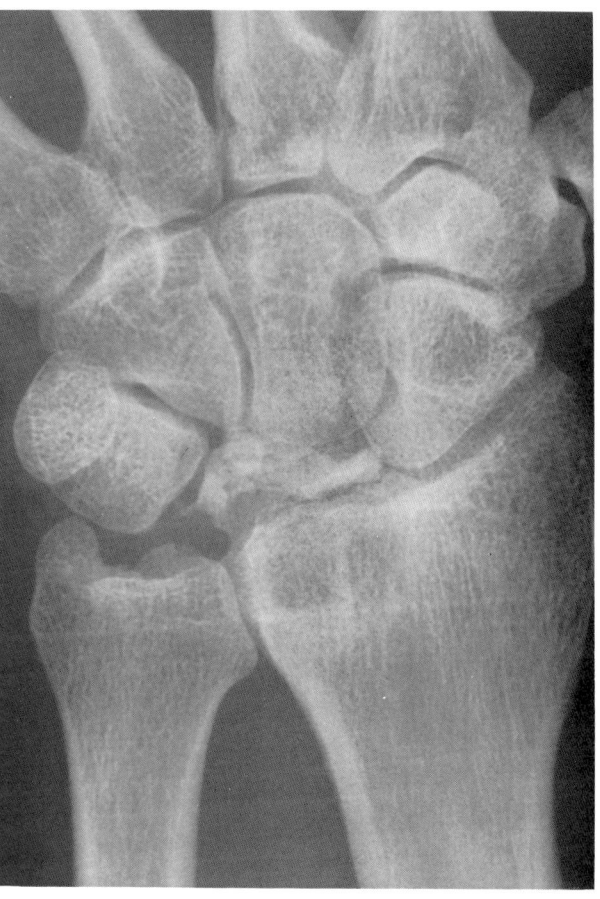

Fig. 20.3 Kienbock's avascular necrosis of lunate. The radial-lunate joint has completely collapsed and is severely painful. Note adjacent radius cyst and rotation of scaphoid

synergistic motion between the scaphoid and lunate (Fig. 20.3).

The triquetrum and the scaphoid are the stabilising pillars for the lunate to work with the radius and the capitate (Fig. 20.4). If the restraining influence of the proximal pole of the scaphoid is lost, the lunate drifts into a dorsal displacement or into a palmar subluxation. Similarly, if the triquetrum's influence is lost, the lunate can drift and become unstable. Since most injuries to the wrist involve the lunate–scaphoid–capitate complex, we shall restrict this chapter to that area.

Although we have come far with the knowledge of wrist mechanics, our present knowledge is based

WRIST INJURIES 303

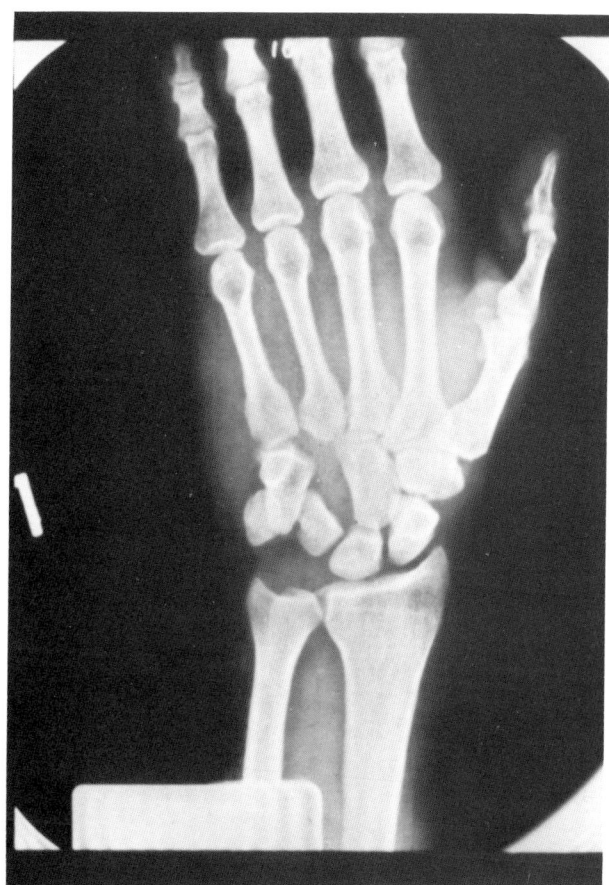

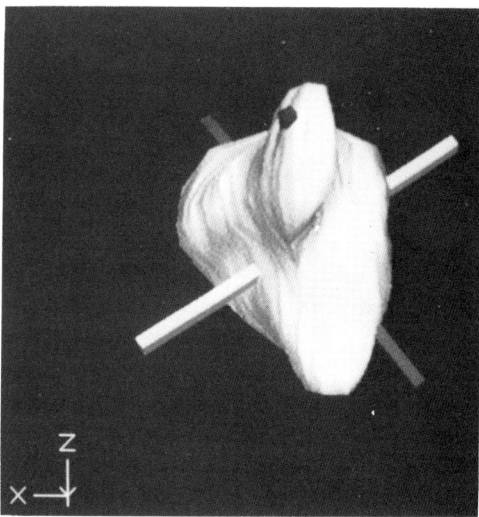

Fig. 20.5 Three-dimensional computed model of carpal hamate generated from CT Scan data. Three principal orthogonal axes obtained by feature extraction analysis traverse the centre of the bone's volume. Changes in the position of the hamate that results from wrist action are represented by changes of the orientation of these axes and can be easily converted to descriptions of translation and angular rotation (Belsole 1985) (reproduced with permission)

Fig. 20.4 Axial subluxation of the carpals through the hamate-capitate joint dislocation. The lunate remains stabilised by the pillar of the triquetrum. A favourable result could be anticipated (Garcia-Elias et al 1985)

mechanics of the wrist, it is important that the surgeon should not embark on an extensive surgical reconstruction based primarily on the radiographs. Many times the wrist can function well for an indeterminate time after an injury despite extensive and forbidding changes on the radiograph (Fig. 20.7).

THE MISSED DIAGNOSIS

The two wrist injuries most frequently missed in the Emergency Room are: 1. scaphoid fractures, 2. lunate and perilunate dislocations. Life threatening injuries from a motorcycle or automobile accident will demand immediate and emergency care, but

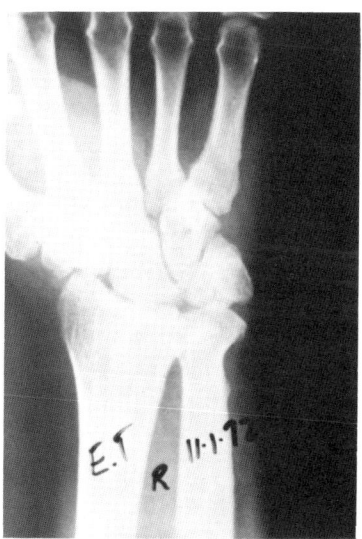

Fig. 20.6 A 55 year old construction labourer who had a proximal row carpectomy 25 years before because of a painful non-union of the scaphoid. He worked daily at heavy construction. Wrist motion and grip strength about 60% of normal wrist. Note that the capitate now occupies the splinate fossa and maintains a satisfactory radio-carpal articulation

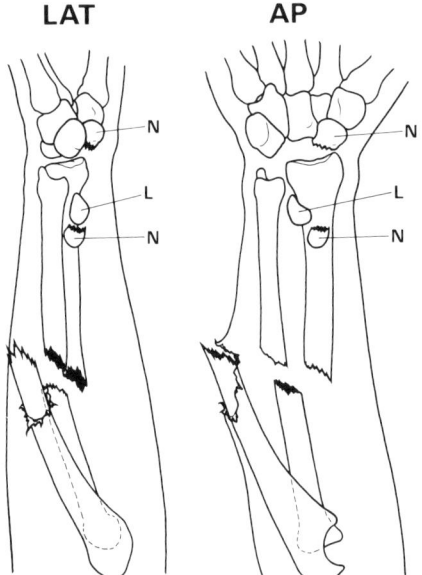

Fig. 20.7 A 22 year old construction worker who fell 20 feet while working. The lunate and proximal navicular were excised. The radius and ulna had compression plating. Despite grip strength and range of motion loss he continued to work as a construction labourer for three years after which he was lost to follow up

after the patient is stabilised, a complete, and thorough examination of the hand and wrist should be performed. Many times this may even necessitate survey radiographs and films of the normal opposite wrist. In the acutely injured wrist the diagnoses are often overlooked due to improper positioning of the radiograph because of the patient's pain or inability to lay the wrist at the proper angle. Confusion results because of the overlapping of the carpals and the number of articular surfaces present. The radiograph is thereby misread or undiagnosed. This leads to unwarranted charges made in some future courtroom scene as the surgeon and radiologist try to cope with this litigious atmosphere. A high index of suspicion on the part of the surgeon and an insistence on repeated accurate films will often cut losses. A shrewd sense of the possible will help prevent non-union of a fracture or a missed dislocation.

Scaphoid fracture

This fracture occurs most frequently in the adult male and if untreated can cause serious complications in wrist mechanics since this bone acts as the stablising link of the wrist between the proximal row of carpals and the distal row. Once this link is broken, the wrist collapses into a zigzag or a concertina deformity (Gilford et al 1943) (Fig. 20.8). Fractures most often occur across the waist of this bone, but if it involves the distal pole, the diagnosis may be missed due to a subtle fracture line. When the fracture involves the proximal pole, a therapeutic problem may occur due to the impoverished blood supply to the end of the scaphoid resulting in non-union or avascular necrosis (Green & O'Brien 1980). It is essential to establish whether the fracture is stable or unstable, whether displaced or undisplaced; this is determined by radiological interpretation (Fisk 1980). The type of injury, whether it be the high velocity impact or simple fall, will aid in assessing ligament and bone injury.

Positioning for the radiograph

After routine wrist views the best position for the scaphoid profile is a posterior-anterior view with the fist clenched and the wrist in ulnar deviation. To determine instability of a fracture this view is compared with one in radial deviation.

An unstable fracture demonstrates a displacement offset greater than 1 mm, a collapse deformity, or a fracture line which is oblique indicating a shear stress force. These injuries imply extensive ligamentous rupture, often due to an incomplete perilunar dislocation or a spontaneously reduced perilunar dislocation.

Treatment of the scaphoid fracture

A *stable fracture* can be treated with cast immobilisation for 8 weeks or if comminuted, a longer time. A short arm cast is used with the wrist in slight palmar flexion and slight radial deviation and the thumb in palmar abduction with the distal joint free. A long arm cast should be utilised if the fracture line is widened or comminuted.

An *unstable fracture* requires open reduction and internal fixation, using Kirschner wires across the fracture site and linking scaphoid to lunate since the lunate and proximal pole of the scaphoid travel together. The distal fragment should be affixed to the capitate to ensure maximum stability. Herbert

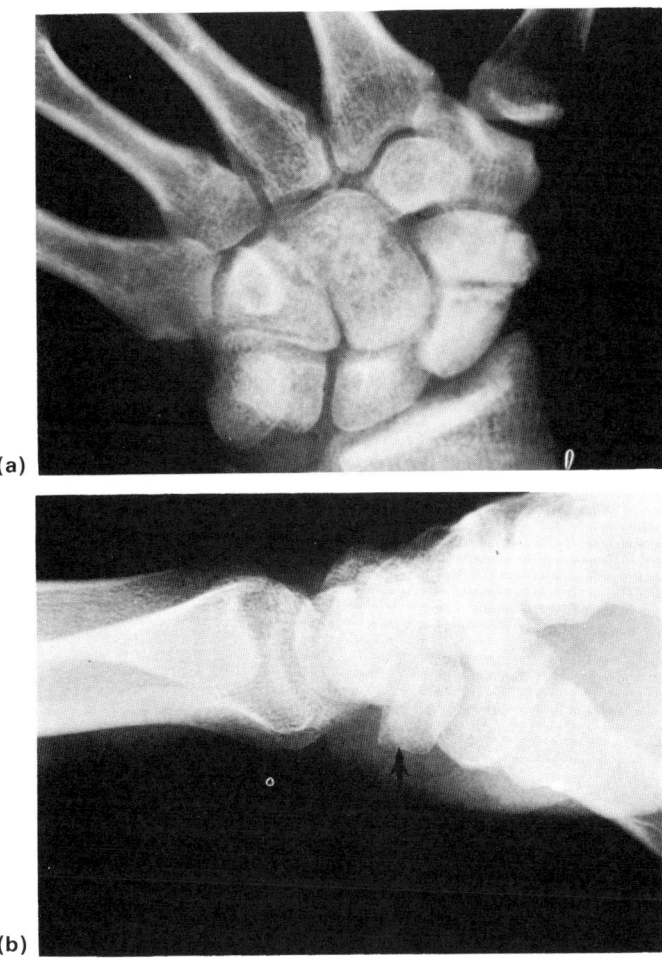

Fig. 20.8 (a) and (b) Non-union of scaphoid with collapse deformity resulting in a vertical position of the scaphoid

(1984) has designed a compression screw which is a superb means of fixing this fracture. However, the unwary and inexperienced surgeon will find this technique difficult and frustrating. It requires practice in the anatomy laboratory. It requires careful exposure of the scaphoid-trapezium joint. It is worth the effort, however.

When the injured wrist is thought to be a 'sprain' and does not improve with splinting over a 2-week period, repeat radiographs should be taken to demonstrate a latent scaphoid fracture.

Non-union of the scaphoid fracture

Almost all stable scaphoid fractures will unite if treated by cast immobilisation immediately after the injury (Stewart 1954). If a non-union is diagnosed, a long arm cast for 6–10 weeks should be tried if no initial treatment was given. With no treatment or delayed treatment the fractures likely to cause significant pain are: 1. the unstable fracture, 2. the displaced fracture, and 3. the proximal pole fracture.

Painful non-union of a scaphoid fracture is the primary indication for surgery. There is now clear evidence that non-union causes post-traumatic arthritic changes, but often is completely asymptomatic until a second injury trips off the pain, perhaps due to abnormal kinematics within the wrist (Ruby et al 1985).

If the non-union of the scaphoid fracture causes

a collapse deformity of the proximal carpal row, the scaphoid tends to turn into a vertical position rather than its normal 45 degree oblique position linking proximal row carpus to distal row (Fig. 20.9). The kinematics of the wrist are thereby distorted and the restraining pillar to the lunate is lost, permitting the lunate to displace, generally in a dorsiflexed position.

Treatment of the non-union

For a collapse deformity of the scaphoid with non-union of the fracture, the palmar approach to the wrist using a modified Russe technique (1960) offers excellent visualisation of the fracture pathology (Fig. 20.10). However, we use a cortico-cancellous bone graft inserted into the site of non-union and the collapse deformity is then wedged open by the graft allowing the scaphoid to resume its normal length as well as its oblique position in the wrist. The distal radius is the source of the graft.

If the non-union is not displaced nor collapsed, either the dorsal approach or the palmar approach can be utilised depending on the surgeon's preference and experience.

For those surgeons proficient in the use of the Herbert screw technique, an additional advantage to this technique is that strong, compressive stabilisation can be added to the open reduction or bone graft procedure (Fig. 20.11).

Electrical stimulation of scaphoid fractures

This relatively new treatment for non-union of scaphoid fractures is still controversial and undergoing evaluation. Early results indicate that the EBI (Electro-Biology, Inc.) bone stimulator is useful if careful patient selection is carried out (Culver 1980).

The fracture site should have less than a 2 mm gap with indistinct margins. This unit should not be used for a displaced fracture, gaps greater than

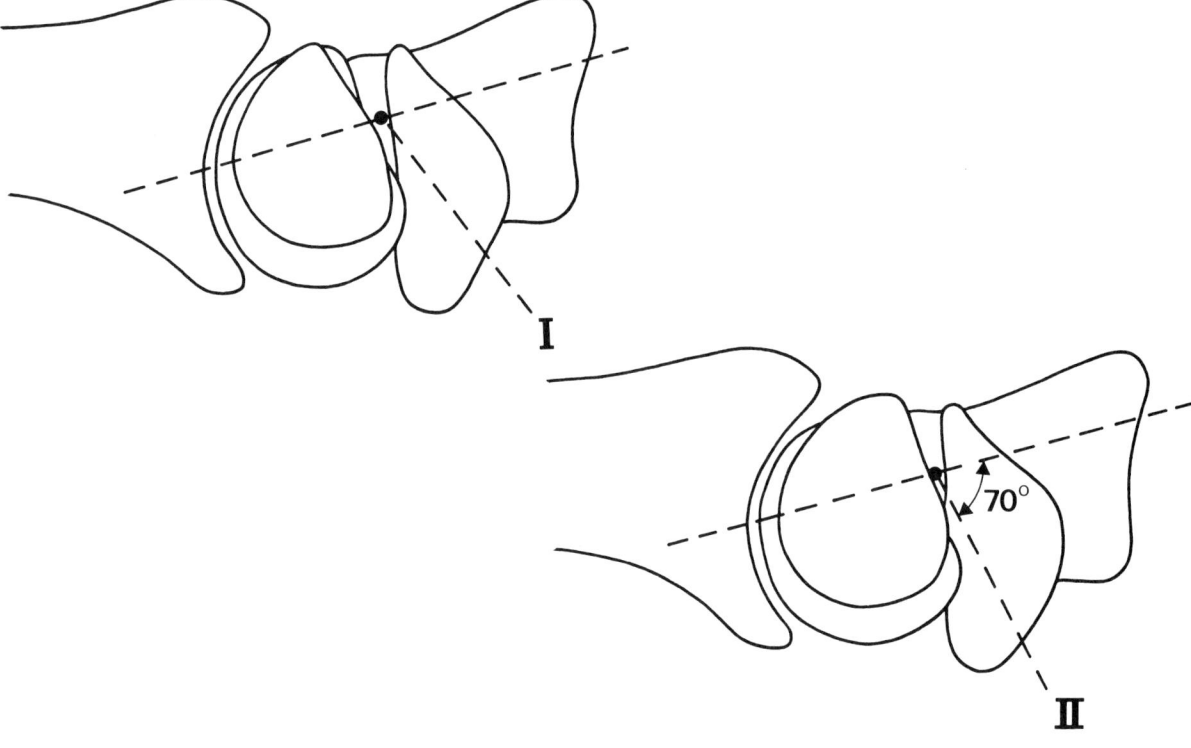

Fig. 20.9 Schematic diagram of the 'hump-back' deformity of the scaphoid with increase in the scapho-lunate angle (personal communication after Linscheid (1986)

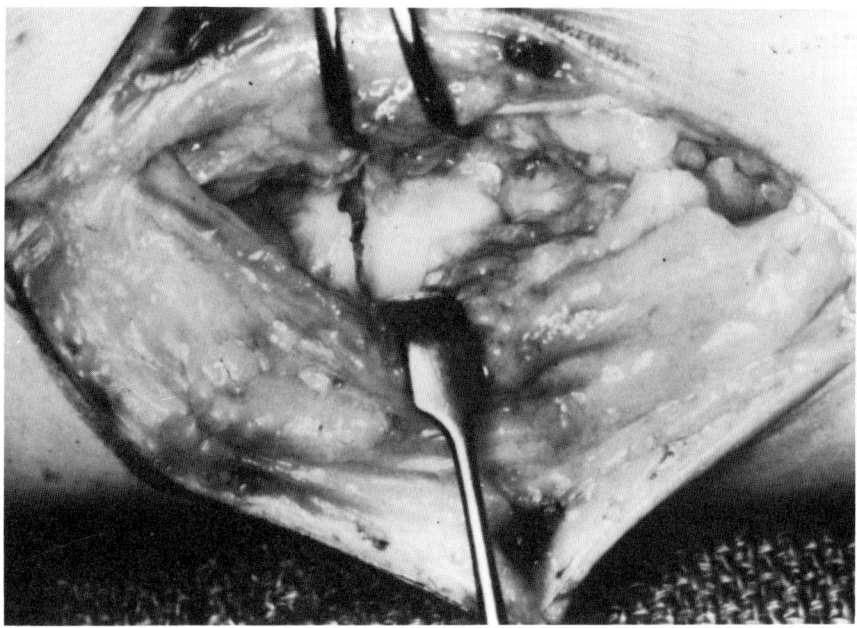

Fig. 20.10 Operative view of a scaphoid non-union, palmar approach. Russe procedure would restore the length of the scaphoid as well as its oblique position connecting the two carpal rows

2 mm, collapsed deformities, or fractures with smooth margins.

The silastic scaphoid implant of Swanson

The silastic spacer has been used since 1969 by Swanson who reports satisfactory results for displaced scaphoid fractures, non-union of the scaphoid, as well as avascular necrosis. Ligament integrity is required for the prosthesis to be stable and effective. A recent report by Peimer (1985) has implicated this prosthesis with silicone synovitis and cyst formation. The use of Kirschner wires through the implant appears to increase these two complications.

Summary

Treatment of scaphoid fracture
—*Recent fracture*
 a. Stable—cast immobilisation
 b. Unstable—open reduction and internal fixation
  —long arm cast

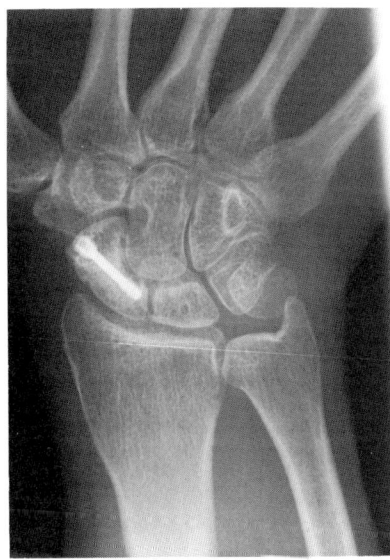

Fig. 20.11 Herbert screw fixation for a non-union of the scaphoid. This patient was immobilised for 18 months prior to a bone graft using a palmar approach. The bone graft failed but Herbert screw compression achieved union

—*Non-Union*
  a. If *untreated*—cast immobilisation for 6–10 weeks
  b. If *previously immobilised*:
     1. Non-displaced—Bone graft procedure, either palmar or dorsal approach
     2. Displaced or collapse deformity—Corticocancellous graft from palmar approach with Herbert screw compression.

Lunate or perilunate dislocation

Lunate and perilunate dislocations are the most common dislocations of the carpals, yet they constitute less than 10% of all carpal injuries. Hyperextension injury to the outstretched hand usually causes this injury. When missed, it is frequently the source of malpractice claims.

In a lunate dislocation, the longitudinal axis of the capitate is colinear with that of the radius, but the lunate is displaced palmarward with its cup tilted volarly ('spilled teacup' sign) disrupting this colinear arrangement (Fig. 20.12 (a)). In the antero-posterior view the lunate assumes a triangular shape instead of its normal quadrilateral shape ('piece of cheese' sign) (Fig. 20.12 (b)). Median nerve compression is often an associated injury, but if closed reduction of the dislocation is carried out early, these neurological symptoms often clear without the necessity of nerve decompression.

Perilunar dislocations are sometimes misdiagnosed in the emergency room and since success in treatment depends on an accurate and early diagnosis, it is essential to study the radiographs carefully. Again the colinear disruption of radius, lunate, and capitate is lost. A precise lateral X-ray film is an absolute necessity and determines this disruption. Closed reduction by traction and manipulation within a few hours of injury is generally successful. Kirschner wire fixation after closed reduction is advisable. Close follow-up with X-ray films at weekly intervals for 3 weeks is necessary to avoid creeping subluxation that often occurs if there is ligament instability. After 2 weeks the dislocation may not be able to be reduced by a surgical procedure and leads to a painful degenerative arthritis. A persistent gap between the scaphoid and lunate of greater than 3 mm is a forbidding diagnostic sign and correlates with significant and often progressive carpal instability. Occasionally, the disruption of energy in this high impact injury will continue through the arcs of the wrist causing disruption in the luno-capitate joint. The carpal instability associated with incongruity between the lunate and triquetrum generally has a more favourable prognosis.

Summary

Treatment of lunate and perilunate dislocation
—*Recent dislocation*
  Closed reduction with traction. Kirschner wire

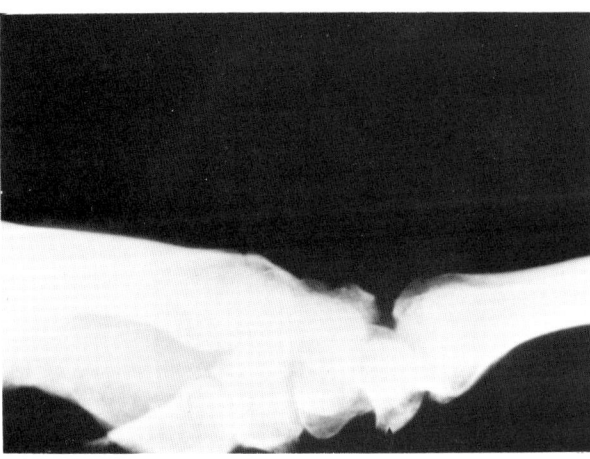
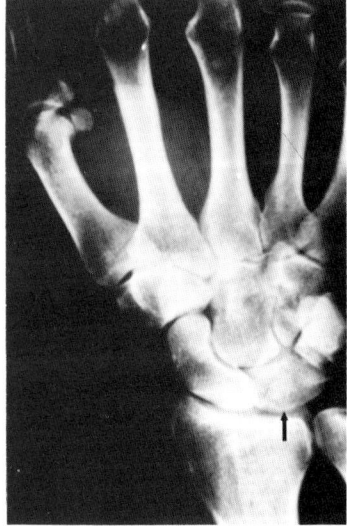

Fig. 20.12 Volar dislocation of the lunate demonstrating the 'spilled teacup' sign on the lateral view (a) and the triangular 'piece of cheese' sign on the AP view (b)

fixation often needed for perilunar dislocation. Weekly post-reduction X-ray examination for 3 weeks.

—*Greater than 2 weeks*
Open reduction through dorsal approach and Kirschner wire fixation.

—*Greater than 6 weeks*
Open reduction should be attempted. Be prepared for proximal row carpectomy or limited wrist arthrodesis.

Trans-scaphoid perilunar fracture dislocation

The majority of perilunar dislocations are accompanied by a fracture of the scaphoid giving evidence to the strong force required to cause this injury. This injury is caused by hyperextension of the wrist with the palm in ulnar deviation with intercarpal supination. Thus, with forced extension and dislocation of the capitate the scaphoid must either fracture or rotate to permit this dislocation between the lunate and capitate. This is due to the relatively fixed territory for each of the carpus. The lunate is relatively fixed to the radius, while the capitate is firmly fixed to the third metacarpal base. The capitate-scaphoid joint is most vulnerable because it is the junction of the fixed axis between hand and forearm. The scaphoid connects the proximal and distal carpal rows so the proximal pole of the scaphoid functions with the lunate and the distal pole functions with the capitate. Thus the fracture force splits the waist of the scaphoid resulting in the trans-scaphoid fracture dislocation.

The trans-scaphoid perilunar fracture dislocation requires early recognition of the dislocation as well as the fracture which in turn requires open reduction and internal fixation. Treatment within the first 24 hours of injury gives a more favourable prognosis (Green & O'Brien 1978). Usually, the recent perilunar dislocation can be reduced by traction but considerable difficulty is encountered in maintaining this position so that open reduction through a dorsal approach is recommended. The dorsal approach gives better visualisation of the reduction and facilitates removal of cartilage fragments and shredded ligaments. However, this dorsal approach is combined with a palmar approach which allows excellent visualisation of the scaphoid fracture. The key to maintenance of the reduction of perilunar dislocation is first to obtain firm stabilisation of the scaphoid fracture. Midcarpal stability is only achieved when there is firm fixation and stability of the scaphoid. The Herbert screw offers strong fixation with compression and therefore braces the midcarpal joint as it spans the proximal row of carpals with the distal carpal row. If Kirschner wires are preferred, the author recommends three wires transfixing the reduced scaphoid fracture to the lunate and capitate. The palmar approach is also used to repair the volar capsule and ligaments. When necessary, the median nerve can be inspected and a decompression performed. A long arm cast including the thumb is applied for 6 weeks, followed by a short arm cast for another 6 weeks or until the scaphoid fracture is healed.

Summary

Treatment of trans-scaphoid perilunar fracture dislocation.
—Dorsal approach to reduce accurately the dislocation combined with *palmar approach* to maintain midcarpal stability by strong fixation of the scaphoid fracture. Use Herbert screw or three Kirschner wires.

Acute scapho-lunate dissociation (rotatory subluxation of the scaphoid)

This injury is often considered to be a 'sprained wrist' and frequently occurs as a result of a fall on the extended hand, although occasionally it has no specific traumatic history. It is characterised by a tear of the interosseous lunate-scaphoid ligament; if the force continues, a tear of the radio-scaphoid-lunate ligament causes complete instability of the carpus. It may become a *dynamic* subluxation recurring hundreds of times as the scaphoid exerts a painful snap palmarward in repeating fashion or it may occur only at the original time of injury and thus cause a static subluxation which will remain with a persistent gap.

If a scapho-lunate dissociation is suspected, an anteroposterior view with the wrist in supination will often increase the scapho-lunate gap (Fig.

20.13). A clenched fist view may also be helpful. A diagnosis of scapho-lunate dissociation is made on the following radiograph features of the AP or PA view (Fig. 20.13):

1. A gap between the scaphoid and lunate greater than 2 mm (the 'Terry Thomas' sign) (Frankel 1977).
2. A foreshortened scaphoid.
3. A double density projection of the cortical waist of the scaphoid (the 'ring' sign).

On the lateral view the scaphoid becomes vertical to the long axis of the radius due to its palmar flexed position. The loss of a stable scaphoid causes instability of the lunate and it tilts dorsally causing a dorsiflexion instability.

If the injury is seen early and diagnosed within the first few days, it is best to reduce the subluxation of the scaphoid to lunate by a dorsal surgical approach. Use 2 or 3 Kirschner wires to fix scaphoid to lunate and to capitate and repair the radio-scaphoid-lunate ligament through an additional palmar incision. The wires should fix the scaphoid at its distal end to the capitate and its proximal end to the lunate as both ends of the scaphoid can be unstable. The wires are cut off outside the skin and bent over. They are left in place for 8 weeks and supported with a short arm cast. Early repair of the ligaments and open reduction are preferred over closed reduction and percutaneous pin fixation because it gives greater stability and a more precise reduction.

If the ligament ruptures are seen late but less than 4 weeks after injury, an open reduction, internal fixation with Kirschner wires, repair of the ruptured ligaments where feasible, and the use of a tendon slip from the extensor carpi radialis brevis to reinforce the repair can stabilise this dissociation.

If the injury is diagnosed after 4 weeks, the triscaphoid arthrodesis of Watson may be necessary. This is a surgical fusion of the scaphoid to the trapezium and trapezoid. This can stabilise the recurrent scaphoid subluxation and yet maintain functional wrist motion. Future arthritic sequelae

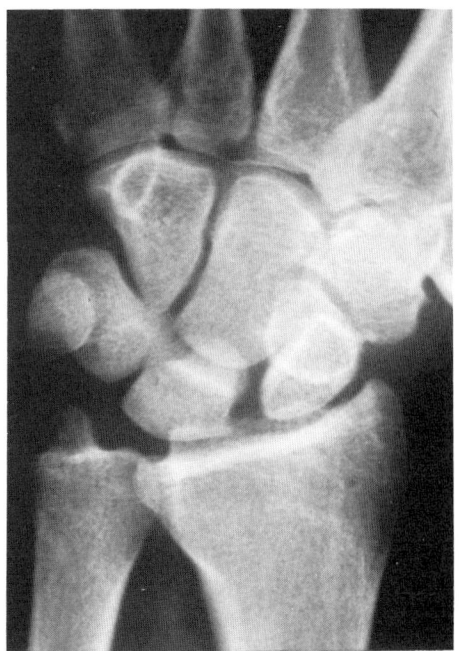

Fig. 20.13 Scapho-lunate dissociation. Note the increased gap ('Terry Thomas' sign) between the scaphoid and lunate. Note also the foreshortened scaphoid and the double density projection of the cortical waist of the scaphoid ('ring' sign)

due to the altered wrist kinematics must be evaluated by the test of time for this surgical procedure.

Summary

Treatment of scapho-lunate dissociation
—*Acute* Occasionally, closed reduction and cast immobilisation.

Generally, open reduction through dorsal approach, repair ligaments, Kirschner wire fixation.
—*Late*
a. *Less than 4 weeks:* Open reduction through dorsal approach, Kirschner wire dixation; reinforce with strip of extensor carpi radialis brevis tendon.
b. *Greater than 4 weeks:* Triscaphoid fusion may be necessary.

REFERENCES

Belsole R 1985 In publication

Campbell R D Jr, Lance E M, Yeoh C B 1964 Lunate and perilunar dislocations. Journal of Bone and Joint Surgery 46B:55–72

Campbell R D Jr, Thompson T C, Lance E M, Adler J B 1965 Indications for open reduction of lunate and perilunate dislocations of the carpal bones. Journal of Bone and Joint Surgery 47A:915–937

Culver J E 1985 American Society for Surgery of the Hand—Correspondence Newsletter

Dobyns J H, Linscheid R L, Chao E Y S et al 1975 Traumatic instability of the wrist. American Academy of Orthopaedic Surgeons Instructional Course Lectures 24:182–199

Dobyns J H 1984 Invited Comment. Journal of Hand Surgery 9A:526

Fisk R L 1980 An overview of injuries of the wrist. Clinical Orthopaedics and Related Research 149:137–144

Frankel V H 1977 The Terry-Thomas sign. Clinical Orthopaedics and Related Research 129:321–322

Garcia-Elias M, Abanco J, Salvador E, Sanchez R 1985 Crush injury of the carpus. Journal of Bone and Joint Surgery 67B:286–289

Gilford W W, Bolton R H, Lambrinudi G 1943 The mechanism of wrist joint with special reference to fracture of the scaphoid. Guy's Hospital Report 92:529

Green D P, O'Brien E T 1980 Classification and management of carpal dislocations. Clinical Orthopaedics and Related Research 149:55–72

Herbert T J, Fisher W E 1984 Management of the fractured scaphoid using a new bone screw. Journal of Bone and Joint Surgery 66B:114–123

Kauer J M G 1974 The interdependence of carpal articulation chains. Acta Anatomica 88:481–501

Moneim M S, Hofammann K E, Omer G E 1984 Transcaphoid perilunate fracture-dislocation result of open reduction and pin fixation. Clinical Orthopaedics and Related Research 190:227–235

Peimer C A 1985 Invasive Silicone Synovitis of the Wrist, Presentation: 40th Annual Meeting, American Society for Surgery of the Hand, Las Vegas

Ruby L K, Stinson J, Belsky M R 1985 The natural history of scaphoid non-union. Journal of Bone and Joint Surgery 67A:428–432

Russe O 1960 Fracture of the carpal navicular. Journal of Bone and Joint Surgery 42A:759–768

Swanson A B 1973 Flexible implant replacement arthroplasty of the scaphoid and lunate bones. In: Flexible Implant Resection Arthroplasty in the Hand and Extremities. C V Mosby Company, St Louis, p 244

Stewart M J 1954 Fractures of the carpal navicular: a report of cases. Journal of Bone and Joint Surgery 36A:998–1006

Taleisnik J 1978 Wrist: anatomy, function and injury. American Academy of Orthopaedic Surgeons Instructional Course Lectures 27:61–87 C V Mosby Company, St Louis

Watson H K, Goodman M L, Johnson T R 1981 Limited wrist arthrodeses. The triscaphoid joint. Journal of Hand Surgery 6:223–233

Watson H K, Ryu J 1984 Degenerative disorders of the carpus. Orthopedic Clinics of North America 15:337–353

Weber E R, Chao E Y S 1978 An experimental approach to the mechanism of scaphoid waist fractures. Journal of Hand Surgery 3:142–148

Weeks P M, Vannier M W, Stevens W G, Gayou D, Gilula L A 1985 Three-dimensional imaging of the wrist. Journal of Hand Surgery 10A:32–39

L. H. Millender and D. A. Bobb

Rheumatoid arthritis

INTRODUCTION

Complications following rheumatoid hand surgery fall into two broad groups. One group represents well known complications such as infection, fractured prosthesis, and recurrent deformities. The second group represents patients who have not necessarily had a complication, however their results are less than expected. This often occurs because of either poor indications or unrealistic goals of surgery. We refer to these unfavourable results as 'the hidden elements' of rheumatoid hand surgery.

In reviewing the results of rheumatoid hand surgery, it is important to consider both the common complications as well as the hidden elements. This can be difficult because standard criteria to evaluate the results of rheumatoid reconstructive surgery do not exist. In this chapter we will consider both the well known complications following rheumatoid reconstruction as well as the hidden elements.

Unfavourable results—hidden elements

Many unfavourable results occur because of poor indications for surgery. In order to minimise this, the surgeon must have a clear understanding for both the indications and the limitations of a given procedure. The patient must understand that his or her hand will never be 'normal'. When evaluating a patient for rheumatoid surgery, four broad categories should be considered. They are 1. pain, 2. appearance, 3. preventing progression, and 4. function. By evaluating patients from this perspective, clearer indications for surgery can be established.

Pain

Most rheumatoid patients primarily complain of pain. It is rather easy to diagnose the cause of pain. When conservative measures are not successful, surgery with arthroplasty or arthrodesis is indicated to alleviate pain. Clearly, the surgeon is on the most solid footing when carrying out surgery for pain and in most cases success can be anticipated.

Appearance

Appearance is another, less frequent, reason for advising rheumatoid hand surgery. This is listed second not because of its importance, but because results are predictable when appearance is the reason for surgery. Deformity and alignment are easily corrected. Nodules can be removed and in general hand appearance can be improved.

The next two areas, preventive surgery and improving function, are the areas where judgement and experience are most necessary. This is where many of the hidden elements occur and where unfortunate results following hand surgery most frequently arise.

PREVENTIVE SURGERY—TENOSYNOVECTOMY AND SYNOVECTOMY

One indication for rheumatoid surgery is to prevent further joint and tendon destruction. The specific complications following tenosynovectomy, synovectomy, and joint reconstruction will be discussed in separate sections. In this section some general comments will be given regarding indications for preventive surgery, in order to prevent unfavourable results.

Tenosynovectomy

In general, both dorsal and flexor tenosynovectomy are acceptable surgical procedures which will prevent the complications of tenosynovitis, especially tendon ruptures. The results of tenosynovectomy have been good. In most series the complications are few and the morbidity low. Therefore, when one presents with dorsal or flexor tenosynovitis which has been persistent and unresponsive to adequate medical treatment, one should expect favourable results from tenosynovectomy.

Synovectomy

In contrast to tenosynovectomy, the results following joint synovectomy are less predictable. Synovectomy will generally alleviate joint pain if there is not excessive joint destruction. Its capacity to prevent further joint destruction is unpredictable.

In general, indications for synovectomy include persistent synovitis limited to few joints, in otherwise healthy patients, with minimal radiographic involvement. These patients may have received temporary relief from steroid injections and rest but have experienced recurrent episodes of synovitis.

The joints where synovectomy is most frequently indicated are the proximal interphalangeal joints to prevent boutenierre deformity, and the wrist, to stop destruction of the carpal bones. Synovectomy has been least effective in the metacarpophalangeal joints because of the many forces causing recurrent deformity (Moberg 1969).

PREVENTIVE SURGERY—INDICATIONS FOR RECONSTRUCTIVE SURGERY

It is accepted that either soft tissue reconstruction or arthroplasty is more successful when carried out prior to extensive instability, deformity, or joint destruction (Millender & Nalebuff 1975a,c).

One of the difficult areas in reconstructive surgery is timing. Although some patients have moderate ulnar drift, and moderate metacarpophalangeal joint subluxations, their function may be adequate for their needs. If they have accomodated to their functional level, arthroplasty may do little more than improve appearance. Additionally, if their grip strength is in the range of 30–40 pounds, they could be weakened after arthroplasty and this of course would be an unfortunate result. Therefore, a 4 to 6 month observation period, looking for progressive disease is indicated prior to performing silastic arthroplasty. However, if the patient is young, has active synovitis, and there has been a rapid progression of the deformity, then one can anticipate continued progression and arthroplasty would be advised at this time.

RECONSTRUCTIVE SURGERY—TO IMPROVE FUNCTION

One area of unforseen results is in attempting surgery on patients with mild deformities who are generally healthy, but frustrated because of a general loss of function. They want to perform activities such as carpentry or athletics but they do not have the strength or endurance. These people, if males, may have grip strengths of 50–70 pounds, compared to 100–110 pounds for a normal person of the same age. Examination may show mild subluxation of the metacarpophalangeal joints, or early wrist or thumb deformity. In this person hand surgery can not restore full function and is not indicated. This person needs to understand his disease, to modify his activities, and to spend time with a well trained hand therapist. Surgery might weaken the patient, frustrate him, and would not produce the desired results.

Another area in which surgery sometimes leads to unforseen results is in the person with a significant amount of destruction affecting many joints, who in spite of his deformities has minimal pain and functions relatively well. Many of these patients are older with fewer demands. In the past we have attempted both metacarpophalangeal joints and proximal interphalangeal joint arthroplasties in patients like this and have been disappointed with the results. Unless there is pain, progressive disease, or a specific reason for the surgery, one should be cautious. Regardless of the result, the change in function will not be dramatic. Unless this is understood, the final result can be disappointing.

The remaining portion of this chapter deals with the unfortunate results in specific areas of rheumatoid hand surgery. These areas include rheumatoid tendon surgery, the radiocarpal joint, the radioulnar joint, the metacarpophalangeal joint, the proximal interphalangeal joint, the rheumatoid thumb, and infected silastic arthroplasties. As each area is developed the hidden elements as well as the unforseen results will be discussed.

RHEUMATOID TENDON SURGERY

Fortunately complications following rheumatoid tendon surgery are not frequent or major. In discussing tendon surgery and its complications, we will discuss dorsal and flexor tenosynovitis and tendon rupture.

Dorsal tenosynovitis

Dorsal tenosynovectomy is effective in preventing tendon rupture. Complications following simple dorsal tenosynovitis are infrequent. They usually involve either an extension lag of the metacarpophalangeal joints or adhesions preventing full digital flexion (Millender & Nalebuff 1975b). Hand therapy is essential in maintaining the results obtained at surgery. The digits are initially splinted in extension to prevent extension lag. Range of motion exercises are begun on the first postoperative day and depending upon the progress, either additional extension or additional flexion is emphasised. If pain or flexor weakness prevents flexion then passive flexion exercises and dynamic flexion splints are added. Alternatively, if significant extension lag persists then a dorsal dynamic splint can be fabricated. Extension lag or flexion contracture is seen more in those patients who have poor tendons at surgery, multiple joint involvement, or a low pain threshold. Generally by the second week patients have a full range of motion if they had full motion preoperatively. It is rare to carry out tenolysis after dorsal tenosynovectomy for rheumatoid arthritis. However, if significant functional impairment exists after 6 months of therapy, tenolysis could be considered (Nalebuff 1969a).

Dorsal tenosynovectomy and tendon transfer

Unfavourable results following tendon transfers are related to the number of tendons that are ruptured, the extent of the tendon involvement, and the type of transfer utilised. For ruptures of the extensor tendons to the fourth and fifth digits, dorsal tenosynovectomy and extensor indicis proprius transfer provides good results. When there are triple or quadruple ruptures, either the flexor digitorum superficialis transfer, palmaris longus intercalated graft, or wrist extensor transfer can be utilised, but the results are less favourable. When extensor tendon ruptures are repaired in association with wrist fusion and wrist extensors are used, excursion can rarely be normal. Wrist extensors have less excursion than the finger extensors, and full digital motion will not be restored. If the transfer is put in tightly, extension is maintained, but there is a subsequent loss of flexion (Nalebuff 1969b).

An additional method is to use the palmaris longus tendon as an intercalated graft following multiple ruptures. In this situation the proximal tendon is identified by making a longer proximal incision. The graft is sutured in tightly to allow for subsequent stretching of the contracted muscle. This method of treatment is not as satisfactory as utilising a normal functioning extensor indicis proprius, but, when three or four ruptures are present it is an alternative to the flexor digitorum superficialis transfer. If one realises the difficulty in regaining full motion after multiple tendon ruptures, then what might have been looked upon as an unforseen result will be more readily accepted (Millender et al 1974).

Extensor tendon ruptures and dislocated metacarpophalangeal joints

One of the most difficult problems to treat is the combination of multiple extensor tendon ruptures associated with dislocated metacarpophalangeal joints. These are severely crippled hands with marked disability. The most unfortunate results follow surgery for these patients. Our general approach is to carry out metacarpophalangeal joint arthroplasty, dorsal tenosynovectomy, distal ulna excision, and tendon transfers, in one stage. Depending on the number of ruptured tendons, and the adequacy of the anastomosis, either early motion is started or immobilisation for 3 weeks is elected. We accept a marked limitation of flexion at the metacarpophalangeal joints with a goal of being able to restore metacarpophalangeal joint alignment, and extension. If the patient has a moderate amount of proximal interphalangeal joint motion then moderate grasp and pinch can be expected.

If one selects to stage the reconstructive procedures, then the metacarpophalangeal joint arthroplasty should be done first, passive range of motion maintained, and then at a second stage, the dorsal tenosynovectomy and tendon transfers can be carried out. The decision to stage the procedures should be related to the experience and ability of the surgeon, as well as the degree of involvement, and expected goals. In general, salvage surgery must be the goal. It can be performed as a single stage, is safe, and will restore a degree of function. It can also be carried out with wrist fusion. We feel this approach is preferable over a two-stage procedure.

Flexor tenosynovitis

Flexor tenosynovitis presents either in the carpal tunnel, the palm, or the digit. Depending upon the anatomical distribution, patients present with various combination of signs and symptoms. These include carpal tunnel syndrome, loss of active with preserved passive flexion, locking and snapping of the digits, and sometimes stiffness of the proximal interphalangeal joint secondary to flexor tenosynovitis. Although results following flexor tenosynovectomy are generally good, unfortunate results do occur. In the majority of cases, unfortunate results are usually related to the severity of the disease. When patients have flexor tenosynovitis without marked infiltration and destruction of the tendons, tenosynovectomy is generally effective in restoring full or near full motion. However, when there is invasion and attenuation with destruction of the tendons, full flexion is not established. Results following flexor tendon ruptures within the digits or multiple flexor tendon ruptures within the wrist and palm are generally not good.

Flexor tenosynovectomy—prevention of complications

Many of the unfortunate results can be prevented by early surgery. Patients with flexor tenosynovitis in contrast to dorsal tenosynovitis develop symptoms and generally are seen by the rheumatologist or surgeon. When steroid injections and medications fail, flexor tenosynovectomy is indicated.

When flexor tendon synovectomy is undertaken, the surgeon must be prepared to do a complete tenosynovectomy of all areas involved. If there is carpal tunnel syndrome with palmar and digital disease, the wrist, palm, and digits must be explored. The surgery for extensive flexor tenosynovitis is demanding, and should not be addressed by one unfamiliar with this type of problem. Failure to carry out complete tenosynovectomy will prevent full excursion of the involved tendons resulting in postoperative adhesions and limited digital flexion.

In some cases, it may be difficult to diagnose the extent of the disease, when a person presents with limited active digital flexion. Patients can have wrist flexor tenosynovitis without carpal tunnel syndrome and failure to remove disease in the carpal canal could prevent restoration of full digital flexion (Nalebuff & Potter 1968).

At the time of surgery one attempts to restore full tendon excursion. The success of this is related to the degree of tendon involvement. There are various techniques which are helpful. An effort must be made to preserve as much pulley mechanism as possible when carrying out digital flexor tenosynovectomy. However, in many cases, a portion of pulley must be excised to allow adequate excursion of the tendon. When it is difficult to obtain full excursion of the diseased tendons through the pulley, one slip of the flexor digitorum superficialis may be excised. The diseased portion of the flexor digitorum profundus can also be excised, being careful not to weaken the tendon. On rare occasions the entire flexor digitorum superficialis may be excised if it is severely diseased and prevents complete flexor digitorum profundus pull through.

When the wrist and proximal palm are explored, the issue of a pulley is not a concern. After the disease is excised one applies traction to the tendon to check for complete excursion. If passive digital flexion is greater than the flexion obtained with traction to the tendon, then additional tenosynovectomy is mandatory. The objective in flexor tenosynovectomy is to establish the same amount of active as passive flexion.

Postoperative management

A well supervised postoperative programme is vital to preserve the flexion obtained at surgery. This programme's success is related to the extent of the disease, the adequacy of tenosynovectomy, the status of the joint, and the ability of the patient to carry out the postoperative rehabilitation. In general, postoperative pain has not been a major problem. Two to three months of a careful hand therapy programme may be required to reach an end result.

Stiff proximal interphalangeal joints associated with flexor tenosynovitis

Proximal interphalangeal joint stiffness can follow digital flexor tenosynovitis and must be diagnosed preoperatively in order to be adequately treated. It must be differentiated from other causes of proximal interphalangeal joint stiffness such as metacarpophalangeal joint subluxation, with swan neck deformity, and intra-articular disease. The mechanism involves a loss of active digital flexion due to flexor tenosynovitis, which may lead to proximal interphalangeal joint stiffness. This is most frequently seen when in addition to flexor tenosynovitis the patients have some degree of proximal interphalangeal joint synovitis, with pain and swelling which prevents them from maintaining passive range of motion.

When seen the major finding may only be proximal interphalangeal joint stiffness, without any evidence of flexor tenosynovitis. When there is no evidence of significant intra-articular disease and when there is no metacarpophalangeal joint subluxation, then one could consider flexor tenosynovitis as a cause. Sometimes flexor tenosynovitis is palpable or there may be more passive than active flexion. When this occurs then flexor tenosynovitis and proximal interphalangeal joint manipulation or proximal interphalangeal joint release can be performed to restore function.

FLEXOR TENDON RUPTURES

The most serious complication of flexor tenosynovitis is flexor tendon rupture. The results following flexor tendon repair are directly related to the number and location of tendon ruptures, and the severity of the flexor tenosynovitis. Flexor tendon ruptures can follow flexor tenosynovitis in the wrist, palm, or the digit. Tendon ruptures can occur from attrition, direct synovial invasion, or ischemic necrosis secondary to increased pressure caused by tenosynovium hypertrophy (Nalebuff 1969).

Flexor tendon ruptures in the carpal tunnel

Most flexor tendon ruptures within the carpal tunnel arise as attrition ruptures. Usually the flexor pollicus longus or the flexor digitorum profundus to the index and middle fingers will rupture by attrition as they glide across the tuberosity of the scaphoid (Mannerfelt & Norman 1969). In this situation flexor tenosynovectomy with an intercalated tendon graft or side to side anastamosis is often satisfactory. However as the number of tendon ruptures increase, the prognosis becomes progressively worse. When excessive or 'malignant' flexor tenosynovitis is associated with multiple tendon ruptures the prognosis is poor. In these cases one can only perform tenosynovectomy and attempt tendon reconstruction with intercalated tendon grafts, side to side repairs, or tendon transfers (Fig. 21.1).

Flexor tendon rupture in the palm and digit

The prognosis of flexor tendon ruptures in the palm and digit again are related to the number and location of tendon ruptures, and the aggressiveness of the tenosynovitis. For isolated flexor digitorum profundus or superficialis ruptures tenosynovec-

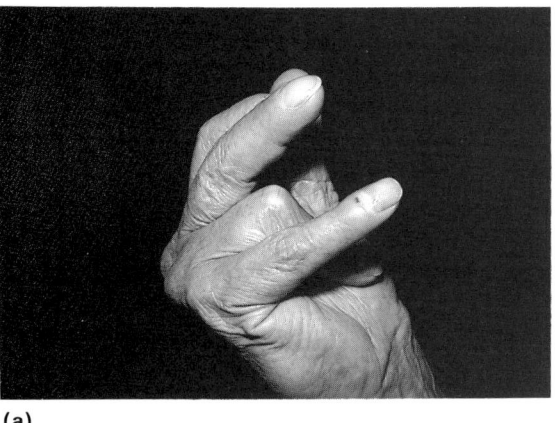 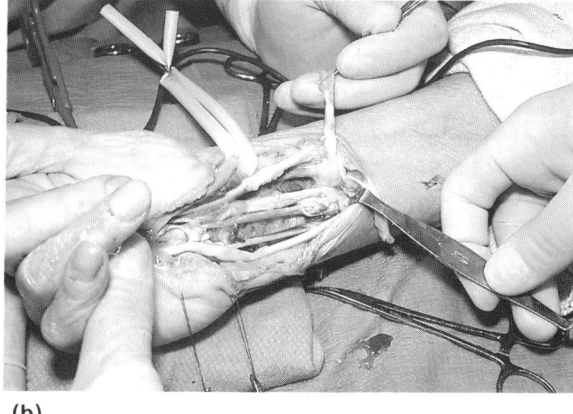

Fig. 21.1 (a) This patient demonstrates multiple flexor tendon ruptures with tenosynovitis at the wrist. (b) Following flexor tenosynovectomy, flexor tendon reconstruction was performed. The prognosis in this situation is only fair.

tomy to prevent further tendon rupture plus tenodesis of the profundus at the distal interphalangeal joint or fusion will restore proximal interphalangeal joint flexion.

Ruptures of the profundus and superficialis within the same digit are the most difficult problems to treat and carry a poor prognosis. In this situation the patients many times will have associated joint disease and stiffness, making restoration of flexion extremely difficult. If the ruptures occur in the palm, an intercalated graft or uncommonly a tendon transfer can be performed as long as passive motion has been maintained and minimal joint disease is present.

However, in most cases, joint disease with limited passive motion is present. The prognosis for restoring active flexion is poor and fusion of the joint in a functional position may be the best approach.

RADIOCARPAL JOINT

The wrist is the foundation of the hand. Wrist involvement can severely affect hand function. Reconstructive wrist surgery is indicated for persistent pain, instability, or deformity that impedes hand function. Reconstructive procedures include wrist fusion, silastic arthroplasty, total wrist arthroplasty, and limited wrist fusion.

Historically, wrist fusion has been the procedure of choice for the rheumatoid wrist. It provides a pain free, stable, and well aligned wrist, with improved hand function. In 1967 Swanson and later Volz & Meuli developed wrist prosthetics which were felt to give all of the advantages of fusion (alignment, stability, etc.) plus preserve and restore motion. Over the years there has been an increasing number of complications associated with these procedures, which has forced us to re-evaluate the rheumatoid wrist and to redefine our indications for surgery.

Silicone rubber wrist prosthesis—prevention of complications

The ideal reconstruction for the rheumatoid wrist would be a prosthesis that would restore alignment, provide stability and motion, alleviate pain, and not undergo recurrent deformity or fracture. This prosthesis however, does not exist. Over the past few years we have learned more about the causes of silicone wrist failures and have narrowed our indications for a silicone prosthesis to decrease the complication rate.

The prosthesis is indicated for patients with persistent pain, low demands, good range of motion, little deformity, good bone stock, and intact tendons. The contraindications include severe instability, deformity, multiple ruptured tendons, and high demands. The high demand patient could range from someone requiring constant use of crutches or walking aids to anyone involved in labour.

Complications are minimised by careful surgical technique which assures proper bone removal, seating of the prosthesis, and careful capsular closure. The success of this procedure relates to capsule and tendon balance. Extensor carpi ulnaris subluxation must be corrected. Postoperative immobilisation should be continued for 4–6 weeks with the goal being to restore 40°–60° of total motion. Too much motion can cause fracture of the prosthesis (Brase & Millender 1985).

Silicone rubber wrist prosthesis: complications

The major complication of a silastic arthroplasty is silastic fracture. Our series of 71 silastic wrist arthroplasties had an average follow up of 68 months. There tended to be an increasing number of fractures with time. The 20% fracture rate demonstrated in this study could be related to several factors. These included poor patient selection, excessive motion and over use. Patients with severe deformity, tendon ruptures, severe instability and poor capsule, tended to do poorly. Implant fracture had a direct correlation with excessive motion. The average wrist motion for the fractured prosthesis group was 68° and for the non-fractured prosthesis group was 48°. 50% of the fractured prosthesis group had motion greater than 75° while only 10% of the non-fractured prosthesis group could obtain that much motion.

We have seen patients who have initially shown excellent results present later with fractures which were felt to be due to overuse. One patient fractured after bike riding and another fractured after using a walker. Platform crutches should be advised for patients with a prosthesis and splints should be used whenever excessive stress will be applied to the wrist.

Almost all patients with fractured prosthesis become symptomatic. They develop increasing pain, weakness, and deformity. The diagnosis is suspected by noting instability and clicking in the physical exam and confirmed by X-ray (Fig. 21.2).

Treatment of fractured prosthesis

Most patients require revision because of pain and disability. In our series 14 were revised to a new prosthesis and 4 were revised to a wrist fusion. After prosthetic revision was carried out, the goal was to perform as tight a capsular closure as possible, immobilise the patient for 6–8 weeks, and restrict motion to a total of 40° if possible. Although revision relieved pain, all patients were weak and considerable functional restriction resulted. Patients who were revised to a wrist fusion had better results than those patients who had a second arthroplasty. If wrist fusion is done, a bone graft is needed. In most cases the revision is carried out in conjunction with metacarpophalangeal joint arthroplasty and the bone from the metacarpal heads is an excellent source of bone graft.

Recurrent deformity after silastic prosthesis

There were 2 patients who developed recurrent radial deformity. This is probably due to an incompetent or ruptured extensor carpi ulnaris and generally is associated with ulnar drift of the metacarpals. When this deformity impedes function or especially if metacarpophalangeal joint arthroplasty's are needed, then one must realign the wrist and this is best done with a fusion, as described in the previous section.

Pain following silastic prosthesis

There are some patients who will have pain following arthroplasty. In Goodman's series it was 16% (Goodman et al, 1980). Sometimes no definite cause for the pain can be determined. All silastic prostheses eventually show collapse or subsidence radiologically, but this is not generally symptomatic. Sometimes pain is associated with involvement of adjacent joints. A rheumatoid flare has been associated with pain. There have been a few patients with pain who were suspected of having fractured prosthesis but it could not be confirmed initially. However, over the next few weeks as instability and deformity progressed, the diagnosis became apparent.

A conservative approach should be undertaken with a period of splinting, alteration of activities, and hand therapy. We have not injected steroids for fear of infection. In most cases unless there is an apparent cause for the pain it will subside in time.

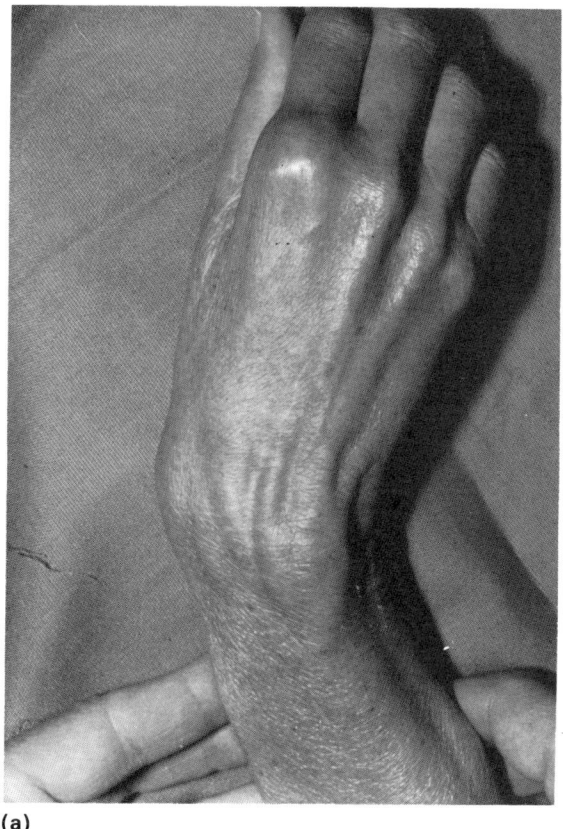
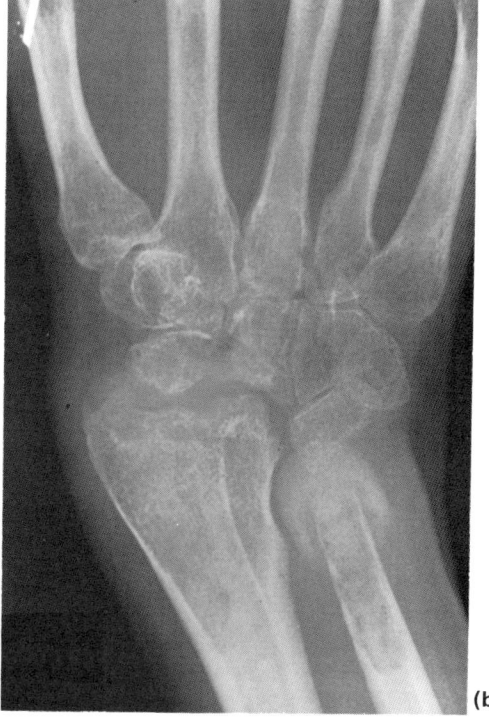
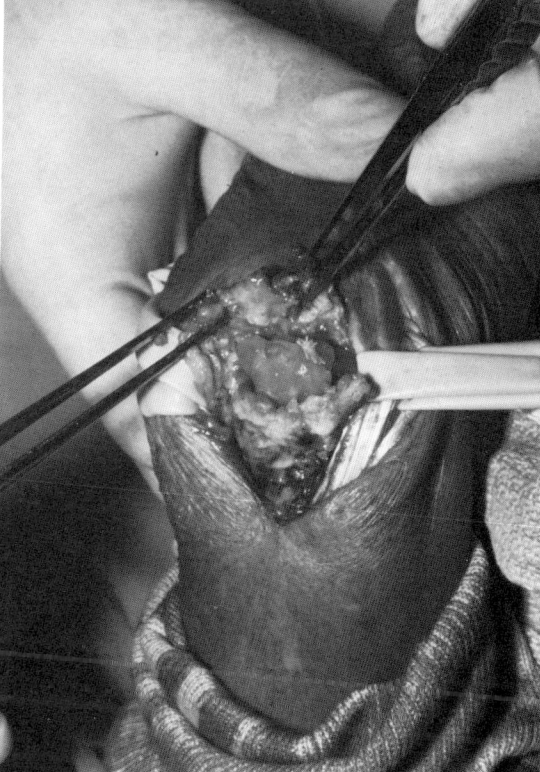

Fig. 21.2 (a) This patient presented with wrist pain 2 years following silicone rubber wrist arthroplasty. Note the ulnar deviation at the wrist. (b) The X-ray demonstrates a fractured wrist prosthesis with ulnar shift of the carpus. Note the cortical erosions beneath the ulnar cap. (c) The fractured wrist prosthesis is identified at the time of revision surgery.

TOTAL WRIST JOINT ARTHROPLASTY

Total wrist joint arthroplasty developed popularity during the 1970s with the prosthetic designs of Meuli and Volz. Since that time design modifications have reduced the incidence of malalignment and prosthetic loosening. However, unforeseen results can occur following total wrist joint arthroplasty including postoperative pain, stiffness, carpal impingement, tendon imbalance, and recurrent deformity.

In our hands silicone wrist arthroplasty has been the preferred procedure leaving us with limited experience using a metal-plastic prosthesis. Beckenbaugh, Linscheid, and others have described the techniques and complications with total wrist arthroplasty and should be referred to before engaging in a reconstructive procedure of this type.

WRIST FUSION

The indications for wrist fusion include patients with total wrist joint involvement, significant instability, and significant deformity which eliminates the possibility of a wrist arthroplasty. The high demand patients are at risk for prosthetic fracture and fusion is best recommended. Another indication for fusion is a painful wrist with only minimal motion. It is unlikely that arthroplasty will restore wrist motion. The patient is generally adjusted to the stiffness and wrist fusion can be performed with less risk.

The surgical procedure is a modification of the technique by Mannerfelt and Clayton in which a Steinman pin is drilled retrograde between the 2nd and 3rd metacarpals and countersunk into the wrist. When this procedure is carried out in conjunction with metacarpophalangeal joint arthroplasty, the pin is inserted through the 3rd metacarpal and countersunk to allow insertion of the prosthesis. Cancellous bone is packed into the metacarpal to prevent protrusion. The wrist is splinted with anterior–posterior splints for 3 to 6 weeks depending upon the amount of stability achieved at surgery (Millender & Nalebuff 1973).

Prevention of complications

In the standard procedure, complications may be associated with pin placement and postoperative pin migration. The most difficult part of the procedure is the introduction of the Steinman pin. The pin must enter a carpus that is often deficient and must exit between the 2nd and 3rd metacarpals. This is a blind drilling and must be accurate. Because of the concern over having the pin penetrate the volar surface of the hand, the tendency is to overcompensate and angle the pin dorsally. The other complication is that the Steinman pin can enter the metacarpal shaft instead of going between the two metacarpals. When either of these situations occur, replacement of the pin must be done. This is difficult because the track has been established. An alternative is to introduce the rod retrograde into the radius to exit dorsoradially and then be driven into the carpus.

Poor Steinman pin placement can be minimised by releasing the soft tissues, so that the hand can be flexed and the carpus brought into the wound. The surgeon then holds the hand with his non-dominant hand and drills with his dominant hand. One can begin with a smaller pin, to assure safe passage, secure a channel, and then introduce the proper sized Steinman pin.

The pin sizes range from 7/64 to 3/16 depending on the size of the medullary canal of the radius. Prior to drilling into the carpus, tap the rod into the radius to determine the proper size and establish a track. After drilling into the carpus the rod should be tapped into the radius and after resistance is encountered back it out 3–4 cm, cut it and countersink it. This prevents having the rod wedged into the radius with the possibility of radial fracture or inability to countersink the rod.

Radial shaft perforations have occurred in our series on several occasions. This was usually recognised at surgery and corrected. However, in one case the Steinman pin perforated the radius, and was not recognised until after surgery. In this case we chose to splint the wrist for several weeks and allow fusion to occur before removing the rod.

Wrist fusion postoperative complications

In the conventional method of wrist fusion, with inadequate bone stock or a loose fitting rod, distal migration can occur. This may result in a painful rod. On occasion the rod may migrate and penetrate the skin. If skin penetration occurs, the rod should be removed. Reintroduction of a pin that has come through the skin is avoided for fear of infection. It can be removed in the office without pain. Once the rod is removed, the wrist is casted. After a rod is removed a fibrous pseudoarthrosis may occur. This is usually asymptomatic and rarely requires additional treatment.

WRIST FUSION IN CONJUNCTION WITH METACARPAL PHALANGEAL JOINT ARTHROPLASTY

When wrist fusion is performed with metacarpophalangeal joint arthroplasty, the Steinman pin is introduced into the shaft of the 3rd metacarpal, which acts to guide the pin into the carpus. Complications of wrist fusion are less with this procedure because the pin travels down the metacarpal, and carpus and is then tapped into the radius. When the rod meets radial resistance it should then be backed out about 2–3 cm, cut off, and then countersunk into the medullary canal. This allows room in the metacarpal for the prosthesis. Sometimes the stem of the prosthesis must be cut if there is inadequate space (Millender & Phillips 1978).

Complications

Complications are uncommon following this procedure. Good fixation is obtained by introducing the rod into the medullary shaft. Stable alignment enhances results following metacarpophalangeal joint arthroplasty. One must prepare the wrist for fusion by opening the joint and removing the cartilage. A blind fusion by just introducing the rod into the medullary canal and into the radius will loosen and fail (Fig. 21.3).

Limited fusions

Nalebuff introduced the concept of limited wrist fusions similar to the limited fusions which have been popularised for trauma by Watson (Nalebuff & Garrod 1984). Either the radio-scapho-lunate joint is fused which will provide about 40–50% of motion in the mid-carpal joint or a mid-carpal fusion is carried out. The appropriate procedure is elected based upon the presence of isolated disease

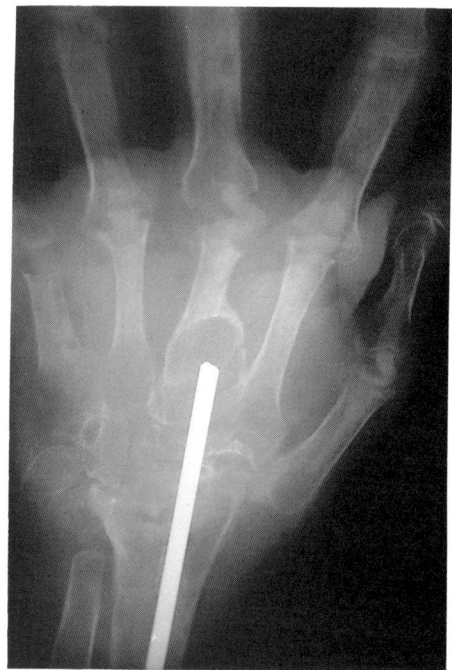

Fig. 21.3 This woman had undergone a 'semi-closed' wrist fusion with metacarpophalangeal joint arthroplasties. The radio-carpal joint had solidly fused. However, motion developed at the carpometacarpal joints causing the Steinman Pin to erode through the dorsal cortex of the third metacarpal.

in either the radio-carpal or mid-carpal joint. The technique is similar to that for fusion following trauma. Most of the problems have been associated with pin placement. It appears that complications can be minimised by not burying the pins under the skin. After the surgery, the wrist is immobilised until solid healing occurs. The pins are removed in 4 to 5 weeks.

Although our experience is limited, the procedure has generally been successful when the indications are specific. It must be utilised for isolated joint destruction. It can not be utilised when there is pan-carpal destruction. Non-union rates have been low. We do not have enough experience at present to state how progression of disease, or increased joint destruction and pain are going to be affected by this procedure.

RADIO-ULNAR JOINT

Involvement of the radio-ulnar joint (caput ulnae syndrome) is a common disability in rheumatoid arthritis and frequently requires surgical correction. The symptoms of this syndrome include radio-ulnar pain, limited radio-ulnar rotation, pain and snapping in radio-ulnar rotation, dislocation of the distal ulna, supination deformity of the hand, and associated tendon ruptures.

Surgical treatment includes distal ulna excision, radio-ulnar synovectomy, reconstruction of the soft tissues, and optional use of the silastic ulnar head prosthesis. Complications of radio-ulnar joint surgery are not common but when present they can cause significant disability and their correction may be difficult.

Complications include persistent pain, especially on rotation, recurrent ulnar subluxation, supination of the wrist, and progressive ulnar translocation of the carpus. Extensor tendon ruptures following distal ulnar excision due to a sharp spike of bone have been reported.

Ulnar head excision—prevention of complications

Most complications are related to soft tissue loss which leads to persistent instability or inadequate reconstruction. Soft tissue reconstruction includes correction of the supination deformity by suturing remnants of the triangular fibrocartilage to the radius thereby realigning the hand to the radius. Often there is little triangular fibrocartilage to use and sometimes a portion of volar capsule or a slip of the extensor carpi ulnaris can be utilised. After this has been corrected then the dorsal subluxation of the distal ulna is corrected by closing tightly the dorsal capsule, relocating the extensor retinaculum, which can also be used to strengthen closure, and relocating the extensor carpi ulnaris.

Postoperative immobilisation is required to allow proper healing. When the deformity and instability is minimal, and a strong closure can be carried out, a well-moulded short anterior and posterior splint is adequate immobilisation. However, when soft tissue closure is inadequate, then wrist support with a long arm cast must be maintained throughout the healing phase.

Ulnar head excision—treatment of complications

Most complications are related to postoperative painful rotation. When these symptoms occur a long period of splinting, gentle range of motion exercises with a well trained hand therapist will often alleviate the symptoms. Often symptoms will decrease with a hand therapy program. No surgery is indicated for 3 to 4 months unless a definite cause for the symptoms can be found.

The big problem is what must one do when the symptoms do not subside? First, what are the causes of the symptoms? If there is gross distal ulnar instability then attempts at carrying out a soft tissue stabilisation procedure utilising extensor carpi ulnaris and local capsule should be attempted. Sometimes the application of a prosthesis will add length or provide a smoother surface for rotation. We generally do not use the distal ulnar prosthesis for routine caput ulnae syndrome excision but occasionally when revising a failed procedure this has eliminated pain. Sometimes the pain is due to radio-ulnar impingement. Revision with ulnar cap is helpful. Sometimes when no cause can be found revision with contouring the distal ulna and application of the cap is helpful. When patients develop carpal translocation, it is not due to ulnar excision, but to destruction of the ulnar triangular fibrocartilage complex. Usually when this occurs radiocarpal fusion or a wrist prosthesis will be needed.

Complications from the ulnar cap

Complications include stem fracture and prosthesis dislocation. Also bony resorption due to periosteal stripping is noted in many cases. When these are asymptomatic nothing needs to be done. When pain, recurrent synovitis, or snapping on rotation occurs, revision with prosthesis removal and soft tissue reconstruction is indicated.

Skin problems and dorsal wrist surgery

All dorsal wrist surgery requires the mobilisation of a radial and ulna skin flap, carried out through a 6–8 cm longitudinal mid-line incision. One of the complications of this surgery is a skin slough. It is usually seen in patients having thin atrophic skin associated with long-term steroid use. The most common cause for this problem is a postoperative haematoma. We advise deflating the tourniquet prior to wound closure to control bleeding. The tourniquet may be re-inflated prior to wound closure to ensure a dry field. In many cases a penrose drain is utilised and removed in 24 hours. Suction drainage does not seem necessary.

If a haematoma develops it must be evacuated, and may require taking the patient back to surgery. Failure to deal with this problem results in wound breakdown, a gaping of the skin, and tendon exposure. In this situation a major complication exists. When this occurs with tendons exposed, daily dressing changes are necessary to allow wound care and allow skin contraction. The other helpful treatment is the application of a frozen pig skin homograph which is changed every 2–4 days. This will protect the underlying tendons. When there is a large gap with multiple tendon exposure there is sometimes partial necrosis of the tendons (Fig. 21.4) (Garner et al 1973).

Our approach to these serious problems is conservative. A skin graft is not applicable because the bed would not accept a graft. A rotation flap has poor marginal skin and carries with it the distinct possibility of having a loss of a large portion of the flap. Additionally, a distant flap would not be feasible in these patients. Using the above described method the skin will contract and close within 2–4 weeks depending upon the size of the defect. Tendon adhesions will develop which can prevent full metacarpophalangeal joint flexion. If the metacarpophalangeal joints are immobilised in extension during this time, the patient will not develop an extension lag. Even with the metacarpophalangeal joints contracted in an extended position, with a good range of proximal interphalangeal joint motion, hand function is not significantly impaired.

METACARPOPHALANGEAL JOINT

The greatest number of complications involving rheumatoid hand surgery occur following metacarpophalangeal joint arthroplasty. This is because metacarpophalangeal joint silastic arthroplasty comprises the largest percentage of rheumatoid surgery and a large number of these will fracture or develop a recurrence of the deformity. In the Mayo Clinic series 29% showed fracture (Beckenbaugh et al 1976).

Fractures are related to the basic instability of the joint, the many forces causing deformity, and the fact that the silicone spacer has no inherent stability.

Many patients will show a mild recurrent ulnar drift, following arthroplasty, which will become stable and is not a problem. However, some of these will progress to a severe ulnar drift which will impede function. With increasing deformity, the prosthesis will generally fracture, then sublux and become painful. Additional problems associated with recurrent deformity with or without fracture is the loss of grip and pinch strength, increasing weakness, and poor appearance.

Causes of complications

The causes of these complications are multiple. One cause of recurrent deformity is wrist imbalance. If there is radial deviation at the wrist joint, which is not corrected, a zigzag deformity of the hand with recurrent ulna drift of the digits will develop following metacarpophalangeal joint arthroplasty (Fig. 21.5). When there is severe preoperative deformity with contractures and poor soft tissues, it is difficult to provide adequate stability and prevent recurrent deformity. Some patients who have strong grip can fracture a prosthesis. This is usually associated with a good capsulo-ligamentous closure and may be due to excessive grip strength or over use. These joints may be completely asymptomatic or they may be associated with a mild change in dexterity and strength. Usually one can note a slight volar subluxation of the proximal phalanx and an instability to anterior posterior stress. X-rays will confirm the fractured prosthesis.

Prevention of complications

Complications are best prevented by performing surgery prior to the development of severe deformity and contracture. This allows complete correction of the deformity. It assures a firm capsular-ligamentous envelope to preserve stability. Swanson has emphasised that success of the operation is related to reconstruction of this strong capsulo-ligamentous envelope. Extensor tendon realignment is carried out. When there is radial wrist

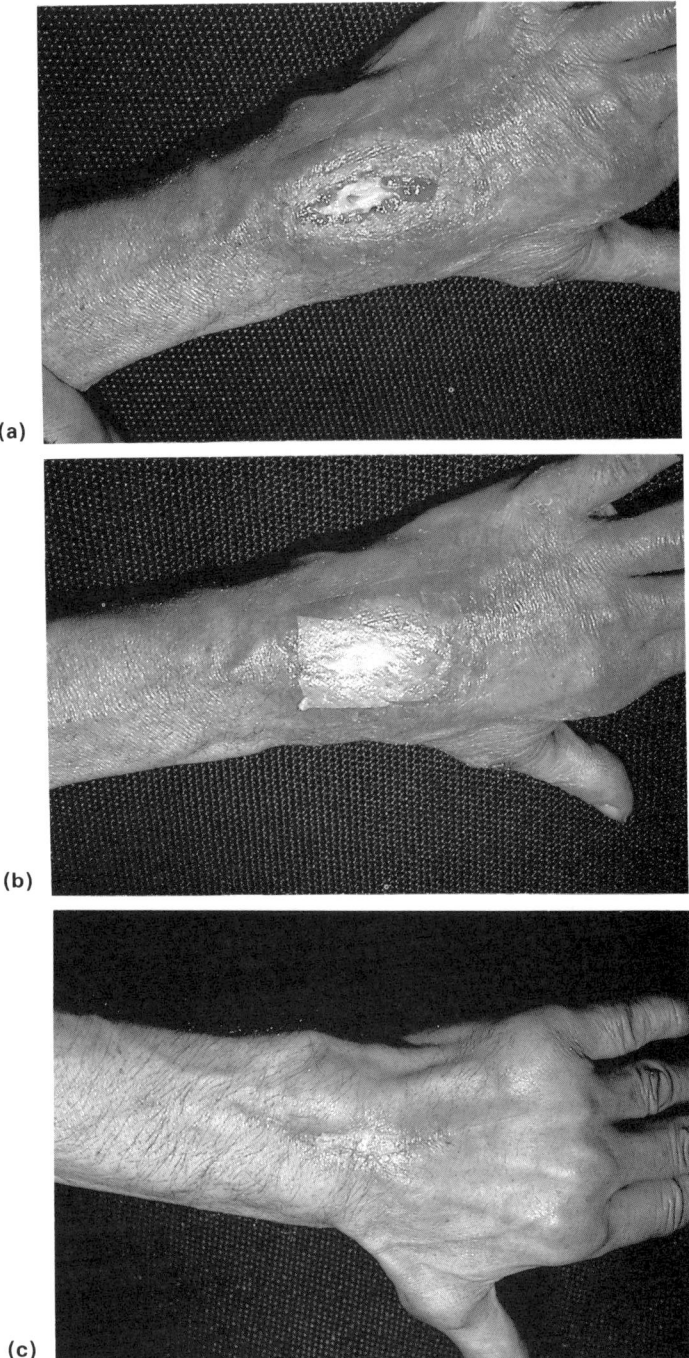

Fig. 21.4 (a) Ten days following dorsal tenosynovectomy this skin slough occurred. Present within the wound are exposed extensor tendons and necrotic tissue. (b) The patient was treated with homograph skin which was changed every 2 to 3 days. (c) The wound has healed in $3\frac{1}{2}$ weeks. Extensor tendon adhesions have left this patient with a 35° extensor lag.

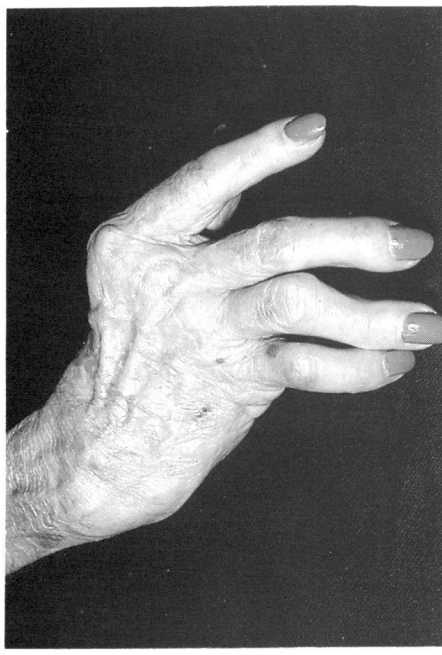 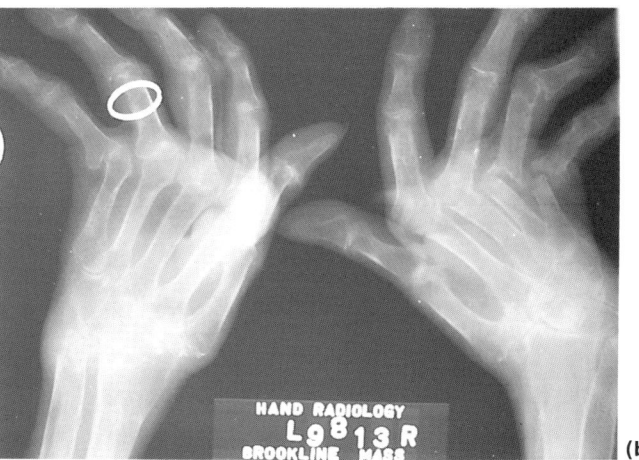

Fig. 21.5 (a) Recurrent ulnar drift has developed following metacarpophalangeal joint arthroplasty. This patient maintained good alignment of her fingers for 2 years following surgery. However, as the wrist began to deteriorate, radial deviation of the wrist eventually led to recurrent ulnar drift of the fingers. (b) The X-ray demonstrates wrist joint destruction with radial deviation. Each of the metacarpophalangeal joint implants is fractured with recurrent ulnar deviation of the fingers.

deviation that is passively correctable, and associated with a ruptured or subluxed extensor carpi ulnaris tendon, then extensor carpi ulnaris repair with an intercalated graft or extensor carpi radialis longus transfer to realign the wrist is indicated.

Some patients present with fixed radial wrist deformities, moderate to severe metacarpophalangeal joint deformities, and poor soft tissues. These problems are harder to correct and predispose to recurrent deformity. If there is significant wrist deformity with pain, then wrist fusion in conjunction with metacarpophalangeal arthroplasty is indicated. Recurrent metacarpophalangeal deformity is infrequent when a well aligned wrist is present. The problem arises in choosing the best procedure for correcting a painless wrist with a fixed radial deformity, and a moderate degree of motion. In this situation, little can be done to realign the wrist. Following metacarpophalangeal arthroplasty, the patients are splinted longer to assure stability. Limited metacarpophalangeal joint motion is accepted. If the proximal interphalangeal joint motion is good then restricting metacarpophalangeal joint motion to 40–50° is probably the best method to prevent recurrent deformity.

In hands with severe deformity and minimal capsule available for reconstruction, the same general approach is followed. One is usually able to align the digits with soft tissue releases and bone resection. In many cases a small sized prosthesis must be inserted because of the narrow medullary canal. After surgery, the metacarpophalangeal joints are immobilised for 2 weeks, proximal interphalangeal joint motion is begun immediately and dynamic splinting is begun after the 2 weeks of immobilisation. The goals in these cases are to obtain 30–50° of metacarpophalangeal joint motion with adequate alignment and stability. If proximal interphalangeal motion is preserved and the wrist is pain free, and well aligned, a moderate degree of function can be restored.

Correction of fracture and recurrent deformity

With fracture and recurrent deformity treatment is based on the patients symptoms and clinical findings (Fig. 21.6). When a fractured prosthesis is asymptomatic or even mildly symptomatic reassurance and observation is often the best treatment (Fig. 21.7). When patients present with recurrent deformity and fractures that are symptomatic, revision is indicated. If the cause was wrist malalignment, one must realign the wrist in order to prevent recurrent digital problems. This usually requires fusion.

Revision arthroplasty for fracture and deformity is technically harder than the original surgery. Like any revision surgery, one is dealing with scar, poor tissue planes, and all components of revision surgery. The goal of revision surgery is to completely correct the deformity, release contracture, resect bone, restore alignment, and reinsert a new prosthesis (Fig. 21.8).

Because a Swanson prosthesis is not fixed, extraction is easy. When the Niebauer prosthesis is being removed the stem is more difficult to extract because of bony ingrowth. After the prosthesis has been inserted any capsular-ligamentous material present is closed.

The postoperative management depends upon the alignment, stability, and soft tissue closure achieved at the time of the revision. In general we would tend to treat these cases like the severe cases and immobilise them longer, attempting to provide a greater degree of stability with less motion and less chance for recurrent deformity.

PROXIMAL INTERPHALANGEAL JOINT—PREVENTION OF UNSATISFACTORY RESULTS

The complications of proximal interphalangeal joint surgery are related to the limitations of our surgical techniques to restore functional range of motion. Because of the intricate extensor and flexor tendon mechanisms and the effects that rheumatoid arthritis has on the joint and tendons, surgical reconstruction is less effective in the proximal interphalangeal joint than any other joint in the hand. A clear understanding of these limitations must be appreciated when one evaluates patients with proximal interphalangeal joint abnormalities. Inappropriate surgery based on inadequate knowledge of these limitations is a frequent cause of unfortunate results.

In considering the proximal interphalangeal joint one should look at four different areas; boutonniere deformity, swan neck deformity, isolated proximal interphalangeal joint destruction, and proximal interphalangeal joint destruction associated with metacarpophalangeal joint involvement.

Boutonniere deformity

Rheumatoid boutonniere surgery must be undertaken with caution because it involves destruction

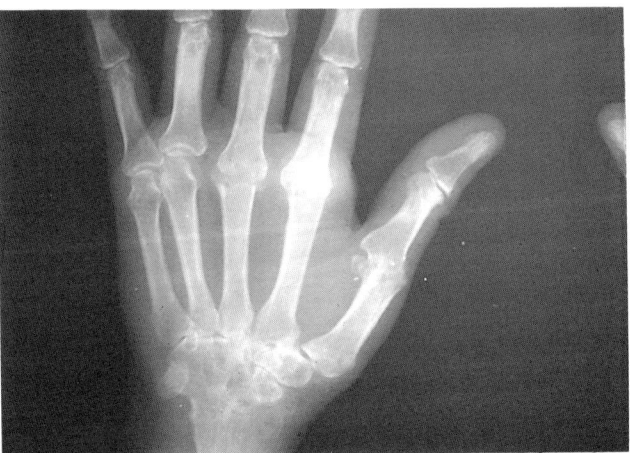

Fig. 21.6 This patient presented with X-rays demonstrating fractured metacarpophalangeal joint arthroplasties in the index and middle fingers. However, he had no pain, no deformity, and no loss of function. Therefore, revision was not necessary.

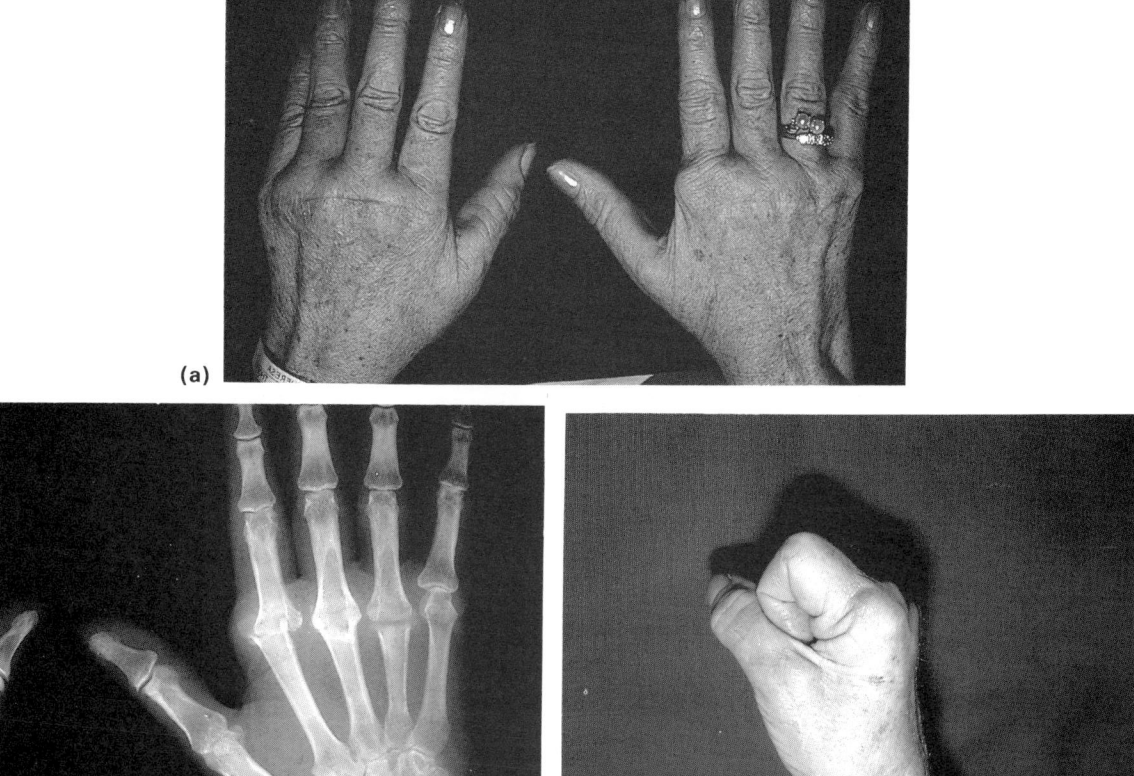

Fig. 21.7 (a) This patient presents with subluxation of the metacarpophalangeal joints to her right index and middle fingers. (b) The X-ray demonstrates fractured metacarpophalangeal joint prosthetics. (c) The patient functions well with this hand. She can make a fist, open and close her hand, and has minimal pain.

of both the extensor mechanism and various degrees of joint involvement. Most boutonniere reconstruction involves synovectomy as well as reconstruction of the extensor mechanism.

When patients have persistent proximal interphalangeal synovitis, or there is a mild stretching of the extensor mechanism, synovectomy is indicated to prevent boutonniere deformity. Boutonniere reconstruction is also indicated for patients with supple boutonniere deformities, especially when it is progressing, and the joint is preserved. In this situation, one should expect good results (Nalebuff & Millender 1975).

The difficult problems and the unfortunate results associated with boutonniere deformities are those associated with severe fixed flexion deformities, especially when the joint is involved. Surgical decisions are difficult and require judgement and experience. In general, if the joint is preserved, and patients have fixed deformities of 45–60°, attempts at releasing these deformities and reconstruction are reasonable. When the deformity is greater than 60–75°, and the joint is involved, the prognosis is guarded. In the ulnar digits where grasp is important, one may elect to correct the distal interphalangeal joint hyperextension, and

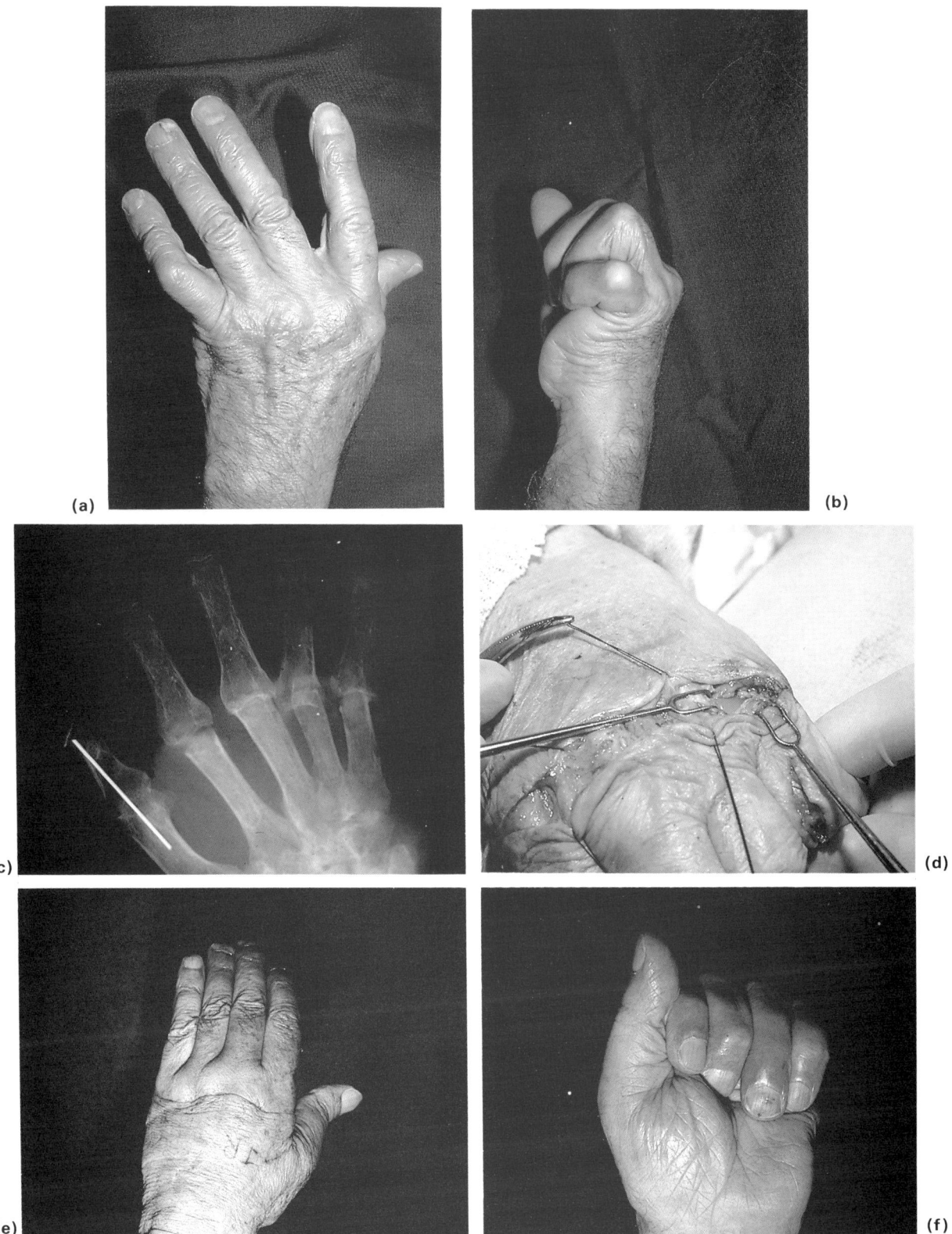

Fig. 21.8 (a) This patient has developed recurrent ulnar drift following metacarpophalangeal joint arthroplasty. (b) Note the deformity while making a fist. (c) The X-ray demonstrates fractured prosthetics in the index and middle finger metacarpophalangeal joints. (d) The patient underwent revision surgery with insertion of new silicone rubber implants. (e) and (f) Postoperatively he has regained a functional range of motion. Note the deformity has been corrected.

leave the proximal interphalangeal joint alone to allow full grasp. This is especially indicated if the joint deformity is not progressive. If the deformity exists in the index and long digits, arthrodesis in a more functional position may be a reasonable choice.

Proximal interphalangeal joint arthroplasty is an alternative in some of these cases. When the joint is destroyed, and boutonniere deformity mild, then arthroplasty would be more successful. However, as the degree of the deformity increases, the results following arthroplasty are less favourable. This is related to many factors, the major ones being the necessity to remove large amounts of bone to restore extension and allow room for the prosthesis. The need to reconstruct a severely attenuated extensor mechanism, and to immobilise the joint during the healing period also makes this procedure less favourable. Because of these factors, the indications for proximal interphalangeal joint arthroplasty are narrow and infrequent.

The other alternative for the severe boutonniere deformity is fusion, but patients would be carefully evaluated prior to recommending fusion. In some patients full flexion is most important, especially with the ulnar digits. They can adapt to a fixed flexion contracture, especially if they have developed compensatory hyperextension in the metacarpophalangeal joints. In these cases the proximal interphalangeal joints should not be fused. When the need is to grasp large objects or when the need for gloves is important, fusion becomes more reasonable. In general fusions are more indicated for the index and middle fingers and less for the ring and small finger proximal interphalangeal joints.

Swan neck deformity

The indications for swan neck surgery are relatively well established and predictable. For supple swan neck deformity with no metacarpophalangeal joint involvement, the flexor digitorum sublimus tenodesis can be carried out in conjunction with tenosynovectomy. This is helpful in correcting the deformity and preventing progression of the deformity (see section on stiff proximal interphalangeal joint and flexor tenosynovitis) (Nalebuff & Millender 1975b).

Most swan neck deformities are associated with subluxation of the metacarpophalangeal joints. The established procedure involves metacarpophalangeal joint arthroplasty with proximal interphalangeal joint manipulation and temporary Kirschner wire fixation. When this is carried out it is generally necessary to expose the flexor tendons in the palm to assure that they have adequate excursion. By correcting the deformity, and providing a moderate range of metacarpophalangeal and proximal interphalangeal joint motion, function is generally improved. When these joints have a severe fixed hyperextension deformity with destruction, manipulation into a functional position, along with metacarpophalangeal arthroplasty is helpful in improving function. The K-wires are left in place for 3–4 weeks to assure that the deformity will not recur. Any flexion which is obtained after the wire is removed is considered a bonus.

Generally metacarpophalangeal joint motion following arthroplasty in these cases is good, because all of the flexor and extensor power is concentrated at the metacarpophalangeal joint level. By placing the proximal interphalangeal joints in a more functional position, general function is augmented.

Proximal interphalangeal joint arthritis with joint destruction

Because our ability to restore motion and improve function is limited in the proximal interphalangeal joint, careful evaluation is required prior to recommending surgery. Most unfortunate results occur when surgical reconstruction is undertaken anticipating an unrealistic result. Many people with flexion deformities or a lack of flexion function quite well. Ill advised surgery can diminish function in these patients. Many rheumatoids have adapted to a certain deformity which has slowly developed over years. Unless one is relatively sure that function can be improved, surgery should be advised with caution.

The main indication for proximal interphalangeal joint surgery is pain. When pain is persistent either arthrodesis or arthroplasty is advised. The indication depends upon the digit and the degree of involvement. In general, arthroplasty is selected when there is less destruction of the bone and extensor tendon mechanism. Fusion is reserved for more severe destruction, deformity, and instability. Additionally, one tries to preserve motion in the ulnar digits to improve grasp. Proximal interphalangeal fusion of the radial two digits may be preferred to maintain pinch.

When patients present with proximal interphalangeal joint deformity, instability, and loss of motion without pain, careful evaluation is necessary prior to recommending surgery. This again, is an area where unfortunate results occur. A careful evaluation to determine the patient's loss, their needs, and their expectations is necessary. When significant impairment exists, fusion, in a functional position, is helpful.

Metacarpophalangeal and proximal interphalangeal joint involvement

The combination of metacarpophalangeal and proximal interphalangeal joint destruction in a rheumatoid patient is a frequent finding. Again, a careful evaluation is necessary to determine the best type of procedure to recommend. In general, proximal interphalangeal joint and metacarpophalangeal joint arthroplasty in the same digit is not successful, and they are infrequently recommended either as a combined procedure or at separate stages. Thus, the decision is to either leave the proximal interphalangeal joint alone, or to fuse the proximal interphalangeal joint in conjunction with metacarpophalangeal joint arthroplasty.

When metacarpophalangeal subluxation is associated with either a severe flexion contracture of the proximal interphalangeal joints, or destruction of the proximal interphalangeal joints, then fusion of the proximal interphalangeal joints with metacarpophalangeal arthroplasty is the recommended procedure. Excellent metacarpophalangeal range of motion is usually established because all of the flexor and extensor power is concentrated at the metacarpophalangeal joint level. For severe deformity, and a salvage type of problem, this combined surgery is recommended.

When there is some preserved motion in the proximal interphalangeal joints we generally accept this, and carry out only metacarpophalangeal arthroplasty. If the proximal interphalangeal joints of the ulnar digits have 40–45° of fixed flexion deformities with full flexion, they should be left alone. If the index or long digit has 40–50° of active flexion, they should also be left alone. If however, the index or long digit has a 60° fixed flexion deformity then one should consider carrying out arthrodesis of the proximal interphalangeal joint along with metacarpophalangeal arthroplasty to improve the patient's pinch.

Technically, a temporary K-wire across the proximal interphalangeal joint, which has a 45–60° fixed flexion deformity, is helpful to restore metacarpophalangeal joint motion in the early postoperative. If a digit has a fixed proximal interphalangeal flexion contracture which is not temporarily pinned, then after the metacarpophalangeal arthroplasty, a claw type deformity can result and limited metacarpophalangeal flexion can occur. Therefore, sometimes, temporary K-wire fixation to allow all the flexor and extensor power to be concentrated at the metacarpophalangeal joint level is appropriate.

DIGITAL FUSIONS

Digital joint fusions comprise a large percentage of rheumatoid hand surgery. They are frequently utilised in the distal interphalangeal joints, thumb interphalangeal joint, and thumb metacarpophalangeal joint. They are also indicated for severe proximal interphalangeal joint deformity and instability. The general indications for fusions are pain, instability, and deformity.

Complications

The complications following digital fusions are associated with problems from Kirschner wires and non-unions. Many times the non-unions are stable, asymptomatic, and provide the same functional result as a solid fusion would. Complications from Kirschner wires are related to pin tract infections, loosening, pain, and tenderness when the pin is buried.

When a Kirschner wire becomes infected, it is immediately removed. Removing the pin generally aborts the infection. If there is cellulitis oral antibiotics should be preserved. It is rare to develop an osteomylitis secondary to a pin tract infection.

More bothersome is the patient with a painful pin which has been buried deep to the skin. This can become difficult especially if the pin is irritating a digital nerve. If the pin cannot be extracted from the dorsum, volar exploration is necessary. Depending on the location of the pin and whether or not the pin can be easily palpated, tourniquet control with adequate operating facilities should be available to avoid injury to the digital nerve.

Another difficult situation arises when the pin migrates and becomes flush with the bone or becomes inbedded in the bone and is unable to be grasped by a needle holder. It may become necessary to take a rongeur and remove some bone around the pin in order to obtain purchase. Another problem to avoid is not grabbing the Kirschner wire head on. When the wire is being removed blindly, if the needle driver grabs the wire from an angle the driver will slip and sometimes a counter force will drive the pin forward, inbedding it into the bone or in the soft tissues.

Non-unions

Non-unions are frequently seen following rheumatoid surgery. Many times a firm fibrous union is painless, stable, and functions as well as a solid fusion. The reason for the high percentage of non-unions is the degree of joint destruction, large amounts of bony resorption, and a lack of good bone stock.

In most cases, digital fusion can be accomplished by standard techniques which include cartilage removal, apposition of cancellous bony surfaces, and firm internal fixation with Kirschner wires. Either a small aluminium splint or a plaster splint can be utilised for additional external fixation until fusion is solid.

When there is adequate bone stock the biggest cause for non-union is failure to completely correct subluxation and maintain firm bony apposition. This may be seen in the thumb metacarpophalangeal joint when the proximal phalanx becomes subluxed volar to the metacarpal. It can also be seen in the severe Type I thumb deformity when the distal phalanx is completely dislocated. When these deformities exist, complete joint release is necessary to provide firm bony contact.

Another problem which leads to non-union is failure to prepare the two bones prior to internal fixation. Many times one bone will show a large cupping deformity and the other bone will show a pencil deformity. Each of these must be corrected. The edges of a cupped bone must be rongeured down to a wide cancellous base. The sclerotic pointed pencil must be removed to obtain healthy bone stock. Shortening is acceptable to obtain firm apposition of the bone. Many times a dowel and cone type of fusion can be used in which the pencil portion is plugged into the dowel to obtain firm apposition and secured with Kirschner wire fixation.

Fusion with severe bone loss

In rheumatoid or psoriatic arthritis with a mutilans component, the amount of bone loss can be enormous. One method that is advocated to stop the severe rapid bone destruction in these joints is to carry out early fusion. When there is significant bone loss, bone grafting is required. Metacarpal heads or bone from a wrist arthrodesis or wrist arthroplasty will make good graft material. If these surgeries are necessary the digital fusions can be easily carried out simultaneously. It is preferable to avoid taking an iliac bone graft in these frail people because of the increased morbidity. And in most cases when bone grafting is needed local bone can be obtained.

There are some occasions where bone stock is needed to restore length. This is most often seen in a thumb with severe bone loss. In these cases a block of iliac graft can be utilised to obtain fusion and restore length. Another method that is helpful is the utilisation of the polypropalene plugs. These plugs are available at different angles and are used as a permanent internal fixation device which will restore a stable joint. Sometimes fusions occur around the device and at other times a firm fibrous union will stabilise the joint.

There are a few cases in which a large amount of bone loss and joint destruction exists, making fusion impossible. We have tried to correct these deformities by removing soft tissue and cartilage and by fixing the joint with Kirschner wires in an attempt to provide a degree of fibrous stability. The amount of stability in these patients has often been minimal and the results of these cases have not been satisfactory.

Correction of non-unions

Rheumatoid digital non-unions should be evaluated differently from non-unions secondary to trauma. Usually a fibrous non-union will be stable, pain free, and functionally acceptable. Even if the non-union demonstrates a degree of motion it may be acceptable. We have found it unnecessary in most cases to re-operate these patients. Additionally, one must realise that the chances for success are less with re-operation and there is a risk for a second non-union. If re-operation is necessary following a failed fusion one probably should use iliac bone graft.

RECONSTRUCTION OF THE RHEUMATOID THUMB

Reconstruction of the rheumatoid thumb is associated with a high degree of success. Unfortunate results are infrequent if indications are proper and expectations are realistic. Interphalangeal joint fusions will restore a pain free, stable, terminal joint (Fig. 21.9). Both metacarpophalangeal fusion and metacarpophalangeal arthroplasties provide pain free stable joints. If metacarpophalangeal arthroplasty is utilised, 20–30° of motion is desired. For basal joint deformity and instability associated with pain, hemi-arthroplasty is the procedure of choice. This provides a stable carpometacarpal joint with acceptable motion. Although function can be improved and pain alleviated, reconstructive surgery can not restore strength or provide a high degree of dexterity.

Prevention of complications

In most cases unfortunate results following thumb reconstruction occur because of poor indications for surgery. When surgery is carried out for persistent pain, instability, or deformity, success can be assured. However, when surgery is attempted to restore a high degree of function, unsatisfactory results occur. Careful preoperative evaluation is necessary to determine the needs, expectations, and realistic goals for the patient.

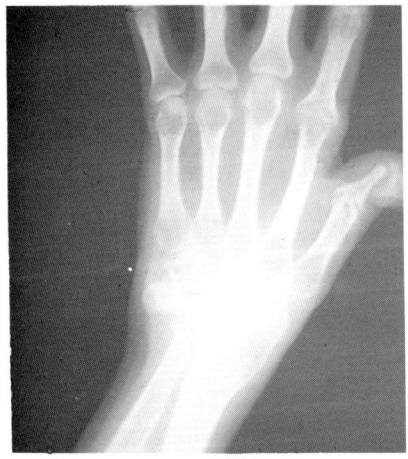
(a)

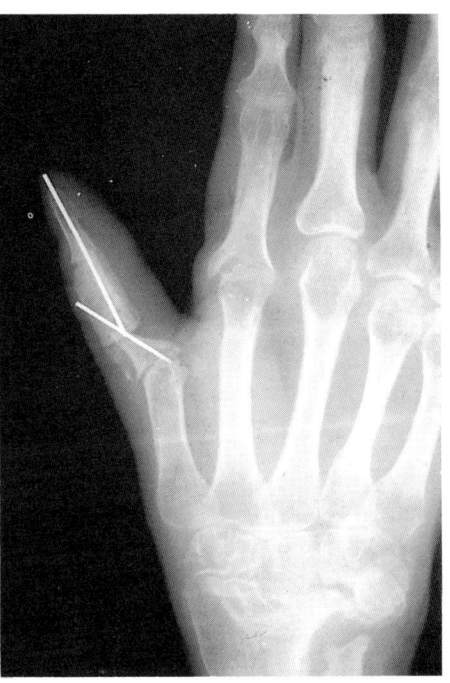
(b)

Fig. 21.9 (a) The thumb in this X-ray is shortened and has an unstable interphalangeal joint with significant bone loss. (b) The interphalangeal joint was fused utilising an iliac bone graft. If the fusion were performed at the time of metacarpophalangeal joint arthroplasty, the resected metacarpal heads could be used as the bone graft.

Two areas where unfortunate results can occur are in fusion of the interphalangeal joint in the thumb and correction of a type III swan neck deformity in the thumb. Often a deformed or unstable interphalangeal joint with a small degree of motion is more functional than a fused interphalangeal joint. Even though it may appear that fusion would be preferable, the patient may have developed substitution methods which are effective and function may decrease if arthrodesis is carried out.

The other area where the severity of the deformity does not parallel the degree of function is in the type III thumb deformity. Many patients with subluxation of the carpometacarpal joint and zigzag collapse patterns of the thumb have acceptable function, and surgery will not improve the condition. Even though the first web space may be narrow because of an adduction contracture, the patients compensate by hyperextending the metacarpophalangeal joint. The patients can grasp moderately sized objects and the preserved metacarpophalangeal and interphalangeal joint motion provides dexterity.

Complications

Complications, as stated, are fortunately infrequent. Non-unions of interphalangeal or metacarpophalangeal joints have been previously discussed. Complications following metacarpophalangeal arthroplasty of the thumb are infrequent. The goal of arthroplasty is to obtain a stable joint with only 20–30° of motion. When there is an incompetent ulnar collateral ligament, failure to reconstruct the ligament can result in lateral instability and this is a relative contraindication to arthroplasty. In these cases fusion is generally selected and by fusing the proximal phalanx in pronation, one can overcome a supination deformity of the carpometacarpal joint.

Carpometacarpal joint complications

Total trapezium excision with silastic trapezial arthroplasty is contraindicated because of the high percentage of dislocations that occur due to poor bone stock and inadequate capsule. To avoid this, a hemiarthroplasty is preferred. Complications are generally technical. Injury to the radial artery can be a significant problem. The radial artery crosses the scapho-trapezial joint deep to the abductor pollicis longus tendon. With severe thumb and wrist deformities, the artery can be injured during trapezial excision. The major complications are related to inadequate correction of the deformity resulting in postoperative subluxation of the prosthesis (Fig. 21.10). The deformity is corrected by releasing the carpometacarpal capsule and resecting the base of the metacarpal. This usually corrects the adduction deformity and rarely is release of the first dorsal interossous necessary. Only a small portion of the trapezium is removed to provide a flat base to accept the hemi-arthroplasty. The trapezium is deformed with dorso-radial collapse. In order to restore a flat base, the medial portion, including the beak and trapezoid articulation, must be removed. After the joint is prepared, the prosthesis is selected and inserted with capsular closure carried out. Shortening of the abductor pollicis longus helps assure stability. Additional surgery, especially stabilisation of the metacarpophalangeal joint of the thumb should be carried out prior to capsular closure. Failure to correct metacarpophalangeal joint hyperextension with either fusion or tenodesis will lead to a recurrence of the subluxation.

Most carpometacarpal hemi-arthroplasties are relatively stable. By shortening the metacarpal there is generally adequate capsule for closure, and

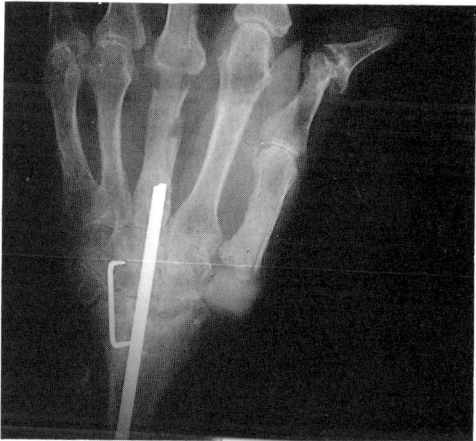

Fig. 21.10 This X-ray demonstrates a dislocated trapezium arthroplasty due to inadequate bone stock and poor soft tissues. Rheumatoid patients should be treated with a hemi-arthroplasty.

subluxation has not been a big problem. This procedure has been successful in alleviating pain and restoring function.

INFECTIONS FOLLOWING SILASTIC ARTHROPLASTY

Infections following silastic arthroplasty are infrequent. Swanson (1972) reviewed his infection rate after 3915 cases, and reports less than a 1% incidence of postoperative infections. Nalebuff and Millender reviewed 2501 silastic arthroplasties and reported an infection rate of 0.48%. This parallels the results of Swanson and points out that silastic arthroplasty has a much lower infection rate than other total joint arthroplasties. The series of Nalebuff and Millender were performed without antibiotics.

Prevention of infections

The most important factors in preventing infection following silastic arthroplasty include avoidance of soft tissue trauma, hematoma, and tight wound closure. These problems are related to proper surgical technique, careful splinting, and postoperative management. We have not found an increased incidence of infection in those patients that were on steroids, or antimetabolites prior to surgery. Additionally, if an open olecranon bursa or an open bunion is present without infection, surgery can be performed with antibiotic coverage. Caution is needed when arthroplasty is performed with an open wound on the same hand. Also if the patient has had a prior total joint replacement, in any major joint, then antibiotic coverage would also be utilised.

The only factor that seemed to be associated with an increased rate of infection was psoriatic arthritis. Active psoriatic skin lesions did lead to an increased incidence of infection. Although one can operate in the face of a mild psoriatic skin lesion, when there are active skin eruptions, surgery should be postponed, and good skin care should be instituted. It should also be mentioned that in the postoperative care with the psoriatic patient, frequent dressing changes should be carried out until the incision heals.

Treatment of infected silastic arthroplasty

Treatment depends upon the joint involved and the severity of the infection. We have seen a few patients who had developed clinical evidence of infection 24–48 hours following surgery. These patients present with an increase in temperature, pain, and swelling, localized to the involved joint. In these patients, satisfactory treatment was obtained with splinting of the involved joint and intravenous antibiotic therapy.

Most infections involved metacarpophalangeal joint arthroplasties and developed on the average within 17 days following surgery. These patients presented with purulent drainage, and in a few cases with X-ray changes. In these cases the prosthesis was removed, the joints were debrided, and the patients received 5 days of intravenous therapy (Fig. 21.11). Following this regimen, they were then converted to oral antibiotics, for approximately 2 weeks. All wounds healed and the patients were left with a stiff resection arthroplasty.

The only situation in which an attempt to replace

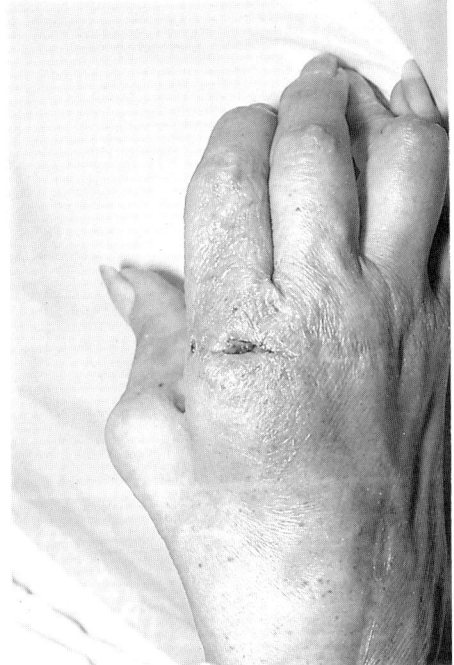

Fig. 21.11 This patient presented 4 weeks following metacarpophalangeal joint arthroplasty with pain, swelling, and purulent drainage from the incision. Treatment included removal of the prosthesis, debridement, and 7 days of intravenous antibiotics, followed by 2 weeks of oral antibiotics. The wound healed without a recurrence of the infection.

a prosthesis would be considered would be in the case of an infected metacarpophalangeal joint in the index finger. In this case a silastic arthroplasty might be inserted to help maintain stability of the joint against lateral pinch. We have done this on a few occasions when there was a late skin breakdown with slight drainage and no evidence of extensive infection. In these cases after debridement a new prosthesis was reinserted and the patients were maintained on intravenous antibiotics for two–three weeks. This has been successful in resolving the problem. The metacarpophalangeal joint of the thumb may also be considered for replacement arthroplasty to further augment stability. Arthrodesis of the metacarpophalangeal joint following infection in the thumb would be difficult because of a lack of bone stock, as well as the presence of soft, infected, rheumatoid bone.

We have not treated an infection involving a silastic arthroplasty of the proximal interphalangeal joint. However, if it was converted to a resection arthroplasty, the goals would be to obtain a stable pseudoarthrosis. We also have not seen a postoperative infection following silastic wrist arthroplasty. However, here also, the prosthesis would be removed, the joint would be debrided, intravenous antibiotics would be instituted, and the wrist would be splinted. If this joint developed into a painful pseudoarthrosis, then a wrist fusion could be performed.

REFERENCES

Beckenbaugh R D, Dobyns J D, Linscheid R L, Bryan R S 1976 Review and analysis of silicone-rubber metacarpophalangeal implants. Journal of Bone and Joint Surgery 58A: 483–487

Brase D, Millender L H 1985 Evaluation of failures after silicone rubber wrist implant arthroplasty. 40th Annual Meeting of the American Society for Surgery of The Hand. January 1985, Las Vegas, Nevada—Proceedings. Journal of Hand Surgery 10A: 427

Garner R W, Mowat A G, Hazelman B L 1973 Wound healing after operations on patients with rheumatoid arthritis. Journal of Bone and Joint Surgery 55B: 134–144

Goodman M, Millender L, Nalebuff E, Phillips C 1980 Arthroplasty of the rheumatoid wrist with silicone rubber: An early evaluation. Journal of Hand Surgery 5: 114–121

Mannerfelt L, Norman O 1969 Attrition ruptures of flexor tendons in rheumatoid arthritis caused by bony spurs in the carpal tunnel. Journal of Bone and Joint Surgery 51B: 270–277

Millender L H, Nalebuff E A 1973 Arthrodesis of the rheumatoid wrist. An evaluation of sixty patients and a description of a different surgical technique. Journal of Bone and Joint Surgery 55A: 1026–1034

Millender L H, Nalebuff E A 1975a Preventive surgery—tenosynovectomy and synovectomy. Orthopaedic Clinics of North America 6: 765–792

Millender L H, Nalebuff E A 1975b Reconstructive surgery in the rheumatoid hand. Orthopaedic Clinics of North America 6: 709–732

Millender L H, Nalebuff E A, Albin R, Ream J R, Gordon M 1974 Dorsal tenosynovectomy and tendon transfer in the rheumatoid hand. Journal of Bone and Joint Surgery 56A: 601–610

Millender L H, Philips C 1978 Combined wrist arthrodesis and metacarpophalangeal joint arthroplasty in rheumatoid arthritis. Orthopedics 1: 43–48

Moberg E 1969 Cartilage lesions. Pp 173–177. In Hijmans W, Paul W D, Herschel H eds. Early Synovectomy in Rheumatoid Arthritis. Excerpta Medica Foundation, Amsterdam, p 173–177

Nalebuff E A 1969a Metacarpophalangeal surgery in rheumatoid arthritis. Surgical Clinics of North America 49: 823–832

Nalebuff E A 1969a Nature and management of flexor tendon nodules in the rheumatoid hand. In Tubiana R ed. La Main Rheumatoide. Expansion Scientifique Francaise, Paris, p 123–128

Nalebuff E A 1969c Surgical treatment of rheumatoid tenosynovitis in the hand. Surgical Clinics of North America 49: 799–809

Nalebuff E A, Millender L H 1975a Surgical treatment of the boutonniere deformity in rheumatoid arthritis. Orthopaedics Clinics of North America 6: 753–763

Nalebuff E A, Millender L H 1975b Surgical treatment of the swan-neck deformity in rheumatoid arthritis. Orthopaedic Clinics of North America 6: 733–752

Nalebuff E A, Potter T A 1968 Rheumatoid involvement of tendon and tendon sheaths in the hand. Clinical Orthopaedics 59: 147–159

Nalebuff E A, Garrod K J 1984 Present approach to the severely involved rheumatoid wrist. Orthopaedic Clinics of North America 15: 369–380

Swanson A B 1972 Flexible implant arthroplasty for arthritic finger joints. Rationale, technique, and results of treatment. Journal of Bone and Joint Surgery 54A: 435–455

22 Osteoarthritis

P. J. Millroy

Primary osteoarthritis occurs commonly in the hands especially at the distal interphalangeal joints and base of the thumb. Hereditary factors are prominent. Women are more commonly afflicted. No cure is known. Surgical treatment is often indicated when conservative treatment has failed or become cumbersome. A succinct review of this condition has been made by Swanson & Swanson (1983). Also arthritic changes in the hands may be post traumatic and may affect any of the joints. Specific joints will now be discussed.

THE DISTAL INTERPHALANGEAL JOINT

Osteoarthritis is common here and is usually due to primary generalised osteoarthritis and less frequently post-traumatic.

Characteristically, there are cycles of pain, remission and final cessation of pain although the joint may be left deformed, angulated and restricted in range. Therefore cosmetic improvement will always be a high patient priority even if not admitted. If pain, loss of function and deformity are severe enough to warrant surgery then arthrodesis is the procedure of choice. Debridement or silicone (condylar) arthroplasty can be considered but the result will often be unsatisfactory functionally and cosmetically.

Problems, prevention and management

1. Position of arthrodesis

This should be discussed in detail with the patient. Most women prefer arthrodesis with only slight flexion or straight. This provides good cosmesis and adequate function. The thumb interphalangeal joint is best straight so that the full tactile area of the pulp can be utilised. It is commonly recommended that the amount of flexion be increased from index across to little to improve the grip but most women do not like too much flexion. In practice, function is adequate with slight flexion including the little and ring finger distal joints.

2. Obtaining bony union

Compared with rheumatoid arthritis, in osteoarthritis the subchondral bone is often sclerotic and must be excised to allow cancellous to cancellous contact. If in doubt about this a bone graft may be required if bone quality and apposition are poor or shortening is severe. A bone graft can be taken out of the distal radius on the dorsal aspect by retracting extensor carpi radialis longus and brevis. Otherwise the olecranon is a satisfactory small donor site.

Delayed and non-union are caused by: 1. Inadequate subchondral bone excision. 2. Distraction at the time of internal fixation. Simple techniques are adequate. Through a dorsal transverse incision carefully placed over the joint line in order to minimise skin retraction, the extensor tendon and collateral ligaments are divided to open out the joint surfaces. Sometimes prior nibbling of an overlying dorsal osteophyte is required. The joint surfaces are excised back to open cancellous surfaces to obtain good apposition in slight flexion. One longitudinal K wire is inserted. The position is carefully checked. The length of K wire in the middle phalanx is checked with a second K wire of the same length. The distal phalanx is then forcefully impacted onto the middle phalanx in the correct rotation. Another K wire can be drilled obliquely across the arthrodesis maintaining compression. Where a silicone hinge arthroplasty of the proximal joint is being done at the same time two oblique K wires will be used.

Intraosseous compression wiring had been effectively used for small joint arthrodesis by my colleagues for many years before it was reported by Lister (1978). It is an excellent technique but is more time consuming and, if necessary, removal is more difficult. The same can be said of lag screw techniques. However, where early use is mandatory these techniques are worthwhile. The Herbert (1984) bone screw provides rigid fixation with compression and without any troublesome screw head. Also the small diameter maintains maximum bone contact (Fig. 22.1). The disadvantages of the Herbert screw are inadequate length of the longest available screw and the price.

3. Skin

In any procedure on the dorsum of the distal joint care of the skin is essential. Minimal flap elevation, loose closure without skin tension and avoidance of haematoma will allow primary healing.

Anaesthesia

In suitable patients with operations limited to one or two joints these procedures can be performed with digital block and a bloodless field provided by a rubber tube tourniquet applied at the base of the finger. No complications have occurred. Otherwise arm block or general anaesthetic will be desirable in multiple joint surgery.

Postoperative care

The patient should be aware of the need for elevation, possible adjustment of bandage tension if pain is severe and throbbing, and the care of pin ends if left exposed. In an 'arthritic' patient the proximal interphalangeal joint should not be immobilised and the patient should be advised to keep this joint and all other upper limb joints fully mobile.

A small aluminium splint is usually applied to protect the arthrodesis once the wound had healed and is maintained until radiographic union is adequate at six to eight weeks. At this time any troublesome pins can be removed. If there is doubt about union the pins can be left in situ longer providing there is no pin track infection. The importance of adequate subchondral excision cannot be overemphasised in obtaining early union.

MUCOUS CYST

This condition is much commoner on the dorsum of the distal joint but may occur around the

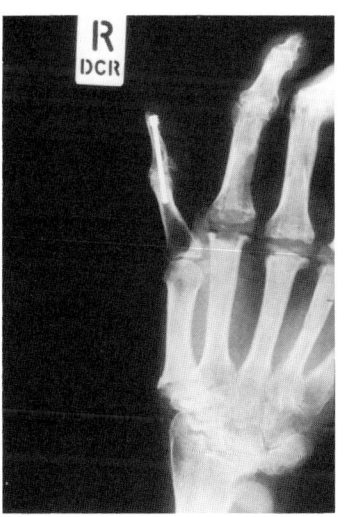
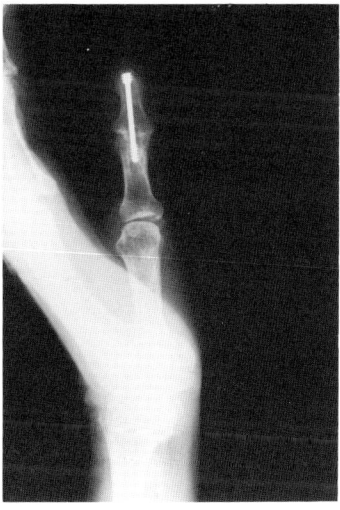

Fig. 22.1 Herbert screw for interphalangeal joint fusion

proximal joint. It is always associated with some degree of osteoarthritis in the adjacent joint. Pressure from a distally sited cyst may cause nail deformity.

Problems, prevention and management

1. The skin cover over the cyst is very thin and needs careful handling. Magnification is advisable. An oblique incision is often best. The less healthy looking skin edge can be excised providing loose closure is possible without tension. Rotation flap is rarely necessary.

2. Recurrence can be common because the underlying osteoarthritis is still present as reported by Dodge et al (1984). Surgery should be performed in a proper outpatient theatre. Local anaesthesia by digital block is adequate. A bloodless field using a properly applied rubber finger tourniquet has caused no complications. Magnification is advisable. A gentle assistant to retract the thin skin edges is desirable. Partial emptying of the cyst by aspiration is technically helpful. Careful excision and avulsion of the cyst wall with synovectomy of the joint and limited debridement will reduce the rate of recurrence to a small percentage. The patient has to understand that osteoarthritis is still present. This may cause joint pain and the cyst may recur. Therefore, occasionally it may be desirable to arthrodese the joint initially or subsequently if recurrence or the osteoarthritis per se are troublesome.

THE PROXIMAL INTERPHALANGEAL JOINT

The approach to the management of arthritis in the proximal interphalangeal joints is usually different in primary generalised osteoarthritis and post-traumatic osteoarthritis. In post-traumatic osteoarthritis the other proximal interphalangeal joints may be normal and thus an arthrodesis or arthroplasty will compare unfavourably. The result will be relatively better when compared to the adjacent arthritic joints in generalised osteoarthritis.

Arthrodesis

An arthrodesis in a single joint that has a normal range of movement of 120° will often cause a disappointing result unless there is a special functional requirement for that finger pulp in a set position with stability. This situation is commonest in the index finger. The patient should understand what an arthrodesis will mean even to the extent of immobilising the proximal joint preoperatively in a light splint with the pulp free.

In post-traumatic arthritis the patient with the other digits normal will often be better served by amputation rather than arthrodesis or even arthroplasty. However, where digits are missing or disabled these procedures help to upgrade function. In my practice, arthrodesis of the proximal interphalangeal joint is a rare operation, but commonest in the index in both types of arthritis.

The techniques for arthrodesis should follow the principles outlined for the distal joint. Tension band wiring can be useful and quick. There is no need for plate and screws. The exact degree of flexion depends on the patient's wishes.

Arthroplasty

Swanson hinge arthroplasty of the proximal interphalangeal joint can provide relatively satisfactory results especially with multiple joint involvement in generalised osteoarthritis. Other implants have not been used by the author except for occasional silicone sponge interposition where bone stock was not adequate for stem insertion.

The problem of single implant arthroplasty in post-traumatic arthritis has been mentioned above. The role of amputation should always be discussed. Also, consideration should be given to perichondrial resurfacing arthroplasty. Seradge et al (1984) reported 36 procedures in the metacarpophalangeal and proximal interphalangeal joints. They recommend this operation in people under 40 years, without systemic disease, without prior infection in the joint and not requiring comcomitant tendon reconstruction. In the proximal joints 55% had good results. The use of this procedure would seem to be more pertinent with other digits missing or disabled.

The same could be said for microvascular free

joint transfer from the foot. The place of this procedure seems uncertain at this time. The author has no experience with this procedure in spite of considerable experience in other free tissue transfers. However, its availability should be kept in mind in exceptional circumstances where other digits are missing and disabled and extensor tendon reconstruction and bone and skin replacement are required and also where perichondrial resurfacing is contraindicated.

Swanson silicone arthroplasty

This procedure is most useful in rheumatoid arthritis and generalised osteoarthritis. Relatively better results are obtained at the metacarpophalangeal level than the proximal interphalangeal level because less range of assessment is satisfactory and stability in the lateral plane is better achieved. Good long term results can be achieved providing the principles as detailed by Swanson (1973a, b) are followed. The implants have now been used for 20 years. The technique and postoperative care will not be elaborated here, but points will be stressed in order to reduce the incidence of unsatisfactory results. Up to four proximal joint arthroplasties with arthrodesis of distal joints can be done in the one operation.

The dorsal approach as recommended by Swanson with careful splitting and detachment of the middle slip gives excellent exposure for preservation of collateral ligaments and radical osteophyte excision. The volar lip of the base of the middle phalanx must be thoroughly excised and smoothed to prevent impingement and implant tear. In osteoarthritis there is often osteophyte formation on the dorsum of the middle phalanx and detachment of the middle slip allows excision and flattening of the whole surface of the base of the middle phalanx. The collateral ligaments need to be detached usually at the proximal phalanx, but in osteoarthritis detachment at the base of the middle phalanx may be advisable for osteophyte removal. Firm reattachment of the collateral ligaments is important in maintaining lateral stability. Ligament reconstruction is rarely required in osteoarthritis.

Reaming needs to be well centralised and widened with power driven pilot burrs and smoothed with a diamond burr. The bone ends need to be smooth with enough gap to prevent compression of the implant. Reaming need not be extreme. All debris should be irrigated from the wound. The size of the implant chosen should not be too wide in the gap or too tight in the stems. The finger should sit straight without lateral deviation before ligaments are reattached, otherwise the bone ends should be revised. Easy passive flexion to 90° should be possible. Collateral ligaments and middle slip are reattached meticulously with sutures through drill holes to allow active and elastic assisted mobilisation within a few days.

Intrinsic contracture is rarely present in osteoarthritis but should be released if necessary. Finally, the palm should be opened routinely and the excursion of the flexor tendons tested. Excursion may be restricted by adhesions from long standing joint stiffness or stenosing tenovaginitis. Lateral or volar approaches to the proximal joint may be used but may be more appropriate in rheumatoid arthritis (Scott & Boswick 1983).

The patient should understand the necessity for continual elevation of the hand above heart level until joint range is maximal, and that active hourly exercises with graduated vigour improves tendon excursion and reduces oedema and periarticular scarring. Passive movements should be used only by way of carefully monitored elastic assistance splinting and will not reduce oedema, not improve tendon excursion nor build up muscle power. Long term maintenance exercises are advised.

Causes and prevention of unsatisfactory results

1. Pain

This is usually not a problem but should be investigated. Early tight dressings should be released, elevation ensured, force of elastic traction adjusted, adequate analgesia and active exercises and the patient will power encouraged. Infection is rare, but should be considered.

2. Stiffness

Osteoarthritis is a stiffening disease and stiffness tends to recur after arthroplasty. Careful technique

340 UNSATISFACTORY RESULTS IN HAND SURGERY

with adequate osteophyte removal, not using too large an implant, making sure tendon excursion is normal and encouragement in meticulous and prolonged postoperative care are essential.

3. Angulation

This should be prevented by parallel resection of bone ends, osteophyte removal, central reaming, good ligament repair and equal lateral band tension.

4. Breakage

Incidence of breakage does not seem to be any higher in the proximal joints than the metacarpophalangeal joints. Smooth parallel bone ends with correct gap and a correctly centred implant, not too big to allow it to jam, will keep the breakage rate to 5% or less. With breakage there is usually a loss of power and alignment. Salvage, if symptoms warrant, can usually be achieved by revision arthroplasty. Silicone small fragment synovitis and bone erosion do not seem to be practical problems at this level in osteoarthritis.

THE METACARPOPHALANGEAL JOINT

Primary generalised osteoarthritis is rare in metacarpophalangeal joints, but can be treated by Swanson arthroplasty. Usually arthroplasty will be indicated in only one or two joints. Careful osteophyte excision is required (Fig. 22.2). Ulna side release is not necessary as in rheumatoid arthritis.

Silicone hinge arthroplasty is usually satisfactory for post-traumatic arthritis. Perichondrial arthroplasty can be considered for the young patient, without prior sepsis and not requiring tendon reconstruction. Arthrodesis is rarely indicated in the finger metacarpophalangeal joints but may be considered after infection.

THE THUMB

Osteoarthritis can affect all joints of the thumb. The basal joint and the interphalangeal joint are usually most severely involved in generalised osteoarthritis whereas osteoarthritis of the meta-

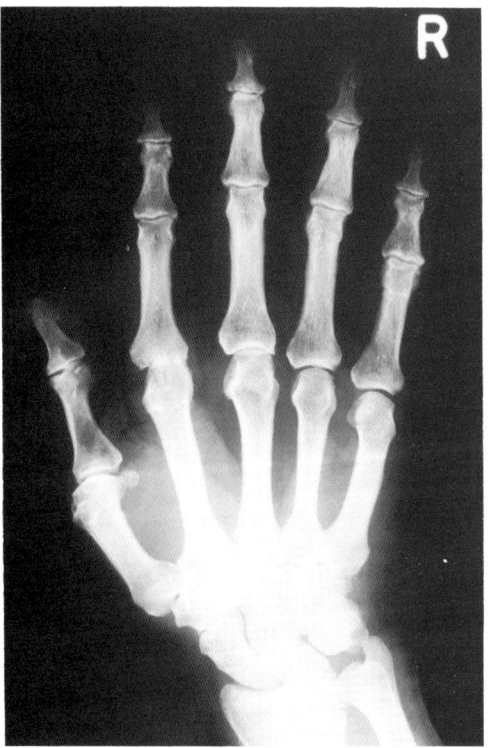 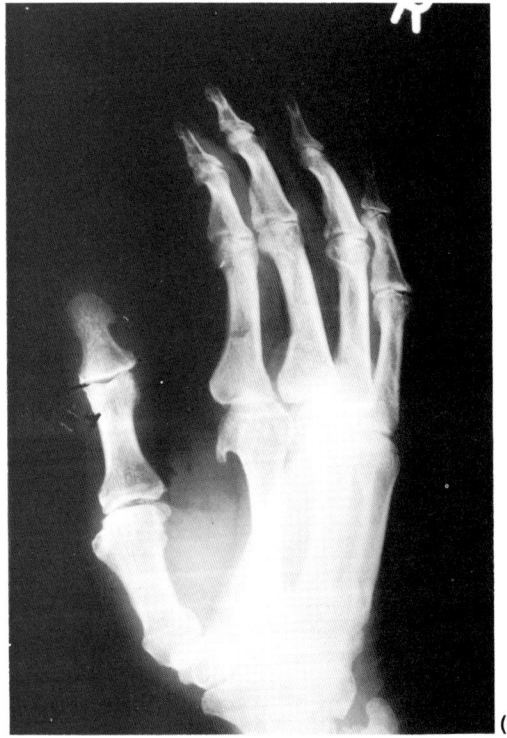

(a)   (b)

Fig. 22.2 (a) and (b) Example of osteoarthritis of the metacarpophalangeal joints of the index and middle fingers

carpophalangeal joint is more commonly post traumatic. However, laxity of the metacarpophalangeal joint is commonly associated with osteoarthritis of the basal joint when the first metacarpal becomes flexed and adducted. In order to maintain span, the metacarpophalangeal joint gradually stretches into hyperextension. It is imperative that the laxity of the metacarpophalangeal joint be corrected at the time of treatment of the basal joint.

In complicated thumb problems stability rather than mobility should be the aim in preventing an unsatisfactory result. For example, if reasonable mobility can be provided at the basal joint, then only rarely would one consider an arthroplasty of the metacarpophalangeal joint rather than arthrodesis even if the interphalangeal joint might require arthrodesis as well.

If it is thought that an arthroplasty of the metacarpophalangeal joint is indicated then only a small range of movement should be aimed for. Swanson silicone hinge arthroplasty with careful collateral ligament repair and longer immobilisation for 4 and up to 6 weeks will provide stability with a useful small range of movement.

Isolated arthritis of the metacarpophalangeal joint or the interphalangeal joint is treated by arthrodesis. Fixing these joints in too much flexion should be avoided. Techniques of arthrodesis of the metacarpophalangeal joint and interphalangeal joint of the thumb are the same as previously described for the finger, including tension band wiring which is useful for metacarpo phalangeal fusion. Ferlic et al (1983) reported results of compression arthrodesis indicating a rapid rate of fusion. The disadvantage is that is may be cumbersome.

The base of the thumb

Generalised osteoarthritis commonly affects the pantrapezial joints and often warrants surgical treatment. Swanson (1981) reported a 48% incidence of arthritis in the trapezium–scaphoid joint in association with arthritis of the trapezium–first metacarpal joint. Therefore, he suggests that total excision of the trapezium will be necessary in most cases to eliminate all arthritic pain. North & Eaton (1983) studied the basal region of the thumb anatomically and radiographically in cadavers. They found that 46% of hands with significant trapezium–first metacarpal disease had degenerative changes in the trapezium–scaphoid joint. If it is certain that only the trapezium–first metacarpal joint is involved treatment may be:

1. Arthrodesis which is usually reserved for younger manual workers especially with post-traumatic arthritis.
2. Arthroplasty with partial trapezium excision.
   a. Tendon interposition.
   b. Silicone interposition.
      i. Burr-hole cover (Ashworth et al 1977).
      ii. Condylar implant (Kessler 1973, Swanson 1981).

The authors 12 cases agree with the excellent results reported by Ashworth et al (1977). The incidence of instability is low. This type of tendon or silicone interposition arthroplasty will not be adequate when:

1. There is fixed flexion–adduction contracture of the first metacarpal.
2. There is pantrapezial arthritis.

The treatment in these situations will be:

Arthroplasty with total trapezium excision
a. Tendon interposition.
b. Silicone trapezium implant.

The author's experience is limited to Swanson implants of which over 100 cases have been done since 1977. Are the results of Swanson trapezium implants better than tendon arthroplasty? Review of the literature does not reveal a definite winner. Amadio et al (1982) compared the results of 25 Swanson implants with 25 tendon spacer procedures. They concluded that the results were similar and satisfactory. In the tendon arthroplasty the long abductor was shortened.

Weilby & Søndorf (1978) reported results following removal of silicone trapezium implants. Here again adequate capsular repair and shortening with invagination of the long abductor as a spacer was used. Excellent salvage was achieved. They state that the results after removal of the implant were better than those following primary excision of the trapezium. In particular strength and stability were better. This has also been the experience of the author.

However in the author's series, four patients have had bilateral procedures—on one side a tendon arthroplasty either primary or salvage and on the other side a stable Swanson trapezium arthroplasty. The latter is preferred by all four patients. Incidentally, two patients had a Swanson trapezium arthroplasty on one side and an arthrodesis on the other. The arthroplasty is preferred.

Providing stability can be achieved it is the author's opinion that the Swanson arthroplasty will result in consistently satisfactory results where total trapezium excision is required. The crux of the matter is *stability* to provide a stable fulcrum to allow near normal movement with strength. Points will be outlined which have been found helpful in achieving this aim.

The anterior approach

An anterior approach is preferred. This is used for all procedures at the base of the thumb providing 'extensile' exposure and allowing strong capsular repair with tendon reinforcement. The radial nerve and artery are not encountered. The palmar branch of the median nerve is easily preserved. The line of incision is shown in Fig. 22.3. If palmaris longus is present the incision can stop at the scaphoid tubercle. If not the incision is extended proximally along the line of flexor carpi radialis. The anterior branch of the radial artery over the scaphoid tubercle is ligated. Abductor pollicis brevis is reflected well ulnarward. Abductor pollicis longus is detached from its insertion and reflected dorsally. The capsule over the front of the trapezium (often poor) is opened transversely and reflected to expose the whole anterior surface of the trapezium and its proximal and distal joints The flexor carpi radialis is located and preserved by nibbling away the lid of its tunnel. The trapezium is excised in pieces, split by an osteotome, and including the osteophyte between the first and second metacarpals. It is important to excise any trapezoid overlying the distal pole of the scaphoid to allow the implant to sit on the whole of the distal pole.

Implant size and loose stem

The metacarpal end is squared and then centrally reamed to allow a loose fit of the implant stem. A tight fit will put more leverage on the implant articulating end and will promote instability. The implant stem can be shortened or narrowed if necessary to ensure a loose fit. Too large an implant will increase tension and reestablish deforming forces and also tend to instability. The wound is carefully irrigated.

Tendon reinforcement

If available the palmaris longus tendon (Jackson 1977) is divided in the forearm through a small incision. The end is pulled out distally at the wrist

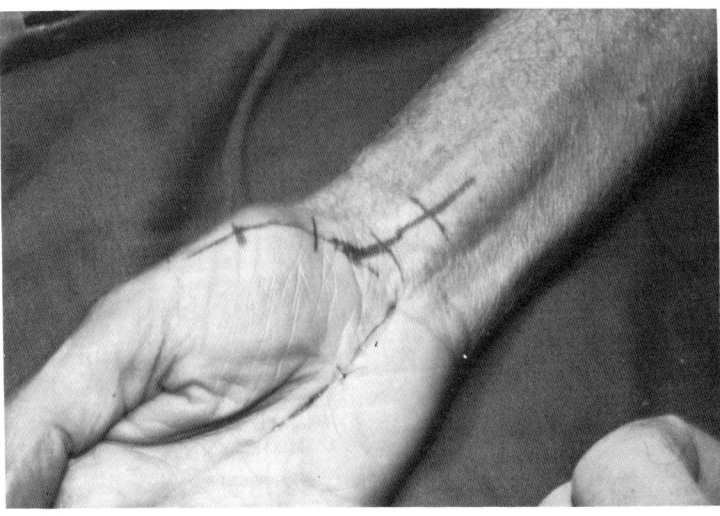

Fig. 22.3 Incision used for anterior approach to the trapezium

crease level preserving the distal insertion. The end is passed into the thumb wound deep to the palmar branch of the median nerve. The dorsal capsule is imbricated and a suture is positioned at the edge of the trapezoid and held.

The implant is then taken from its packet and inserted correctly with minimal handling. The thumb is held in abduction. The palmaris longus or a strip of flexor carpi radialis left attached at its insertion is then passed to the previously held suture at the trapezoid edge around the middle of the implant. Firmly anchored here, the tendon strip is then passed back over the implant and attached to the edge of the flexor carpi radialis. The remains of the capsule are carefully closed snugly, especially along the scaphoid edge. Stability is tested. The long abductor is reattached to the metacarpal base via a suture through a drill hole already prepared. The abductor brevis is replaced and loosely sutured at its edge. Skin is closed. The thumb is immobilised with the first metacarpal abducted. It is well known that the metacarpophalangeal joint must not be hyperextended.

Postoperative care

Immobilisation is continued for six weeks allowing full mobility of the thumb interphalangeal joint and all fingers. After six weeks the thumb is mobilised, but forceful grip is not allowed for another eight weeks.

Correction of metacarpophalangeal joint hyperextension

Persisting hyperextension will provoke implant instability early during immobilisation and also late as the first metacarpal deforms again into flexion (Fig. 22.4).

In mild deformity the metacarpophalangeal joint should be pinned for 6 weeks in moderate flexion. In moderate to severe deformity firm volar capsulodesis is required sometimes with tendon graft reinforcement and the joint is pinned for 6 weeks in moderate flexion.

In severe deformity where strong repair is not feasible or the joint degenerate, arthrodesis is performed.

Correction of adduction

This is usually released by trapeziectomy and appropriate squaring of the metacarpal base and selecting a smallish implant. However, at times through a separate incision on the ulnar side of the metacarpal the fascia overlying the adductor needs to be released. Occasionally partial release of the adductor insertion is required. Temporary pin

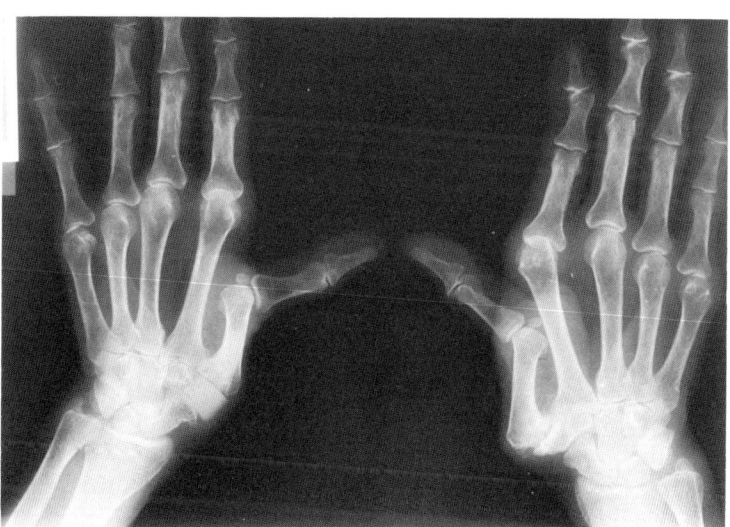

Fig. 22.4 An unusual case of implant stability in spite of recurrence of metacarpal adduction and metacarpophalangeal hyperextension

fixation of the implant is occasionally advisable leaving the pin end under the skin.

Carpal tunnel compression of the median nerve

This condition commonly accompanies osteoarthritis at the thumb base. It should always be considered as a cause of part of the symptom complex and wasting and weakness of the abductor pollicis brevis. If indicated, median neurolysis should be done at the time of thumb surgery. If thenar wasting is gross, opposition tendon transfer may be prudent to rebalance the thumb.

Arthrodesis of the base of the thumb

This procedure is reserved for the patient requiring heavy use of the thumb when it is certain that arthritis is limited to the trapezium–first metacarpal joint. The aim is to obtain:

1. Early solid fusion without disturbance of adjacent joints by cancellous to cancellous contact as stressed by Carroll & Hill (1973). A bone graft may be occasionally necessary if shortening is extreme or bone quality poor. Fixation by 2 K wires or lag screw is adequate. The Herbert screw as shown in Fig. 22.5 provides good fixation with compression but without compromising adjacent joints.
2. The position of fixation of the first metacarpal needs to be precise. Eaton & Littler (1969) recommend the first metacarpal diverging from the second at 35 to 40 degrees palmar and 20 degrees of radial abduction, the relationship assumed when a fist is made. This fist position allows precise positioning intraoperatively. This position is also recommended by Stark et al (1977). Their review confirms the excellent results of arthrodesis with few complications.

A rationale for the management of osteoarthritis at the base of the thumb has been proposed in order to minimise unsatisfactory results. Where indicated the Swanson trapezium implant has provided excellent results in the authors series with a low (4%) incidence of instability. If this procedure is not being done frequently it is recommended that the other methods be used in order to minimise complications and still achieve a reasonable result.

ARTHRITIS AT THE TRAPEZIUM–SCAPHOID JOINT

Arthritis isolated to the trapezium–scaphoid joint without detectable carpal instability of the scaphoid and without significant involvement of the trapezium–first metacarpal joint is a distinct if somewhat uncommon entity. Crosby et al (1978) reported a series of 49 hands of 34 patients, but this series included cases with carpal instability and pantrapezial arthritis where trapezium–scaphoid arthritis was the preponderant part. They refer to the scanty literature on the topic. Watson & Hempton (1980) reported a series of 13 arthrodeses of the scaphoid–trapezium–trapezoid joints, seven of which were for localised arthritis.

If it can be certain by clinical and radiographic investigation, including carpal instability views, that this is an isolated entity and is the cause of significant symptoms then localised arthrodesis is the treatment of choice. Injection of long-acting local anaesthetic into the joint can be a useful diagnostic test, and a pointer to management especially where there may be a degree of pantrapezial arthritis. Arthrodesis can be done by dorsal or volar approach. The latter is preferred by the author. A bone graft is essential to maintain correct carpal relationship and length. Fixation with compression using Herbert bone screw achieves rapid union. Arthrodesis with correct scaphoid reduction is also advocated for arthritis with scaphoid instability providing the radioscaphoid joint is in good order. The patient with a solid fusion in correct position will have a stronger grip and pinch and will not notice any postoperative loss of movement. However, compared with normal, there will be 20% loss of flexion and extension and 33% loss of radial and ulnar deviation (Watson & Hempton 1980).

A recent referral indicates an unsatisfactory result (Fig. 22.6). A silicone trapezium arthroplasty had been performed for trapezium–scaphoid arthritis secondary to long-standing scaphoid instability. The patient still complains of wrist pain and restricted range of movement with obvious synovitis. Arthrodesis of the scaphoid–trapezium–trapezoid joints with the scaphoid reduced would have been the preferred treatment.

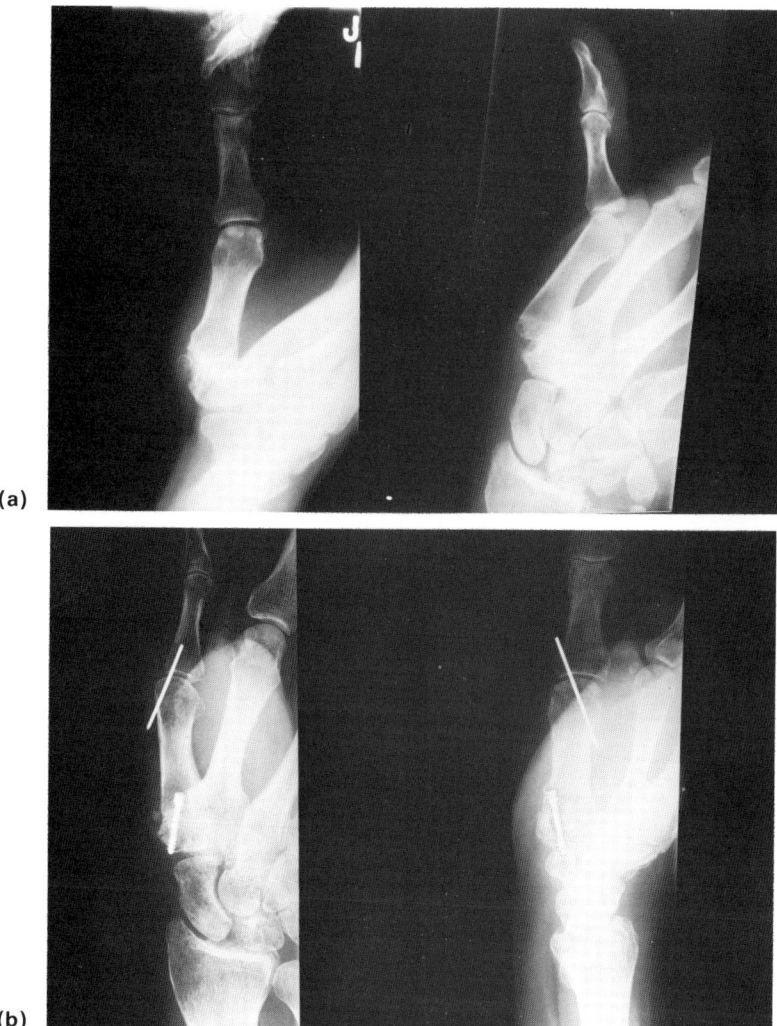

Fig. 22.5 (a) Preoperative radiograph showing severe osteoarthritis of base of thumb with associated deformities. (b) The patient (a surgeon) would have no other treatment but arthrodesis. Herbert screw provided excellent fixation. Union is proceeding well at 7 weeks. Temporary fixation at metacarpophalangeal joint is used after palmar capsulodesis

THE INFERIOR RADIO–ULNAR JOINT

Primary osteoarthritis is rare here but traumatic arthritis is common after injury such as fracture, ligamentous disruption, and length discrepancy.

Unsatisfactory results are not uncommon after excision of the lower end of the ulna (Darrach's Operation). Too much bone excision produces hypermobility of the proximal end of the ulnar with impingement on the radius, new bone formation, limited rotation, weakness, and, in rheumatoid arthritis, tendon rupture and ulna carpal shift. Silicone capping can alleviate some of these problems but can result in synovitis, implant dislocation and tear.

The Lauenstein operation will significantly reduce the incidence of unsatisfactory results. This procedure has received scanty attention in the literature. Steindler (1946) ascribed this procedure to Carl Lauenstein of Germany in 1890 (Fig. 22.7).

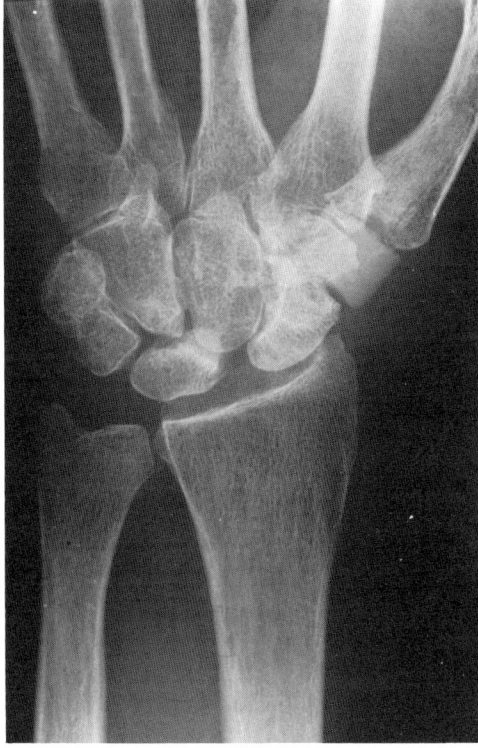

Fig. 22.6 See text for details

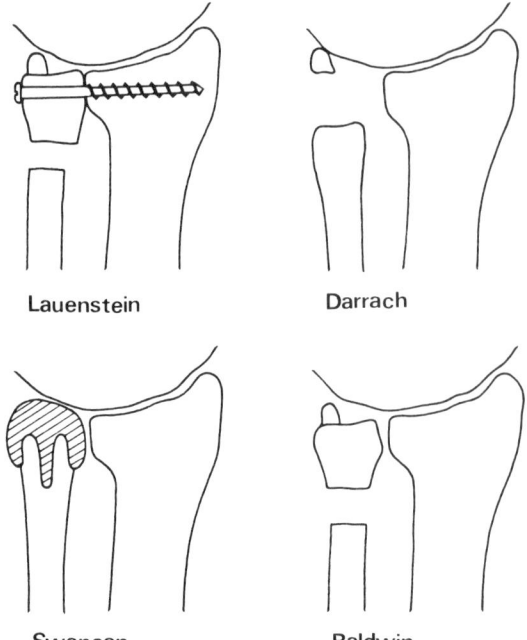

Fig. 22.7 Illustration of alternative procedures available. The Lauenstein is preferred. The Baldwin operation does not include fusion of the inferior radio-ulnar joint

Briefly it involves arthrodesis of the inferior radio-ulnar joint with ulnar length corrected. A permanent pseudarthrosis is fashioned 2 cm proximally in the lower ulna by excision of enough bone with its periosteum to leave a 1 cm gap through which pronator quadratus is pulled and anchored. If this muscle is of poor substance an anchovy of tendon can be used such as a strip of extensor carpi ulnaris. Adequate stability of the proximal end of the ulna should be maintained by limiting gap size to 1 cm and careful soft tissue repair. Because firm bone fixation of the ulna to the radius is obtained with a lag screw, early mobilisation into pronation and supination is advised at no later than 2 weeks postoperatively.

Since 1981 the author has performed 24 Lauenstein operations. Thirteen of these to the end of 1983 have been reviewed. All were pain-free during normal activity though two experienced discomfort with heavy use. These two patients, a labourer and a boilermaker, were unable to resume their former occupations despite strong stable wrists with full rotation. Pronation and supination were improved in all cases and were normal in most. New bone formation has not occurred at the pseudarthrosis. Strength has been maintained or improved. Loss of strength is a common complaint after excision of the lower end of the ulna.

REFERENCES

Amadio P C, Millender L H, Smith R J 1982 Silicone spacer or tendon spacer for trapezium resection arthroplasty—comparison of results. Journal of Hand Surgery 7:237–244

Ashworth C R, Blatt G, Chuinard R G, Stark H H 1977 Silicone-rubber interposition arthroplasty of the carpo-metacarpal joint of the thumb. Journal of Hand Surgery 2:345–357

Carroll R E, Hill N A 1973 Arthrodesis of the carpo-metacarpal joint of the thumb. Journal of Bone and Joint Surgery 55B:292–294

Crosby E B, Linscheid R L, Dobyns J H 1978 Scaphotrapezial trapezoidal arthrosis. Journal of Hand Surgery 3:223–234

Dodge L D, Brown R L, Niebauer J J, Relton McCarroll Jnr H 1984 The treatment of mucus cysts: Long term follow-up in sixty two cases. Journal of Hand Surgery 9A:901–904

Eaton R G, Littler J W 1969 A study of the basal joint of the thumb. Treatment of its disabilities by fusion. Journal of Bone and Joint Surgery 51A: 661–668

Faithfull D K, Herbert T J 1984 Small joint fusions in the hand using the Herbert bone screw. Journal of Hand Surgery 9B: 167–168

Ferlic D C, Turner B D, Clayton M L 1983 Compression arthrodesis of the thumb. Journal of Hand Surgery 8: 207–210

Jackson I T, St Onge R A 1977 Use of palmaris longus tendon to stabilise trapezium implants. The Hand 9: 42

Kessler I 1973 Silicone arthroplasty of the trapeziometacarpal joint. Journal of Bone and Joint Surgery 55B: 285–291

Lister G 1978 Intraosseous wiring of the digital skeleton. Journal of Hand Surgery 3: 427–435

North E R, Eaton R G 1983 Degenerative joint disease of the trapezium: A comparative radiographic and anatomic study. Journal of Hand Surgery 8: 160–167

Scott F A, Boswick J A 1983 Palmer arthroplasty for the treatment of stiff swan-neck deformity. Journal of Hand Surgery 8: 267–272

Stark H H, Moore J F, Ashworth C R, Boyes J H 1977 Fusion of the first metacarpo trapezial joint for degenerative arthritis. Journal of Bone and Joint Surgery 59A: 22–26

Steindler A 1946 The Traumatic Deformities and Disabilities of the Upper Limb. Thomas, Illinois

Swanson A B 1973a Implant resection arthroplasty of the proximal interphalangeal joint. Orthopedic Clinics of North America 4: 1007–1027

Swanson A B 1973b Flexible Implant Arthroplasty in the Hand and Extremities. C V Mosby Co, St Louis

Swanson A B, Swanson G de Groot, Watermeier J J 1981 Trapezium implant arthroplasty. Journal of Hand Surgery 6: 125–141

Swanson A B, Swanson G de Groot 1983 Osteoarthritis in the hand. Journal of Hand Surgery 8: 669–675

Watson H K, Hempton R F 1980 Limited wrist arthrodeses 1. The triscaphoid joint. Journal of Hand Surgery 5: 320–327

Weilby A, Søndorf J 1978 Results following removal of silicone trapezium metacarpal implants. Journal of Hand Surgery 3: 154–156

23 Dupuytren's disease

The dilemma of doing too little or too much is exemplified in the treatment of Dupuytren's disease. If the surgeon does a limited operation there is a good chance that joint contracture will not be fully corrected or that recurrent contracture will appear soon thereafter. If a radical or extensive fasciectomy is performed morbidity may be prolonged or even permanent limitation of flexion and extension may occur. Therefore the surgeon must evaluate his patient carefully and choose an operation that is appropriate for the patient and for the severity of disease affecting the hand.

SELECTION OF THE PATIENT FOR OPERATION

It is not possible with any accuracy to determine preoperatively how well a patient will do after an operation for Dupuyten's disease. However certain factors should be considered. Age is not of much help. Both the very young and very old do well or badly although disease at a young age usually suggests an aggressive form of disease which has a tendency to recur. It is often said that women do less well than men. This is not entirely true. The incidence of complications following operation is similar in the sexes and not statistically different (males 16%; females 19%—McFarlane 1985). However sympathetic dystrophy and loss of finger flexion are more common in women (Tubiana et al 1981, McFarlane 1985). Therefore caution is advised in selecting female patients for operation.

Diabetes mellitus, epilepsy and alcoholism are three diseases that are associated with Dupuyten's disease. Clearly, diabetes is not an unfavourable prognostic factor. The majority of diabetics who have Dupuyten's disease do not consult a surgeon because their disease never reaches the stage of disabling joint contracture (Noble et al 1984). However epileptic and alcoholic patients, seen by the surgeon because of Dupuytren's disease, have severe and extensive involvement (Fig. 23.1). They require radical surgery (and often skin grafting) to remove the disease and correct joint contracture. Often they have neither a favourable mental outlook nor an optimal physical condition to tolerate an extensive operation. The dilemma is that a lesser operation is of little or no value to the patient (Fig. 23.2).

Patients with debilitating disease, primarily cardiovascular and pulmonary disease, can be helped considerably by minor operations. Subcutaneous and open fasciotomy are effective in correcting metacarpophalangeal joint contracture for as long as 5 years (Rowley et al 1984). Fasciotomy to correct proximal interphalangeal joint contracture is less satisfactory (Watson 1984). Fasciotomy can be performed under local anaesthesia and is associated with little or no morbidity. The initial results are so good that it is tempting to treat all patients in this manner.

Another consideration is to identify the patient with 'Dupuytren's Diathesis', a term introduced by Hueston (1963). These patients develop Dupuytren's disease at an early age, usually in the third or fourth decade, other members of the immediate family are also involved, the disease is extensive and bilateral, and ectopic deposits on the dorsum of the hand (knuckle pads), the penis (Peyronie's disease), and the soles of the feet (plantar fibromatosis) are often present. Fre-

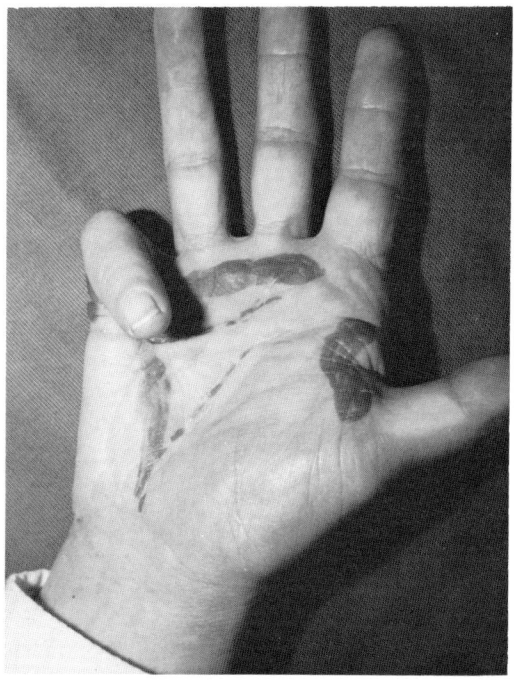

Fig. 23.1 The right hand of a 57 year old alcoholic who has had previous operations on both hands. The left hand is involved similarly and he has plantar fibromatosis. The dotted lines incidate previous incisions. He is not a good candidate for operation

quently these patients have already been operated upon only to have early recurrence of the disease. It is rare for a patient to have all of these unfavourable diatheses factors but when two or three factors are noted, the surgeon must realise (and so inform the patient) that it will be difficult to control the disease, even by very radical surgery. There is good evidence that radical excision of overlying skin as well as fascia (dermofasciectomy) is useful in controlling the disease in patients with a strong diathesis (Hueston 1984, Tonkin et al 1984).

INDICATIONS FOR OPERATION

Because Dupuytren's disease is a benign process, and because the rate of progression is unpredictable, it is not necessary, nor wise, to operate upon a patient simply because the disease is present. It is important to explain the nature of the disease to the patient, pointing out that it is not related to cancer or poor health. Furthermore, the morbidity following operation and the time involved in regaining full use of the hand must be mentioned. With this information some patients with severe disease and extensive contractures may decide not to have an operation. One should never tell a patient that they must have an operation. It is this very patient who will have an unsatisfactory result.

A nodule in the palm may concern the patient, and the nodule may be tender, but if the nature of the disease is explained to the patient the pain invariably disappears and treatment is unnecessary (Fig. 23.3). Only occasionally is a nodule so large that its removal alone is justified. Extensive skin involvement in the palm occasionally justifies early operation but almost always an operation is advised because of finger joint contracture.

The metacarpophalangeal joint is most frequently contracted. Fortunately contracture at this joint can be corrected by operation, regardless of the duration or severity of the contracture. Usually a contracture of about 30 degrees at the metacarpophalangeal joint causes enough annoyance to justify operation.

Contracture at the proximal interphalangeal joint is difficult to correct, regardless of the duration or severity of the contracture, so an operation should be advised as soon as a contracture is apparent.

The distal interphalangeal joint is involved in Dupuytren's disease. Occasionally a flexion contracture occurs, usually in the little finger. The contracture is not severe nor disabling but it is surprisingly difficult to correct (Millesi 1967). It is due to disease in the retrovascular cord of Thomine (1972). More frequently a hyperextension deformity is present and again is seen most often at the distal interphalangeal joint of the little finger. The hyperextension may be passively correctable, in fact corrected by the patient when fully flexing the finger, or it may be fixed. A fixed hyperextension deformity is always associated with severe flexion contracture at the proximal interphalangeal joint and is a sign that it will be very difficult, if not impossible, to fully correct the flexion contracture at the proximal interphalangeal joint.

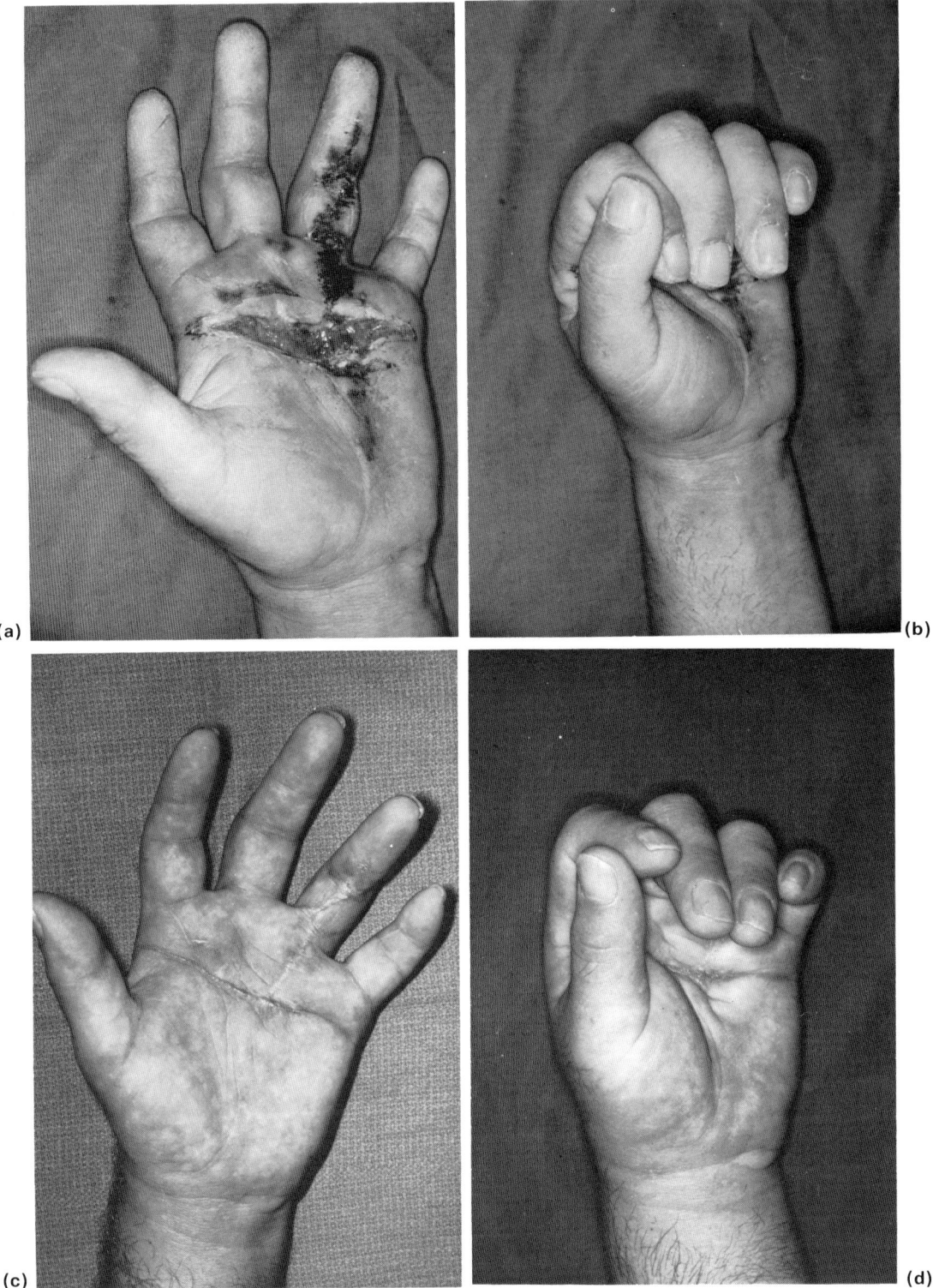

Fig. 23.2 (a) and (b) The appearance of the left hand of a 31 year old epileptic who has received anticonvulsive therapy since age 18. An extensive fasciectomy in the palm and ring finger was performed. The palmar wound was left open. One week postoperatively he has an acceptable range of flexion and extension. (c) and (d) Three months postoperatively he has not improved in spite of splinting and therapy. Even though he had no pain or other signs of sympathetic dystrophy, he was admitted to hospital for more intensive therapy and sympathetic blocks. (e) and (f) One year postoperatively he has persistent flexion contracture at the proximal interphalangeal joints of all fingers of 30 to 45 degrees but can now make a firm fist. He was unable to work as a labourer for 6 months after operation

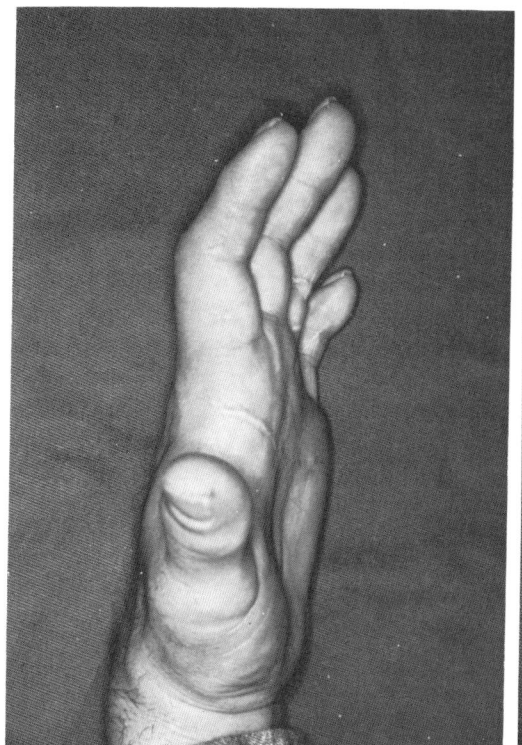
(e)

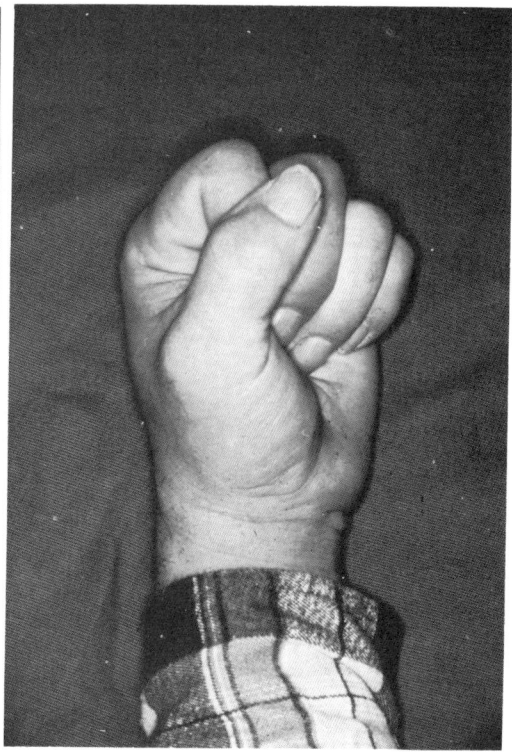
(f)

Almost always, patients with Dupuytren's disease are able to make a firm fist, that is, they have full flexion. Occasionally a patient will have limitation of full flexion, even though they have not had a previous operation. These patients often have distal joint hyperextension. It is wise to record this lack of flexion preoperatively so that any postoperative limitation of flexion can be properly assessed.

CHOICE OF OPERATION

Many operations have been described (Hueston 1982, McFarlane 1982). Rather than be restricted to one or two procedures the surgeon has far more latitude if the operation is considered in three parts—1. the skin incision, 2. the incision or excision of fascia, and 3. the wound closure. With this approach a type of skin incision is not tied to whether the fascia is simply incised or radically excised or the management of the fascia need not dictate whether the wound is sutured, grafted or left open to heal by second intention.

INTRAOPERATIVE CONSIDERATIONS

The anaesthetic

A regional block is the anaesthetic of choice. An infraclavicular block is best because there is no risk of pneumothorax but the anaesthetist may prefer a supraclavicular block. The value of a regional block over a general anaesthetic is that it provides a sympathectomy effect. If a long acting agent is used this effect may last more than 24 hours and this is a first and extremely important step in the prevention of reflex sympathetic dystrophy. An intravenous block is not recommended. Local anaesthesia is appropriate for fasciotomies and other less extensive operations.

The tourniquet

The possibility of tourniquet paralysis is always present in treating Dupuytren's disease. Many patients have peripheral neuropathy or the potential for it because of associated alcoholism or diabetes mellitus. The tourniquet pressure that

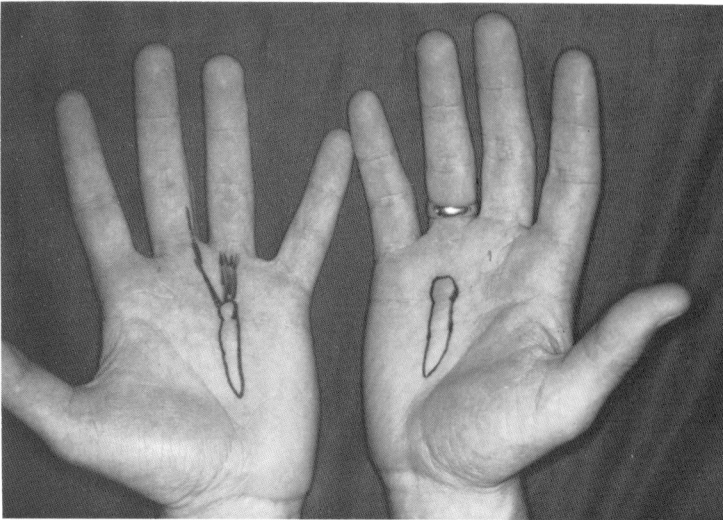

Fig. 23.3 This 26 year old man first noticed thickening in the palm one year before. He associated the thickening with strengthening exercises at his health club and wondered if he should cease this activity. There was no family history of Dupuytren's disease or other diathesis factors. The disease was explained to him. He was advised that he should not have an operation now, that he should not restrict his activities but that he would likely develop joint contracture within 10–15 years

would be tolerated by normal nerves can damage these susceptible nerves. A tourniquet pressure of 33.3 kPa (250 mmHg) is satisfactory. The tourniquet gauge should be checked before each operation to be sure that it is recording the actual pressure in the system. Usually the dissection can be completed in about one hour and therefore the tourniquet can be released, haemostasis obtained and the wounds closed. If the dissection will take longer, the tourniquet should be released for about 15 minutes each hour.

The incision and exposure of the diseased fascia

The dissection and removal of the diseased fascia is the essential part of the operation, but the planning of the skin incision in relation to the extent of the underlying disease is extremely important. Time spent marking the incision(s) with a pen is well worthwhile to be sure that the incision will provide adequate exposure to the underlying fascia. This is done before the tourniquet is inflated.

The skin incision should be just deep enough to expose the diseased fascia. In the proximal palm the incision will pass through the skin and a variable layer of fibrofatty tissue before the fascia is encountered and in this area the skin can be dissected off the underlying fascia without concern for its vascularity and subsequent viability. There are good sized vessels that perforate the palmar aponeurosis to supply the skin and these vessels should be preserved if they do not interfere with excision of the diseased fascia.

In the distal palm and proximal part of the finger there is little or no fibrofatty tissue between the skin and the diseased fascia. There is, however, a plane between the skin and the fascia but this plane can only be found with the aid of a magnifying loupe and developed with sharp scalpel dissection. When the skin has been dissected from the diseased fascia it will be very thin and may be devascularised but it is necessary to perform this dissection in order to remove disease and prevent recurrence. If, at the completion of the dissection when the tourniquet is released, the viability of the skin is in question one of two options are available. The skin of doubtful viability can be excised and the area covered by a full thickness skin graft, or the skin can be treated as a free graft and held firmly in place with a bolus dressing. The latter procedure is extremely useful and usually 'saves' skin that would otherwise necrose (Fig. 23.4).

Haemostasis

Haemostasis is essential to an uneventful postoperative course. It is accomplished by using sharp dissection throughout, using a magnifying loupe (about four power) during the dissection, and cauterising even the smallest vessels with fine tipped bipolar coagulation forceps. Even the small vessels encountered during the skin incisions are coagulated. The commonest cause of a haematoma in the palm is failure to identify the vessels in the distal palm passing to the dorsum of the hand. These vessels are often cut during the difficult dissection in the distal palm. Within the finger large veins are encountered immediately deep to the skin and should be cauterised when cut. Dissection within the finger is essentially the exposure of the neurovascular bundles. Many branches of the digital arteries must be cut. They are easily identified with loupe magnification and should be cauterised at least 2 mm from the main artery in order to prevent intimal damage to the digital artery. With careful attention to haemostasis there will be very little bleeding when the tourniquet is released, prior to wound closure.

Exposure of the neurovascular bundle and excision of the diseased fascia

Preservation of both the arteries and nerves of the palm and digits is essential to a good result. Division of a nerve is an immediate problem to the patient. Arterial injury is more subtle but is manifested by cold intolerance and trophic change. If either structure is divided, it should be repaired. In the palm the arteries and nerves are reasonably safe from injury because they are deep to the diseased fascia. However at the palmar-digital junction and in the digit various cords of diseased fascia pass deep to and around the neurovascular bundle. The nerve and artery are never 'imbedded' in the diseased fascia; there is always a plane of dissection but at times this plane is difficult to develop. Again, loupe magnification is extremely helpful. An aid to dissection at the palmar-digital junction is to hold the adjacent digits apart. This manoeuver places the neurovascular bundles and the diseased fascia under tension and makes it much easier to dissect the nerve and artery from the fascia. A clear understanding of the normal and altered anatomy of the fascia at the palmar-digital junction and within the finger is essential if injury to the artery and nerve is to be avoided (McFarlane 1974).

After the skin has been elevated to expose the underlying fascia the neurovascular bundles should be exposed the full length of the incision. It is easier to find the bundle near the distal interphalangeal joint where it is superficial, and follow it proximally. When both neurovascular bundles are exposed the dissection is almost complete. It is then a simple matter of removing all of the tissue between the bundles and on either side of the bundles.

When operating upon a digit with recurrent contracture it is extremely difficult to isolate the artery and nerve. The structures are not only involved with recurrent diseased tissue but also with scar tissue from the previous operation (Fig. 23.4(b)). Loupe magnification is essential for this dissection. Also the state of the neurovascular bundles should be evaluated preoperatively. Numbness on one or other side of the digit indicates previous division of a digital nerve and therefore it is likely that the digital artery was cut as well. Cold intolerance might also suggest diminished arterial supply to the digit and a digital Allen's test might indicate lack of digital artery flow on one or other side. Under these circumstances it is essential that the remaining digital artery be preserved or gangrene of the finger may occur.

Failure to gain full extension

As stated above it should always be possible to fully correct a flexion contracture at the metacarpophalangeal joint. However it is not always possible to fully correct a contracture at the proximal interphalangeal joint (Legge & McFarlane 1980). If, after removing all of the diseased fascia from the finger, the joint does not fully extend, the first consideration is that all of the fascia has not been excised. In turn the areas of the central, lateral and

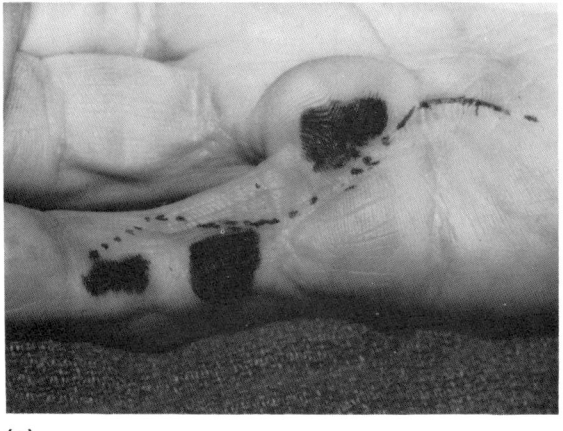
(a)

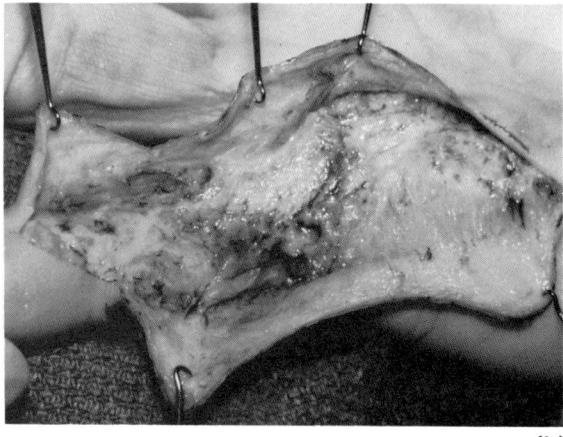
(b)

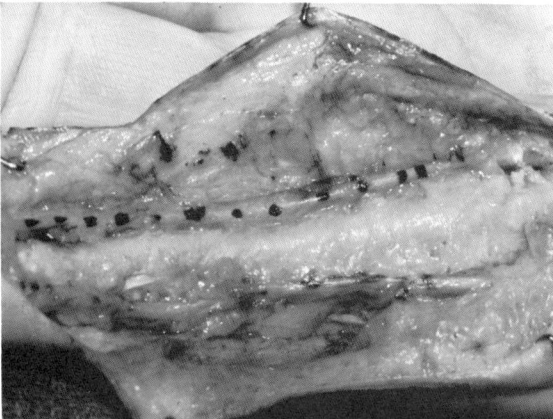
(c)

Fig. 23.4 This 59 year old school custodian had an operation on his right hand 6 years previously. He said that the finger came out straight initially but hard lumps appeared and the finger bent again. (a) The appearance of the finger at the second operation. A sinuous incision was used previously as shown by the dotted line and recurrent disease is marked by dye. Note that the recurrent disease involves the base of the curved flaps. (b) The original incision has been used but the skin flaps have been developed very thin in order to be able to remove the disease fascia. The tissue is a combination of recurrent disease and scar tissue. (c) Both neurovascular bundles have been exposed and the disease tissue removed. In addition to that tissue adherent to skin there was also a lateral cord arising from the abductor digiti minimi tendon and a spiral cord on the radial side. The cause of this patient's recurrence was failure to remove all of the diseased cords and to carefully disect the skin off the underlying fascia. (d) It would have been prudent to perform a dermofascietomy. However the skin flaps were retained and supported by a bolus dressing. A pretendinous cord to the thumb was removed at the same operation. (e) The bolus dressing was removed 10 days postoperatively. The skin is barely viable. (f) and (g) Three months later the wounds are healed and he has full extension and full flexion

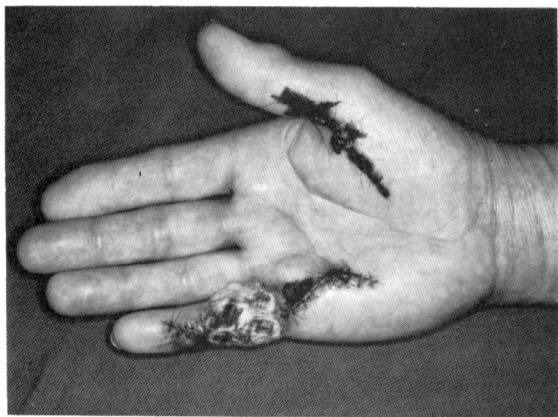
(d)

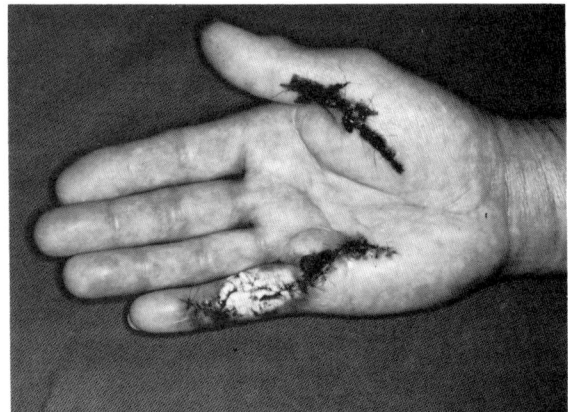
(e)

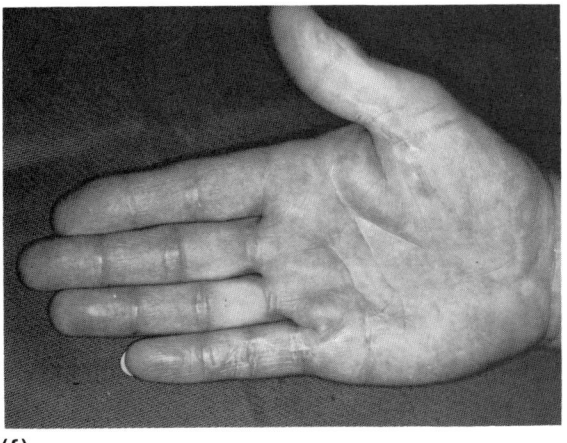
(f)

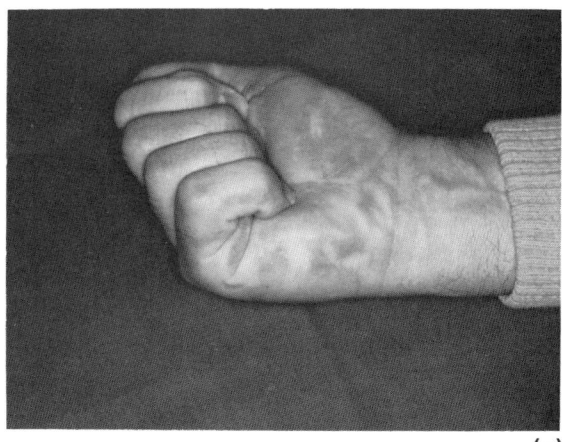
(g)

spiral cords on both sides are examined and if no diseased tissue remains, the persistent contracture may be due to a retrovascular cord which as the name implies, lies dorsal to the neurovascular bundle in the region of the proximal interphalangeal joint.

If all of the diseased fascia has been removed and the joint will not extend, the next structure to examine is the flexor tendon sheath. Frequently the tendon sheath is foreshortened. Simple incision of the sheath and gentle extension of the digit will often correct the residual contracture but the joint should never be forcefully extended. Occasionally one sees a patient with recurrent Dupuytren's disease and yet hyperextension (swan neck deformity) at the proximal interphalangeal joint. The deformity is the result of forceful extension at the previous operation. Release of some of the capsular structures about the proximal interphalangeal joint may be considered. Release of the check rein ligaments (Watson et al 1979) is a relatively simple procedure and may correct the contracture. Excision of portions of the collateral ligament (Curtis 1954) requires more experience but is often successful, but any procedure on the proximal interphalangeal joint should be undertaken with caution. It is much better to accept as much as 30 degrees of flexion contracture rather than correct this contracture surgically and find later that the patient cannot fully flex the finger. Also, residual flexion at the proximal interphalangeal joint can often be corrected or at least improved by postoperative splinting and therapy. It should be the exception and not the rule to violate the capsular structures about the proximal interphalangeal joint.

In spite of all of these considerations there are many patients in whom full extension is obtained at the proximal interphalangeal joint at operation and yet they gradually develop a flexion contracture in the postoperative period in spite of normal wound healing, adequate splinting and close observation by the therapist and the surgeon (Fig. 23.5). This is an unsolved problem that is especially common in the little finger. In Table 23.1 the pre- and post-operative results from a large series of patients are tabulated (McFarlane 1985). The results of treatment in the little finger at the proximal interphalangeal joint are poor compared to those at other joints. One should forewarn the patient that a contracture at the proximal interphalangeal joint is not likely to be fully corrected (Fig. 23.6).

On occasion the surgeon is confronted with the problem of a disabling degree of flexion contracture at the proximal interphalangeal joint that has not responded to the appropriate surgical procedures. Solutions to this problem are not ideal but consist of amputation, proximal interphalangeal joint fusion and replacement arthroplasty. Amputation is not recommended and is performed only if the patient insists upon this treatment. Fusion is a reasonable solution but replacement arthroplasty accomplishes the same goal of correcting the flexion contracture but at the same time provides a few degrees of flexion and extension at the proximal

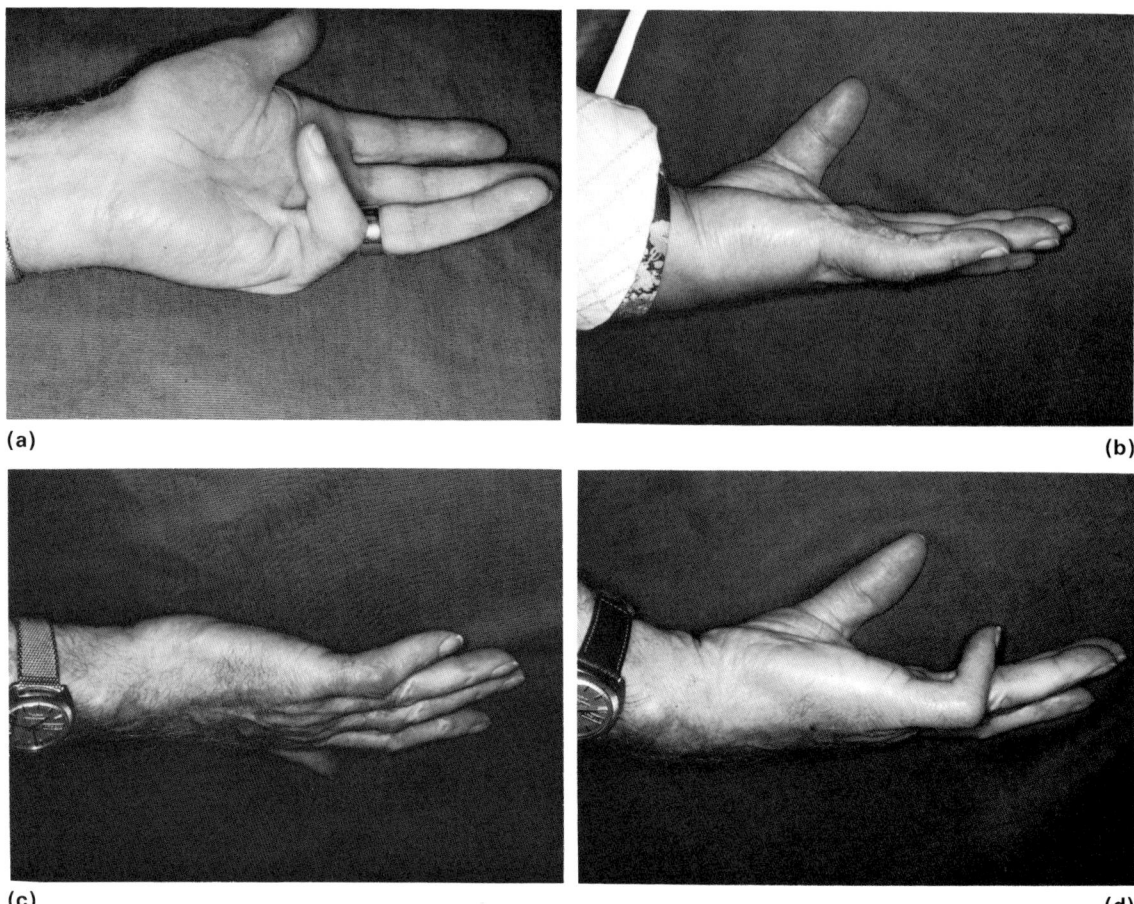

Fig. 23.5 (a) The left hand of a 75 year old retired executive who first noticed his finger pulling down 2 years before. There was 75 degrees of contracture at the metacarpophalangeal joint and 70 degrees at the proximal interphalangeal joint. At operation the metacarpophalangeal joint was easily corrected by excising a pretendinous cord. The central and retrovascular cords were clinically diseased and excised but the proximal interphalangeal joint contracture was not completely corrected. Incision of the flexor tendon sheath did not improve flexion but nothing further was done. (b) Three months postoperatively under the supervision of the therapist the patient could almost completely extend his finger. (c) Six months postoperatively he had flexion contracture of 40 degrees. (d) Two years postoperatively the proximal interphalangeal joint was flexed to 85 degrees but there was no flexion contracture at the metacarpophalangeal joint. There was no palpable Dupuytren's disease. This unexpected result is due to scar contracture

interphalangeal joint. Replacement arthroplasty is the treatment of choice when it is not possible to regain extension and retain flexion by other means.

Closure of the wound

Because the viability of the skin cannot be predicted before the fascia is excised, it is best to delay the design of Z-plasty flaps until after the removal of the fascia. In this way areas of very thin skin can be excluded from the design of the Z-plasties. Although it is desirable to place Z-plasties at the palmar and interphalangeal creases, they should be moved proximally or distally to avoid areas of avascular skin. This latitude in dealing with areas of avascular skin is lost when a zigzag or sinuous incision is used. The surgeon may find that the base of a triangular or C-shaped flap that was created at the time of the initial incision is the very area where the diseased fascia is adherent to the overlying skin (Fig. 23.4(a)). Usually the surgeon will leave this fascia in order to preserve the blood

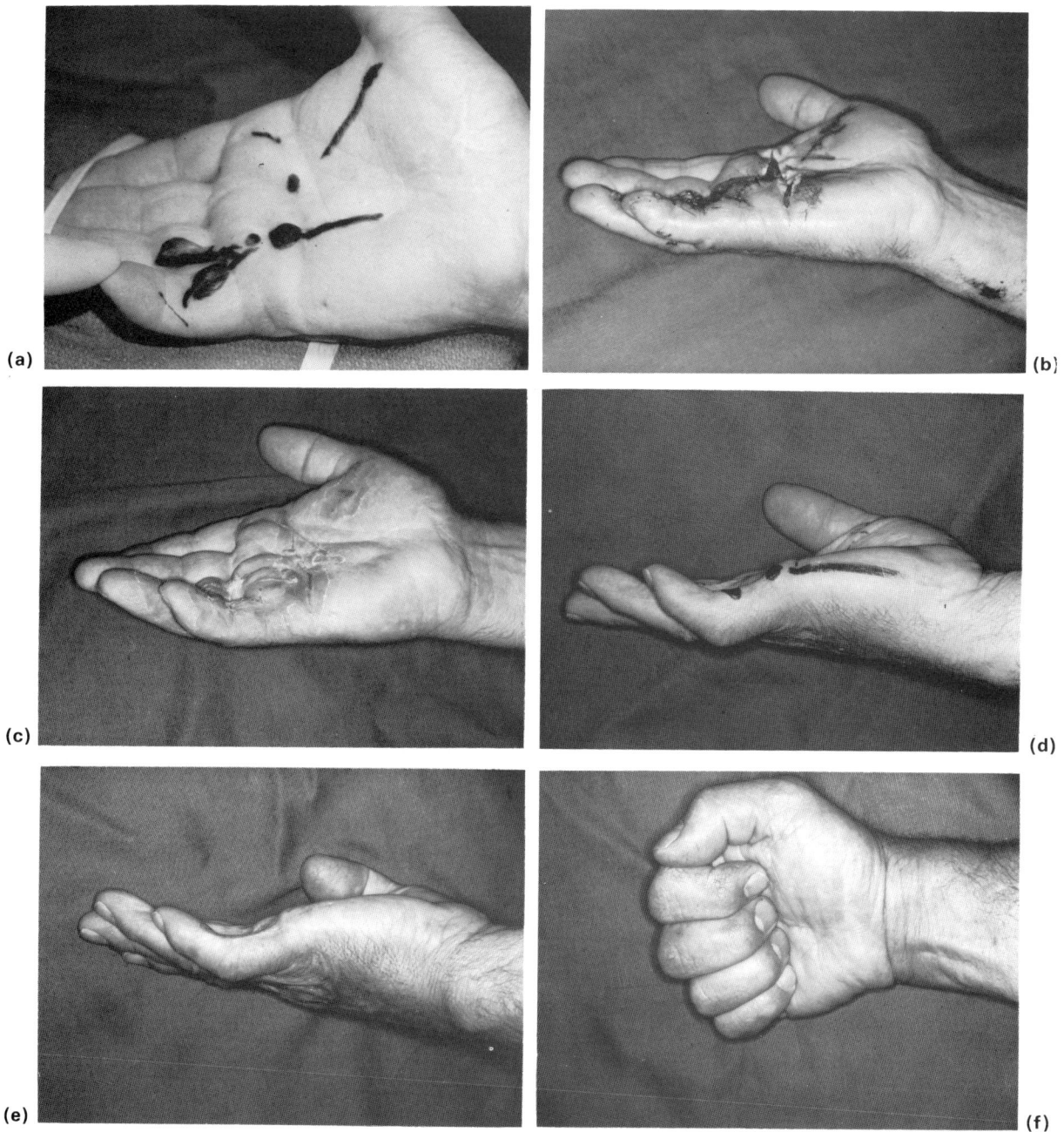

Fig. 23.6 (a) The right hand of a 49 year old railroad engineer showing extensive disease in the little finger which had been present for many years. The left hand was more severely involved. Knuckle pads were present on both hands. His mother and one sister had Dupuytren's disease. At operation an extensive fasciectomy was performed in the palm, the little and ring fingers. (b) and (c) The wounds healed without incident and he returned to work 6 weeks after operation. By that time the little and ring fingers were almost straight. (d) One year later the little finger had flexed to 65 degrees at the proximal interphalangeal joint. An ulnar lateral cord was palpable. (e) and (f) A dermofasciectomy was performed 2 years after the first operation. Four years after the second operation the contracture is static at 45 degrees and he has full flexion. This patient illustrates the difference between the palm and fingers and also between the little and ring fingers. Recurrent disease and recurrent contracture are very common in the little finger

Table 23.1 The correction of flexion contracture in each joint in each finger in 1202 operations at 6–18 months postoperative

	Little			Ring			Middle		
	N	Pre	Post	N	Pre	Post	N	Pre	Post
MP joint	258	44.1 ± 24.8*	3.2 ± 11.1	251	36.3 ± 20.0	2.5 ± 8.4	126	28.1 ± 16.3	2.3 ± 7.5
Outcome†									
Perfect	84%	42.8 ± 24.1	0	86%	34.3 ± 18.9	0	87%	27.9 ± 15.9	0
Improved	13%	54.9 ± 25.3	14.3 ± 11.2	12%	52.5 ± 20.4	15.3 ± 14.0	10%	31.1 ± 20.8	14.8 ± 8.1
Same/Worse	3%	31.4 ± 31.5	46.4 ± 35.9	2%	22.0 ± 16.8	29.0 ± 21.3	3%	25.0 ± 17.3	27.5 ± 20.6
PIP joint	263	52.9 ± 25.2	27.2 ± 23.0	138	49.5 ± 26.5	16.9 ± 21.0	42	39.6 ± 21.6	20.8 ± 21.5
Outcome									
Perfect	19%	46.5 ± 23.8	0	45%	41.7 ± 24.1	0	36%	30.3 ± 14.3	0
Improved	56%	63.2 ± 21.3	28.8 ± 17.4	42%	64.3 ± 22.8	29.0 ± 18.2	43%	50.4 ± 20.7	26.4 ± 13.4
Same/Worse	25%	34.9 ± 22.7	44.9 ± 23.3	13%	28.2 ± 19.8	36.2 ± 22.7	21%	33.7 ± 25.6	44.2 ± 22.1
DIP joint	52	26.9 ± 17.0	8.8 ± 17.0	23	32.8 ± 28.1	4.0 ± 10.5	6	18.3 ± 16.0	9.2 ± 20.1
Outcome									
Perfect	56%	20.9 ± 15.2	0	82%	29.5 ± 23.8	0	66%	12.5 ± 5.0	0
Improved	33%	38.6 ± 15.4	16.6 ± 7.7	9%	87.0 ± 4.2	32.5 ± 17.7	17%	10.0	5.0
Same/Worse	11%	23.0 ± 13.7	29.7 ± 8.9	9%	10.0 ± 7.1	14.0 ± 1.4	17%	50.0	50.0

	Index			Thumb		
	N	Pre	Post	N	Pre	Post
MP joint	27	23.3 ± 15.2	4.6 ± 9.3	16	19.6 ± 11.6	8.8 ± 17.2
Outcome						
Perfect	78%	21.1 ± 12.2	0	69%	21.5 ± 11.2	0
Improved	11%	45.0 ± 26.0	20.0 ± 10.0	6%	35.0	30.0
Same/Worse	11%	16.7 ± 5.8	21.7 ± 2.9	25%	10.4 ± 7.1	27.5 ± 24.0

* Mean ± Standard Deviation
† Perfect—the flexion contracture was completely corrected. Improved—the flexion contracture was less but not completely corrected. Same/Worse—there was no correction or the flexion contracture was worse.

supply to the flap. This is a frequent cause of recurrence. It is for this reason alone that a midline longitudinal incision (later altered by two or three Z-plasties) is preferred to a zigzag or sinuous incision.

If a transverse incision is used in the palm or digit one has the choice of closing it, or covering the defect with a free skin graft, or of simply leaving the incision open. The open palm technique of McCash (1964) is now an accepted procedure and the principle has been extended to apply to transverse incisions in the digits. It is highly recommended as a technique that reduces morbidity due to haematoma, skin necrosis and infection.

POSTOPERATIVE COMPLICATIONS

Haematoma, skin necrosis and infection

This triad usually occur together because a haematoma compromises the circulation to skin that is barely viable and infection follows necrosis of the skin. As mentioned, accurate haemostasis during the entire operation will prevent a haematoma. If a haematoma develops, it should be evacuated. If the haematoma is in the palm it is likely to be extensive and it is best to return the patient to the operating room, open the incision, evacuate the haematoma and control the bleeding. Attempts to evacuate the haematoma on the ward or in the office are usually unsatisfactory.

Necrosis of portions of small triangular flaps can often be prevented by attention to detail at operation and by treating these flaps as free grafts and applying a bolus dressing. If necrosis occurs it is best to continue dressing the wound and splinting the hand until the wounds are healed rather than considering skin grafting of small areas. With prolonged splinting, the final results may be satisfactory. If more extensive skin necrosis occurs then a split thickness skin graft should be applied as soon as possible to prevent scar contracture. The final result under these circumstances is not likely to be satisfactory.

Pain and swelling

It is best to keep the patient in the hospital overnight following operation so that there is assurance that the hand will be elevated. With the application of a firm dressing, a splint, and elevation of the hand, pain and swelling should be minimal. If it is not the cause of the pain can be attended to whether it be a tight dressing, a haematoma or the onset of sympathetic dystrophy. It is our custom to remove the initial dressing on the first postoperative day and apply a thermoplastic splint under the direction of the hand therapist that holds the involved digits in extension. Thus the postoperative therapy begins on the first day, but more important the wounds are inspected.

Reflex sympathetic dystrophy and limitation of flexion

Limitation of flexion is a feature of sympathetic dystrophy but occurs with all complications. It is indeed an index of morbidity and if prolonged beyond 8–10 weeks of operation becomes a complication per se. One should not expect the patient to be able to flex the fingers immediately after operation and in fact too much flexion before the wounds are healed may be detrimental (Fig. 23.7). One should look for progressive increase in the range of flexion and expect the fingertips to touch the palm within 3 weeks of operation. Full flexion to the distal crease of the palm may not be accomplished for 3 or 4 months after operation. There need be no concern as long as progress is made but the patient must be reassured that full flexion will be regained.

Sympathetic dystrophy is a dreaded complication of any hand operation but is perhaps most common after fasciectomy (Fig. 23.8). The incidence is unknown because lesser degrees of dystrophy are common. Well established sympathetic dystrophy occurs after 4% of operations. The incidence is significantly greater in women than men occurring twice as often in females (3.5% males; 7.2% females–McFarlane 1985). Two val-

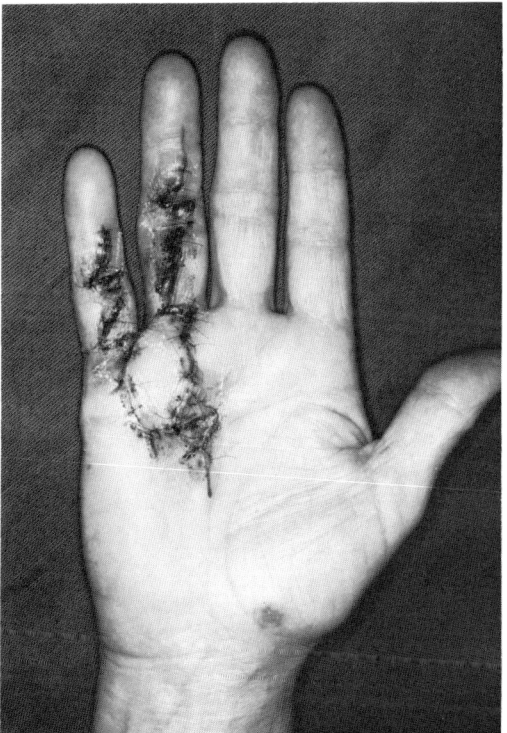
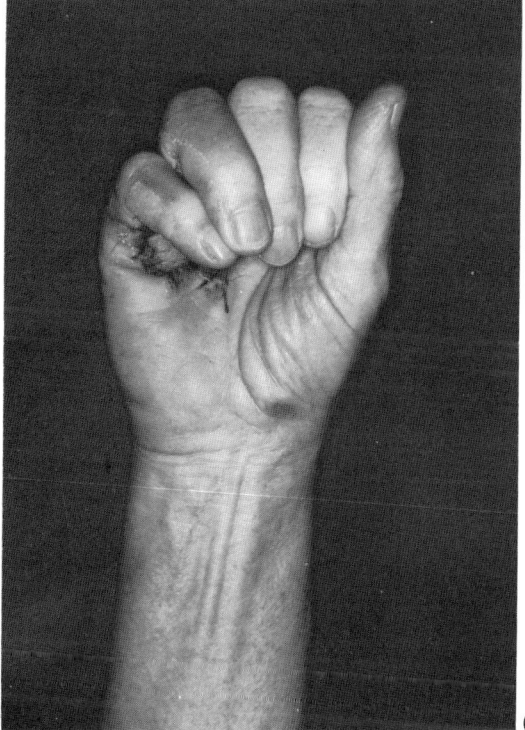

Fig. 23.7 (a) and (b) The right hand of a 66 year old salesman who was operated upon 2 weeks previously. He has almost full extension and the expected degree of flexion

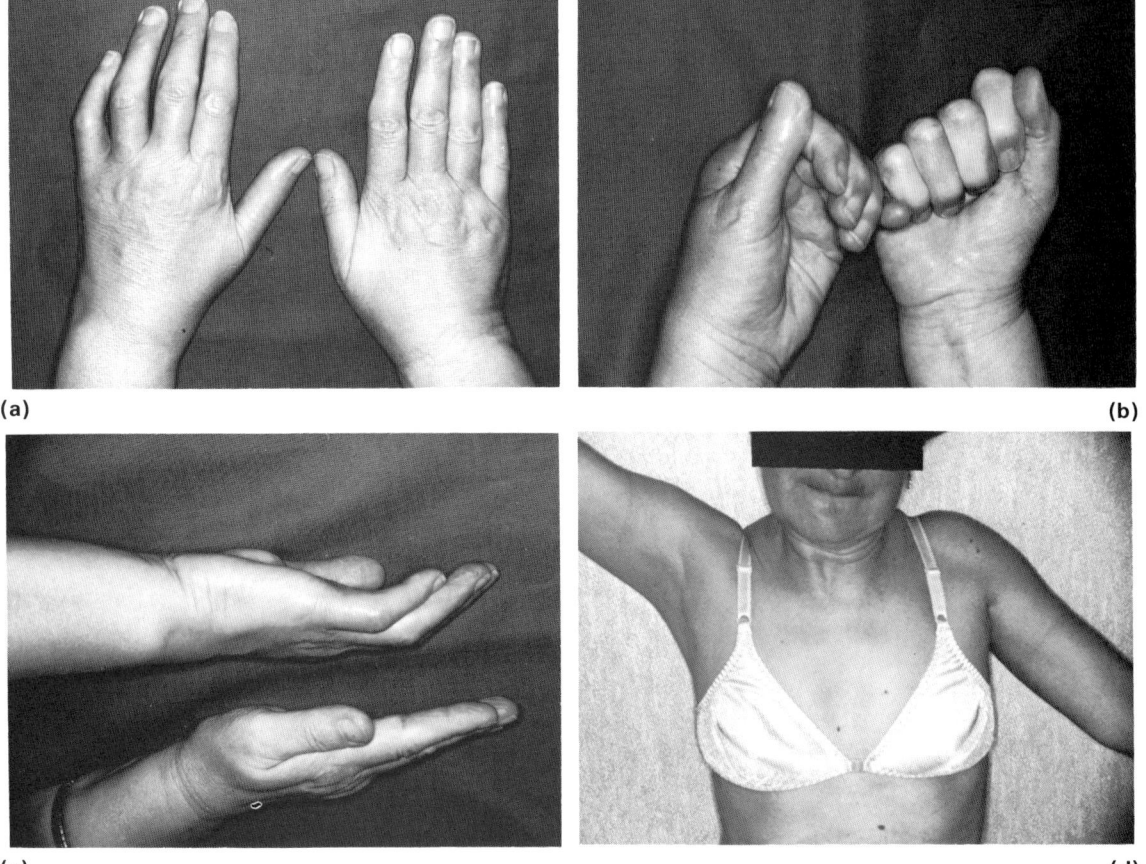

Fig. 23.8 This 53 year old female cook was seen because of painful trigger fingers and thumb but also had 20 degrees of contracture at the proximal interphalangeal joint of the left little finger. She was an insulin dependent diabetic. The left hand was operated upon first releasing the trigger thumb and index finger and performing an extensive fasciectomy on the little finger. A similar operation was performed on the right hand 2 weeks later. The presence of sympathetic dystrophy in the left hand was not appreciated for 6 weeks postoperatively. (a)–(c) To show the swelling and loss of movement in the left hand. (d) Limitation of shoulder abduction should have been detected sooner

uable preventative measures are the use of regional block anaesthesia, especially with long acting agents, to provide a sympathectomy effect and observation of the patient overnight to be sure that the hand is elevated and pain and swelling are minimal. Any intra or postoperative complication can trigger the onset of sympathetic dystrophy. If pain and swelling persist the patient should remain in hospital or be readmitted to hospital and receive repeated sympathetic blocks or quanethidine infusion as well as appropriate sedation and hand therapy. One should look for pain and limitation of shoulder abduction as this may be an early sign of sympathetic dystrophy.

In spite of all of these precautions some patients will appear 2 or 3 weeks after operation with severe sympathetic dystrophy. It is extremely difficult to treat these patients and they are likely to have pain, swelling and limitation of movement for many months and may never regain full finger flexion.

Recurrence and extension of disease

Recurrence means that diseased fascia reappears within the area of operation whereas extension refers to disease appearing beyond this area. It is appropriate to consider both as a postoperative complication because to some extent both are preventable. Recurrence is prevented by meticulous removal of all diseased fascia. This is relatively easy in the palm but difficult in the finger. Extension is prevented by removing all fascia that is clinically diseased, that is, performing a sufficiently extensive operation in the first instance.

In the same way that the indications for and the type of operation are different in the palm and finger, the significance of recurrence and extension are different in these two areas. In the palm recurrent disease infrequently causes metacarpophalangeal joint contracture and therefore does not require treatment. Extension of disease in the adjacent ray is likely to progress to metacarpophalangeal and/or proximal interphalangeal contracture and require operation in the usual way (Fig. 23.9).

Recurrence in a finger invariably causes proximal interphalangeal joint contracture, in fact, the joint may not have been fully corrected at the first operation. It is due to leaving diseased fascia on the skin flaps or, more frequently, failing to remove all of the diseased cords and potentially diseased bands of fascia in the finger (Fig. 23.4). Recurrence in the finger is best prevented by a radical fasciectomy and as mentioned previously a dermofasciectomy may be needed.

Often persistent or recurrent proximal interphalangeal joint contracture is due to scar contraction caused by the tissue trauma of the fasciectomy (Fig. 23.5). This is a dilemma of treatment which is as yet unsolved but scar contracture can, to some degree, be controlled by prolonged splinting. There is a biological variable which is most apparent in patients with a strong Dupuytren's diathesis. There are also those patients, who are not identifiable preoperatively, who produce more scar tissue than others.

Recurrence and extension are all too frequent in the thumb web (Fig. 23.10). This is due to a failure to realise that three cords converge on the base of the thumb—the pretendinous cord, the transverse fibres of the palmar aponeurosis and the natatory cord (Tubiana & Defrenne 1976). Also disease in the thumb is often removed 'en passant' after a difficult digital dissection and an adequate fasciec-

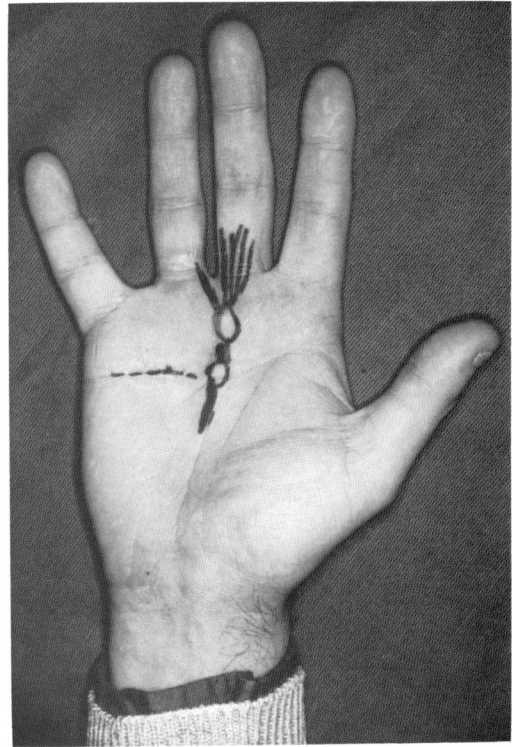

Fig. 23.9 This 34 year old soldier had two previous operations on the right hand. The first operation was performed to remove a tender lump and the second operation because the lump became larger. This is an example of operating too early. He now has extension of disease and 25 degrees of contracture at the metacarpophalangeal of the middle finger

tomy is not performed. Recurrence and extension are disabling because thumb extension and abduction are compromised.

CONCLUSIONS

The problems associated with the treatment of patients with Dupuytren's disease are greater than one might expect. However, a satisfactory result and a satisfied patient can be obtained with attention to the details of choosing an appropriate operation for each patient, careful operative technique and close postoperative follow-up.

362 UNSATISFACTORY RESULTS IN HAND SURGERY

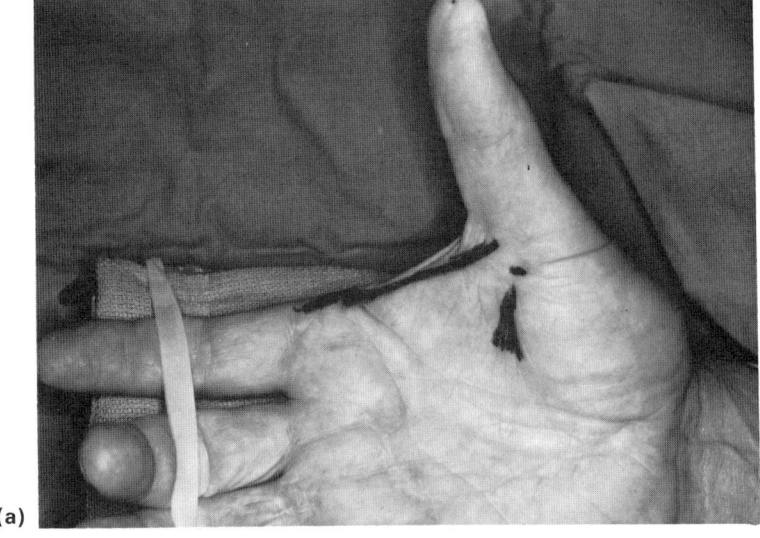

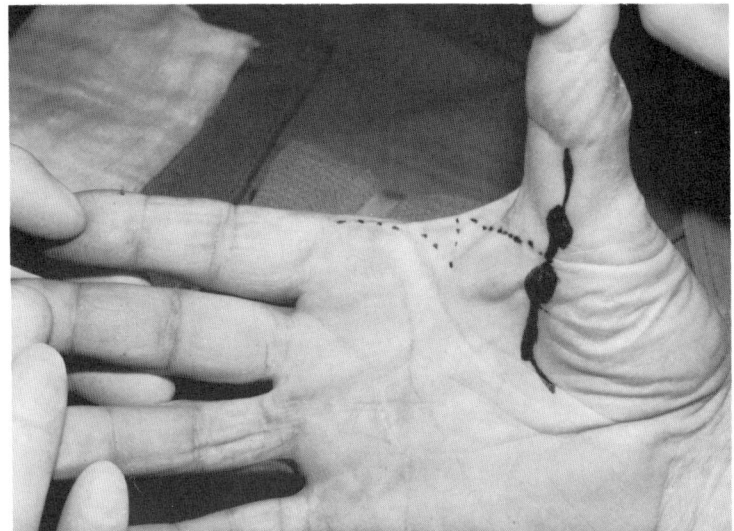

Fig. 23.10 (a) and (b) The right hand of a 58 year old manager in which a thumb web contracture was corrected by excising the natatory cord and the termination of the transverse fibres of the palmar aponeurosis. The dotted lines indicate the two digital nerves to the thumb and the radial digital nerve to the index finger. (c) and (d) Seven years later he requested further treatment and the pretendinous cord to the thumb was excised. This tissue should have been removed at the first operation

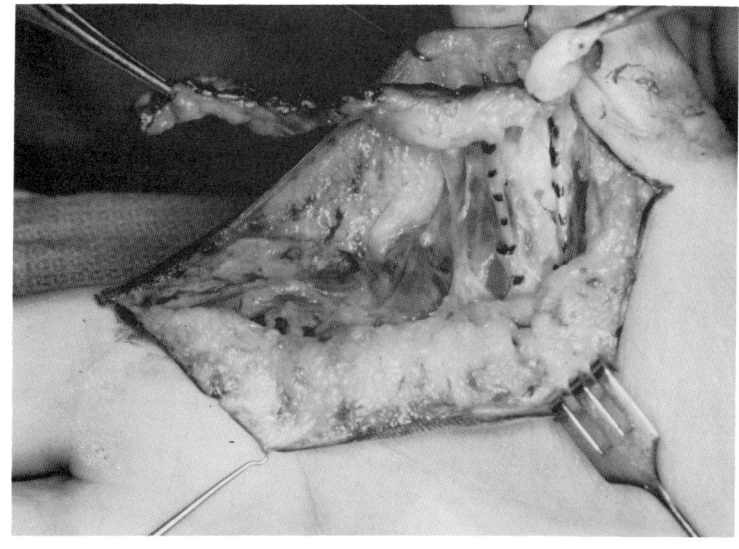

(c)

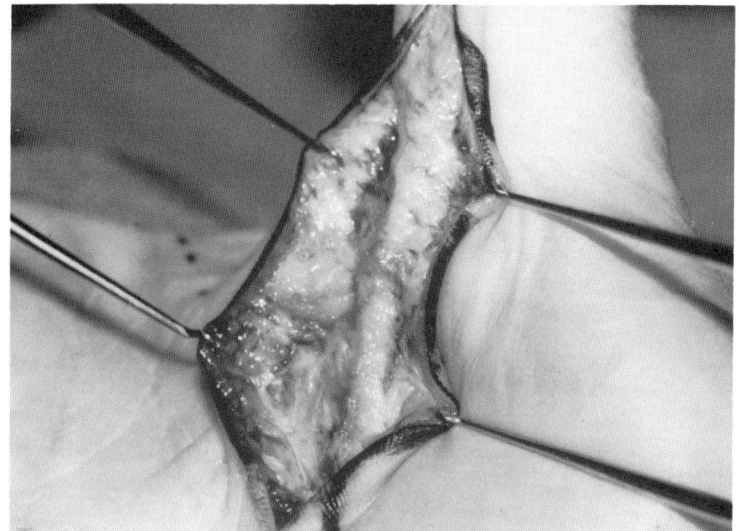

(d)

REFERENCES

Curtis R M 1954 Capsulectomy of the interphalangeal joints of the fingers. Journal of Bone and Joint Surgery 36A: 1219

Hueston J T 1963 Dupuytren's Contracture. E and S Livingstone Ltd, Edinburgh and London

Hueston J T 1982 In: Flynn J E ed. Hand Surgery, Williams and Wilkins, Baltimore, p 797–823

Hueston J T 1984 Dermofasciectomy for Dupuytren's disease. Bulletin of the Hospital for Joint Diseases Orthopedic Institute 44: 224

Legge J W H, McFarlane R M 1980 Prediction of results of Dupuytren's contracture. Journal of Hand Surgery 5: 608

McCash C R 1964 The open palm technique in Dupuytren's contracture. British Journal of Plastic Surgery 17: 271

McFarlane R M 1974 Patterns of the diseased fascia in the fingers in Dupuytren's contracture. Plastic and Reconstructive Surgery 54: 31

McFarlane R M 1982 In: Green D P ed. Operative Hand Surgery. Churchill Livingstone, New York. p 463–498

McFarlane R M 1982 In: Strickland J W, Steichen J B eds. Difficult Problems in Hand Surgery. C V Mosby, St Louis, p 389–398

McFarlane R M 1985 Dupuytren's Disease Study of the International Federation of Societies for Surgery of the Hand. Unpublished data

Millesi H 1967 Uber die Beugekontraktur des Dislalen Interphalangealgelenkes im Rahmen einer Dupuytrenschen Erkrankung. Brun's Beitrage zur Klinischen Chirurgie 214: 399

Noble J, Heathcote J G, Cohen H 1984 Diabetes mellitus in the aetiology of Dupuytren's disease. Journal of Bone and Joint Surgery 66B:322

Rowley D I, Couch M, Chesney R B, Norris S H 1984 Assessment of percutaneous fasciotomy in the management of Dupuytren's contracture. Journal of Hand Surgery 9B:163

Thomine J M 1972 Le Fascia Digital—development et anatomie. In: Tubiana R ed. La Maladie de Dupuytren, 2nd edn. Expansion Scientific Francais, Paris

Tonkin M A, Burke F D, Varian J P 1984 Dupuytren's contracture: a comparative study of fasciectomy and dermofasciectomy in one hundred patients. Journal of Hand Surgery 9B:156

Tubiana R, Fahrer M, McCullough C J 1981 Recurrence and other complications in surgery of Dupuytren's contracture. Clinics in Plastic Surgery 8:45

Watson J D 1984 Fasciotomy and Z-plasty in the management of Dupuytren's contracture. British Journal of Plastic Surgery 37:27

A. O. Narakas

24 Brachial plexus

In order to grasp and shape the world around him, man has been given an exquisite tool, the hand. To perform this task he was gifted with the shoulder, a joint with an unequalled range of movement and an elbow to extend the reach of the hand. The human brain devotes a few trillion neurones to command the upper limb through half-a-million myelinated and unmyelinated axons grouped in an entity we call the brachial plexus, which consists of nerve trunks, divisions, cords and terminal branches. These axons are of unequal value and their central connections differ widely in quantity and quality. For instance, there is no doubt today that the number and volume of neurones in the spinal cord, and particularly in the brain linked with the function of the shoulder, are greater than of those devoted to the elbow, the hand having by far the greatest. The ulnar and median nerves, terminal branches of the brachial plexus, have immensely richer central connections than an axillary or a musculo-cutaneous nerve. The latter effects quite simple work: primarily, it flexes the elbow or supinates the forearm; secondarily, it contributes to the stabilization of the humeral head (long portion of the biceps) and the scapula (short portion). The sensibility it provides to the forearm is far less discriminative than the tactile gnosis a human hand can offer. Nor is the motor function of that nerve nearly as sophisticated as the play of our fingers. Therefore, surgical restoration of a normal or near normal function in the upper extremity of a patient with a brachial plexus lesion will depend on the nervous pathways affected; those of the musculo-cutaneous, suprascapular, axillary nerves will be far easier to repair and will regenerate more satisfactorily than those of very demanding nerves, such as the ulnar and median, and, to a lesser extent, of the radial. This hierarchy has to be borne in mind when considering prognosis after repair. Nature and extent of injury play a definite role. When a trunk is sharply cut, little nervous tissue is lost, less than when a bullet severs a trunk, and much less when a rupture is caused by a traction injury. Timing and quality of repair, i.e. age of the patient and of the lesion, also play an important role.

Therefore, it must be realized from the start that good results in brachial plexus surgery can be obtained only when:

1. The lesion is limited in extent and is affecting nervous pathways which are not connected to sophisticated motor or sensory functions.
2. The lesion is benign, such as caused by sharp laceration or compression which is not of long duration.
3. Blood supply to the injured nerves is not impeded, as in fibrosis after irradiation, and the limb is well-perfused, presenting no ischaemic or fibrotic segments.
4. Tendinous, skeletal, muscular structures in the limb are healthy or have been properly treated and no deformities or contractures are present.
5. Injury has not affected the neurones in the spinal cord themselves so that they are able to produce sprouts and grow neofibres. This is more likely to occur in distal than in proximal injuries.

We will examine these different factors in order to avoid pitfalls in treatment and be confronted with a result which is worse than expected. Realism must be a rule. There are goals beyond our reach.

At the current state of the art we cannot restore hand intrinsic muscle function by suturing or grafting the median or ulnar nerve fascicles in the brachial plexus of an adult. Other goals can only be partially reached, such as flexion and extension of the digits.

The restoration of function of a simple articulation, such as the elbow or even the wrist, will be far easier to achieve than obtaining full range of motion in a shoulder, which requires the harmonious activity of at least a dozen muscles.

The aims of repair have to follow a guideline: reconstruct the less demanding function first.

At present, this way of thinking gives the following priorities in a total brachial plexus palsy:

1. Elbow flexion
2. Adduction in the shoulder (thoraco-humeral pinch)
3. Shoulder stability
4. Protective sensibility in forearm
5. Shoulder abduction, forward elevation and external rotation
6. Wrist flexion or stability
7. Protective sensibility in some parts of hand
8. Elbow extension
9. Wrist extension
10. Adduction of thumb (key pinch)
11. Flexion of fingers
12. Extension of thumb and fingers

Thumb opposition is the coronation of hand function. To aim for it in total brachial plexus lesions is not useful nor realistic. When many nervous pathways are destroyed, only a few of these goals can be reached.

PROBLEMS IN DIAGNOSIS

Because in the past brachial plexus injuries (BPI) were not common and little could be done for them, their diagnosis and their treatment remained surrounded by an aura of irrationality, which only started to disappear a decade ago. Experience, gained in the last 20 years with over 1100 plexopathies of various origins, has shown that diagnosis has been impeded or rendered incomplete by the following facts:

1. In traumatic injuries (by far the most common are traction lesions), the circumstances of the accident were not well analysed, i.e. a guess was not made on kinetic energies which produced injury. Only violent trauma can cause a brachial plexus rupture and/or root avulsion. A motorcycle or car accident dislocating a shoulder has a totally different significance with regards to the severity of nerve lesions from a fall from one's own height. Even the latter may have different consequences on the axillary nerve, for example, if the fall was with the arm in abduction and internal rotation (likelihood of rupture) or in adduction against the thorax (likelihood of a simple contusion, which will recover in a matter of weeks or months). People over 60 years may 'fracture' their axillary artery or cause damage to the intima of the vessel with interruption of circulation by a simple fall, while this never happens in young patients. The nerve damage will be minor in the former even if it causes a complete palsy, it will be major in the young sustaining a severe accident because the artery is more elastic than the nerve. If it ruptures, the nerves are very likely to have ruptured also.

2. The neurological deficits are not noted initially because the patient is unconscious or because there are several life-threatening injuries which focus the attention of casualty doctors. Often, even in common shoulder dislocations, the patient being perfectly conscious, neither he nor the doctor who reduced the dislocation are able to tell afterwards if the deltoid and/or other muscles were paralysed prior to reduction. This may have some legal consequences and is paramount for the decisions to be taken concerning the treatment: a violent accident causing a dislocation with immediate palsy is likely to have caused ruptures of nerve trunks, even root avulsions requiring surgical intervention. On the contrary, no prior palsy to reduction, an easy relocation of the humeral head followed by palsy, is likely to have caused a minor nerve stretch injury (neuropraxia or a second-degree injury according to Sunderland) which will recover without surgical intervention on nerves.

3. Compartment compression syndromes of the upper limb from deltoid down to the hand are not diagnosed within the safe period (six hours) or are diagnosed too late, when muscles have suffered irreparable damage. Even if nerves are not severely injured and are able to recover spontaneously without any surgical repair, their regeneration will be impeded by ischaemic, fibrosed muscles which never become functional again, even when reinnervated. This happens when the upper limb has been submitted to severe blunt trauma, to a crush (e.g. conveyor belt, mountaineer's rope, arm caught in a mechanical device) and when fractures of humerus and both bones of the forearm occur.

4. Vascular damage may go unrecognized, particularly when the limb is well perfused through intact collateral channels (periscapular etc.). In the hours after emergency admission, a wrong positioning of the patient on the operating table or in the ward may impede the precarious vascular balance, resulting in compartment ischaemia (flexors or extensors of the digits) which will be recognized only when it is too late.

5. Massive root avulsions may produce a partial Brown-Séquard syndrome, which will escape diagnosis in the severely injured patient, particularly because the lower extremity on the same side as the BPI will be fractured and the patient will have a thoracic or abdominal trauma. This partial syndrome goes then unrecognized for years, even by the surgeons operating on the brachial plexus as it happened four times to the author, i.e. in half of the patients with that syndrome. Repair of the plexus in these cases may be doomed to failure particularly when using intercostal nerves.

6. Bernard–Horner syndrome (the name of Pourfour du Petit should be added as he was the first to describe, in 1727, the anatomical bases which are responsible for it) is not seen because of trauma to the face or orbit or because it is not expected; anisocoria may be interpreted as a sign of CNS involvement.

In obstetric palsy common obstacles for full history and diagnosis are inaccuracies of observations done in the perinatal period:

1. Several months down the line, nobody knows if at that time the child could or could not move (flex, even less extend) his fingers. The culpabilized obstetrician has hardly seen the baby, the paediatrician has no idea how to examine a baby with an obstetric palsy, nurses and parents, doctors and physiotherapists notice only the paralysed shoulder and elbow. The neuropaediatrician will be more concerned with possible brain damage. He will have very little experience with obstetric palsy because it is rare in countries advanced enough to have neuropaediatricians.

2. Nobody will be able to tell if the elbow of the baby was in permanent extension because of the still active triceps or because of the weight of the limb which was put along the body or kept there by the action of a still-functional lower part of the pectoralis major which may be spared in C5–C6–C7 lesions.

3. Parents and medical personnel will sometimes not be aware if at the start Bernard–Horner syndrome was present.

4. In long-standing cases, very often little information is available on the calendar of recovery, i.e. at what age the child started to flex his elbow, extend his wrist, actively abduct his shoulder and to what extent. The abnormal pattern of motion attracts more attention than the deficits of isolated muscles. Nobody will, for example, notice that the deltoid is still totally paralysed in a child who abducts his arm with the help of a recovered supraspinatus.

In penetrating wounds initial localized deficits will not be noticed because compensating mechanisms are present, because pain and shock limit possibilities of testing, and because function of articulations is not well-understood by a majority of doctors in casualty departments. A severance of the musculo-cutaneous nerve may escape attention because the brachio-radialis as well as forearm muscles can easily produce an elbow flexion. An axillary nerve lesion goes unnoticed because the supra-spinatus in conjunction with other muscles, such as the pectoralis major, maintain a full arm abduction. The contrary may happen. Axillary nerve severance is diagnosed, but not the injury to the supra-scapular nerve. Paralysis of finger extension can be compensated by a combination of wrist flexion and activity of intrinsic muscles of the hand.

In post-radiation plexopathy it is always difficult to define when the first symptoms started, the daily and total dosage of irradiation received and the various fields irradiated. As the latency between radiotherapy and first symptoms may extend for years, initial documents may be lost and the radiotherapist involved will never know of the late complication. The possibility of associated slow-growing metastases is not considered. A carpal or a cubital tunnel syndrome is diagnosed, but the plexopathy induced by radiation and the thoracic outlet syndrome associated initially with it, remain unrecognized because the whole limb was not examined until electrophysiological examinations were performed. In the above mentioned and in various other plexopathies, particularly in thoracic outlet syndromes, the diagnosis is missed initially because only distal peripheral neuropathies are taken into account, two level lesions are forgotten and anatomical anomalies at the cervico-thoracic outlet and in the arm are not considered.

PITFALLS IN CLINICAL EXAMINATION

We have already mentioned some trick movements which may foul accurate diagnosis. BPI cases must be examined systematically, bearing in mind CNS and concomitant PNS lesions. In traction lesions, occurring through violent trauma, injury to brain and spinal cord have to be remembered, as well as metastases localized in these structures in a patient presenting with radiation plexopathy. The same applies to obstetric palsies and BP lesions of unknown origin. Clinical examination is then paramount because the localization of the lesion, i.e. at the level of the CNS, at the roots, in the spinal cord or above, will determine the therapeutic decisions. The author has been impressed in this respect, during his 20 years of experience, by the accuracy of descriptions made by neurologists, probably because these specialists are educationally orientated towards observation and diagnosis and the inadequacy or limitations of the clinical picture of the same patient given by surgeons, who are educated not to speculate but, in the limited scope of possible treatment, to make immediate therapeutic decisions. For this purpose, they may consider more what they know than what they do not know.

Examination of patients with BP lesions may overlook the following signs (from proximal to distal):

1. An anisocoria, particularly difficult to notice in people with dark eyes; thus, a partial or a transient Horner syndrome may be missed and not related to loss of hand function. On the other hand, there will always be a member of the family to certify that the patient has always had one 'smaller eye' thus denying a sign essential to diagnosis.

2. Atrophy and weakness of deep muscles of the neck innervated by the posterior ramus of upper roots, a finding which must arouse suspicion of C5–C6–C7 radicular involvement confirmed by palsy of rhomboids and serratus anterior.

3. Fractures of the posterior arc of the first rib and transverse process of C7 speak in favour of lower root avulsion. In these fresh cases, paralysis of the sympathetic fibres will produce anhidrosis of the hand, until the avulsed spinal ganglions, still capable of function, recover from the initial shock.

4. Scapular winging accepting various interpretations. It is absent in total paralysis and will appear in active forward elevation of the arm only in partial or complete paralysis of the long thoracic nerve, provided muscles inserted on the coracoid process are active and tilt the scapula forward. The medial border will be prominent in palsies of the trapezius and rhomboids and the inferior tip will stand out when the arm is at rest along the thorax when there is a contracture limiting internal rotation, a fact seen often in long-standing obstetric palsy. The passive and active humero-scapular angle (lateral border of scapula-axis of humerus) is an item useful to record.

5. Downward subluxation of the humeral head will be noted in deltoid paralysis only if there is an associated palsy of the supra-scapular nerve or, in the elderly, a rotator cuff rupture. Absence of $40°$ to $60°$ initial abduction in the shoulder cannot be explained by an axillary nerve palsy alone. Young patients may even present with an apparently full ROM with a complete deltoid paralysis. An internally rotated humerus by palsy of external rotators cannot be abducted more than $60°$.

6. Chronic drooping of the shoulder may cause a secondary thoracic outlet syndrome in longer

standing cases in the absence of initial involvement by lesions of the lower trunk.

7. Joint contractures require radiological investigation to diagnose ectopic bone formation and spasticity will point immediately to an upper motor neurone lesion which can be the sole cause of paralysis or associated with a BP injury.

8. In complete musculo-cutaneous nerve lesions, flexion of the elbow is possible by the brachio-radialis and other forearm muscles as previously explained.

9. Supination of the forearm is full even when the biceps is paralysed if forearm muscles are intact. Pronation seems normal when pronator teres is totally paralysed but other muscles inserted on the medial epicondyle and the pronator quadratus are functional.

10. Numerous trick movements to compensate for deficits in wrist and finger function may go unnoticed, though they will not escape the attention of a hand surgeon. Clawing will appear only if some digital flexors are still active.

11. Mobility of diaphragm which can easily be checked by percussion is seldom tested by examiners. Phrenic nerve function has to be ascertained.

12. Sensory testing has to be approximate but accurate and distinguished in total anaesthesia, thermo analgesia, disturbed sensation and normal sensation. The affected areas have to be mapped out on the extremity. Discrepancies with motor function have to be submitted to more close scrutiny in order to explain them.

Experience has shown that the best way to record all findings is to use some kind of chart which reminds the examiner to test all functions of the limb, not forgetting the passive and active ROM, circumferential measures to evaluate muscular wasting and recording of radial and ulnar pulses in order to not forget the vascular condition of the limb. Often traumatic BP injuries co-exist with soft-tissue and bone injury, particularly fractures of radius and ulna which limit passive function by alteration of bone alignment, interosseous membrane and muscle fibrosis or tendinous adherences. Ectopic bone formation may be present around the shoulder and elbow. Clavicular, upper rib, scapular, proximal fractures of the humerus and their consequences have to be integrated to assess properly the condition of the paralysed upper extremity.

Assessment of function is a real challenge in obstetric palsy, particularly in babies or young children. Scapulo-thoracic and scapulo-humeral functions are intimately interrelated. The minimal and maximal scapulo-humeral active angle has to be noted in order to evaluate real abduction, elevation and rotation in the shoulder. Joint contraction causing a limitation of internal rotation results in winging of the scapula with the limb at rest. Contractures in the upper portion of the capsule and underdevelopment of the rotator cuff muscles limit adduction and external rotation, the child compensating this deficit with the scapulo-thoracic joint.

Numerous synkinesias produce distorted motional patterns which may deform the humeral head in conjunction with growth retardation of affected segments. Muscular imbalance will dislocate the radial head, produce persistent forearm pronation or supination.

It is very difficult to assess intrinsic hand muscle function in a small child and the tendency is to neglect to describe accurately the altered grasp.

Children with obstetric palsy do not realize their handicap before kindergarten or school age. They have been born with an extremity different from the contralateral and they use it at their best. They do not miss what they never had. Therefore, they are not handicapped as long as they are not put in competition with other, normal, children and less affected than their parents. Clinical examination should allow on the one hand to establish their functional deficits and on the other, what they have made of residual function; pitfalls consist of neglecting one or the other aspect.

In any other progressive or partial palsy of any origin, the extraordinary compensating mechanisms for lost function have to be taken into account. All muscles have two insertions. Normally there is a preferential function, e.g. the triceps extends the elbow. But because the triceps has a subglenoidal insertion, it can act as a humeral adductor or a posterior elevator. Flexors and extensors of wrist and fingers can act as elbow flexors. These accessory and inverted ancillary functions gain in importance with progressions of paralysis masking it partially.

SPECIAL INVESTIGATIONS

It is a common error in a cervical myelogram to look only for meningocoeles. The negative outline of rootlets, their absence and depressions in the vertebral canal are more important than a pouch filled with contrast medium which means hardly anything more than a rupture in the dural cul-de-sac. Combination of myelography with CT scan allows a better representation of the position of the spinal cord within the medullary canal, shows possible spinal cord lesions and continuity or interruption of anterior or posterior roots. These findings have always to be consistent with the results of the clinical examination, which still has the precedence.

Electrophysiology is very useful if its limitations are recognized. It shows preferentially the activity of nerve fibres most sensitive to stimulation. Function of other fibres may go unnoticed unless differential recordings are performed, separating fast from slow-conducting fibres and giving an approximation of their relative numbers. In total loss of function, it is not possible by electrophysiology alone to distinguish between axonotmesis not requiring surgical repair and neurotmesis. Sensory evoked potentials cannot be recorded in infraganglionic lesions and will be found in root avulsion only when the spinal ganglion cells have recovered from trauma. As in myelography, clinical judgement prevails when discrepancies are noted. In severe injuries and after surgical repair, all electrophysiology can tell is that reinnervation has or has not occurred but not to what functional extent with regards to muscle power, ROM and harmony of movement. It may show that sensory conduction is present but tell little of the message conveyed to the brain.

PITFALLS DURING OPERATIVE PROCEDURES

Surgical exploration has two specific aims: visual control of the pathology and the best possible repair.

To achieve both, an almost bloodless field with wide exposure is required. Subcutaneous and subfascial infiltrations with a vasoconstricting solution, elevation of the upper half of the patient by 30° to 60°, meticulous haemostasis with bipolar coagulation and detailed knowledge of the anatomy of the region will allow the surgeon to achieve his tasks.

The following sources of bleeding have to be avoided or controlled:

1. Small vessels on top, in and under the platysma colli, as well as in between the lobules of fat-covering the plexus. Many gather at each pole of lymphatic ganglions which are imbedded in the subfascial fat.

2. Small vessels running together with the cervical sensory rami and the phrenic nerve, particularly at the top of the incision where the scaleni meet.

3. Transverse vascular bundles crossing the plexus.

4. Ascending vessels which cross the spinal nerves close to or inside the intervertebral foramina. In particular, to coagulate the veins may be insufficient and may damage the nerve; compression by a micro-pack into the foramen may hinder repair.

5. Bleeding of arterioles in the epineurium, particularly in the proximal segments of spinal nerves and trunks, has to be stopped using very fine micro-coagulation forceps.

6. The same applies to arterioles between the fascicles when nerves have been trimmed for repair. A nerve holder or a rubber band can be used as a 'tourniquet' around the trunk to help to identify the bleeding vessel which always retracts about 0.5–1 mm into the stump unless fixed by interfascicular scar. This prevents it from collapsing spontaneously and ceasing to bleed. Presence of such a scar means that the trimming was not sufficient; so it must be excised and the surgeon will again meet the former situation.

7. In the area where the axillary nerve enters the quadrangular space, the supra-scapular nerve approaches the scapular notch, the musculocutaneous nerve enters the coraco-brachialis, and vessels accompany them. Their bleeding is very disturbing and sometimes difficult to stop. The same applies to the veins and arterioles between the lateral and posterior cords.

Identification of nerve stumps may be difficult.

The proximal stumps C5, C6 and C7 are often put by trauma in a vertical position, along the spine and are hidden by scaleni and scar. They must be found to be repaired. Distal stumps are retracted medially by scar, adherent to the subclavian artery and the venous cistern just behind the medial-third of the clavicle. Avulsed roots coil up on themselves and the distal portion of the ruptured upper trunk hides behind the clavicle. The supra-scapular nerve has to be found and may serve as a guide. Not infrequently, it may be injured at or behind the scapular notch. The proximal stump of the axillary nerve may coil up behind the posterior cord or even the clavicle and the distal stump can be fixed in the quadrangular space or posterior to it, necessitating an axillary and a posterior approach. Injury to circumflex vessels has to be avoided.

When ruptured at its origin, the distal musculo-cutaneous nerve may retract into the arm as much as 10 cm and will be difficult to find under the short portion of the biceps. The distal stump of the radial nerve accompanied by the deep humeral artery may be very tricky to locate, particularly in infraclavicular plexus lesions with axillary artery rupture which was repaired in an emergency. Confusion occurs when the origin of the terminal branches of the plexus is not situated in the axilla but more distally. The median nerve may form a common trunk with the musculo-cutaneous nerve or half of it. It is even possible that the median and ulnar nerves have a common trunk for several centimetres. The medial cord can be displaced laterally by scar while the posterior cord slides under it. In such cases, the former is mistaken for the latter. A two- or three-level injury has to be identified and repair planned accordingly.

Erroneously, the author has grafted the ruptured upper trunk and waited in vain for return of function in cases where he did not recognize at operation that the supra-scapular nerve was ruptured at the scapular notch or avulsed from muscle, the musculo-cutaneous nerve ruptured in the coraco-brachialis, and the axillary in the quadrangular space. In a few other cases, where myelography was misleading, roots were avulsed but remained in the foramen while the upper trunk was ruptured. Useless nerve grafting was carried out.

Errors in repair

Harvesting of both sural nerves before complete exploration of the brachial plexus, i.e. knowing what the lesions are and which repair is possible, and proceeding to intercostal nerve transfers onto the musculo-cutaneous nerve without ascertaining *de visu* that C5 and C6 are avulsed from the spinal cord, cannot be justified. The author has even seen two cases of obstetric palsy (lesions in this condition are exclusively supra-clavicular) in whom both sural nerves were harvested, then the axilla explored, no lesion found and the young patient closed, telling the parents that the child will heal spontaneously!

Insufficient trimming of stumps, and calculating grafts too short, so that they have to be put in under tension (liberated stumps may retract 2–3 cm), are other errors. Not isolating fascicular groups in the distal stump so that grafts will be connected to interfascicular scar and not nerve tissue, putting suction drains near the grafts, not reinserting the pectoralis major tendon when it has been severed for exposure, letting persist a non-union of or a grossly deformed clavicle are other errors which will jeopardize a possible repair.

Disputable choices in repair

There are choices in repair which lack logic without being entirely wrong. If supra-scapular nerve repair is abandoned, there is little sense in repairing the fascicles leading to the axillary nerve. No grafts should be wasted on the latter if in the future a shoulder arthrodesis is planned. If proximal nerve stumps are available, some of the anterior thoracic nerves for the pectoralis major should be repaired; otherwise, the very useful humero-pectoral 'pinch' will not be restored and will rely on the weight of the arm alone. There is little sense in using only one intercostal nerve per avulsed root or a terminal branch. The author has seen patients in whom one intercostal nerve was used for each of the musculo-cutaneous and the axillary nerve and one for the lateral origin of the median!

A complete reconstruction plan associating nerve repair and measures such as arthrodeses, tenodesis and muscle transfer have to be made. Performing the latter, it must be realized that only strong muscles can be used with independent or synkinetic function (e.g. biceps–triceps synkinesia after plexus repair), that pectoralis major, latissimus dorsi transfers and Steindler's procedure will yield mostly partial results for reasons too numerous to be discussed here and that shoulder control is essential for a hand to be used. Intrinsic muscle activity will never recover in adults after plexus repair, when the fascicles of the ulnar and median nerves have been interrupted. The activity and independence of forearm muscles will be limited in these cases so that transfers for wrist and finger imbalance will be impossible or will be deemed to partial failure by crossing to many unstable joints unless secure stabilizing procedures (arthrodeses, very strong tenodeses) are done.

Postoperative treatment

Severe BPI affect mostly young people at the start of their economic independence. The irreparable loss of most of the functions of the upper extremity is a severe blow to them and jeopardizes their future. Only in about 15% of the cases can a good result be expected from repair. All other patients will remain handicapped. Change of occupation, learning a new trade or even return to work as early as possible is the best cure for pain syndromes which often accompany root avulsions and the best quarantee of resuming a normal life without wasting time for a questionable result. Outside short periods for physiotherapy to improve already regained muscle function or a possible surgical intervention to add one, there is no reason at all to wait for the result of plexus repair before returning to active life. The worst consequence of a plexus injury is lost independence. People with a partially or completely paralysed upper extremity can study, do a variety of jobs, drive a car or another vehicle, enjoy sports of all kinds. They learn to iron out their handicap and the more they succeed in overcoming the social consequences of their injury, the happier they are.

Index

Abdominal flap, 179
Abductor tendons, in de Quervain's syndrome, 56–57
Abscesses, 42, 43–44
Accessory collateral ligaments, joint stiffness and, 27, 33, 34
Acrosyndactyly, 76, 82, 83, 86
Acrylic oyster splints, 198
Actinomycosis, 49
Active exercise, joint stiffness and, 28, 29–30
  first web contracture, 38
  MP joint, 31–32
  PIP joint, 33, 36, 37
Adhesions
  skin, 27
  tendon, 27, 31, 256–257
Amputations, 140–156, 194
  complications: implications, 140
  osteomyelitis and, 49
  painful stump, 140–150
    bony irregularities, 147
    nail deformities, 147, 150
    neuroma pain, 140–147
  tendon problems, 150–156
    intrinsic plus deformity, 151, 155
    lumbrical plus finger, 151
    management of flexors, 155–156, 246–247
    profundus tendon blockage, 150–151
    quadriga syndrome, 150–151
    unsatisfactory skin cover, 156
Analgesics, 226
Antidepressants, 226
Apert's syndrome, 76
Aponeurotic fibroma, juvenile, 56
Arteriography, 221–222
Arthrodesis
  boutonniere deformity, 329
  digital joints
    bone loss, severe, 331
    complications, 330–331
    non unions, 331, 332
  DIP joint, 336–337
  MP joint, 332, 333, 340
  osteoarthritis and, 336–337, 338, 340, 341, 344, 346

PIP joint, 329–330, 338
  with MP arthroplasty, 330
  radio-ulnar joint, 345–346
  swan-neck deformity, 329–330, 332
  thumb, 332, 333, 343, 344
  trapezium-scaphoid joint, 344
  wrist joint, 320–321
    complications, 320–321
    with MP joint arthroplasty, 321, 325, 326
Arthroplasty
  boutonniere deformity, 329
  carpometacarpal joint, 333–334
  hemiarthroplasties, 333–334
  indications for, 313
  infections: silastic arthroplasties, 334–335
  MP joint, 315, 321, 323, 325–326, 329, 330
    with PIP fusion, 330
    thumb, 332, 333
    with wrist fusion, 321, 325
  osteoarthritis and, PIP joint, 329–330, 338–340
  radiocarpal joint, 317–319
  radio-ulnar joint, 322, 345
  silastic wrist prosthesis, 317–320
  swan-neck deformity, 329
  Swanson silicone, 339, 340, 341
  thumb, 332, 333–334, 341–344
  total wrist joint, 320
  trapezium-scaphoid joint, 341–344
  volar plate, 293
Articular cartilage and joint stiffness, 25, 27
Articular fracture, 27, 295–296
Atasoy method, 169, 171
Atypical mycobacteria, 49
Autogenous nerve grafts, 210–211
Avulsion flaps, 175, 179
Avulsion injuries
  DIP joint, 254–255
  PIP joint, 255–256

Baldwin operation, 346
Bennett's fracture, 296, 298–300
Bernard–Horner syndrome, and brachial plexus injury, 362

Biceps-to-triceps transfer, 278, 280
Bilhaut-Cloquet procedure, 102, 108
Bite wounds, 48–49, 294
Boeck's sarcoidosis, 49
Bone graft
  bone lengthening, 116–117
  non-union of fractures, 286, 306
  rheumatoid bone loss and, 331
  thumb reconstruction, 116–117
Bone lengthening
  distraction, 116–117, 206
  ulna, 94
Bone stimulation, electrical, 286, 306–307
Boutonniere deformity
  arthrodesis, 329
  arthroplasty, 329
  management, 254–255, 326–327, 329
  splintage, 251, 254–255
  rheumatoid arthritis and, 326–327, 329
Bowstringing, 242, 252
Brachial plexus injury
  diagnosis, 366
  errors in repair, 371
  operative procedures, 370
  post-operative treatment, 372
  special investigations, 370
Bridge graft, Bunnell's, 241
Brown-Sequard syndrome, and brachial plexus injury, 367
Brucellosis, 49
Brunner incision, 235
Bunnell
  bridge graft, 241
  double right angle suture, 236
  figure-of-eight suture, 235, 241
  pulley advancement, 268
  tendon graft procedures, 236–237
  test, for intrinsic tightness, 22
Burns, 187–207
  damage to deep structures, 189–194
    muscle, 193–194
    nerves, 192–193
    open joints, 194
  electrical burns, 191, 192–193, 198
  high tension, 193–194

Burns (contd)
  extension of skin destruction, 188–189
    chemical burns, 189
    infection, 188–189
    vascular embarrassment, 189
  scar contractures, 194–205
    dorsal, 201, 203
    flexion, 199, 201
    prevention, 198–199
    proximal limb, 203–204
    restriction of scar tissue, 194, 196, 198
    surgical release, 199–204
    underlying orthopaedic abnormalities, 204–205
    web space, 199
  swelling, 187–188, 193–194
    compression, 187–188
    immobility, 188
    persistent oedema, 188
  tissue loss, 205–206
    deepening of first web space, 206
    distraction bone lengthening, 206
    free toe transfer, 206
    ray transfer, 206

Cable graft: nerves, 210
Calcification, heterotopic, 204
Candidiasis, 49
Capener splint, 33, 168
Caput ulnae syndrome, 321–323
Carpal tunnel syndrome, 59–63
  applied anatomy, 59–60
  complications, 60–61
  decompression, 60–63
Carpometacarpal joint hemiarthroplasties, 333–334
  thumb duplication and, 106
  thumb fracture, 299, 300
Cellulitis, management, 42, 44
Centralisation of carpus, 91–94
Central slip injury, 254–255
  re-insertion, 255
Cervical radiculopathy, 222
Chemical burns, 189
Children
  burn patients, 198
  juvenile aponeurotic fibroma, 56
  operations on, 41
  recurring digital fibrous tumour, 56
  see also specific conditions
Clam digger posture see Intrinsic plus posture
Club hand, 89–100
  correction of wrist deformity, 91–94
  operative treatment, 91–100
  pollicisation, 94–100
  potential complications of radial absence, 89–91
  premature fusion of ulnar epiphysis, 93–94
  recurrence of deformity, 93
  ulnar lengthening, 94
Coccidiomycosis, 49

'Cocked hat flap', 116
Codeine, 226
Collar stud abscess, 44, 47
Collateral ligaments
  joint stiffness and, 27, 31, 32, 33, 34, 36–37
    accessory ligaments, 27, 33, 34
    in MP extension contracture, 31, 32
    in PIP extension contracture, 36–37
    in PIP flexion contracture, 33, 34
    in thumb duplication, Type I, 104
    thumb fracture and, 295–296
Colles fractures, tendon injury, 252
Compartment compression, syndrome, and brachial plexus injury, 372
Compartmental infection, 44
  deep space infection, 46–47
Compartmental syndrome see Volkmann's ischaemic contracture
Conjoint tendon repair, 255–256
Consent, informed, 3–4, 225
Continuous passive motion (CPM) devices, 33, 36, 37
Counselling/explanation, 3–4
  club hand, 90
  Dupuytren's contracture, 349
  nerve compression lesions, 225
  syndactyly, 65–66, 86–87
  tetraplegia, 275
  thumb duplication, 102
  thumb reconstruction, 109
Crane method, 179, 181, 183
Cross-finger flap, 168, 171, 179, 217
  technique, 162, 183
Cross-forearm flap, 171, 179
CT, computed tomography scans, 222, 302
Cysts
  epidermoid, 56
  mucous, 54–55, 337–338
  nail, 147, 150
  sebaceous, 56
  see also Ganglia

Darrach's operation, 345
Decompression
  burns, 187–188
  nerves, 56, 59–64, 220–230
  tendons, 56–59
Degloved thumb, 167, 183
De Quervain's syndrome, 56–58
  surgical anatomy, 57
  treatment, 57–58
Deltopectoral flap, 192
Dermatofibroma, 55–56
Dermodesis, in mallet finger, 256
Desmoid tumours, 56
Digital joint fusions (rheumatoid), 330–332
  non-unions, 331, 332
  with severe bone loss, 331
Dilantin, and pain relief, 226
Discrimination tests, sensory, 213

Dislocations see Fractures and dislocations
Distal interphalangeal (DIP) joint
  arthrodesis, 336–337
  avulsion fractures, 254–255
  dislocation, 287
  extensor tendon injury and, 251, 255–256
  mallet deformity, 251, 255–256, 287, 289
  osteoarthritis, 336–337
  Type I thumb duplication and, 104
Distal phalanx
  thumb duplication and, 102, 103–104
Distal phalanx fractures, 285–289
  dislocation, 287
  mallet deformities, 287–289
  thumb, 295
  transverse, 285–286
Distal suture technique, 234, 238–239
Distraction bone lengthening, 116–117, 206
Dorsal wrist ganglion, 52
Double crush syndrome, 222
Double ischaemic insult, 15–16
Double pedicle flap, 171, 203
Dressings
  burns and, 188–189
  routine skin graft, 162
  syndactyly and, 85
Drug abuse, 226
Dupuytren's disease, 348–363
  indications for operation, 349, 351
  operative considerations, 351–358
  patient selection, 348–349
  post-operative complications, 358–361
  recurrence and extension of disease, 360–361
  results, 358
Dysesthesia, 224
Dynamic splinting, 29, 32, 33, 36, 37, 325

Ectopic hair, skin grafts and, 80
Ectrosyndactyly, 86
Elbow
  burn contracture: release, 203, 204–205
  club hand and, 89–90, 91
  repair in tetraplegia, 278, 280
  ulnar neuropathy, 229
Electrical bone stimulation, 286, 306–307
Electrical burns, 191, 192–193, 198
  high tension, 193–194
Electrocautery with neurectomy, 143–144
Electrodiagnosis: nerve compression lesions, 221
Electromyography, 221
Elevation, joint stiffness and, 25–26
Ellipsoid infarct, 20
'End feel' of stiff joint, 31
Epidermal cysts, 56

Epineurectomy, indications for, 228
Epineurial suture, 209–210
Epineurotomy, 62
Epiphyseal closure, in syndactyly, 82–83, 85
Eponychia, 43–44
Escharotomy, burns and, 187–188
Explanation *see* Counselling/Explanation
Exsanguination, tourniquet and, 9–10
Extension contracture, 31–33, 36–37
    splinting and, 32, 36, 37
    surgical release, 32, 36–37
Extensor digitorum communis, lesions, 253
Extensor indicis proprius, tendon transfer, 252–253
Extensor pollicis longus, injury and, 252
Extensor retinaculum, wrist injury and, 252
Extensor tendon
    in thumb duplication, 103–104, 105, 106
    in thumb reconstruction, 124
    toe to thumb transfer and, 135
Extensor tendon injuries, 250–257
    anatomy and pathomechanics, 250–251
    boutonniere deformity and, 251, 254–255
    burns and, 189, 191, 194
    de Quervain's syndrome and, 56–58
    DIP joint, 251, 255–256
    joint stiffness and, 27
    lesions associated with skin loss, 257
    MP joint, 250, 253–254
    PIP joint, 250–251, 254–255
    problems over bony shafts, 256–257
    reasons for repair failure, 251–252
    ruptures and MP joints, 314–315
    wrist joint and, 250, 252–253
Extrinsic muscles in management of contractures, 20–21

Factitious disorders, 3
Fascial spaces, infections and, 43, 46–47
Fascicular bundle suture, 210
Fasciectomy, in Dupuytren's disease, 352–353
Fasciotomy
    burns and, 193–194
    delayed, 20
    Dupuytren's disease and, 352–353, 355
    Volkmann's ischaemic contracture, 18–20
Felon, surgical treatment, 45
Fibroblasts, tumours of, 55–56
Fibroma, juvenile aponeurotic, 56
Fibrosarcomas, 56
Fibrous tumour, recurring, 56
Fish-mouth suture technique, 238, 245
Flag flap, 173

Flexion contractures
    burn patients, 198–199, 201
    deformity *see* Club hand
    splinting, 33, 36
    surgical release, 34–35
Flexor pollicis longus, loss, 241
Flexor profundis loss with normal superficialis, 241
Flexor sheath contracture, 35
Flexor tendon
    carpal tunnel syndrome, 59–63
    thumb duplication and, 103, 104–105, 106
    thumb reconstruction, level IV, 124
    toe to thumb transfer and, 135
    trigger finger/thumb, 58–59
Flexor tendon injury, 232–248
    amputation and, 246–247
    flexor pulley system, 233
    reconstruction, 246
    general principles, 232, 247–248
    joint stiffness and, 25, 27–28
    primary tendon repair, 232–236
        delayed, 234
        flap necrosis, 235
        joint contracture and, 236
        profundus avulsion, 234–235
        rupture, 235
        wound infection, 235
        zones 1 and 2, 233–236
        zones 3–5, 236
    ruptures, 316–317
        carpal tunnel, 316
        palm and digit, 316–317
    tendon grafting, 236–246
        Bunnell bridge graft, 241
        factors influencing result, 237–241
        indications for, 237
        staged grafts, 244–246
        unsatisfactory results, 241–244, 245–246
Flexor tenosynovectomy, 62, 313, 315–317
Flexor tenosynovitis, 315–317
Fluidotherapy, 38
Fractures and dislocations, 281–300
    acute scapho-lunate dissociation, 309–310
    aetiology, unsatisfactory results, 281–285
        mobilisation, 284–285
    articular, 27, 295–296
    Bennett's fracture, 296, 298–300
    distal phalanx, 285–289
    lunate/perilunate dislocation, 308–309
    metacarpal, 293–295
    middle phalanx, 289
    osteochondral: diagnosis, 27
    proximal phalanx, 289–293
    Rolando's fracture, 296, 298–299
    scaphoid, 301–308
    thumb, 295–300
    trans-scaphoid perilunar fracture dislocation, 309
    wrist injuries, 301–310

F-response technique, 221
Fungal infections, 49
Furuncle, 44

Ganglia, 50–55
    complications, 50–51
    dorsal wrist, 52
    mucous cysts, 54–55, 337–338
    operative treatment, 51–2
    volar retinacular, 53–54
    volar wrist, 52–53
General considerations, 1–4
    minor surgery and infections, 40–43
Giant cell tumour, 55
Grafts *see* Bone graft; Skin grafts; Flexor tendon, tendon grafting
Groin flap, 167–168, 179, 192, 257

Haematoma, post-operative, 322–323, 358
    skin grafts and, 158, 169, 177
Heat treatment modalities, joint stiffness and, 26, 28–29, 33, 38
Hemiarthroplasty of thumb, 333–334
Herbert screw technique, 306, 309
Histiocytoma, fibrous, 55
Hooked nail deformity, 147
Hyperaesthesia
    amputations and, 141, 144, 145
    nerve injury, 215
    thumb reconstruction and, 110, 112, 113
Hyperextension deformity of thumb, 95, 97, 99, 124, 212
Hyperpigmentation of skin grafts, 79, 161
Hypertrophic scar, in de Quervain's syndrome, 57, 58
Hypesthesia, 110

Incisions
    hand infections and, 42–43
    nerve decompressions and, 56
Inclusion cysts, 56
Infections
    bite wounds, 48–49, 294
    burns, 188–189
    digital fusion pins and, 330
    silastic arthroplasty, 334–335
    skin grafts, 159, 169, 177, 181
    tendon injury, 235, 246, 252
Infections in minor surgical procedures, 40–49
    chronic infections, 49
    complications, 42
    felon, 45
    fungal infection, 49
    incisions, 42–43
    prevention, 41–43
    sites, and specific infections, 43–49
    skin infections, 44
    space infections, 44
        deep space infections, 46–47
Intrinsic minus posture, 20

Intrinsic muscle contracture
　management, 21–22, 36, 37
　release, 21–22
Intrinsic plus posture, 21, 26, 27–28, 151, 155
Intrinsic tendon tightness, 27–28
Ischaemia
　pollicisation and, 95–96, 97
　rebound, 15–16
　tourniquets and, 8, 9
　see also Volkmann's ischaemic contracture

Joint jack, 33
Joint contractures
　tendon repairs and, 236, 241–242, 263–264
　tetraplegia and, 276
　see also Joint stiffness
Joint injury, burns and, 194, 204
Joint reconstruction in thumb duplication, 104–105, 106
Joint stiffness, 24–39
　development, 24–25
　evaluation, 26–28
　prevention, 25–26
　treatment, 28–38
　　established contractures, 31–39
　　first web contracture, 37–38
　　MP joint extension contracture, 31–36
　　PIP joint extension contracture, 36–37
　　PIP joint flexion contracture, principles of, 28–31
　　results, 38
　see also Remedial treatment
Jumbled hand, 69

Kessler locking suture, 233, 234, 235
Kinematics of wrist, 301–303
Kutler technique, 169, 171

Lateral pinch repairs, in tetraplegia, 280
Lateral slip injury, 255
Lauenstein operation, 345–346
Lipoma, 55
Littler's depiction of thumb reconstruction, 122, 123
LMB wire foam splint, 33
Lumbrical plus syndrome, 151, 242, 244
Lunate/perilunate dislocations, 308–309
Lymphangitis, 42

Mallet deformity, 251, 255–256, 287, 289
Malingering patients, 3
Mania operativa, 147, 227
Massage, joint stiffness and, 28, 33, 38
Median nerve
　and brachial plexus injury, 371

in club hand, 90–91
compression at wrist, 229
　carpal tunnel syndrome, 59–63
neurolysis, 62
palsy, 211, 217–218
Metacarpal
　abduction-pronation-recession osteotomy, 127, 129
　fractures
　　Bennett's, 296, 298–300
　　dorsal angulation, 293–294
　　intra-articular, 294–295
　　metaphysis, 294
　　oblique, 294
　　Rolando's, 296, 298–299
　　rotational deformity, 294
　　shaft and neck, 294
　　thumb, 296, 297
　lengthening, 116–117
　thumb reconstruction, 115–121, 121–124
Metacarpophalangeal (MP) joint
　arthrodesis, 332, 333, 340
　arthroplasty, 315, 321, 323, 325–326, 329, 330
　　with PIP fusion, 330
　　thumb, 332, 333
　　with wrist fusion, 321, 325
　bite wounds and, 48–49
　dislocated, and tendon ruptures, 314–315
　extension contracture, 31–33
　　non-operative treatment, 31, 33
　　splints and, 32, 33
　　surgical release, 32–33
　extensor tendon injury, 250, 253–254
　　dorsal hood repair, 254
　reconstruction, 104–105, 126
　in rheumatoid arthritis, 314–315, 320, 321, 323, 325–326, 332, 333
　　rheumatoid with PIP involvement, 330
　in swan-neck deformity, 329
　thumb injury, 296
　toe to thumb transfer and, 134
Microsurgical reconstruction see Toe to thumb transfer
Middle phalanx, transverse fractures, 289
Minnesota Rate of Manipulation Test, 30
Mucous cyst, 54–55, 337–338
Munchausen-type patient, 147, 227
Muscles
　burn injuries, 193–194
　evaluation in tendon transfers, 260–261, 262–263
　internal splints, 211–212
　intrinsic, contractures, 21–22, 36, 37
　sliding procedure, 20, 21
　tetraplegia and, 274–280
　tourniquets and, 9
　transplantation, 21
　see also Volkmann's ischaemic contracture

Mycobacterial infections, 49
Myelography, 222

Nail/nail bed
　fracture of distal phalanx, 286
　infections, 43–44
　mucous cysts and, 54
　nail spurs and cysts, 43–44, 147, 150
　parrot-beak or hooked nail deformity, 147
　skin grafts and, 171
　syndactyly and, 82
　thumb reconstruction and, 102, 104, 110, 111, 132
Narcotics and pain relief, 226
Nerves, 209–218
　conduction velocity determination, 221
　neuroma-in-continuity, 216
　pain problems, 213–216
　palsied hand, 216–218
　re-education techniques, 211–213
　reflex sympathetic dystrophy, 214–216
　sensory reconstruction, 217–218
　stimulation, diagnostic, 17
　suture techniques, 209–211
Nerves, compression lesions, 220–230
　causes of unsatisfactory results, 222–225
　counselling and consent, 225
　diagnosis, 221–222, 225
　　differential diagnosis, 222–223
　epineurectomy, indications for, 228
　median nerve at wrist, 229
　multiple procedures, 227
　non-surgical modalities, 225–226
　operative management, 226–230
　pain management, 226
　pathology, 220–221, 222–224
　preoperative management, 225–226
　radial nerve, 230
　sites, 220
　thoracic outlet syndrome, 228
　transposition of nerves, 228, 230
　ulnar neuropathy at elbow, 229
　see also Nerve injuries
Nerve injuries
　burns, 192–193
　carpal tunnel syndrome, 59–63
　de Quervain's syndrome, 57–58
　entrapments, 56, 59–64
　incisions for decompression, 56
　joint stiffness and, 28
　tourniquets and, 8–9, 10–12
　trigger finger/thumb, 58–59
　ulnar nerve compression at wrist, 63
Neurectomy, 143–144
Neurofibroma, 222
Neurolemmomas, 222
Neurolysis, median, in carpal tunnel syndrome, 62
Neuroma
　de Quervain's syndrome and, 57, 58
　neuroma-in-continuity, 216

pain, in amputation stump, 140–147
　clinical presentations, 141
　conservative treatment, 143
　histology, 140–141
　operative treatment, 143–144, 147
　prevention, 141, 143
　syndactyly and, 80
　thumb repair and, 110, 133
Neurovascular bundles, syndactyly and, 80–81
Neurovascular island flaps, 110, 117, 171–173, 183, 217
Niebauer prosthesis, 326

Obstetric palsy, and brachial plexus injury, 371, 372
Oedema
　burns and, 187–188
　inflammatory, 42
　joint stiffness and, 24, 25–26, 28–29
　perineurial, 214
　in treatment of club hand, 92
Orthotics, nerve lesions and, 225–226
Osteoarthritis, 336–346
　arthrodeses, 336–337, 338, 340, 341, 344, 346
　arthroplasty, 338–340, 341–344, 345
　DIP joint, 336–337
　inferior radio-ulnar joint, 345–346
　MP joint, 340
　mucous cyst and, 337–338
　PIP joint, 338–340
　thumb, 340–344
　trapezium-scaphoid joint, 344
Osteochondral fractures, diagnosis, 27
Osteomyelitis, 49
Osteoplastic thumb reconstruction, 117, 119
Osteotomy, abduction-pronation-recession of metacarpal, 127, 129

Pain
　amputation stump, 140–147
　infection and, 42, 43
　joint stiffness and, 24, 26, 29
　nail deformities, 147, 150
　nerve lesions, 213, 216, 226
　post-operative, 41
　rheumatoid arthritis, 312, 318
　see also Neuroma
Palsied hand, 216–218
　sensory reconstruction, 217–218
"Paradoxical extension", 151
Paresis, tourniquet paralysis, 8, 10, 12
Paresthesias, nerve lesions and, 222
Paronychia, 43–44
Parrot-beak nail deformity, 147
Pedicle flaps, 173–185
　avulsion flaps, 175, 179, 181
　bulky flaps, 179, 181, 183
　faulty suturing, 177
　poor sensory innervation, 183
　unsatisfactory results
　　origin, 173–175
　　prevention, 175–179
　　treatment, 179–185
　vascular supply and viability, 175
　see also Skin grafts; specific flaps
Perilunate/lunate dislocation, 308–309
Phalangisation see Web deepening
Pigmented villonodular synovitis, 55
Poker finger, 79, 86
Poland's syndrome, 86
Pollicisation
　club hand, 94–100
　　appearance, 97, 99
　　bony fusion at base of thumb, 99
　　length of thumb, 97
　　neurological complications, 96–97
　　skin healing, 97
　　vascular complications, 95–96
　thumb reconstruction in congenital deficiency, 126–127, 129
　traumatic loss and
　　level II, 114–115
　　level III, 119, 121
　　level IV, 122–124
　　level V, 124, 126
　　Littler's depiction, 123
　　management of skeleton, 122, 124
　　skin incision and web reconstruction, 122
　　vascular compromise, 122
Polysyndactyly, 69, 86
Post-traumatic arthritis, 338, 340
Profundus tendon
　avulsion, 234–235
　blockage, 150–151
　lumbrical plus finger, 151
Proximal interphalangeal (PIP) joint
　arthrodesis, 329–330, 338
　　with MP arthroplasty, 330
　arthroplasty, 293, 329–330, 338–340
　avulsion fractures, 255–256
　boutonniere deformity, 254–255, 326–327, 329
　contraction in primary tendon repair, 236
　dislocations, 291–293
　　dorsal, 291, 292–293
　　fracture, 292–293
　　volar, 291–292
　extension contractures, 36–37, 38
　　non-oprative treatment, 36, 37
　　surgical release, 36–37
　flexion contractures, 33–36, 38
　　burns and, 202–199
　　non-operative treatment, 33–34, 36
　　surgical release, 34–35
　osteoarthritis, 338–340
　rheumatoid arthritis and, 316, 326–330
　　arthritis with joint destruction, 329–330
　　fusion, 329
　　MP involvement, 330
　stiff, with flexor tenosynovitis, 316
　swan-neck deformity and, 329–330
Proximal limb contractures, 203–204

Proximal phalanx
　dislocations, 291–293
　fractures, 289–293
　　intercondylar, 291
　　neck of phalanx, 291
　　oblique, 291
　　rotational deformity, 291
　　transverse, 289
　injury, thumb reconstruction, 111–115, 115–121
　thumb duplication, Types I and II, 103–105
Proximal suture technique, 238–239
Psoriatic arthritis, and infections, 334
Psychotherapy, pain and, 226
Pulley reconstruction, 246, 264, 267–268
Pyoderma, 44
Pyogenic granuloma, 44

Quadriga syndrome, 150–151

Radial
　aplasia, congenital, 127, 129
　nerve compression, 230
　palsy, 211, 217–218
　sensory flaps, 110, 111
　see also Club hand
Radiocarpal joint, arthroplasty, 317–319
Radiology see X-rays
Radio-ulnar joint
　arthrodesis, 345–346
　arthroplasty, 322, 345
　osteoarthritis, 345–346
　rheumatoid arthritis, 321–323
Raynaud's disease, 261
Ray transfer, burns and, 206
Rebound ischaemia, 15–16
Reflex sympathetic dystrophy, 2, 26, 214–216, 224, 359–360
Remedial treatment, joint stiffness
　active exercise programme, 28, 29–30, 31–32, 33, 36, 37, 38
　elevation, 25–26
　'end feel', prognosis and, 31
　evaluation, 29–30, 37
　heat and cold modalities, 26, 28–29, 33, 38
　massage, 28, 33, 38
　oedema and, 24, 25, 26, 28–29
　pain and, 26
　passive exercise, 29, 31, 33, 36
　patient motivation and, 28, 30, 32
　splinting, 26, 29, 31–32, 33, 36, 38
　TENS, 26, 33, 38
Retinacular ligaments, 34, 37
Rheumatoid arthritis, 312–335
　considerations, 312
　digital fusions, 330–332
　flexor tendon ruptures, 316–317
　infections following arthroplasty, 334–335
　MP joint, 323–326

Rheumatoid arthritis (contd)
  PIP joint, 326–330
  radiocarpal joint, 317–319
  radio-ulnar joint, 321–323
  reconstructive surgery
    improvements of function, 313–314
    indications for, 313
    thumb, 332–334
  silastic wrist prosthesis, 317–319
  total wrist joint arthroplasty, 320
  wrist fusion, 320
    with MP joint arthroplasty, 321
Rod implants, tendon grafts and, 244–246
Rolando's fracture, 296, 298–299
Rotatory subluxation of scaphoid, 309–310
Russe technique, 306

Scaphoid fracture, 304–308
  acute scapho-lunate dissociation, 309–310
  non-union, 305–306, 308
  silastic implant of Swanson, 307
  trans-scaphoid perilunar fracture dislocation, 309
Scar contracture, hypertrophic, 57, 58
  see also Burns, scar contractures
Sebaceous cyst, 56
Secondary gain, 224–225
Sensitivity
  discrimination tests, 213
  reconstruction, palsied hand, 217–218
  sensory re-education, 212–213
  skin grafts, 159, 161, 168, 169, 171
  tendon transfer and, 261–262
  tetraplegia, 276
Septic arthritis, 253, 294
  treatment, 48
Septic tenosynovitis, 47–48, 49
Serial casting splints, 33, 38
Silastic arthroplasty
  infections and, 334–335
  Swanson arthroplasty, 326, 339, 340, 341–344
    scaphoid implant, 307
  wrist prosthesis, 317–319
    fractured, 318
Silver sulphadiazine, 189
Skin flaps, in syndactyly
  skin coverage, 77–78
  surgical design, 68–70
  web flap design, 73–74
  see also Skin grafts; Thumb reconstruction
Skin grafts
  syndactyly and
    donor sites, 75, 76, 77, 78
    full thickness graft, 76–78
    nail-cuticle distortion, 82
    partial thickness graft, 75–76
    see also Skin flaps
  tendon injury and, 257

thumb duplication and, 106
thumb reconstruction and, 110, 113, 116, 117
toe to thumb transfers, 133, 135
Skin grafts, unsatisfactory results, 158–173
  amputations, 156
  contracture, 159, 168, 171
  cosmetic considerations, 161, 169, 173
  deep structure involvement, 161
  dressing technique, 162
  graft failure, 158–159, 161–162, 167–168, 169
  hypersensitivity, 159, 161, 168
  infection, 159
  instability, 159, 168, 169, 171
  lack of sensation, 161, 168, 171–173
  management, 169–173
  mechanical factors, 159, 168
  origins, 158–161
  prevention, 161–169
  vascularity of graft bed, 158, 161–162, 169, 171
  see also Pedicle flaps
Skin loss, and tendon injury, 257
Skin release, PIP contractures, 35, 37
Sliding transposition flap, 171
Somatoform disorders, 3
Somatosensory evoked potential, 221
Spasticity, of tetraplegia, 274, 275
Splints
  dynamic, 29, 32, 33, 36, 37, 325
  joint stiffness and, 26, 29, 31–32, 33, 36, 38
  internal muscle splints, 211–212
  serial casting, 33, 38
Sporotrichosis, 49
Steinman pin, 320, 321
Stener lesion, 296
Streptococcus infection, 42, 159
Subonychia, 43–44
Sulfamylon, 189
Sutures
  materials, 81–82, 235
  nerve suture techniques, 209–211
  primary tendon repair, 233, 234–235
  syndactyly and, 81–82
  tendon grafting, 238–239
  see also specific sutures
Swan neck deformity, 239, 244, 255, 287–289
  arthrodesis, 329–330, 332
  arthroplasty, 329
  surgery, 329–330
Swanson arthroplasty, 326, 339, 340, 341–344
  scaphoid, 307
Swanson procedure, 346
Swelling, burns and, 187–188, 193–194
  see also Oedema
Sympathectomy, 215
Symphalangism, 86
Syndactyly, 65–87
  classification, 65

contractures, 66–70
  correction, 71–87
  counselling, 65–66, 86–87
  distal migration of web space, 72–74
  dressings and splints, 85
  epiphyseal closure and angulations, 82–83, 85
  factors in unsatisfactory results, 65–70
  individualisation, overzealous, 86
  nail/cuticle distortion, 82
  neuroma, 81
  neurovascular bundles, 80–81
  post-burn, 199
  secondary, 70
  skin coverage, 75–78
  surgical design, 67–70
  suture material, 81–82
Synovectomy, rheumatoid arthritis and, 312–313
Synovitis, 246
  pigmented villonodular, 55

Tangential excision, in deep burn, 196
Tegretol, in pain relief, 226
Tendons
  adhesions, joint stiffness and, 27, 31
  burns and, 189, 191, 194
  entrapments, 56–59
  grafts see Flexor tendon injury, tendon grafting
  problems following amputations, 150–156
  rheumatoid, surgery, 314–316, 317
  see also specific tendons and conditions
Tendon transfers, 259–273
  immobilisation, 269, 271, 273
  joint mobility, 263–264
  muscle evaluation, 260–261, 262–263
  palsied hand, 216, 217
  patient evaluation, 259
  physical therapy, 273
  route of transfer, 264, 267–269
  sensibility, 261–262
  skeletal integrity, 260
  tendon insertion, 269
  tissue status, 259–260
Tenolysis, 30, 242, 257, 314
Tenosynovectomy, 49, 57, 58, 312–313, 315–317
  dorsal, 314
    with tendon transfer, 314
  flexor, 62, 313, 315–317
Tenosynovitis
  dorsal, 314
    with tendon transfer, 314
  flexor, 315–317
  pigmented nodular, 55
  septic, 47–48, 49
  stenosing, 56–58
Tenotomy, 255
Tenovaginitis, stenosing see Trigger finger/thumb
Terminal phalanx injury, 109–111

Tetraplegia, 274–280
  causes of unsatisfactory results, 275–280
  classification, 277–278
  condition of muscles, 275
  defects in surgical procedure, 278, 280
  functional tests, 276
  patient evaluation, 275–278
Thoracic outlet syndrome, 221, 222, 228
Thrombosis, tourniquets and, 9
Thromboxane, tissue levels, 194
Thumb
  arthrodeses, 332, 333, 343, 344
  arthroplasty, 332, 333–334, 341–344
  degloved, 167, 183
  first web contracture, 37–38, 199
  fractures, 295–300
    Bennett's, 296, 298–300
    distal phalanx, 295
    intra-articular, 295–296
    metacarpal, 296, 297, 298–300
    Rolando's, 296, 298–299
    trapeziometacarpal dislocations, 300
  osteoarthritis, 340–344
  osteoplastic reconstruction, 117, 119
  release of burn contractures, 199
  rheumatoid, reconstruction, 332–334
  'thumb stall', 116
  trigger thumb, 58–59
  see also Pollicisation, club hand
Thumb duplication, 101–108
  classification, 101
  results, 107–108
  surgical considerations, 102, 108
  surgical techniques, 102–106
    Type I deformities, 102–104
    Type II deformities, 104–105
    Type III deformities, 105–106
Thumb reconstruction, conventional, 109–129, 137–138
  congenital deficiency, 126–127, 129
  considerations and classification, 109, 137–138
  traumatic loss, 109–126
    level I, 109–111
    level II, 111–115
    level III, 115–121
    level IV, 121–124
    level V, 121–126
  see also Toe to thumb transfer
Tine's sign, 227
Tissue pressure, measurement, 17
Toe to digit/thumb transfer, burns and, 206
Toe to thumb transfer, microsurgical, 129–136
  congenital absence of thumb, 135–136
  donor site dissection, 133
  donor site morbidity, 132, 133–134
  errors in surgery, 133
  great toe transfer, 130, 132, 134
  management of complications, 135
  partial toe transfer, 132
  planning procedure, 132–133
  post-operative care, 135
  recipient site errors, 133–135
  second toe to thumb transfer, 132, 134–135
  sensory reconstruction and, 217
  wrap-around flap, 135, 217
Tourniquets, 5–12
  complications, 8–9, 10–12
  contraindications, 9
  exsanguination, 9–10
  hazards and malfunctions, 5–7
  historical aspects, 5
  intra-operative bleeding, 10, 12
  occlusion time and pressure, 10
  paresis (paralysis syndrome), 8, 10, 12
  system types, 5, 7–8, 12
Transcutaneous electrical nerve stimulation (TENS), 26, 33, 38, 215–216, 226
Trans-scaphoid perilunar fracture dislocation, 309
Transposition, of decompressed nerves, 228
Trapeziometacarpal joint
  capsulotomy, 115
  dislocations, 300
  loss and reconstruction, 124, 126
Trapezium excision, 115, 341, 342, 343–344
Trapezium-scaphoid joint
  arthrodesis, 343, 344
  arthroplasty, 341–344
  osteoarthritis, 341–344
Triamcinolone injection, 242
Trigger finger/thumb, 58–59
  surgical anatomy, 58
Tumours, 49–56
  classification, 49–50
  nerves and, 222

Ulna
  in club hand syndrome
    development, 91
    operative treatment, 91, 92–94
    prehension and, 90
    premature fusion of lower epiphysis, 93–94
    ulnar lengthening, 94
  head, excision, 322
Ulnar nerve
  and brachial plexus injury, 371
  compression at wrist, 63
  neuropathy at elbow, 229
  palsy, 211, 217–218

Venous thrombosis, tourniquets and, 9
Volar
  advancement flaps, 110
  retinacular ganglion, 53–54
  wrist ganglion, 52–53
Volar plate, 25
  arthroplasty, 293
  injury in thumb fracture, 295–296
  joint stiffness and, 27
  in PIP flexion contracture, 33–35
Volkmann's ischaemic contracture, 14–22
  causes, 16
  clinical features, 16–17
  diagnosis, 16–17
  management of contractures, 20–22
  pathophysiology, 14–16
  prevention, 16
  treatment
    non-operative, 18
    surgical, 18–20

Webs
  contracture (first), 37–38
    surgical release, 38
  reconstruction
    congenital deficiency, 126
    thumb, 113–114
    see also Syndactyly
  spaces
    deepening, in burn patient, 206
    release of burn contracture, 199
Wolfe graft, burns and, 199, 203
Work simulator, 30
Wrap-around flap, 132, 133, 135, 217
Wrist injuries, 301–310
  acute scapho-lunate dislocation, 309–310
  kinematics of wrist, 301–303
  lunate/perilunate dislocation, 308–309
  scaphoid fractures, 304–308
  trans-scaphoid perilunar fracture dislocation, 309
Wrist joint
  arthroplasty, 320
  arthrodesis, 320–321
    with MP joint arthroplasty, 321, 325, 326
  extensor tendon injury, 250, 252–253
  osteoarthritis, 345–346
  radiocarpal joint, 317–319
  radio-ulnar joint, 321–323
  rheumatoid arthritis and, 317–323
  silastic wrist prosthesis, 317–320
  ulnar nerve compression, 63
  see also Club hand

Xanthoma, fibrous, 55
Xerography, 221
X-rays
  compression lesions, 221–222
  fractures, 282
  wrist fractures, 302–303, 304, 308

Z-plasties, 30, 71, 74, 103, 106, 113–114, 356, 358